MICROBIOLOGY SERIES 3

Series Editor: Dr. Ajit Varma

MICROBES
Health and Environment

Editors

Ashok K Chauhan
Founder President
Ritnand Baldeo Education Foundation,
NOIDA, India

Ajit Varma
Amity Institute of Herbal and
Microbial Studies,
NOIDA, India

I.K. International Publishing House Pvt. Ltd.
New Delhi • Mumbai • Bangalore

Cover page photograph depicts protoplast production from symbiotic fungus *Piriformospora indica*. The regenerated cells conserved their plant growth promotion activities and enhanced the maize root proliferation. Interaction of fungus with medicinal herbs leads to excessive production of secondary metabolites

Published by

I.K. International Publishing House Pvt. Ltd.
S-25, Green Park Extension
Uphaar Cinema Market
New Delhi - 110 016 (India)
E-mail : ik_in@vsnl.net

Branch Offices

A-6, Royal Industrial Estate, Naigaum Cross Road
Wadala, Mumbai - 400 031 (India)
E-mail : ik_mumbai@vsnl.net

G-4 "Embassy Centre", 11 Crescent Road, Kumara Park East
Bangalore - 560 001 (India)
E-mail : ik_bang@vsnl.net

ISBN 81-88237-51-5

First Reprint 2007

Published by Krishan Makhijani for I.K. International Publishing House Pvt. Ltd., S-25, Green Park Extension, Uphaar Cinema Market, New Delhi - 110 016 and Printed by Rekha Printers Pvt. Ltd., Okhla Industrial Area, Phase II, New Delhi - 110 020.

Foreword

The future of biological and planetary sciences lies in understanding the role microbes play in shaping the earth and its inhabitants. *Microbes: Health and Environment* reflects the world of microbes and their diversified nature, one that is unlikely to fit into any division of modern biology. Yet another milestone in the evolution of the world of microbes, the volume offers an important basis for discussion, criticism and hence progress.

The contributors in the volume are leading authorities from varied backgrounds, focused on the diverse areas of research on microbes. They come from differenι government laboratories, universities, IITs and industries, actively involved in basic, applied and industrial research.

I am convinced that the volume will be a boon to the undergraduate and postgraduate students of biological sciences, plant sciences, microbiology, bioinformatics, biotechnology, environmental science and soil science, besides scientists, whether in academia, industry or government. The present book provides a continuing organized report of an exciting facet of biology, which would contribute in shaping the intellectual calibre and industry. I hope the readers will find it as exciting as the contributors who wrote the following chapters.

Asis Datta

Director, NCPGR, New Delhi

Preface

For more than three billion years, microbes have mediated critical processes that allow higher organisms to evolve. These creatures dominate the Earth's biodiversity particularly in oceans, where they account for ninety per cent of the biomass. Scientists estimate that there are about one million bacteria and ten million viruses per milliliter of ocean water, and about one billion bacteria per gram of sediment. They possess great metabolic diversity and this characteristic has great biological significance. Modern researchers have revealed more novel characteristics of microorganisms, which are on the threshold of large-scale application to overcome many of the problems that we are facing today such as food, energy, medicine and environmental degradation. Probing, monitoring and modifying the activities of microorganisms have become easier in the last few decades with the growing knowledge gathered through molecular biology techniques leading to their efficient applications in agriculture, forestry, environmental industry and medicine. This book is a collection of large information gathered through novel work of researchers on the impact of microbes on our health and immediate environment.

This book gives a comprehensive account related to all the above themes. The book contains altogether seventeen chapters and each focuses on the title of the book. The first chapter gives an introduction about the classification of microbes and its impact on our health and environment. The preceding three chapters define the association between plants and microbes. Microbes, for example, bacteria and fungus have a symbiotic association with plants that assist them in obtaining nutrients and water and may protect them against diseases. Besides these, there is an increase in its active constituents. This book also emphasizes the need for conservation of these medicinally important plants and gives relevant bibliography for the benefit of academicians and industrialists. The next two chapters describe cyanobacteria which besides its well documented use as bio-fertilizer in conjunction with rice crop, has also been exploited for the production of valuable compounds, such as pigments, pharmaceuticals and as biological agents in bioremediation and reclamation of saline-alkali soils. The other chapters deal with the role of microbes on soil degradation.The following chapter gives an outlook on how the neurotoxin botulinum which is a potentially lethal biological agent can be used as a medicine for several neuromuscular disorders. It also stresses upon its unique characteristics including exclusive substrate specificity and localized action.

Microbes play a very important role in the field of agriculture. Functions of association between plants and PGPR benefit crops by stimulating plant growth, or by reducing the damage from soil-borne plant pathogens, the biological component of the soil ecosystem, and in particular the role of plants within the soil ecosystem and the types of effects that they can confer on both PGPR and soil processes. Another example is about the symbiotic relationship of fungi and bacteria (Arbucular Mycorrhizal Fungi) which markedly improves the nodulation and nitrogen fixation by interaction with *B. japonicum,* a legume bacterium, mainly by providing the high phosphorus requirement for the fixation process. The book also covers the importance of Fungus protoplasts, which serve as a potent tool for fungal biotechnology research. Microbes also help in combating pollution, ie., adding phytase to the animal diet not only improves the bio-availability of proteins and minerals, but also plays an important role in combating environmental phosphorus pollution in the areas of intensive live stock population. The preceding chapter also gives a brief outlook on reduction of toxicity by understanding the detoxification mechanisms that exist in living organisms and tailoring them through genetic engineering. Biotechnological application of microbial xylanase has been shown to make a significant contribution towards healthier environment by reducing the environmental loadings of paper mill effluents.

The main objective of this volume is to highlight the developments and achievements in the field of microbes.

We express my heartfelt gratitude to all the contributors for their overwhelming support and cooperation.

Editors

Contents

List of Contributors

A. Arunachalam, Restoration Ecology Laboratory, North Eastern Regional Institute of Science and Technology, Nirjuli 791109, Arunachal Pradesh, India

A. Babbar, Central Council for Research in Ayurveda and Siddha, Janakpuri, New Delhi 110058, India.

A. C. Kharkwal, Amity Institute of Herbal and Microbial studies, Amity University, NOIDA, 201303, UP, India

A. Das, Amity Institute of Herbal and Microbial studies, Amity University, NOIDA, 201303, UP, India

A. K. Chauhan, AKC House, E 27, Defence Colony, New Delhi 110024, India

A. Suresh, Indian Agricultural Research Institute, New Delhi 110012, India

A.Varma, Amity Institute of Herbal and Microbial Studies, Amity University, NOIDA-201303, UP, India

B. D. Kaushik, Indian Agricultural Research Institute, New Delhi 110012, India

B. Li, University of Massachusetts Dartmouth, 285 Old Westport Road, Dartmouth, MA 02747, USA

B. N. Prasad, Tribhuvan University, Kirtipur, Katmandu, Nepal

B. R. Singh, University of Massachusetts Dartmouth, 285 Old Westport Road, Dartmouth, MA 02747, USA

B. Singh, Delhi University, South Campus, Benito Juarez Road, New Delhi 110021, India

C. S. Nautiyal, National Botanical Research Institute, Lucknow, UP, India

D. B. Sahoo, Delhi University, Delhi 110007, India

Djajadi, University of Western Australia, 35, Sterling Highway, Carwley, 6009, WA, Australia

E. Kothe, Jena University, Jena, Germany

G. Ebena, Jena University, Jena, Germany

G. S. Lavekar, Central Council for Research in Ayurveda and Siddha, Janakpuri, New Delhi 110058, India

H. Kharkwal, Amity Institute of Herbal and Microbial studies, Amity University, NOIDA 201303, UP, India

J. Paul, School of Life Sciences, Jawaharlal Nehru University, New Delhi 110067, India

K. Arunachalam, Restoration Ecology Laboratory, North Eastern Regional Institute of Science and Technology, Nirjuli 791109, Arunachal Pradesh, India

K. Bhatnagar, Amity Institute of Herbal and Microbial Studies, Amity University, NOIDA, 201303, UP, India

K. Shrivastava, Restoration Ecology Laboratory, North Eastern Regional Institute of Science and Technology, Nirjuli 791109, Arunachal Pradesh, India

K. Abbott, University of Western Australia, 35, Sterling Highway, Crawley, 6009, WA, Australia

M. Rai, Amravati University, Amravati 444602, Maharashtra, India

P. Kaur, Delhi University, South Campus, Benito Juarez Road, New Delhi 110021, India

R. Ade, Amravati University, Amravati 444602, Maharashtra, India

R. Biswas, Department of Biochemical Engineering and Biotechnology, Indian Institute of Technology, New Delhi 110016, India

R. Hampp, University of Tuebingen, Auf der Morgenstelle 1, Tuebingen 72076, Germany

R. Prasad, Amity Institute of Herbal and Microbial studies, Amity University, NOIDA, 201303, UP, India

R. Prasanna, Centre for Conservation and Utilization of Blue Green Algae, New Delhi 110012, India

S. Adhikari, Delhi University, South Campus, Benito Juarez Road, New Delhi 110021, India

S. K. Sharma, Centre for Food Safety Applied Nutrition, US Department of Food and Drug Administration, College Park, MD 20740, US

K. S. Prasad, School of Environmental Sciences, Jawaharlal Nehru University, New Delhi 110067, India

S. Mishra, Department of Biochemical Engineering and Biotechnology, Indian Institute of Technology, New Delhi 110016, India

S. Nayak, Centre for Conservation and Utilization of Blue Green Algae, New Delhi, India

S. Neupane, Tribhuvan University, Kirtipur, Kathmandu, Nepal

T. Hurek, Cooperation Laboratory, Max Planck Institute for Marine Microbiology, University of Bremen FB 2, Leobener Str. NW2, Bremen 28359, Germany

T. Satyanarayana, Delhi University, South Campus, Benito Juarez Road, New Delhi 110021, India

T-wchang, University of Massachusetts Dartmouth, 285 Old Westport Road, Dartmouth, MA 02747 USA

V. S. Bisaria, Department of Biochemical Engineering and Biotechnology, Indian Institute of Technology, New Delhi 110016, India

V. Sahai, Department of Biochemical Engineering and Biotechnology, Indian Institute of Technology, New Delhi 110016, India

Impact of Micro-organisms on Environment and Health

AK CHAUHAN[1], A DAS[2], H KHARKWAL[2], AC KHARKWAL[2] and A VARMA[2*]

The future of biological and planetary sciences lies in understanding the role the microbes play in shaping this earth and its inhabitants. Life originated with microbes, and all forms of life are derived from microbes. They thrived for billions of years before any plants or animals existed, and continue to be the most abundant form of life on earth. Microbes generate more than half the oxygen we breathe in, excavate huge underground caverns, contribute mightily to the changes in our climate, and make up the largest mass of living things on earth. It is not an exaggeration to state that they are everywhere and often in very large number. Micro-organisms permeate the soil, water, and air of our planet. They created the atmosphere, turned bare rock and lava into soil, made possible the eventual evolution of larger life-forms, and continue to dominate the lives and functions of all living plants and animals. In today's world microbes hold their significance in the survival of world ecosystem, such as their role in global warming as well as the role of microbes in biotechnology.

Some microbes cause diseases; others are essential to agriculture for food production or for industry to carry out chemical transformation. Life without higher organisms is possible, but not without microbes. It's no wonder that ours has been called the planet of the microbes. These striking realities of life on earth are not widely appreciated as yet. The public perception of microbes as undesirable vermin – 'germs' should best be

1. AKC House, E-27 Defense Colony, New Delhi 110024

Amity Institute of Herbal & Microbial Studies, Block 'A', Amity Campus, Sector 125, Noida, UP 201303

* Corresponding author: ajitvarma@aihmr.amity.edu

eradicated. At present, concerns for *bio-terrorism* alert the people to the hazards of the agents of disease, but people are not generally aware of the global importance of microbes. Commonly, the study of microbes is either neglected or is relegated to a special academic niche.

For agriculturalists, the greatest interest in micro-life is in the complex communities of micro-organisms that are part of the soil. One gram (the same weight as a small paperclip) of healthy soil can contain between one and ten billion micro-organisms. Microbes present underground, when spread over the surface of the earth, would make a layer five feet thick. Invisible soil microorganisms on same piece of land can outweigh the livestock per hectare (2.4 acres) by factors of 10 or 100 times! Communities of bacteria, fungi, algae, protozoa, and other micro-organisms aerate the soil, make nutrients available to plants, purify drinking water and air channels, maintain soil structure, and recycle nutrients and organic matter that allow vegetation to grow. Every chemical transformation that happens in soil involves micro-organisms. Some micro-organisms excrete enzymes and other nutritions substances that stimulate plant-feeding. Micro-organisms provide a living reserve of nutrients like nitrogen and sulphur that would otherwise be easily leached. A healthy population of soil micro-organisms can also maintain ecological balance, preventing the onset of major problems from the viruses or other pathogens that live in the soil.

Thousands of species of micro-organisms have been recognized and named, but the number of unknown species is estimated to be in the millions. Almost every time, microbiologists search in a soil sample, they discover a previously unknown species. A few that are known to be of benefit to agriculture and forestry are listed below:

Mycorrhizae: Fungi that associate symbiotically with the roots of many kinds of plants, acting as a conduit for soil nutrients. Many scientists believe it was trees' association with these fungi that enabled them to colonize large tracts of land, giving rise to the forests.

Other Endosymbionts: An axenically cultivable mycorrhiza-like fungus has recently been described from the rhizosphere soil samples of xerophytic plants growing in north-west Rajasthan. The fungus was named *Piriformospora indica* based on its characteristic pear-shaped chlamydospores. According to the analysis of 18S rDNA and the ultrastructure of the septal pore, its phylogenetic relationship is within the Hymenomycetes (Basidiomycota). *P. indica* tremendously improves the growth and overall biomass of diverse hosts, including legumes, medicinal and economically important plants. Pronounced growth promotional effect was also seen with terrestrial orchids. The fungus promises to be a potential orchid mycorrhizal fungus. The fungus also provides protection when inoculated to the tissue culture raised plantlets by overcoming the 'transient transplant shock' on transfer to the field rendering almost 100% survival. The fungus forms inter- and intracellular hyphae in the root cortex, often differentiating into dense hyphal coils (arbuscule-like structures), spore and vesicle-like structures. Like 'AM fungi', hyphae multiply within the host cortical tissues and never traverse through the endodermis. Likewise, they also do not invade the aerial portion of the plant (stem and leaves). Fungus has a wide host range from herbs, shrubs and woody trees. The fungus could be mass multiplied on cheap and simplified medium. The fungus has great potential for application in agro-forestry, flori-horticulture, arboriculture, viticulture and especially for better establishment of tissue culture-raised plants that is much needed for the application in plant industry thus would open up numerous opportunities for the optimization of plant productivity in both, managed and natural ecosystems, while minimizing risks of environmental damage. Infecting crops with a fungus could be an alternative to genetically modifying them to boost yields, say scientists. In research published in the Proceedings of the National Academy of Sciences, USA (Waller et al. 2005), they showed that barley infected with fungus *Piriformospora indica* had three key advantages over uninfected plants. Apart from being able to grow in salty conditions, the infected barley yielded up to 11 per cent more grain, mainly because each plant had more seed-heads than uninfected barley. It naturally infects the roots of plants growing in the same environment. Scientists found that the fungus could be used to improve the stress and pathogen resistance of other plants that are difficult to genetically modify. It can easily be grown on a large scale and could become a new tool for sustainable agriculture (Verma et al. 1998; Varma et al. 1999; Varma et al. 2001; Pham et al. 2004 and Prasad et al. 2005). The properties of the fungus, *Piriformospora indica*, have been patented (Varma A and Franken P, 1997, European Patent Office, Muenchen, Germany. Patent No. 97121440.8-2105, Nov. 1998). The culture has been deposited at Braunsweich, Germany (DMS No.11827) and National Bureau of Agriculturally Important Micro-organisms (NBAIM), PUSA New Delhi.

Another endosymbiont namely *Geosiphon pyriformis* (Kütz.) v. Wettstein which is the only known fungus forming endosymbiosis with cyanobacteria, *Nostoc punctiforme* (Schussler and Kluge 2001; Schussler and Wolf 2005). At hyphal tips the coenocytic soil fungus forms unicellular, multinucleated 'bladders', about 1-2 mm in size, harbouring the cyanobacteria. The cyanobacterium can be cultivated without the fungus, whereas the fungus is an obligate symbiont. The fungus is capable of incorporating various strains of *N. punctiforme*. Provided compatibility of the *Nostoc* strain with the fungus, each single event of incorporation results in the formation of one typical *Geosiphon* bladder.

Rhizobia: These are bacteria that live in nodules on the roots of nitrogen-fixing plants, gathering the atmospheric nitrogen for plants like legumes. Actinobacteria is a kind of bacteria whose members break down the difficult-to-digest cellulose of trees on forest floors. Some kinds of actinobacteria, like *Frankia*, can also fix atmospheric nitrogen and can form nitrogen-fixing nodules with non-leguminous plants like alder trees.

Endophyte: It is an organism that lives within a plant for at least part of its life without causing apparent disease. Endophytes are ubiquitous and have been found in nearly all plants studied to date. Endophytic bacteria are capable of systemic infection and colonization of inner tissues of plants, without causing symptoms of any plant disease. In grasses, nitrogen-fixing bacteria such as *Azoarcus* sp. or *Herbaspirillum seropedicae* colonize the root cortex and, to a lesser extent, the vessels. In most cases they cannot be isolated root-free indicating that they are ecologically dependent on the host plant. Our model system consists of a pioneer plant, Kallar grass, which grows luxuriantly on low-fertility soils in the Punjab of Pakistan, and *Azoarcus* sp., *diazotrophs* abundant inside its roots and expressing nitrogenase gene(s) therein. In *gnotobiotic culture*, these bacteria are also capable of infecting rice seedlings (Reinhold-Hurek and Hurek 1998; Egener and Reinhold-Hurek 2000).

Cyanobacteria (blue-green algae): These tiny entities can photosynthesize, and some hundred strains of cyanobacteria are also able to fix nitrogen from the air. This enables them to colonize and thrive on barren areas, such as immediately following a lava flow—or even a nuclear blast! They are important in the early stages of pioneering harsh conditions. Some forms of cyanobacteria have also been used traditionally in rice production to fix nitrogen for rice crops. Several photosynthetic anaerobic (anoxybiont) serve as azotroph.

Lichens: These are symbiotic beings that are combinations of fungi and algae. Lichens can break down solid rock, releasing phosphates and nitrates, which generate food for plant's roots.

Others: Several diverse groups of fungi, bacteria, yeasts, algae, protozoans, and many more play crucial roles in maintaining the health and integrity of soil, and productivity of the land.

Microbes can either be a cause or remedy for environmental problems and are increasingly used for bioremediation to counteract the effects of human activity on the earth's natural system. There are many opportunities to use microbes to create new ways of doing old things, or to generate valuable new sources for human society like biodegradable, renewable microbial plastics which do not cause environmental problems.

Micro-organisms are used in nutrient recycling, in food, feed, biodegradation, pollution control, waste water treatment, biosynthesis and medicines. When plants and animals take up nutrients, they are not available to other living organisms. When the plants and animals die, the nutrients remain in the carcasses. If the dead substances, or detritus, are not broken down by microbes, those nutrients will never become available for help to sustain the life of other organisms. There are a finite amount of nutrients available in the environment and we cannot simply make more. The nutrients that are trapped in detritus must be released for continuity of life on the earth. It is the microbial population of the environment that is responsible for this nutrient recycling.

Micro-organisms are naturally found in foods, since there is no environment where some type of microbes cannot live. Live cells, dead cells and cellular byproducts, all have specific use in some kinds of food. These include such products as fermented meats and some dairy products. Microbes have been used for centuries to provide us with food. Bread is the result of a *microbial fermentation* of sugar to produce carbon dioxide—the bubbles that make bread rise. We owe our beer and wine to similar little yeast that convert sugar into alcohol for our consumption. Yoghurt and cheese are produced by bacterial fermentation of the sugar lactose present in milk. Microbes such as *phytoplankton* also serve as the nutrient source that indirectly feeds all *marine animals*. Microbial symbioses with plants allow them to grow strong and increase productivity - sometimes they are even essential for plant's survival. Microbes can also spoil foods and in some cases actually cause disease in humans.

Microorganisms are responsible for getting rid of the waste generated by industry and households. They detoxify acid mine drainage and other toxins that we dump into the soil and water. The nutrients gained from the breakdown of these products then go to feed plants or algae, which in turn feed all animals.

When we flush things down the drain or the toilet, they go to a septic system or waste water treatment plant at the end of the line. After primary mechanical treatment and aeration microbes remove organic materials from the filthy water that flows into these systems and, eventually, water is safely returned to the rivers and streams. The *methane* produced during treatment can even be used to generate heat or electricity for the operation.

We have discovered that microorganisms are useful for making things as well. Products such as xanthan gum (a food thickener) are harvested from their bacterial producers. Most of our vitamin B12, riboflavin, and vitamin C are produced by bacterial fermentation. Approximately 70% of antibiotics currently in use are also the product of microbial fermentation.

In pollution control, researchers are using bacteria that metabolize methane gas to clean up hazardous waste dumps and landfills. These methane-eating bacteria make an enzyme that can break down more than 250 pollutants into harmless cells. By piping methane into the soil, researchers can increase growth of the bacteria that normally live in the polluted soil. More bacteria means faster pollution break up. Also, bacteria are being used as one of the tools to clean up oil spills. These bacteria eat the oil, turning it into carbon dioxide and other harmless by-products.

Fungi, including *black mushrooms, actinomycetes* and bacteria, are an important source of medicine, including many antibiotics such as *penicillin* and *tetracycline, anti-tissue rejection drugs* for organ transplants, *cancer drugs*, and *anti-inflammatory products*. These are the medicines to fight-off harmful bacteria that cause sore-throats, ear infections, *diarrhoea* and other discomforts. Scientists have changed the genetic material of bacteria and yeasts to turn them into medicine. They inject genes, for medicines they want to make, into the microbe cells, as if adding new building information to the microbe's cell DNA. The scientists then grow the microbes in huge containers called *fermenters* where they reproduce into billions, all making new medicines.

Due to their tremendous usages, microbes are being used in different industries like health, *pharmaceuticals*, biotech, distillery, agriculture, horticulture etc. We highlight here some of the major usages of microbes in the chapters selected for the book.

Mushrooms are actually a fungus some of which can be cultivated and also be found growing wild in many regions of the world. They are *saprophytes* and play a role in the decomposition of organic matter in the biosphere. But most importantly, mushrooms have a high food value and can be used as a substitute for protein rich foods in human diet. Periods of severe food shortages cause famines, but protein deficiencies are manifested in malnutrition observed in many poor communities of developing nations. The cultivation or resourceful search for protein rich foods must be a goal in the struggle to combat malnutrition. With protein contents that may be as high as 60 per cent, source of vitamins B, D and the minerals potassium, selenium, copper, phosphorus and with health benefits such as the enhancement of body *immunity systems*, mushrooms are good food-source that could be part in any food security programmes. At present, about two thousand species (belonging to thirty different genera) of mushrooms are either consumed fresh or dried to make into soups, sauces and other food products, although all mushrooms are not edible. Out of the two thousand or so edible species of mushrooms, only eighty have been artificially cultivated around the world.

Humans depend on having a microbial population, called micro-biota in the body, for normal body functioning. There are normally ten times more microbial cells in a human body than human cells. The useful bacteria that live on and in the human body protect humans from the harmful invaders. Without the useful bacteria, the harmful ones can slip in and easily cause problems in humans. Human digestion has also evolved to use bacteria for assistance, allowing it to gain nutrition from plant polysaccharides that the body's own enzymes will not degrade. Microbes are used for altering the active ingredients or compounds in medicinal plants. Plants are also nature's medicine. Studies state that between 25 to 50 per cent of all the medicines prescribed worldwide today come from plants or are based on chemicals found in plants. According to the World Health Organization, nearly 70 per cent of the earth's 6.2 billion people rely on plant-based traditional medicines to relieve pain, to heal wounds and to prevent or cure diseases.

Recently fungus *Piriformospora indica* was found to enhance the anti-oxidants in *Baccopa monnieri* and *Baccosides* (memory plus ingredients). A patent entitled '*Piriformospora indica* - a symbiotic fungus promotes biomass of *Bacopa monnieri*, enhances the antioxidant activity and bacoside concentration' has been filed to seek the protection of this discovery from European, North American countries and the countries of Indian subcontinent. *Bacopa monnieri* is a plant of great economic importance and is known to be used as nerve tonic, adaptogen, *antioxidant*, *antimicrobial*, *antifungal*, *sedative*, *cardio tonic*, *anticonvulsent*, *antidepressant* and useful for cancer patients experiencing pain. The fungus *P. indica* is documented to promote plant growth and protects the host against root pathogens and insects. Fungus root colonization promoted the plant growth and enhanced antioxidant activity and the active ingredient bacoside by several folds. Symbiotic fungus, *P. indica*, enhances the plant biomass, antioxidant activity and bacoside concentration in *Bacopa monnieri* (Russo and Borrelli 2005).

Often in dealing with land that has been cleared of natural vegetation and depleted of micro life, modern farmers have tried to improve productivity by adding soluble fertilizers. However, given the increasing recognition of the role of micro-organisms, the way the future may focus on fostering land, when necessary, reintroducing healthy populations of micro-life in the soil to enhance productivity. The use of mycorrhizae, cyanobacteria and rhizobia inoculants has become almost standard in forestry and agriculture. Other ways to increase productivity with micro-life are being researched and practiced world-wide. These techniques range from simply bringing in small amounts of healthy soil to inoculate new plantings in degraded areas, to the manufacture and application of special biostimulants to feed and encourage micro life, or to introducing blends of selected beneficial micro-organisms to be used in nursery or field production. The importance of *arbuscular fungi* for plant development and health is now widely demonstrated. However, although it is more and more evident that they are not only an integral part of many cultivated plants but also an essential component of soil fertility, their rational use in plant production is still in its infancy. Because of their role as *bioregulators, biofertilizers*, and *biocontrol agents*, they represent potentially important tools for new orientations in agriculture. A disadvantage of *micropropagation*, the most powerful technique for cloning plant species, is the high mortality rate during the transfer of *in vitro* plantlets to *ex vitro*. Inoculation of plantlets with AMF during acclimatization has been recommended for reducing the stress of acclimatization, providing faster growth and better establishment of micropropagated plants. *Piriformospora indica* promises to be an excellent candidate for biological hardening of micropropagated plantlets as the fungus rendered more than 90 per cent survival rate of the transferred plantlets of *Nicotiana tabacum* L. and *Bacopa monniera*. Recent experiments on the tissue culture-raised coffee (*Coffea arabica* L.) plants have shown very promising results.

Manipulating and engineering the *rhizosphere* of plants to elicit benefits such as suppression of soil-borne crop diseases, phyto-remediation, optimization of nutrient supply, production of plant growth promoting substances, and improvement of plant-soil-water relations offers a powerful, new way forward for land management. Practical manipulation and engineering of the rhizosphere can, however, only be facilitated by the development of a better understanding of biological interactions in the root environment and the generation of reliable models that explain and predict the dynamics of rhizosphere populations and their interactions. Immunological, biochemical and molecular methods in combination with X-ray computed topographic, isotopic and more traditional, taxonomic approaches now provide powerful tools to evaluate the population dynamics and function of the micro flora and micro fauna at scales relevant to resolving biological interactions in the root environment.

Fungal protoplasts represent the finest cell system and offer exciting possibilities in the field of somatic cell genetics, strain improvement by mutagenesis, fusion and transformation, membrane research, investigations on the effects of different chemical substances on fungal cells, production of metabolites and secretery proteins and studies of the different steps and structures dealing with cell-wall synthesis. Protoplast is the term used to describe the *osmotically fragile* cells completely devoid of cell-wall residues. Formation of protoplasts from mycorrhizal fungi present several impediments, not generally encountered with other fungi (Singh 2002; Varavallo et al. 2004; Zhao et al. 2004).

Plant root exudates not only provide the essential resources to sustain the abundant and diverse rhizosphere microbial community, but also contain the chemical signals which influence interactions in the rhizosphere at a range of trophic levels. Such interactions range from the direct effect of specific compounds diffusing from roots on the germination of spores to the effects of *parasitic nematodes* influencing the composition of root exudates which trigger changes in the pathogenic/saprophytic stages of fungi in the rhizosphere. Such studies will lead to the identification of a range of bio-active compounds, with opportunities for wealth creation, and to increased fundamental understanding of plant, microbial and micro faunal processes and signalling mechanisms.

In the great majority of natural communities, the primary producers depend heavily on micro-organisms. Some of the microbes are symbionts, as in the case of mycorrhizae and nitrogen fixers; others are free-living, but nevertheless linked tightly to the well-being of the primary producers. These include the organisms that decompose and mineralize organic detritus, others that promote plant growth and suppress plant pathogens, and some that build soil structure. Intentional introduction of the beneficial micro-organisms sometimes makes the difficult plant species easier to grow. *Plant growth-promoting Rhizobacteria* (*PGPR*) include a range of organisms that live in close association with roots. PGPR are of great potential importance, and their culture and modes of action are the subject of active research. The possible mechanisms by which PGPR aid plant growth include suppression of root pathogens through chelating of iron or production of antibiotics, fixation of nitrogen, and production of plant hormones. PGPR are synergistic with mycorrhizae in stimulating plant growth, and PGPR may stimulate root colonization by mycorrhizal fungi. There has been some success with PGPR in agriculture, and commercial preparations are likely to become available.

Another group of microbes are plant viruses which represent an important class of plant pathogen that collectively is responsible for billions of dollars in food and fibre crop losses annually. Accordingly, the studies of plant viruses represent an important area of research for sustaining agricultural systems. A general lack of understanding of the fundamental steps of viral infections has hindered the development of novel anti-virus strategies. Plant viruses can also be valuable for biotechnological applications i.e., for the production of commercially-important protein pharmaceuticals, such as vaccines.

In the field of chemical technology, where manufacture of a variety of products on large scale has resulted in serious effluent and hazardous waste disposal problems, the need for safer and 'environmental friendly' technologies has become imminent. This has resulted in scientists attempting to learn from natural processes, and therefore a new aspect of microbiology and biotechnology has rapidly emerged. Micro-organisms perform their myriads of biochemical reactions under ambient conditions with little or no toxic and hazardous by-products. Therefore enzyme alternatives to polluting chemical technologies, which began initially as an idea, have reached realistic proportions, whereby they can be considered as worthwhile and practical technologies of the future. One such area is the pulp and paper industry where the quantities of raw materials processed are huge, as well as the use of naturally hazardous chemicals are also large. *Xylanases* enzymes are used as effective bio-reagents to achieve bio-bleaching in place of poisonous chlorine compounds used for pulp brightness of a high order in the manufacture of high-quality paper products.

Microorganisms are used in large-scale heap or tank aeration processes for the commercial extraction of a variety of metals from their ores or concentrates. These include copper, cobalt, gold and, in the past, uranium. The *metal solubilization-* processes are considered to be largely chemical with the micro-organisms providing the chemicals and the space (exopolysaccharide layer) where the mineral dissolution reactions occur. The remarkable adaptability of biomining micro-organisms is assisted by several of the processes being continuous-flow systems that enable the continual selection of micro-organisms that are more efficient at mineral degradation. Adaptability is also assisted by the processes being open and non-sterile thereby permitting new organisms to enter. This openness allows for the possibility of new genes that improve cell fitness to be selected from the horizontal gene pool. Bioleaching processes are carried out at a range of temperatures from ambient to a demonstration plant that has been operated at 80°C. As would be expected, the types of iron- and sulphur-oxidizing microbes present differ depending on the temperature range. The types of microbes found in processes that operate from ambient to 40°C, tend to be similar irrespective of the mineral, as are those within the temperature ranges of 45–55°C and 75– 80°C.

Phytase is a *phosphohydrolytic enzyme* that initiates the stepwise removal of phosphate from phytate. Supplemental microbial phytase in diets for swine and poultry has become an effective tool for improving bioavailability of phytate-phosphorus to these food producing animals, reducing dietary inorganic phosphorus supplementation, and controlling manure phosphorus excretion in complying with environmental regulation. Several commercial phytase enzymes have been available, but none of them is completely satisfactory.

The common people normally only hear about micro-organisms in terms of viruses or harmful bacteria, to be battled with soap, disinfectants, and other weapons in our modern arsenal. However, in general the functions of most microorganisms are benign or very much to our benefit, and to destroy them would be to destroy ourselves. The human body, for example, is teeming with micro life—about 10% of the average human body weight is made up of micro-organisms! Each square centimeter human skin hosts an average of 100,000 bacteria, maintaining the health of the skin, and countless millions occupy our intestines. Our vital abilities to breathe and digest food are all intricately linked to the micro-organisms that reside within us and make our life possible. The web of life depends on this vast network of micro-organisms. Recognizing the numerous invaluable functions of microbes should decrease the germ phobia. Micro-organisms are everywhere - a largely unseen world of activities that helped to create the biosphere and that continue to support the life processes on earth. So, Welcome to the Microbial World. In fact, we are part of it!

REFERENCES

Egener T, Reinhold-Hurek B (2000) Endophytic expression of *nif* genes of *Azoarcus* sp. BH72 in rice roots. *Mol. Plant-Microbe Interact* 12: 813-819

Pham GH, Singh An, Malla R, Kumari R, Prasad R, Sachdev M, Luis P, Kaldorf M, Tatjana P, Harrmann S, Hehl S, Declerck S, Buscot F, Oelmuller R, Rexer KH, Kost G and Varma A (2004) Interaction of *P. indica* with Other Micro-organisms and Plants. In: Varma A, Abbott L, Werner D and Hampp R (eds) *Plant Surface Microbiology*. Springer-Verlag, Germany, pp 237-265

Prasad R, Pham GH, Kumari R, Singh A, Yadav V, Sachdev M, Peskan T, Hehl S, Oelmuller R and Varma A (2005) Sebacinaceae: Culturable Mycorrhiza–like Endosymbiotic Fungi and their Interaction with Non-transformed and Transformed Roots. In: Declerck S, Strullu DG, Fortin JA (eds) *In Vitro Culture of Mycorrhizae*. Springer-Verlag, Germany, pp 291-312

Reinhold-Hurek B, Hurek T (1998) Life in grasses: diazotrophic endophytes. *Trends Microbiol.* 6: 139-144

Russo A, Borrelli F (2005) *Bacopa monniera*, a reputed non-tropic plant: an overview. *Pytomedicine* 12: 305-317

Schussler A, Kluge M (2001) *Geosiphon pyriforme*, an endocytosymbiosis between fungus and cyanobacteria, and its meaning as a model system for arbuscular mycorrhizal research. In: Hock B (ed) *The Mycota IX*. Springer, Germany, pp 151-161

Schussler A, Wolf E (2005) *Geosiphon pyriformis*-a Glomeromycotan Soil Fungus forming endosymbiosis with cyanobacteria. In: Declerck S, Strullu DG, Fortin JA (eds) *In Vitro Culture of Mycorrhizae*. Springer Germany, pp 271-287

Singh A (2002) Intergeneric hybridization between a yeast strain and a plant growth promoting endophytic fungus by isolation, fusion and regeneration of somatic protoplasts, PhD Thesis, JNU, New Delhi

Varavallo MA, de Queiroz MV, Pereira JF and de Araujo EF (2004) Isolation and regeneration of *Penicillium brevicompactum* protoplasts. Acta Scientiarum. *Biological Sciences*. 26: 475-479

Varma A, Singh A, Sudha, Sahay N S,Sharma J, Roy A, Kumari M, Rana D, Thakran S, Deka D,Bharti K, Hurek T, Blechert O, Rexer KH, Kost G, Hahn A, Maier W, Walter M, Strack D and Kranner I (2001) *Piriformospora indica*: An Axenically culturable Mycorrhiza-Like endosymbiotic fungus In: Hock B (Ed) *The Mycota IX*. Springer, Berlin, pp 151-161

Varma A, Verma S, Sudha, Sahay N, Britta B, Franken P (1999) *Piriformospora indica* – a cultivable plant growth promoting root endophyte with similarities to arbuscular mycorrhizal fungi. *Applied and Environmental Microbiology,* USA, 65: 2741-2744

Verma S, Varma A, Rexer Karl-Heinz, Hassel A, Kost G, Sarbhoy A, Bisen P, Buetechorn P and Franken P (1998). *Piriformospora indica* gen-nov, a new root colonizing fungus. Mycologia-USA, 90: 895-909.

Waller F, Achatz B, Baltruschat H, Fodor J, Becker K, Fischer M, Heier T, Huckelhoven R, Neumann C, Wettstein DV, Franken P and Kogel KH (2005) The endophytic fungus *Piriformospora indica* reprogrammes barley to salt stress tolerance, disease resistance, and higher yield. *Proceedings of the National Academy of Sciences of the United States of America* 102: 13386-13391

Zhao K, Zhou D, Ping W and Ge J (2004) Study on the preparation and regeneration of protoplast from taxol-producing fungus *Nodulisporium sylviforme. Nature and Science* 2: 52-59.

Synergism Between Medicinal Plants and Microbes

A DAS[1], R PRASAD[1], K BHATNAGAR[1], GS LAVEKAR[2] and A VARMA[1]

1. INTRODUCTION

Micro-organisms exist in every niche of our biosphere and occupy a peculiar place in the human view of life. Microbes receive little attention in our general texts of biology. They are largely ignored by most professional biologists and are virtually unknown to the public except in the contexts of disease and rot. Yet, the workings of the biosphere depend absolutely on the activities of the microbial world. A handful of soil contains billions of microbial organisms; there are so many different types that accurate numbers remain unknown. We know so little about microbial biology, despite it being a part of biology that looms so large in the sustenance of life on this planet. The reason for our poor understanding of the microbial world lies in the fact that microbes are tiny, individually invisible to the eye. Micro-organisms are organisms of microscopic or submicroscopic size and we need a microscope to see them. The lower limit of our eye's resolution is about 0.1 to 0.2 mm or 100-200 μm. Most microbes range in size from about 0.2 to the 200 μm in upper limit, although some fruiting bodies of fungi can become much larger. The mere existence of microbial life was recognized only relatively recently in history, about 300 years ago, with Leeuwenhoek's invention of the microscope. Microbes like

1. Amity Institute of Microbial and Herbal Studies, Amity University, Block A, Amity Campus, Sector 125, NOIDA, Uttar Pradesh, India,
E-mail: ajitvarma@aihmr.amity.edu

2. Central Council for Research in Ayurveda & Siddha, 61-65 Institutional Area, Opp. D Block, Janakpuri, New Delhi 110058, India, E-mail: indiaccrasdir1@nic.in

non-descript rods and spheres are difficult to classify by morphology under microscope, the way that large organisms had always been related to one another. It was not until the late 19th century and the development of pure-culture techniques that microbial organisms could be studied as individual types and characterized to some extent, mainly by nutritional criteria. However, the pure-culture approach to the study of the microbial world seriously constrained the view of microbial diversity because most microbes defy cultivation by standard methods. Moreover, the morphological and nutritional criteria used to describe microbes failed to provide a natural taxonomy, ordered according to evolutionary relationships. Molecular tools and perspective based on gene sequences are now alleviating these constraints to some extent. Even the early results are changing our perception of microbial diversity.

Microbes were present on earth 3.5 to 4 billion years ago, and they've been evolving and expanding into new environments ever since. Replicating quickly, exchanging genetic material with each other and with other organisms, bacteria and archaea have become ubiquitous. Not only are they everywhere, but these tiny organisms also manipulate the environments in which they live. Their presence has driven the development of new ecosystems, some of which allowed for the evolution of more complex organisms. Without micro-organisms, the recycling of essential nutrients on earth would halt. Micro-organisms are the principal drivers of the global elemental cycles. Microbes communicate; some generate the signals for the formation of metabolically diverse communities. Some use sophisticated signalling to establish complex relationships with higher organisms.

A large part of all micro-organisms live in soils, sediments, aquifers and geological formations where they mineralize the organic compounds originating mainly from photosynthetic primary production.

2. MICROBES AS THE FIRST ORGANISMS

No one knows for certain where life began. Hot springs and volcanic (*hydrothermal*) vents on the ocean floor, however, may represent the kinds of environments where cellular life began. Before the ozone layer formed, the surface of earth was exposed to strong radiation. Thus, most of the earth's earliest organisms probably developed beneath the terrestrial surface or in the oceans. It's likely that these early microbes adapted to the high temperatures associated with abundant volcanic activity. Geological turmoil resulted in the accumulation of carbon dioxide in the atmosphere.

Sometime later, about 2 or 2.5 billion years ago, gaseous oxygen began to appear. Unlike the carbon dioxide, oxygen came about because of microbes. Microbes, similar to today's cyanobacteria, were present at that time. This fact is based on the presence of fossilized microbial mats consisting of the layers of *filamentous prokaryotes* and trapped sediment that date back to that time. *Stromatolite-forming bacteria* obtained carbon from carbon dioxide and got their energy by photosynthesis, splitting water to generate oxygen gas in the process. These organisms brought the oxygen level in earth's atmosphere to about ten per cent of what it is present today which was enough to allow the evolution of oxygen-using organisms. Gaseous oxygen also contributed to the formation of the ozone layer, which blocks UV radiation. New terrestrial habitats were now open for an evolving diversity of microbes.

3. DIVERSITY OF LIFE

Biological diversity, also called 'biodiversity', consists of all of the plants, animals, and micro-organisms that make up the spectacular variety of life on earth. In the 19th century, evidence began to accumulate and various schemes were proposed to classify living organisms with three, four, or more kingdoms. The scheme most often used currently divides all living organisms into five kingdoms: *Monera* (bacteria), *Protista*, Fungi, *Plantae*, and Animalia. Two basic cell lines also have appeared during evolutionary history. These lines, termed prokaryotic cells and eukaryotic cells, differ primarily in the complexity of their cell-structure. Five kingdoms scheme co-existed with scheme dividing life into two main divisions, i.e. the prokaryotes that are bacteria, etc. and the eukaryotes that are animals, plants, fungi, and protists (Prescott et al.1996). In general, prokaryotic cells are smaller than eukaryotic cells, and they lack special structures such as a nucleus and organelles. Organelles are small membrane-bound cell structures that perform specific functions in eukaryotic cells.

Although biologists have found the system of five kingdoms and two basic cell types to be a valuable method of classification, recent studies in molecular biology have provided a more accurate view of the relationships and origins of cells. It has been determined that certain types of molecules in cells, called small ribosomal ribonucleic acid (rRNA), provide a 'living record' of the evolutionary history of an organism. Analysis of this molecule in prokaryotic and eukaryotic cells indicates that certain unusual cells called archaea (originally archaebacteria) are so different from the other two groups that they should be included in a separate super kingdom. The difference between the structure of prokaryotes and eukaryotes is so great that it is considered to be the most important distinction among groups of organisms. Most prokaryotes are bacteria, and the two terms are often treated as synonyms. However, Woese has proposed dividing prokaryotes into the bacteria and archaea (originally eubacteria and archaebacteria) because of the significant genetic differences between the two. This arrangement of eukaryote, bacteria, and archaea is called the three-domain system.

Viruses are not cellular and are therefore called particles rather than organisms. They are included in microbiology because of their small size and close relationship with cells. However, they are of considerable biological importance. Therefore, excluding the viruses, there are two types of micro-organisms: prokaryotes, and eukaryotes. Prokaryotes (from Old Greek pro- before + karyon nut, referring to the cell nucleus, + suffix -*otos*, pl. *-otes*; also spelled 'procaryotes') are organisms without a cell nucleus (= karyon), or indeed any other membrane-bound organelles, in most cases unicellular (in rare cases, multicellular). This is in contrast to eukaryotes (also spelled 'eucaryotes'), organisms that have cell nuclei and may be variously unicellular or multicellular.

All prokaryotes are microorganisms, but only some eukaryotes are micro-organisms. The bodies of most micro-organisms consist of either a single cell or just a few cells. Because of their role in diseases, certain animals such as helminth worms and insects, many of which can be seen with naked eyes, are also considered in the study of micro-organisms. Even in its seeming simplicity, the microscopic world is every bit as complex and diverse as the macroscopic one. There is no doubt that micro-organisms also outnumber macroscopic organisms by a factor of several million. So, what were once called 'prokaryotes' are far more diverse than anyone had suspected. The Prokaryotes are now divided into two domains, the Bacteria and the Archaea, as different from each other as either is from the Eukaryota, or eukaryotes (Fig. 1). None of these groups are ancestral to the others and each shares certain features with the others as well as having unique characteristics of its own.

4. METHODS FOR CLASSIFYING MICROBIAL DIVERSITY

4.1 Morphological Diversity

Morphological diversity of micro-organisms are based on its morphological features, structures etc. With the help of microscope, it can be distinguished into prokaryotic/eukaryotic and some obvious prokaryotic differences but it is insufficient to distinguish microbe types that appear the same.

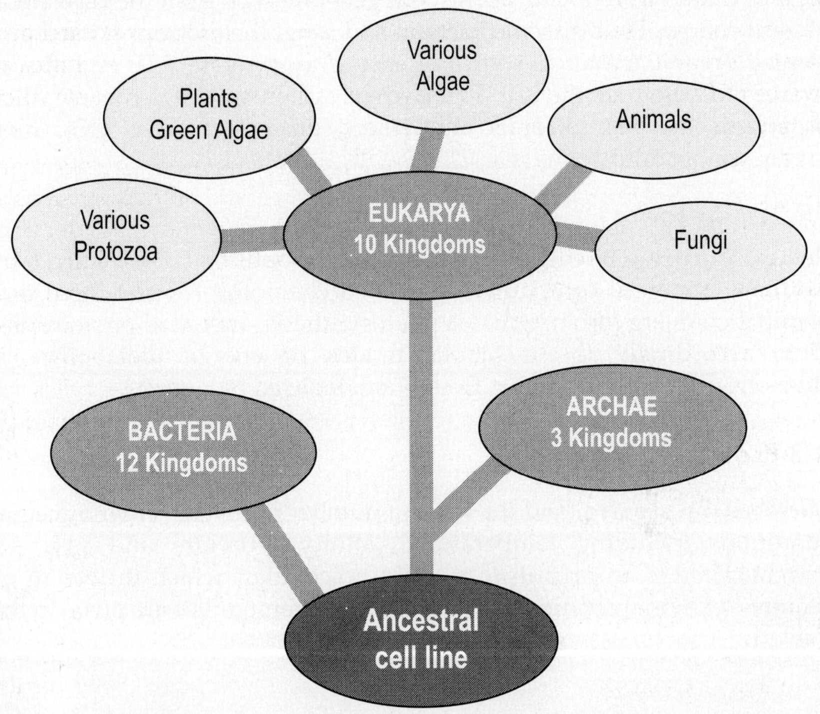

Fig. 1 A system for representing the origins of cell lines and major taxonomic groups as proposed by Carl Woese and colleagues. They proposed three distinct cell lines placed in superkingdoms called domains. The first primitive cells called progenotes were ancestors of both lines of prokaryotes (Domains Bacteria and Archaea) and the archaea emerged from the same cell line as eukaryotes (Domain Eukarya)

4.2 Metabolic Diversity

Metabolic differences on the basis of biochemical differences (based on enzymological studies) can help further to distinguish microbial diversity.

4.2.1 Carbon Source

Micro-organisms are classified as *autotrophs* or *heterotrophs* based on whether or not they require pre-formed organic matter. Autotrophs derive energy from either light absorption (*photoautotrophs*) or oxidation of inorganic molecules (*chemoautotrophs*). In most of the light reactions the bacteria are fixing carbon dioxide into organic carbon, just as green plants do. Some photosynthetic bacteria (*photoheterotrophs*) require pre-formed organic matter as reducing agents, but generate ATP from the absorption of light energy. Finally, some bacteria and fungi (heterotrophs) used pre-formed organic matter as source of energy to generate ATP and also as source of carbon for the cell. Thus, when carbon source is organic, then organisms are heterotrophs and when carbon source is CO_2, then organisms are autotrophs (Fig. 2).

4.2.2 Energy Source

Energy source can be chemicals or solar. Autotrophs that obtain energy by oxidizing chemical compounds are called chemotrophs, and those that obtain their energy from light, via photosynthesis, are called phototrophs. Thus accordingly the metabolic modes of energy metabolism is chemotrophy or phototrophy. Details are depicted in Figure 3.

4.3 Ecological Diversity

Microbes can survive (and thrive) in a number of diverse environmental conditions including temperature, salinity, pressure and pH. An extremophile is an organism, usually unicellular, which thrives in or requires 'extreme' conditions. Examples of extremophiles are given in the Table 1.

4.3.1 Temperature

Micro-organisms can tolerate temperature range of –5°C to 118°C. Micro-organisms may be hyperthermophile or psychrophile. A hyperthermophile is an organism that thrives in extremely hot environments that is, hotter than around 60°C. The optimal temperatures are between 80°C and 110°C. Most hyperthermophiles micro-organisms are extremophile and are found within the domain archaea, though some bacteria and cyanobacteria are able to tolerate temperatures of around 70°C, e.g., *Pyrolobus*. Many hyperthermophiles are able to withstand other environmental extremes for instance, high acidity or radiation levels.

A *psychrophile* is a type of organism which thrives at what is considered to be unusually cold temperatures. They can be contrasted with thermophiles which thrive at unusually hot temperatures. There are generally considered to be two groups of psychrophiles: 'classic' psychrophiles and a second group that are sometimes referred to as psychrotrophs by food microbiologists. Classic psychrophiles are those organisms having a growth temperature optimum of 15°C or lower and do not grow in a climate beyond a maximum temperature of 20°C. They are largely found in icy places (such as in Antarctica) or at the freezing bottom of the ocean floor.

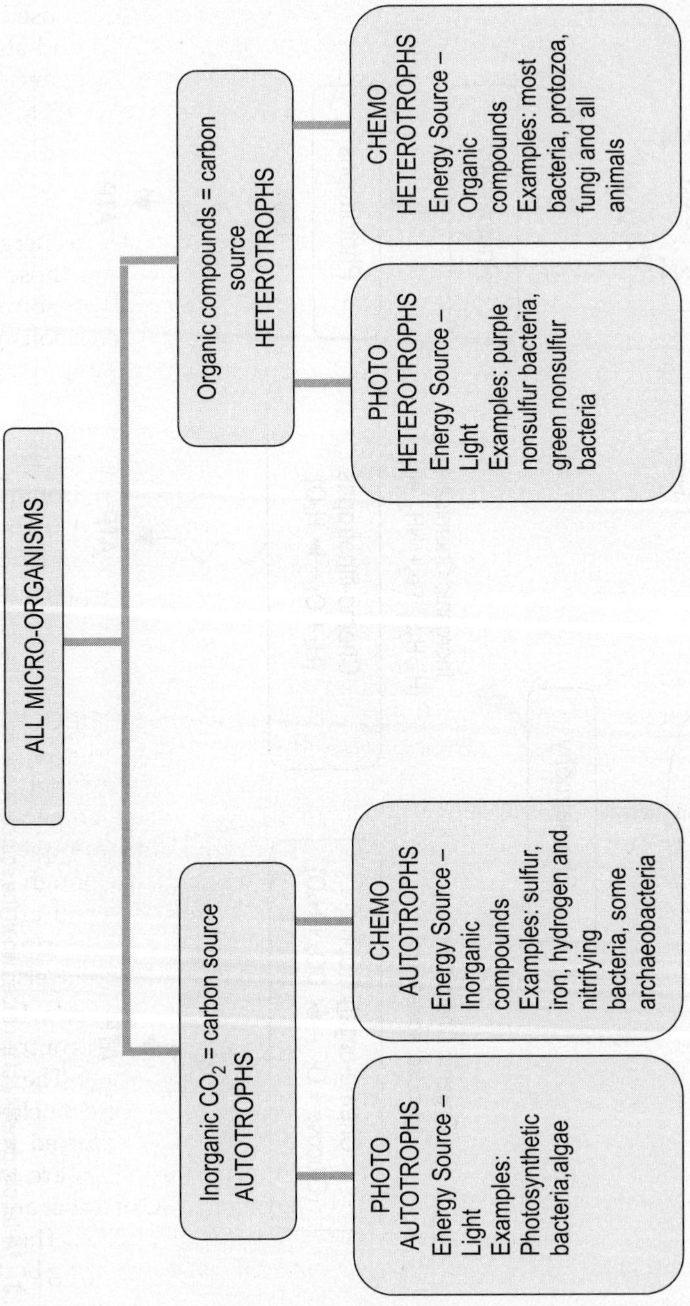

Fig. 2 The main types of energy capturing metabolism

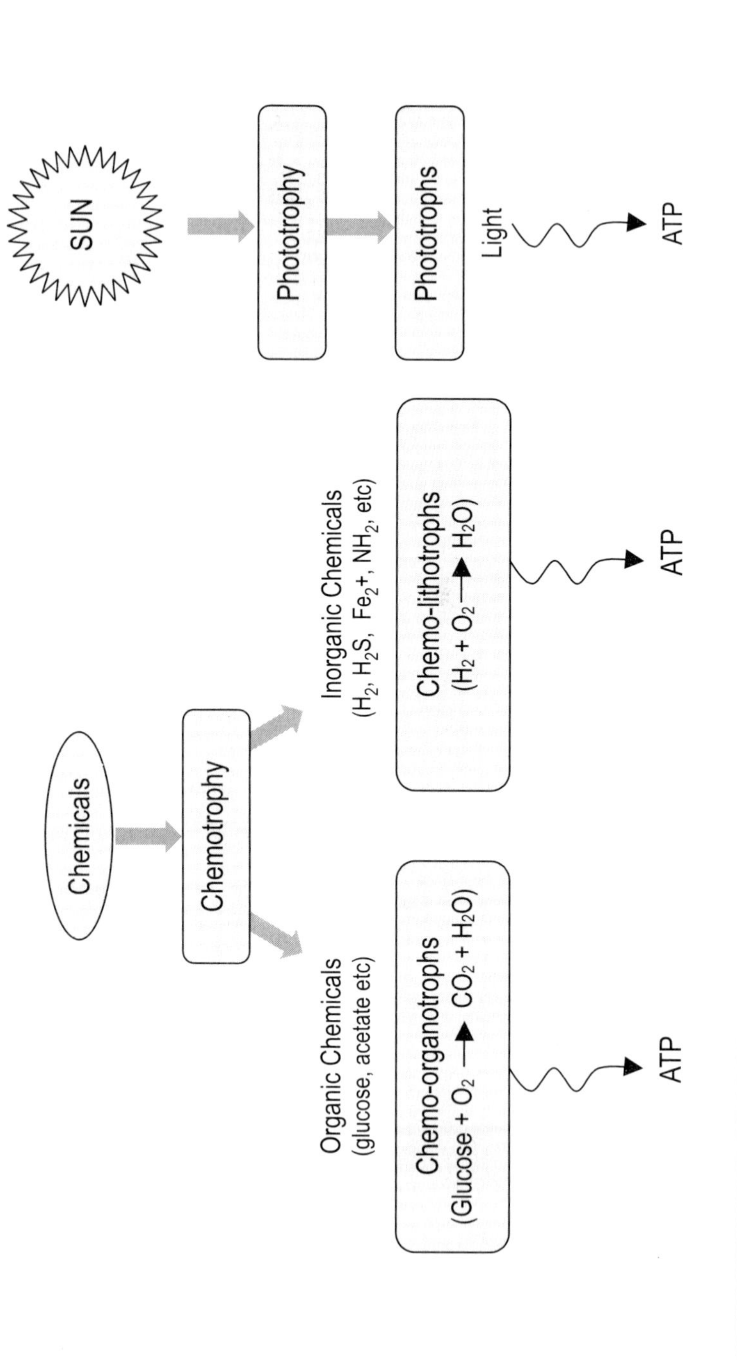

Fig. 3 Metabolic diversity of microbes when the source of energy is either chemicals or solar

Table 1 Example of Extremeophiles

Extreme	*Descriptive term*	*Genus/Sp*	*Domain*	*Habitat*	*Minimum*	*Optimum*	*Maximum*
Temperature							
High	Hyperthermophile	*Pyrolobus fumarii*	Archaea	Hot undersea Hydrothermal vents	90°C	105°C	113°C
Low	Psychrophile	*Polaromonas vacuolata*	Bacteria	Sea- ice	0°C	4°C	12°C
pH							
Low	*Acidophile*	*Picrophilus ashimae*	Archaea	Acid hot springs	–0.06	0.7 Thermophile 60°C	4
High	*Alkaliphile*	*Natronobacterium gregory*	Archaea	Soda lakes	8.5	10 Halophile 20% salt	12
Pressure	*Barophile*	MT41 (Mariana Trench)	Bacteria sediments	Deep ocean	500 atm	700 atm	>1000 atm
Salt (NaCl)	*Halophile*	*Halobacterium salinarum*	Archaea	Salterms	15%	25%	32% Saturation

4.3.2 Salinity

Micro-organisms can tolerate high amount of salt concentrations in freshwater, saltwater or even present in Dead Sea e.g., *Halobacterium salinarum.*

Halophiles are extremophiles that thrive in environments with very high concentrations of salt (at least 0.2 M [molar]). The name comes from Greek for 'salt-loving'. The extreme halophiles or halobacteria, a group of archaea, require at least 2 M of salt and are usually found in saturated solutions. These are the primary inhabitants of salt lakes and inland seas, such as the Dead Sea, where they tint the sediments bright colours.

4.3.3 pH

Micro-organisms can tolerate pH ranging between 0-11. They can be acidophile or alkaliphile. Micro-organisms that can live in an acidic environment are acidophile.

Organisms that prefer or can tolerate alkaline conditions, typically in the range of pH 8-11, are alkaliphile.

4. 3. 4 Pressure

Micro-organism which grows best (or can only grow) in high-pressure environments, such as deep-sea environments are barophile.

4.4 Genetic Diversity

Gene sequences are done with the help of tools of molecular biology, DNA sequencing etc. DNA sequencing allows the comparison of genes from different microbes.

5 SOME OF THE SELECTED IMPORTANT MICROBES

5.1 Archaea

The archaea resemble bacteria to a great extent, so much so that they were once thought to be a weird group of bacteria. However, when their ribosomal RNA was sequenced, scientists found that they bore no close relationship to the bacteria and were, in fact, more closely related to the eukaryotes. For a long time they were referred to as archaebacteria, but to emphasize their distinctness, these are now called Archaea. Cell-wall chemistry was one of the first phenotypical characteristics to distinguish archaebacteria from eubacteria (Kandler and Konig 1985; Kandler and Konig 1993). Archaeans are among the earliest forms of life that appeared on earth billions of years ago. It's now generally believed that the archaea and bacteria developed separately from a common ancestor nearly four billion years ago. Millions of years later, the ancestors of today's eukaryotes split off from the archaea. Thus, while archaeans resemble bacteria and have some genes that are similar to bacterial genes, they also contain other genes that are more like what is found in eukaryotes.

They have also been called Extremophiles in recognition of the extreme environments in which they have been found.

5.1.1 Properties of Archaea

The archaea represents a mixture of traits which are characteristic of the other prokaryotes, the bacteria and those found in eukaryotes. Characteristics are tabulated in the Table 2.

5.1.2 Types of Archaea

There are three main types of archaea: the crenarchaeota, which are characterized by their ability to tolerate extreme temperature and acidity; the euryarchaeota, which include methane-producers and salt-lovers; and the korarchaeota, a catch-all group of archaeans about which very little is known. Among these three main types of archaea are some sub-types, which include:

Methanogens are those archaeans that produce methane gas as a waste product of their 'digestion' or process of making energy, e.g., *Methanococcus, Methanobacterium* (Akca et al.2002).

Halophiles are those archaeans that live in very saline environments, e.g. *Halobacterium, Natrinobacterium*.

Table 2 Summarisation of some Eukaryotic and Bacterial Traits in Archaea

Eukaryotic Traits	*Bacterial Traits*
• DNA replication machinery	
• Histones	
• Nucleosome-like structures	• Single, circular chromosome
• Transcription machinery	• Operons
• RNA polymerase	• No introns
• TFIIB	• Bacterial-type membrane transport channels
• TATA-binding protein (TBP)	
• Translation machinery	• Many metabolic processes
• Initiation factors	• Energy production
• Ribosomal proteins	• Nitrogen-fixation
• Elongation factors	• Polysaccharide synthesis
• Poisoned by diphtheria toxin	

Thermophiles are those archaeans that live at extremely hot temperatures.

Psychrophiles are those archaeans that live at unusually cold temperatures.

Acidophiles are those archaeans which live at low pH (as low as pH 1 and who die at pH 7)

Alkaliphiles are those archaeans which thrive at a high pH. The archaeon *Natronococcus occultus* survives optimally in extremely alkaline biotopes with a pH value between 9.5 and 10.0 and a salt concentration around 3.5 mol/l (Niemetz et al.1997)

5.1.3 Economic Importance of the Archaea

Because they have enzymes that can function at high temperatures, considerable effort is being made to exploit the archaea for commercial processes such as providing enzymes to be added to detergents (maintain their activity at high temperatures and pH); an enzyme to convert corn starch into dextrins. Archaea may also be enlisted to aid in cleaning up contaminated sites, e.g. petroleum spills.

5.2 Bacteria

All prokaryotes have long been grouped together in one kingdom, Monera. However, strong new evidence indicates that there are actually two distinct groups of prokaryotes: Bacteria (or Eubacteria) and Archaea (or Archaebacteria) (Fig. 1).

Bacteria are found everywhere in water, soil, and even air. These small prokaryotic cells, typically from 0.2 to 1 μm in length, are capable of living in boiling water, frozen ground, acid volcanoes, and at the bottom of the ocean. They can reproduce by doubling with a generation time of 20 minutes, or survive for centuries in a resting stage. In natural waters (lakes, streams, oceans) their generation time is around 1 day. In soils they live in a film of water around plant roots or other particles, and their activity is dependent on the temperature and the amount of available moisture. In general, bacteria are found in concentrations of 10^6 cells/ml of water in surface waters, and 10^9 cells/ml of soil in soils and sediments.

5.2.1 Properties of Bacteria

Bacteria are prokaryotic (no membrane-enclosed nucleus), contain no mitochondria or chloroplasts. They have a single chromosome with a closed circle of double-stranded DNA and with no associated histones.If flagella are present, they are made of a single filament of the protein flagellin; there are none of the '9+2' tubulin-containing microtubules of the eukaryotes. Ribosome of bacteria differ in their structure from those of eukaryotes. They have rigid cell-wall made of *peptidoglycan*. The plasma membrane is a phospholipid bilayer but contains no cholesterol or other steroids. Mitosis is absent and mostly they reproduce asexually. Sexual reproduction, very different from that of eukaryotes and meiosis, is absent. Many bacteria form a single spore when their food supply runs low. Most of the water is removed from the spore and metabolism ceases. Spores are so resistant to adverse conditions of dryness and temperature that they may remain viable even after fifty years of dormancy.

5.2.2 Types of Bacteria

Until recently classification has done on the basis of such traits as:

- Shape
  - Bacilli: rod-shaped
  - Cocci: spherical
  - Spirilla: curved walls
- Ability to form spores
- Method of energy production (glycolysis for anaerobes, cellular respiration for aerobes)
- Nutritional requirements
- Reaction to the Gram stain.

5.2.2.1 Gram Staining

The Gram stain is named after the 19th century Danish bacteriologist who developed it.

In gram staining the bacterial cells are first stained with a purple dye called crystal violet. Then the preparation is treated with alcohol or acetone. This washes the stain out of Gram-negative cells. Then to view them requires the use of a counter stain of a different color (e.g., the pink of safranin). Bacteria that are not decolourized by alcohol/acetone wash are Gram-positive.

Although the Gram stain might seem to be an arbitrary criterion to use in bacterial taxonomy, it does, in fact, distinguish between two fundamentally different kinds of bacterial cell-walls and reflects a natural division among the bacteria. A table of the staining characteristics for some common bacteria of medical importance is given below in Table 3. More recently, genome sequencing, especially of their 16S ribosomal RNA (rRNA), has provided new insights into the evolutionary relationships among the bacteria.

Table 3 A Table of the staining characteristics for some common bacteria of medical importance is given below

	Gram positive	*Gram negative*
Cocci (round)	*Staphylococcus* (in clusters)	*Neisseria* (in pairs)
	Streptococcus (in chains)	*Moraxella* (in pairs)
Bacilli (rod-like)	*Listeria*	*Enterobacteriaceae* (coliforms)
	Bacillus	*Escherichia coli*
	Corynebacterium	*Klebsiella*
		Salmonella
		Shigella
		Proteus
		Pseudomonas
		Haemophilus
		Bordetella
		Legionella
		Campylobacter (spiral)
		Helicobacter (spiral)
	Clostridium (anaerobic)	*Bacteroides* (anaerobic)

5.2.3 Economic Importance of Bacteria

Bacteria may be pathogens, such as *Clostridium tetani*. These bacilli are the pathogens responsible for causing tetanus in humans. Nitrogen-fixing bacteria (such as *Rhizobium* sp) inhabit the root-cells of plants in the legume family (Fabaceae). These moneran sybionts convert gaseous nitrogen from the atmosphere (N_2) into usable 'fixed' nitrogen (ammonia, nitrite and nitrate), which can be absorbed by the roots and used by the plant to manufacture protein and nucleic acids. Industrial enzymes are also produced by bacteria, e.g. protease is produced by *Bacillus subtilis* (Ingraham and Ingraham 2000).

5.3 Algae

The algae (singular *alga*) comprise several different groups of living organisms usually found in wet places or water bodies and capture light energy through photosynthesis, converting inorganic substances into simple sugars. Algae were traditionally regarded as simple plants, and some are closely related to the higher plants. Others appear to represent different protist groups, alongside other organisms that are traditionally considered more animal-like (protozoa).

The eukaryotic algae (those with compartmentalized cells) are part of a diverse group of organisms called protists. The kingdom Protista (once included partly in the animal kingdom and partly in the plant kingdom) is now divided into a number of as yet not adequately circumscribed kingdoms. The prokaryotic algae (the cyanobacteria) are included with bacteria in the kingdom Monera.

5.3.1 Properties of Algae

Reproduction in algae may be isogamous, anisogamous, or oogamous. Female gametangia are not enclosed by a wall of sterile cells as in higher cryptogams. Mostly autotrophic (photosynthetic) pigments are variable and are the basis of classification; all have chlorophyll a; some have b, others c; all have accessory pigments of some kind, e.g., phycocyanin (bluish), phycoerythrin (reddish), carotenes (yellow-brown), xanthophylls (brown).

Some algae are heterotrophic (get energy from non-photosynthetic sources also). Algae have great variations in size; they may be unicellular 3-10 μm (microns) to giant kelps up to 70 meters long and growing at up to 50 cm per day, found in mostly aquatic situations (need water to reproduce and, generally, to photosynthesize).

Algae are found just about everywhere on earth: in the sea, in our rivers and lakes, on soils and walls, in animals and plants (as symbionts - partners collaborating together); in fact, just about everywhere where there is light with which to photosynthesise.

5.3.2 Types of Algae

Algae have traditionally been classified on the basis of:

- Colour (photosynthetic pigments)
- Storage material
- Flagella
- Cell-wall

Being aquatic, algae are marine, freshwater and terrestrial. Terrestrial algae are effectively surviving in an aquatic environment on land. Algae may be planktonic or benthic; planktonic or floating algae. For micro-algae, these often have strange shapes which help the algae suspend as well as serve an anti-predation role. Benthic algae are attached algae. These are algae anchored to the substratum. Major algal forms are tabulated in the Table 4.

5.3.3 Algae and Symbioses

Algae frequently form part of a symbiosis with other organisms. In these symbioses, the algae photosynthesise and supply photosynthates to their

Table 4 Major Algal Forms

Group	*Common Name*	*Niche*	*Major Accessory Pigment*	*Reserve*	*Flagella (a)*	*Remarks*
Chlorophytes	Green algae	m/f/t; varied	Chl b	starch	(2)	Most diverse group
Euglenophytes	Euglenoids	m/f; planktonic	Chl b	β 1-3 glucan	2	Proteinaceous pellicle instead of wall; facultative autotrophs
Phaeophytes	Brown algae	m; benthic	fucoxanthin (carotenoid)	β 1-3 glucan (laminarin), mannitol	(2)	Usually macro-algae
Chrysophytes	Golden-brown algae (incl. diatoms)	m/f; planktonic	Fucoxanthin (carotenoid)	β 1-3 glucan	(1 - 3)	Diatoms with SiO_2 walls
Rhodophytes	Red algae	m; benthic	Phycoerythrin	floridean starch	0	Usually macro-algae
Pyrrophytes	Dinoflagellates	m/f; planktonic	Peridinin (carotenoid)	form of starch	2	Internal cellulose wall
Cyanobacteria	Blue-green bacteria	m; planktonic	Bacterial chlorophyll, phycocyanin and phycoerythrin.	glycogen granules, cyanophycin granules	0	Responsible for nitrogen fixation on land and in water

NOTES:

m = marine f = freshwater t = terrestrial

(a) implies if present

host. The host organism is then capable of deriving some or all of its energy requirements from the alga. Examples include:

a) Lichens - a fungus, is the host, usually with a green alga or a cyanobacterium as the symbiont. Both, fungi and algae found in lichens are capable of living independently.

b) Corals - several algae form symbiotic relationship (zooxanthellae) with corals. Notable amongst these is the dinoflagellate *Symbiodinium*, found in many hard corals. The loss of *Symbiodinium* or other zooxanthellae from the host leads to coral bleaching.

5.3.4 Economic Use of Algae

Marine algae, as primary producers, are ecologically important, and economically have been used as food and medicines for centuries. Today, various species of marine algae provide not only food but also produce extracts such as agar, carrageen, and alginates. These extracts are used in numerous food, pharmaceutical, cosmetic, and industrial applications.

Algae, the major food of fish (and thus indirectly of many other animals), are a keystone in the aquatic food chain of life; they are the primary producers of the food that provides energy to the whole system. They are also important to aquatic life in their capacity to supply oxygen through photosynthesis. *Seaweeds*, e.g. the kelps (kombu) and the red algae *Porphyra* (nori), have long been used as a source of food, especially in Asia. Both cultivated and naturally growing seaweeds have been harvested in the Pacific Basin for hundreds of years. Kelps are also much used as fertilizer, and kelp-ash is used industrially for its potassium and sodium salts. Other useful products of algae are agar and carrageen, which are used as a stabilizer in foods, cosmetics, and paints.

5.4 Actinomycetes

Actinomycetes dominate the microbial life in soil where they play a major role in decaying dead organic matter. Many of them have turned out to be the source of valuable antibiotics, including streptomycin, erythromycin, and tetracycline.

5.4.1 Properties of Actinomycetes

The actinomycetes are prokaryotic, aerobic, Gram-positive bacteria that assemble themselves in branching filaments, which resemble the roots of a plant or tree. They are primarily found in soil, and are very widely distributed. They have the ability to break down many different varieties of organic compounds and are crucial in the mineralization of organic matter. Actinomycetes are so important because of their ability to produce antibiotics. Actinomycetes actually produce most of the naturally occurring antibiotics used in medicines today.

5.4.2 Types of Actinomycetes

The actinomycetes are divided into several families

(i) The family Actinomyceteae comprises of two genera: Actinomyces and *Nocardia*. A few species are pathogenic. *A.israelii* causes actinomycosis in man, *A.bovis* in cattle.

(ii) The family Mycobacteriaceae has a single genus, *Mycobacterium*, which contains several pathogenic species causing diseases such as leprosy and tuberculosis.

(iii) The family Streptomyceteae comprises several organisms found in the soil. They are rarely pathogenic. In contrast, several species of the genus *Streptomyces* produce antibiotics. Erythromycin is produced by *Streptomyces erythreus*, Streptomycin by *S. griseus*, Aureomycin by *S. aureofaciens*, Oleandomycin by *S. antibioticus*, Spiramycin by *S. ambofaciens*.

Sometimes the name 'Actinomycetes' is used restrictively for members of the genus *Actinomyces* only, instead of all members of the Actinomycetales.

5.4.3 Economic Importance of Actinomycetes

Actinomycetes are the primary decomposers of tough plant materials like bark, newspaper and woody stems. They are especially effective at attacking tough, raw plant tissues (cellulose, chitin, and lignin), softening them up for their less enterprising relatives. Actinomycetes are so important because of their ability to produce antibiotics. Actinomycetes actually produce most of the naturally occurring antibiotics used in medicines today.

Although most actinomycetes are free-living microorganisms, there are a few that are pathogens. *Actinomyces israelii*, for example, causes skin and mouth lesions at wound sites. The lesions usually drain pus, which contains the telltale yellow sulphur granules produced by *Actinomyces israelii*. Other Actinomyces species, mainly *Actinomyces viscosus* and *Actinomyces naeslundii*, have also been isolated in large number on teeth that have undergone significant decay. These species are early colonizers of teeth surfaces in the formation of plaque.

5.5 Fungi

Fungi are an important group of multicellular eukaryotic organisms comprising a meshwork of thread-like filamentous cells joined end-to-end.

The whole body of a fungus is called the mycelium. Fungi are non-photosynthesising, heterotrophic organisms that derive their energy from a saprophytic or parasitic existence. They are unicellular amoeboid, or filamentous, never having the leaves, stems, and roots–characteristic of higher plants. Reproduction occurs by sexual or asexual spore formation.

5.5.1 Properties of Fungi

Most fungi grow as tubular filaments called hyphae. An interwoven mass of hyphae is called a mycelium. The walls of hyphae are often strengthened with chitin, a polymer of N-acetylglucosamine. The linkage between the sugars is like that of cellulose and peptidoglycan, and produces the same sort of structural rigidity. Fungi are heterotrophic i.e. these organisms are dependent on preformed organic matter for growth and energy. Most fungi are saprophytes, feeding on dead or decaying material, getting nourishment from the surroundings (often first digested by secreting enzymes). This helps to remove leaf litter and other debris that would otherwise accumulate on the ground. Thus, they perform a crucial role in nature by decomposing dead organisms and releasing their nutrients for reuse by the living organisms. Nutrients absorbed by the fungus then become available for other organisms which may eat fungi. Many fungi are parasitic, feeding on living organisms without killing them. Ergot, corn smut, Dutch elm disease, and ringworm are all diseases caused by parasitic fungi. Most fungi are multicellular, but some, the yeasts, are simple unicellular organisms probably evolved from multicellular ancestors.

Fungi usually grow best in environments that are slightly acidic (a pH measurement of 5 or so). They can grow on substances with very low moisture. Fungi are present all over the world, in marine as well as terrestrial environments. Most fungi are capable of asexual and sexual reproduction. Asexual reproduction is by fragmentation or spore formation. Those that reproduce sexually produce gametes in specialized areas of the hyphae called gametangia. The gametes may be released to fuse into spores elsewhere, or the gametangia themselves may fuse. In some cases dikaryons (*di*=two, *karyo*=nucleus), which are found only among fungi, result when unspecialized hyphae fuse but their nuclei remain distinct part of the life cycle.

5.5.2 Types of Fungi

Fungi are divided into the Oomycota ('lower fungi'), with cellulose cell-walls, and the Eumycota ('true fungi'), with chitin cell-walls.

Eumycota are divided into: Zygomycetes, Ascomycetes, Basidiomycetes, and Deuteromycetes.

(i) Zygomycetes have thick-walled resting sexual spores called zygospores formed from the fusion of neighboring gametangia; their asexual spores are produced in a sporangium and are called sporangiospores. There is no distinguishable male or female. Zygomycetes includes black bread mold and molds, such as those of the genus *Glomus,* that form important symbiotic relationships with plants. Most are soil-living saprobes that feed on dead animal or plant remains. Some are parasitic of plants or insects.

(ii) Ascomycetes produce sexual spores (ascospores) in a sack-like body called an ascus; their asexual spores are produced externally, borne on a conidiophore. Ascomycetes include yeasts, the powdery mildews, the black and blue-green molds, edible types such as the morel and the truffle and species that cause diseases in plants like Dutch elm disease, chestnut blight, apple scab, and ergot. There are over 50,000 species, about 25,000 of which occur only in lichens. In ascomycetes, the hyphae are subdivided by porous walls through which the cytoplasm and the nuclei can pass. Their life cycle is a complex combination of sexual and asexual reproduction.

(iii) In *Basidiomycetes,* two hyphae fuse to form a *dikaryotic mycelium* (a mycelium in which both nuclei remain distinct). These mycelia differentiate into reproductive structures called basidia that make up the basidiocarp (the body popularly known as the mushroom cap). The nuclei then fuse and undergo meiosis, creating spores with one nucleus each. When these spores germinate, they produce hyphae, and the process begins again. Some notable Basidiomycetes are the cultivated, edible mushroom that finds its way into pizza, soups, etc., *Amanita muscaria* which forms a beautiful mushroom but deadly when eaten, Smuts which parasites the important crops like wheat, oats, and rye, Rusts such as wheat black stem rust (*Puccinia graminis*) and white pine blister rust.

(iv) Deuteromycetes comprise a miscellaneous assortment of fungi that do not fit neatly in other divisions; they have in common an apparent lack of sexual reproductive features. Also called Fungi Imperfectii, the group includes species that help create Roquefort and Camembert cheeses that cause diseases in plants and in animals (e.g., athlete's foot and ringworm), and that produce penicillin. A number of the fungi classified as Deuteromycetes have been found to be asexual stages of species in other groups, and some classification schemes consider the Deuteromycetes a class under Ascomycota.

5.5.3 Fungi and Symbioses

Fungi form mutually beneficial symbiotic relationship with another organism, for example mycorrhizae and lichens.

5.5.3.1 Mycorrhiza

The association of fungus and root of a vascular plant is called a mycorrhiza. Mycorrhiza, the nutritional symbiosis between fungi and plants, has been found in 85% of higher plant genera. Silver Birch can form root associations with up to 100 different fungi, notably Fly Agaric. The plant benefits by more-efficient mineral (nitrogen and phosphorus) uptake. The fungus benefits by the sugars translocated to the root by the plant.

5.5.3.2 Lichens

Lichens are products of a symbiosis between a fungus and autotrophic green alga or cyanobacterium (the '*photobiont*') or in some cases with both. The fungal partner (the '*mycobiont*') in most lichens (98% of them) is an Ascomycete. Zygomycetes make up the remainder. The relationship is often characterized as mutualistic i.e., both partners benefit. Lichens secrete a variety of unusual chemicals; some of these probably assist in the breakdown of rock substrates. Some 15,000 species of lichenized fungi are known, and perhaps 20% of fungi, mostly Ascomycetes, are lichenized.

5.5.4 Economic Use of Fungi

Fungi are often directly involved in our lives. Some of these relationships are beneficial, some harmful. Fungi are valuable economically as a source of antibiotics, of vitamins, and of various industrially important chemicals, such as alcohols, acetone, and enzymes, as well as for their role in fermentation processes as in the production of alcoholic beverages, vinegar, and cheese and bread dough. Yeasts are necessary for bread baking, and humans eat many fungi, such as the mushrooms. They are extremely important in soil renewal, through the decomposition of organic matter (humus). Fungi are also important in agriculture and food production; mycorrhizal fungi render increased disease-resistance to some plants. Many medical applications of fungi have recently been discovered, especially antibiotics produced by fungi. The first among these is penicillin, possibly the most important non-genetic medical breakthrough of the last century. Fungi are good sources of dyes. Certain mushrooms provide excellent surfaces for painting or etching.

Most fungi are decomposers, breaking dead organisms down into detritus and returning inorganic nutrients to the ecosystem. Many fungi have enzymes that work to 'rot' or 'digest' the cellulose and lignin found in the wood of trees. The lignin is an important source of carbon for many organisms. As such, fungi are also extremely adaptable, and can break down many substances, including some toxic pollutants. This adaptability also accounts for the presence of fungi in many different environments around the world.

Even though certain fungi are recyclers of dead wood, they can also be very harmful to living trees. Thus, some fungi are parasitic and cause devastating plant infections; though only about fifty species are known to harm animals. Such diseases are called mycoses or fungal infections. Some molds in particular, release toxic chemicals called *mycotoxins* that can result in poisoning or death. Various fungi can also cause serious damage to fruit harvests and other crops. Serious agricultural pests, parasitic fungi such as the rusts and the smuts can ruin entire crops, especially affecting cereals such as wheat and corn. Dutch elm disease, chestnut blight, rust, smut, certain mildews and ergot are caused by various fungi. The water mold *Phytophthora infestans* was the cause of the late blight of potatoes that resulted in the Great Potato Famine in Ireland (1845–49).

5.6 Slime Mold

Slime mold or slime fungus, a heterotrophic organism once regarded as a fungus but later classified with the Protista. In a recent system of classification based on analysis of nucleic acid (genetic material) sequences, slime molds have been classified in a major group called the eukarya (or eukaryotes), which includes plants and animals.

5.6.1 Types of Slime Molds

There are two groups of slime molds, the plasmodial slime molds of the phylum (division) *Myxomycota* and the cellular slime molds of *Acrasiomycota*.

There are about 65 cellular and 500 known plasmodial slime mold species, found in forests and sometimes lawns throughout the world. In a few species the plasmodium, under favourable conditions, may cover an area of several square feet. A slime mold is the cause of clubroot, a disease of cabbage and related plants.

5.6.1.1 Plasmodial Slime Molds

The plasmodial slime molds (myxomycetes) are a group of fungus-like organisms usually present and sometimes abundant in terrestrial ecosystems. The myxomycete life cycle involves two very different trophic (feeding) stages, one consisting of uninucleate amoebae with or without flagella, and the other consisting of a distinctive multinucleate structure, the plasmodium. Myxomycete plasmodia typically occur in cool, moist, shady places such as within crevices of decaying wood, beneath the partially decayed bark of logs and stumps, and in leaf litter on the forest floor. Under favourable conditions, the plasmodium gives rise to one or more fruiting bodies containing spores. The spores of myxomycetes are for most species apparently wind-dispersed and complete the life cycle by germinating to produce the uninucleate amoeboflagellate cells.

Plasmodial slime molds, like *Physarum*, are basically enormous single cells with thousands of nuclei. They are formed when individual flagellated cells swarm together and fuse. The result is one large bag of cytoplasm with many diploid nuclei. The fruiting bodies produced by Myxomycetes are somewhat suggestive to those produced by higher fungi, although they are considerably smaller (usually no more than 1-2 mm tall). Although large enough to be seen with the naked eye, they are best observed with a hand lens or under a stereomicroscope. Only then can their intricate nature be fully appreciated. Fruiting bodies may take the shape of tiny goblets, globes, plumes, or other shapes more difficult to describe. Some occur in tightly packed clusters, while others are scattered or even solitary. Many of the more intricate forms have a spore case held aloft on a delicate stalk, but others are attached directly to the substrate by their bases. These 'giant cells' have been extremely useful in studies of cytoplasmic streaming (the movement of cell contents) because it is possible to see this happening even under relatively low magnification. In addition, the large size of the slime mold 'cell' makes them easier to manipulate than most cells.

There are approximately 1000 recognized species of Myxomycetes. The majority of species are probably cosmopolitan, but a few species appear to be confined to the tropics or subtropics and some others have been collected only in temperate regions. Myxomycetes appear to be particularly abundant in temperate forests, but at least some species apparently occur in any terrestrial ecosystem with plants (and thus plant detritus) present. Most of what is known about the assemblage of Myxomycetes associated with particular types of terrestrial ecosystems has been derived from studies carried out in temperate regions of the northern hemisphere. In these forests, Myxomycetes are associated with a number of different microhabitats. These include coarse woody debris on the forest floor, the bark surface of living trees, and forest floor leaf litter. Each of these microhabitats tends to be characterized by a distinct assemblage of Myxomycetes.

5.6.1.2 Cellular Slime Molds

The cellular slime molds spend most of their lives as separate single-celled amoeboid protists, but upon the release of a chemical signal, the individual cells aggregate into a great swarm. Cellular slime molds are thus of great interest to cell and developmental biologists, because they provide a comparatively simple and easily manipulated system for understanding how cells interact to generate a multicellular organism. There are two groups of cellular slime molds, the *Dictyostelida* and the *Acrasida*, which may not be closely related to each other.

5.7 Mycoplasmas

Mycoplasmas have the distinction of being the smallest living organisms. They are so small (0.1 µm) that they can be seen only under the electron microscope. They are pleuropneumonia-like organism. Mycoplasmas are obligate parasites, i.e., they can live only within the cells of other organisms. They are probably the descendants of Gram-positive bacteria who have lost much of their genome — now depending on the gene products of their host. Thus any of numerous parasitic, pathogenic micro-organisms of the genus *Mycoplasma* that lack a true cell wall, are Gram-negative, and need sterols such as cholesterol for growth.

5.8 Virus

A virus is a microscopic non-living parasite that infects cells in biological organisms. Viruses are obligate intracellular parasites; they can reproduce only by invading and controlling other cells as they lack the cellular machinery for self reproduction. The term virus usually refers to those particles which infect eukaryotes (multi-celled organisms and many single-celled organisms), whilst the term bacteriophage or phage is used to describe those infecting prokaryotes (bacteria and bacteria-like organisms). A virus is basically a tiny bundle of genetic material—either DNA or RNA—carried in a shell called the viral coat or capsid, which is made up of bits of protein called capsomeres. Some viruses have an additional layer around this coat called an envelope. *Bacteriophages* are viruses that infect bacteria. They are used in gene technology to transfer foreign DNA that has been spliced into their nucleic acid into bacterial cells. The bacteria then acquire the ability to carry out the function of that particular gene and make specific proteins.

Viruses are found on or in just about every material and environment on earth from soil to water to air. They are basically found anywhere. There are three virus shapes: polyhedral, rod and complex. Viruses are neither unicellular nor multicellular organisms; they are somewhere between being living and non-living. Viruses have genes and show inheritance, but are reliant on host cells to produce new generations of viruses. Examples of virus diseases in humans are measles, chicken pox, flu and AIDS.

5.9 Protozoa

Protozoa are defined as single-celled eukaryotic organisms that feed heterotrophically and exhibit diverse motility mechanisms. Protozoa are also important as parasites and symbionts of multicellular animals.

5.9.1 Types of Protozoa

Protozoa have traditionally been divided on the basis of locomotion, although this is no longer believed to represent genuine relationships. The groups are:

(i) Flagellates (or *Mastigophora*)
(ii) Amoebae (or *Sarcodina*)
(iii) Sporozoans (or *Sporozoa, Apicomplexa*)
(iv) Ciliates (or *Ciliophora*)

Most protozoans are too small to be seen with the naked eyes - most are around 0.01-0.05 mm, although forms up to 0.5 mm are still fairly common - but can easily be found under a microscope. Protozoa are ubiquitous throughout aqueous environments and the soil, and play an important role in their ecology. A few are also important parasites. Protozoa are infamous for their role in causing disease, and parasitic species are among the best-known protozoa. For example, *Microsporidia* comprise a unique group of obligate, intracellular parasitic protozoa. *Microsporidia* are amazingly diverse organisms with more than 700 species and 80 genera that are capable of infecting a variety of plant, animal, and even other protist hosts. Since 1985, however, physicians have documented an unusual rise in worldwide infections in AIDS patients caused by four different genera of microsporidia (*Encephalitozoon, Nosema, Pleistophora* and *Enterocytozoon*).

5.9.2 Key Features of Protozoa

Protozoa are unicellular organisms belonging to a number of different phyla. Most of them are motile and heterotrophic. Food is digested within a food vacuole. Excess water is eliminated by means of a contractile vacuole.

5.9.2.1 Features of Flagellates

Flagella are the locomotor or food-capturing organelles.

5.9.2.2 Features of Amoeba

Pseudopodia are the locomotor or food-capturing organelles and skeletal structures are highly developed in this group.

5.9.2.3 Features of Sporozoans

Ring like, tubular, and filamentous organelles at the apical end of the body are a distinguishing feature of these parasitic protozoa.

5.9.2.4 Features of Ciliates

Cilia are present at some stage in the life cycle. Two types of nuclei are present which are macronucleus and micronucleus.

5.9.3 Economic Use of Protozoa

Some protozoa are harmless or even beneficial symbionts. A bewildering array of ciliates, for example, inhabit the rumen and reticulum of ruminates and the caecum and colon of equids. Little is known about the relationship of the ciliates to their host, but a few may aid the animal in digesting cellulose.

Polluted water often has a rich and characteristic protozoan fauna. The relative abundance and diversity of protozoa are used as indicators of organic and toxic pollution. (Cairns et al. 1972; Foissner 1987; Niederlehner et al. 1990; Curds 1992).

6. UTILITY OF MICROBES

Microorganisms are defined as 'living organisms too small to be seen with naked eyes'. The microorganisms have profound influence on all aspects of the earth and its residents, e.g. recycling of nutrients, decomposition, formation of minerals etc. For billions of years microbes have extensively shaped the development of the earth's habitats and the evolution of other life forms. It is understandable that scientists searching for life on other planets first look for signs of micro-organisms. Microbes can be found nearly everywhere, from deep in the earth's crust to the polar ice caps and oceans, to the bodies of plants and animals. Being mostly invisible, the actions of micro-organisms are usually not as obvious or familiar as those of larger plants and animals. They make up for their small size by occurring in large numbers and living in places that many other organisms cannot survive. Above all, they play central roles in the earth's landscape that are essential to life. Among the members of huge group of micro-organisms are bacteria, fungi, protozoa, algae, viruses, and parasitic worms. There are many kinds of relationships between micro-organisms and humans; most are beneficial, but some are harmful.

6.1 Microbial Involvement in Energy and Nutrient Flow

Microbes are deeply involved in the flow of energy and food through the earth's ecosystems. At the producer end of this range is photosynthesis, formation of food using energy derived from sun. Photosynthetic micro-organisms, including algae and Cyanobacteria, account for more than 50% of the earth's photosynthesis. In addition to serving as the basis for the food chains in the ocean and fresh water, these micro-organisms also contribute the major portion of oxygen to the atmosphere.

Another process that helps keeping the earth in balance is the process of biological decomposition and nutrient recycling. Decomposition involves the breakdown of dead matter and wastes into simple compounds that can be directed back into the natural cycles of living things. If it were not for multitudes of bacteria and fungi, many chemical elements would become locked up and unavailable to organisms. In the long-term scheme of things, micro-organisms are the main force that drives the structure and content of the soil, water, and atmosphere. Decomposers play strategic and often very specific roles in the cycling of elements such as nitrogen, sulphur, phosphorus, and carbon between the living and non-living environment.

The temperature of the earth is regulated by '*greenhouse gases*,' such as carbon dioxide and methane that create an insulation layer in the atmosphere and help retain heat. Much of this gas is produced by microbes living in the environment and the digestive tracts of animals.

Recent estimates propose that, based on weight and numbers, up to 50% of all organisms exist within and beneath the earth's crust in sediments, rocks, and even volcanoes. These are mostly primitive microbes that can survive high temperatures and nutrient extremes. It is increasingly evident that this enormous underground community of microbes is a significant influence on weathering, mineral extraction and soil formation.

6.2 Symbiotic Associations of Microbes

Microbes have also developed symbiotic associations with other organisms that are highly beneficial to the participating members. Microbes form inter-relationships with animals, notably represented by the stomach of cattle, which harbor a rich assortment of bacteria to digest the complex carbohydrates of the animal diets. Other microbes become normal flora that serve as barriers to infectious agents. Bacteria and fungi live in complex associations with plants that assist them in obtaining nutrients and water and may protect them against disease. Some of the examples are discussed below.

6.2.1 Mycorrhizae

Mycorrhizae are a symbiotic relationship between fungi and plants. Mycorrhizal fungi live on the roots of plants and provide inorganic nutrients and resistance to some pathogens, to the plants in exchange for organic sugars. The first colonization of land by plants was facilitated, if not made possible, by the ability of mycorrhizal fungi to uptake nutrients from hostile soil.

Most plants rely on a symbiotic fungus to aid them in acquiring water and nutrients from the soil. The specialized roots which the plants grow and the fungus which inhabits them are together known as mycorrhizae, or 'fungal roots'. The fungus, with its large surface area, is able to soak up water and nutrients over a large area and provide them to the plant. In return, the plant provides energy-rich sugars manufactured through photosynthesis. Arbuscular Mycorrhizal Fungi belong to a single order, the Glomerales (Morton and Benny 1990), which include all the species capable of living symbiotically with plants. The bulk of known species belong to the family *Glomaceae* (Pirozynski and Dalpe 1989) which includes the genera *Glomus* and *Sclerocystis*. *Piriformaspora indica* is another novel endophytic root colonizing fungus which is potential candidate to serve as biofertilizer, bioprotector, bioregulator, bioherbicide/weedicide, environmental stresses (chemical and physical) and an excellent source for the hardening of the tissue culture raised crops/plants.

6.2.2 Lichens

The lichens are fungi living in symbiotic relationships with algae or cyanobacteria. They consist of algae or bacteria trapped in the fungal hyphae. Though the details of this relationship are not completely understood, the fungus typically provides water and minerals for the algae or bacteria in exchange for organic food from photosynthesis. The photosynthetic species in lichens are actually capable of living by themselves, but the fungal species depend on their counterparts for survival. Lichens can reproduce asexually when small reproductive units, consisting of both fungi and algae or bacteria, break off from the lichen and are carried by the wind to other locations; they can also reproduce sexually through independent sexual reproduction of both, parts and a reattachment. Due to the effectiveness of the mutualist relationship in lichens, they can grow in the most inhospitable of terrestrial habitats, and often serve as key organisms in the primary succession of a habitat.

6.3 Role of Microbes in Environment

Another way of tapping into the unlimited potential of micro-organisms is the relatively new science of bioremediation. This process involves the introduction of microbes into the environment to restore stability or to clean up toxic pollutants. Bioremediation is required to control the massive levels of pollution from industry and modern living. Microbes have a surprising capacity to break down chemicals that would be harmful to other organisms. Agencies and companies have developed microbes to handle oil spills and detoxify sites contaminated with heavy metals, pesticides, and other chemical wastes. The solid waste disposal industry is interested in developing methods for degrading the tons of garbage in landfills, especially man-made plastics and paper products. One form of bioremediation that has been in use for some time is the treatment of water and sewage.

When we flush things down the drain or the toilet, they go to a septic system or waste water treatment plant at the end of the line. After primary mechanical treatment and aeration microbes remove organic materials from the filthy water that flows into these systems and, eventually, water is safely returned to the rivers and streams. The methane produced during treatment can even be used to generate heat or electricity for the operation. Since clean freshwater supplies are rapidly dwindling worldwide, it will become even more important to find ways to reclaim polluted water. Thus, micro-organisms are responsible for getting rid of the waste generated by industry and households. They detoxify acid mine drainage and other toxins that we dump into the soil and water. The nutrients gained from the breakdown of these products then go to feed plants or algae, which in turn feed all animals. Researchers are using bacteria that eat methane gas to clean up hazardous waste dumps and landfills. These methane-munching bacteria, or methanotrophs, (*meth-an-oh-trofs*) produce an enzyme that can break down more than 250 nasty pollutants into harmless molecules. By piping methane into the soil, we can increase growth of the methanotrophs that normally live in the polluted soil. Soil microbes are used as indicators of ecosystem pollution by heavy metals.

6.4 Improving Productivity of Land with Microorganisms

Due to deforestation, land has been cleared of natural vegetation and depleted of microlife. Modern farmers have tried to improve productivity by adding soluble fertilizers. However, given the increasing recognition of the role of micro-organisms, the way the future may focus on fostering and, when necessary, reintroducing healthy populations of microlife in the soil to enhance productivity. The use of mycorrhizae and *Rhizobium* inoculants has become almost standard in forestry and agriculture. Other ways to increase productivity with microlife are being researched and practiced worldwide. These techniques range from simply bringing in small amounts of healthy soil to inoculate new plantings in degraded areas, to the manufacture and application of special biostimulants to feed and encourage microlife, or to introducing blends of selected beneficial micro-organisms to be used in nursery or field production.

6.5 Applications of Microorganisms of Versatile Chemical Machines

It is clear that micro-organisms have monumental importance to the earth's operation. It is this very diversity and versatility that also makes them an excellent saviour for solving human problems. By accident or choice, humans have been using micro-organisms for thousands of years to improve life and even to mould civilizations.

6.5.1 Food

The use of microbes to create products is the science of biotechnology. This science of technology relies on the chemical reactions of microorganisms to produce a variety of foods and manufactured materials through a process called fermentation. Yeasts, a type of microscopic fungi, supply the necessary reactions to make bread, alcoholic beverages, and vitamins. Microbes have been used for centuries to provide us with food. Bread is the result of a microbial fermentation of sugar to produce carbon dioxide - the bubbles that make bread rise. We owe our beer and wine to similar little yeast that convert sugars into alcohol for our consumption. Yogurt and cheese are produced by bacterial fermentation of lactose, the sugar in milk. Some specialized bacteria have unique capacities to ferment milk products, pickle foods, and even to mine precious metals from raw minerals. Microbes, such as *phytoplankton* also serve as the nutrient source that indirectly feeds all marine animals and microbial symbioses with plants allow them to grow strong and increase productivity - sometimes they are even essential for plant survival.

6.5.2 Production of Drugs

Microbes are also employed to synthesize drugs (antibiotics and hormones) and to mass-produce enzymes for industry and amino acids for health supplements. Fungi and bacteria produce powerful antibiotics such as penicillin and tetracycline. These are drugs we use to fight off nasty bacteria that cause sore-throats, ear infections, diarrhoea and other discomforts. Scientists have changed, or engineered the genetic blueprints of bacteria and yeasts to turn them into mini medicine-making factories. They stick genes for medicines they want to make-say, insulin for diabetes- into the microbial cells, as if adding new building information to the microbe's blueprint. The scientists then grow the microbes in huge containers called fermenters where they reproduce into billions, all making insulin. Most of our vitamin B12, riboflavin, and vitamin C are produced by bacterial fermentation. Approximately 70% of antibiotics currently in use are also the product of microbial fermentation.

6.5.3 Production of Industrial Products

Micro-organisms are useful for making products such as xanthan gum (a food thickener) which are harvested from their bacterial producers. Micro-organisms are a rich source of enzymes that have many commercial use. Some of the examples of enzymes are diastase, cellulase, collagenase, invertase, protease produced respectively from *Aspergillus oryzae*, *Trichoderma konigi*, *Clostridium histolyticum*, *Saccharomyces cerevisiae*, *Bacillus subtilis* (Ingraham and Ingraham 2000). Scientists have discovered bacteria in bat guano, which is rich in ammonia, and are very efficient in the nitrification process. In the near future these organisms may be used to remove nitrogen from industrial waste before it reaches our lakes and rivers.

Genetic engineering is a newer area of biotechnology that manipulates the genetics of microbes, plants and animals for the purpose of creating new products and genetically modified organisms. One powerful technique for designing new organisms is termed recombinant DNA. This technology makes it possible to deliberately alter DNA and to switch genetic material from one organism to another. Bacteria and fungi were some of the first microorganisms to be genetically engineered, because they are so adaptable to changes in their genetic makeup. Recombinant DNA technology has unlimited potential in terms of medical, industrial and agricultural use. Microbes can be engineered to synthesize desirable proteins such as drugs, hormones, enzymes and physiological substances. Among the genetically unique organisms that have been designed by bioengineers are bacteria that contain a natural pesticide, viruses that serve as vaccines, pigs that produce human hemoglobin, and plants that do not ripen too rapidly. The techniques also extend to the characterization of human genetic material and diseases.

6.6 Microbes Affect Human Health

We depend on having a microbial population, called our micro biota, for our health. There are normally 10 times more microbial cells in a human body than human cells. The good bacteria that live on and in protect us from the bad invaders that might come our way. Without the good bacteria, the bad ones can slip in and easily cause problems. Our own digestion has also evolved to use bacteria for assistance, allowing us to gain nutrition from plant polysaccharides that our own enzymes will not degrade. This is one of the reasons why taking antibiotics can lead to episodes of diarrhoea - we have disrupted our natural gut biota.

6.6.1 Infectious Diseases and the Human Condition

Humanity is plagued by nearly 2,000 different microbes that can infect human body and cause various diseases. Infectious diseases still devastate human populations worldwide, despite significant strides in understanding and treating them. The most recent estimates from the World Health Organization (WHO) point to a total of 10 billion new infections across the world every year. There are more infections than people because many people acquire more than one infection. Infectious diseases are also the most common cause of death in much of humanity.

The worldwide death toll is about 13 million people, and many of these diseases are preventable by drugs and vaccines. Those hardest hit are residents in countries where access to adequate medical care is lacking. One-third of the earth's inhabitants live on less than $1 per day, are malnourished, and are not fully immunized. Adding to the overload of infectious diseases, we are also witnessing an increase in the number of new (emerging) and older (re-emerging) diseases. *AIDS, hepatitis C*, and viral encephalitis are examples of recently identified diseases that cause severe mortality and morbidity are currently on the rise. To somewhat balance this trend, there have also been some advances in eradication of diseases such as polio, measles, leprosy and certain parasitic worms. It is significant that, in addition to known infectious diseases, many other diseases are suspected of having a microbial origin. A connection has been established between of certain kinds of cancers and viruses, between diabetes and the coxsackie virus, and between schizophrenia and a virus called the borna agent. Mounting scientific evidence strongly links them to some forms of cancer, coronary artery disease, diabetes, multiple sclerosis, autism and chronic lung diseases.

A further health complication from infectious diseases is the increasing number of patients with weakened defenses that are kept alive for extended periods. They are subjected to infections by common microbes that are not pathogenic to healthy people. There is also an increase in microbes that are resistant to drugs. It appears that even with the most modern technology available to us, microbes still have the 'last word,' as the great French microbiologist Louis Pasteur observed.

Newly identified diseases that are becoming more prominent are termed emerging. A list of twenty most common emerging diseases that have been diagnosed over a span of 30 years is given in Table 5. Some of them were associated with a specific geographic site (Ebola fever),

Table 5 A list of prominent emerging diseases over a span of 30 years

Microbe	*Source*	*Disease*	*Year of Emergence*
Lassa fever virus	Rodents	Lassa fever	1969
Monkey pox virus	Monkeys, rodents	Monkey pox	1970
Marburg virus	Monkeys?	Hemorrhagic fever	1975
Ebola virus	Monkeys?	Hemorrhagic fever	1977
Legionella bacteria	Water	Legionnaire's disease	1977
Human T-cell virus	Humans	Lymphoma, leukemia	1980
Staphylococcus *bacteria*	Humans	Toxic shock syndrome	1981
Human immuno-deficiency virus	Humans	AIDS	1981
Escherichia coli bacteria	Cattle	Hemolytic uremic syndrome	1982
Borrelia bacteria	Ticks	*Lyme disease*	1982
Helicobacter bacteria	Humans	Peptic ulcers	1983
Hepatitis C virus	Humans	Hepatitis, liver diseases	1989
Hantavirus syndrome	Mice	Respiratory distress syndrome	1993
Hendra virus	Bats	Encephalitis	1994
Cryptosporidium protozoa	Water	Diarrhoea, enteric disease	1994
Ehrlichia bacteria	Ticks	Arthritis, muscle pain	1995
New variant CJD prion	Cattle	*Creutzfeldt-Jakob disease*	1996
Nipah virus	Bats	Encephalitis, pneumonia	1998
Arenavirus	Woodrats	Respiratory distress	1999
West Nile virus	Mosquitoes	*Encephalitis*	1999

whereas others were spread across all continents (AIDS). Older diseases that have been known for hundreds of years and are increasing in occurrence are termed re-emerging. Among the diseases currently experiencing resurgence are tuberculosis, influenza, malaria, cholera, and hepatitis B. Many factors play a part in emergence, but fundamental to all emerging diseases is the formidable capacity of micro-organisms to respond and adapt to the alterations in the individual, community and environment.

6.6.2 Microbes have Bothered us for Millennia

Microbes have probably always caused diseases in humans. Since ancient times, historians have documented some of those diseases, and present-day archeologists and microbiologists are discovering evidences of infectious diseases in prehistoric human skeletons.

Smallpox, which is caused by a variola virus, was described in ancient Egyptian and Chinese writings. According to some researchers, over the centuries smallpox was responsible for more deaths than all other infectious diseases combined. It killed millions of people over thousands of years before being eradicated late in the 20th century by worldwide vaccination. The last case of smallpox was recorded in 1977.

The protozoan parasite *Plasmodium* causes malaria, a tropical disease that, usually, is transmitted to humans during the bite of the *Anopheles* mosquito. In ancient times, this disease was mentioned in Egyptian writings called hieroglyphics and was described in detail by the Greek physician Hippocrates. Malaria ravaged invaders from the Roman Empire. Though rare in the United States, malaria remains a serious public health threat worldwide. It kills 3 million people each year, most of whom are children.

Evidence on a 1300 B.C. Egyptian stone engraving shows that poliomyelitis (polio) has been around since ancient times. In the 1990s, public health officials launched a massive international vaccination campaign to eradicate the poliovirus, which causes paralysis and can be deadly.

6.6.3 Microbes can Make us Sick

According to health care experts, infectious diseases caused by microbes are responsible for more deaths worldwide than any other single cause. They estimate the annual cost of medical care for treating infectious diseases in the United States alone is about $120 billion.

The science of microbiology explores how microbes work and how to control them, and it seeks ways to use that knowledge to prevent and treat the diseases that microbes cause. The 20th century saw an extraordinary increase in knowledge about microbes. Microbiologists (scientists who study microbes) and other researchers scored many successes in learning how microbes cause certain infectious diseases and how to combat those microbes.

Unfortunately, microbes are much better adapting to new environments than people. On earth for billions of years, microbes are constantly challenging human newcomers with ingenious new survival tactics. Our life is precious to us. We want to live a long time and stay as healthy as possible. We do not want to be limited by diseases the genes we were born with, and also we want to conceal the obvious signs of aging. So, our expectations are high. Drugs or medicines should be highly effective in low doses and should not cause harmful side effects. We need new drugs or medicines to be developed to protect us from threats like HIV, SARS, influenza and heart attacks. There is a growing demand too for 'Lifestyle' drugs too that will affect our appearance, removing wrinkles from our skin, keeping our weight down and restore our hair colour. Hence, the responsibility rests largely on the shoulders of those scientists who know how to design and synthesize molecules that have therapeutic actions on our bodies.

7. WHAT ARE DRUGS AND MEDICINES?

A drug or medicine is a product that:

- Is intended or marketed for use in the diagnosis, cure, mitigation, treatment, or prevention of disease, illness, injury or pain;
- Is applied to the human body or ingested or inhaled by humans;
- Is not an appliance or device; and
- Is not food.

An appliance or device is an instrument, apparatus, implement, machine, contrivance, implant, chemical, or other similar or related product that does not achieve its primarily intended purposes through chemical action within or on the body and which is not dependent upon being metabolized for the achievement of its primarily intended purposes.

Thus, a drug is any substance that can be used to modify a chemical process or processes in the body, for example to treat an illness, relieve a symptom, enhance a performance or ability, or to alter states of mind. The word 'drug' is etymologically derived from the Dutch/Low German word 'droog', which means 'dry', since in the past most drugs were dried plant parts. During the past century, advances in medications have enabled doctors to cure many diseases and save lives.

Thousands of years ago, the Chinese were taking *Ginkgo* to keep aging minds sharp. In ancient Greece, women used the herb Queen Anne's lace as a contraceptive. And for centuries, Native Americans used echinacea to fight infections. Herbal medicines have been used by every human society to treat one ailment or another, and archeologists have even discovered remnants of herbal remedies in 60,000 year old Neanderthal burial sites.

8. SOURCES OF DRUGS OR MEDICINES

Drugs are obtained from many sources. Many inorganic materials, such as metals, are chemotherapeutic. Hormones, alkaloids, vaccines, and antibiotics come from living organisms; even today many are extracted from plants and other drugs are synthetic or semi-synthetic. Synthetics are often more effective and are easier to prepare in standardized units. The techniques of genetic engineering are being applied to the production of drugs; genetically engineered livestock that incorporate human genes are being developed for the production of scarce human enzymes and other proteins. Some medicines are produced in a laboratory by mixing together a number of chemicals. Forty percent of all prescriptions dispensed are for substances derived from plants, animals or micro-organisms, and a few medicines are even biologically engineered by inserting genes into bacteria that make them produce the desired substance. The list of wonder drugs originated from wild species includes aspirin for pain relief (from meadowsweet), penicillin for antibiotics (from the *Pencillium* fungi), digitoxin for cardiac treatment (from common foxglove), L-dopa for Parkinson's disease (from velvet bean), taxol for ovarian cancer (from the Pacific yew), and quinine for malaria (from yellow *Cinchona*).

For most of the 20th century, American physicians enamoured by synthetic drugs and influenced by pharmaceutical advertising were quick to dismiss herbs as crude and unproven folk remedies. That's now starting to change. New scientific evidence supports the benefits of herbal medicines, and more consumers are opting for natural and nontoxic treatments. Traditional medicines are used by about 60 per cent of the world's population. These are not only used for primary health care in rural areas and in developing countries, but also in developed countries as well as where modern medicines are predominantly used (Kamboj 2000). In western world also, the use of herbal medicines is steadily growing with approximately 40 per cent of population reporting use of herb to treat medical illnesses within the past year (Bent and Ko 2004). Demand for medicinal plants is increasing, in both developing and developed countries, due to growing recognition of natural products being non-narcotic, having no side-effects, easily available at affordable prices and sometime the only source of health care available to the poor. Public, academic and government interest in traditional medicines is growing exponentially due to the increased incidence of the adverse drug reactions and economic burden of the modern system of medicine (Dubey *et al* 2004). As per World Health Organization (WHO) estimates, almost 80% of the population of developing countries relies on traditional medicines, mostly plant drugs, for their primary health care needs. Also, modern pharmacopoeia still contains at least 25% drugs derived from plants and many others which are synthetic analogues built on prototype compounds isolated from plants.

Studies state that between 25-50 per cent of all the medicines prescribed worldwide today come from plants or are based on chemicals found in plants. These drugs further furnish the template for 90 per cent of modern synthetic drugs. According to the World Health Organization, nearly 70 per cent of the earth's 6.2 billion people rely on plant-based traditional medicine to relieve pain, to heal wounds, and to prevent or cure diseases.

9. WHAT IS HERBAL MEDICINE?

All plants produce chemical compounds as part of their normal metabolic activities. These can be split into two categories - primary metabolites, such as sugars and fats, found in all plants; and secondary metabolites found in a smaller range of plants, some only in a particular genus or species. The autologous functions of secondary metabolites are varied, for example as toxins to deter predation, or to attract insects for pollination. It is these secondary metabolites which can have therapeutic actions in humans, and which can be refined to produce drugs. Some examples are insulin from the roots of dahlias, morphine and codeine from the poppy, digoxin from the foxglove. Aspirin, perhaps the most common drug for treating headaches, originally came from willow bark. Quinine, used to prevent malaria infections, was once obtained from the bark of a Peruvian tree. Vinblastine, a drug used to treat leukemia, comes from periwinkle plants, and digitalis, a heart stimulant, is still made from pressed foxglove leaves.

9.1 Examples of Herbal Medicines

Examples of some commonly used herbal medicines:

- Artichoke and several other plants have been associated with reduced total serum cholesterol levels in preliminary studies(Thompson and Ernst 2003).
- Black cohosh and other plants that contain phytoestrogens (plant molecules with estrogen activity) have been found to have some benefits for treatment of symptoms resulting from menopause (Kronenberg and Fugh-Berman 2003).
- Echinacea extracts have been shown to limit the length of colds in some clinical trials, although some studies have found it to have no effect (Block and Mead 2003).
- Garlic has been found to lower total cholesterol levels, mildly reduce blood pressure, reduces platelet aggregation, and has antibacterial properties.

- St John's wort has been found to be more effective than placebo for the treatment of mild to moderate depression in some clinical trials (Gupta and Moller 2003).

10. WHAT IS THE HISTORY OF HERBAL MEDICINE?

Plants had been used for medicinal purposes long before recorded history. For example, ancient Chinese and Egyptian papyrus writings describe medicinal plant uses. Indigenous cultures (e.g., African and Native American) used herbs in their healing rituals, while others developed traditional medical systems (e.g., Ayurveda and Traditional Chinese Medicine) in which herbal therapies were used systematically. Scientists found that people in different parts of the globe tended to use the same or similar plants for the same purposes.

In the early 19th century, when methods of chemical analysis first became available, scientists began extracting and modifying the active ingredients from plants. Later, chemists began making their own version of plant compounds, beginning the transition from raw herbs to synthetic pharmaceuticals. Over time, the use of herbal medicines declined in favour of pharmaceuticals.

Recently, the World Health Organization estimated that 80% of people worldwide rely on herbal medicines for some aspect of their primary healthcare. In the last twenty years, increasing public dissatisfaction with the cost of prescription medications, combined with an interest in returning to natural or organic remedies, has led to an increase in the use of herbal medicines. In Germany, roughly 600 to 700 plant-based medicines are available and are prescribed by approximately 70% of German physicians.

11. HOW DO HERBS WORK?

For most herbs, the specific ingredient that causes a therapeutic effect is not known. Whole herbs contain many ingredients, and it is likely that they work together to produce the desired medicinal effect. Many factors decide how effective an herb will be. For example, the type of environment (climate, bugs, soil quality) in which a plant grew will affect its components, as will how and when it was harvested and processed.

12. HOW ARE HERBS USED?

Herbal medicine and conventional medicine have three important differences:

12.1 Use of Whole Plants

Herbalists generally use unpurified whole plant extracts containing several different compounds. They claim that these can work together such that the effect of the whole herb is greater than the summed effects of its components. They also claim that toxicity is reduced when whole herbs are used instead of isolated active ingredients ('buffering'). Although two samples of a particular herbal drug may contain several active compounds in different proportions, practitioners claim that this is not generally problematic.

12.2 Herb Combining

Several different herbs are used together. Practitioners say that combinations of plants improve efficacy and reduce adverse effects.

12.3 Different Diagnostic Approach

Herbal practitioners use different diagnostic principles than conventional practitioners. For example, they might observe the under functioning of a patient's systems of elimination. A diuretic or laxative combination of herbs might be prescribed alongside herbs with anti-inflammatory properties.

13. MEDICINAL PLANTS IN INDIA

India is endowed with a rich wealth of medicinal plants. These plants have made a good contribution to the development of ancient *Indian materia medica*. One of the earliest treatises on Indian medicine, the Charak Samhita (1000 B.C), records the use of over 340 drugs of vegetable origin. Most of these continue to be gathered from wild plants to meet the demand of the medical profession. Thus, despite the rich heritage of knowledge on the use of plant drugs, little attention has been paid to grow them as field crops in the country till the latter part of the nineteenth century.

In general, agronomic practices for growing poppy, isabgol, senna, cinchona, ipecac, belladonna, ergot and a few others have been developed and there is now localized cultivation of these medicinal plants commercially. The average annual foreign trade in crude drugs and their phytochemicals is between 60 and 80 million rupees and this accounts for a little over 0.5 per cent of the world trade in these commodities. A list of annual demand of thirty two prioritized medicinal plants is given in Table 6.

Table 6 List of Annual Demand of 32 Prioritized Medicinal Plants
Source: National Medicinal Plants Board, Ministry of Health and Family Welfare, Government of India

Annual Demand of 32 Prioritized Medicinal Plants				
S.No.	*Species*	*Demand (in tonnes)*		*Annual Growth Rate (%)*
		2001-2002	*2004-2005*	
1	Amla	22729.5	41782.9	22.5
2	Ashok	7051.3	10724.2	15.0
3	Ashwagandha	7028.7	9127.5	9.1
4	Atis	270.1	448.4	18.4
5	Bael	5381.2	7084.5	9.6
6	Bhumi amalaki	2212.6	2985.3	10.5
7	Brahmi	3822.5	6621.8	20.1
8	Chandan	635.2	1073.1	19.1
9	Chirata	965.2	1284.7	10.0
10	Daru haridra	1187.3	1829.4	15.5
11	Giloe	2258.3	2932.6	9.1
12	Gudmar	N.A.	N.A.	N.A.
13	Guggal	1505.0	2548.9	19.2
14	Isabgol	N.A.	N.A.	N.A.
15	Jatamansi	674.9	866.8	8.7
16	Kalihari	65.4	100.5	15.4
17	Kalmegh	2005.0	2197.3	3.1
18	Kesar	N.A.	N.A.	N.A.
19	Kokum	N.A.	N.A.	N.A.
20	Kuth	1414.1	1826.3	8.9
21	Kutki	220.3	317.0	12.9
22	Makoy	2077.9	2192.2	1.8
23	Mulethi	873.4	1359.8	15.9
24	Patharchur	37.8	60.8	17.2
25	Pippali	3992.5	6280.4	16.3
26	Safed Musali	N.A.	N.A.	N.A.
27	Sarpgandha	423.6	588.7	11.6
28	Senna	6462.5	11677.3	21.8
29	Shatavari	10924.7	16658.5	15.1
30	Tulsi	3296.8	5402.9	17.9
31	Vatsnabh	322.3	3426.8	30.0
32	Viavidang	N.A.	N.A.	N.A.

The curative properties of drugs are due to the presence of complex chemical substances of varied composition (present as secondary plant metabolites) in one or more parts of these plants. These plant metabolites according to their composition, are grouped as alkaloids, glycosides, cortico-steroids, essential oils, etc. The alkaloids form the largest group, which includes morphine and codein (poppy), strychnine and brucine (nux vomica), quinine (*Cinchona*), ergotamine (Ergot), hypocyamine (*Belladona*), scolapomine (*Datura*), emetine (ipecac), cocaine(coco), ephedrine (Ephedra), reserpine (*Rauwolfia*), caffeine (tea dust), aconitine (*Aconitum*), vascine (vasaca). Santonin (*Artemisia*), lobelin (*Lobelia*) and a large number of others. Glycosides form another important group represented by digoxin (foxglove), stropanthin (*Strophanthus*), glycyrrhizin (liquorice), barbolin (*Aloe*), sennocides (*Senna*), etc. Cortico-steroids have come into prominence recently and diosgenin (*Dioscorea*), solasodin (*Solanum* sp.), etc. command a large world demand these days. Some essential oils such as those of valerian (*kutch*) and peppermint also possess medicating properties and are used in pharmaceutical industry. However, it should be stated in all fairness that our knowledge of the genetic and physiological make-up of most of the medicinal plants is poor and we know still less about the biosynthetic pathways leading to the formation of active constituents for which these crops are valued. A summary of comparative study of some of the selected prioritised medicinal plants of India is given in the Table 7.

14. INTERACTION OF MEDICINAL PLANTS WITH MICROBES

The roots of almost all higher plants are known to form mutualistic symbioses with fungi. These are termed mycorrhizae (Brundrett 1991). Fungi of very diverse kinds, belonging to all the major groups, take part in mycorrhizae. Based on morphology and the species involved, several different types are recognized. Fungi associated with roots can help the plant to get phosphate and other nutrients from the soil. These mycorrhizal associations are of two kinds which are known as endomycorrhizae and ectomycorrhizae. Endomycorrhizae invade the root tissues and often occur in herbaceous plants whereas ectomycorrhizae that form a sheath of mycelium around the root and often occur in woody plants. Any natural ecosystem normally contains a mixture of types of mycorrhizal associations.

The main mycorrhizal response is one of increased efficiency of mineral uptake especially of poorly mobile ions and there is a voluminous literature dealing with the nutritional benefits that plants derive from mycorrhizal associations. Mycorrhizae are also involved in the transfer of

Table 7 Summary of comparative study of some selected prioritised medicinal plants of India

S.No.	*Name*	*Botanical Name (Family)*	*Parts used*	*Habit*	*Constituents*	*Demand in tonnes (2004-2005)*	*Habitat (in India)*
1.	Amla	*Emblica officinalis* (Euphorbiaceae)	Fruits	Tree	Rich source of *Ascorbic acid*	41782.9	Tropical Eastern Asia
2.	Shatavari	*Asparagus racemosus* (Liliaceae)	Roots and leaves	Woody climber	*Shatavarins, Isoflavones, asparagamine, racemosol*	16658.5	Tropical N. India
3.	Senna	*Cassia angustifolia* (Leguminosae)	Dried leaves and pods	Tree	*Sennoside* A and B	11677.3	Tamil Nadu
4.	Ashok	*Saraca indica* (Leguminosae)	Bark	Tree	*Haematooxylin, leucopelargonidin* (extracted from bark)	10724.2	Almost throughout India, C. and E. Himalayas, N.E. India
5.	Ashwagan *-dha*	*Withania somnifera* (Solanaceae)	Whole plant	Evergreen shrub	*Withaferin,* anaferin, tropine	9127.5	M.P.
6.	Bael	*Aegle marmelos* (Rutaceae)	Fruits, root bark, leaves	Tree	Non reducing sugar, ABA, *marmelosin*	7084.5	Throughout India
7.	Brahmi	*Bacopa monniera* (Scrophulariaceae)	Whole plant	Herb	*Bacosides,* brahmine	6621.8	Throughout tropical India (S. India)

Contd.

Table 7

S.No.	Name	Botanical Name (Family)	Parts used	Habit	Constituents	Demand in tonnes (2004-2005)	Habitat (in India)
8.	Pippali	*Piper longum* (Piperaceae)	Dry spike	Climber or under shrub	Piperine	6280.4	N.E. India, S. India, central Himalayas to Assam
9.	Tulsi	*Ocimum* sp. (Labiatae)	Leaves	Perennial herb	Essential oils, tannins and vitamins	5402.9	Throughout India
10.	Vatsnabh	*Aconitum ferox* (Ranunculaceae)	Tuberous roots	Herb	Pseudaconitine, benzyl aconitine	3426.8	Indian Himalayas alpine region
11.	Bhumi amalaki	*Phyllanthus amarus* (Euphorbiaceae)	Whole plant	Annual herb	Phyllanthin, hypophyllanthin	2985.3	S. India
12.	Giloe	*Tinospora cardifolia* (Minispermaceae)	Leaves, stems	Big Climber	Berberine, gilonin giloin, tinosporon etc.	2932.6	Tropical India
13.	Guggal	*Commiphora mukul* (Burseraceae)	Gums	Small tree	Guggulipids, Guggulsterone	2548.9	Karnataka, Rajasthan, Deccan and Gujarat.
14.	Kalmegh	*Andrographis paniculata* (Acanthaceae)	Whole plant	Annual herb	Andrographolide, kalmeghin (maximum in leaves)	2197.3	S. India

Contd.

Table 7

S.No.	*Name*	*Botanical Name (Family)*	*Parts used*	*Habit*	*Constituents*	*Demand in tonnes (2004-2005)*	*Habitat (in India)*
15.	Makoy	*Solanum nigrum* (Solanaceae)	Whole plant (leaves, fruits)	Annual herb	Solanine, saponin, fruit has trigogenin,	2192.2	All over India
16.	Daru haridra	*Berberis aristata* (Berberidaceae)	Roots, stem, bark, fruits	Erect spinous shrub	Barberine	1829.4	Assam, Bihar. Himalayan region
17	Kuth	*Saussurea lappa* or *S. costus* *(Compositae)*	Tuberous roots	Perennial herb plant (3m)	Saussuine etc.	1826.3	E. Himalayas
18.	Mulethi	*Glycyrrhiza glabra* (Leguminosae)	Roots and rhizome	Herb	Glycyrrhizic acid	1359.8	Sub Himalayan tracts
19.	Chirata	*Swertia chirata* (Gentianaceae)	Whole plant	Herb	Gentianine, swerchirin, chiratin, ophelic acid etc.	1284.7	Temperate Himalayas
20.	Chandan	*Santalum album* (Santalaceae)	Wood	Small tree	Essential oils	1073.1	Andhra Pradesh, Bihar, Karnataka, Madhya Pradesh, Maharashtra and Tamilnadu.
20.	Jatamansi	*Nardostachys grandiflora* or	Rhizome	Perennial herb	Valerenic acid, valeopotrites	866.8	Sikkim, Bhutan

Contd.

Table 7

S.No.	*Name*	*Botanical Name (Family)*	*Parts used*	*Habit*	*Constituents*	*Demand in tonnes (2004-2005)*	*Habitat (in India)*
		Valerian wallichi (Valerianaceae)					
21	Sarpagan -dha	*Rouvolfia serpentina* (Apocynaceae)	Roots	Perennial herb	55 alkaloids (reserpine, ajamaline, ajalalicine) etc.	588.7	Himmalayan foothills, peninsular India
22.	Atis	*Aconitun heterophyllum* (Ranunculaceae)	Root	Herb	Atisine, heteophylsive etc.	448.4	Alpine and subalpine zone of Himalayas
23.	Kutki	*Picrorhiza kurroa* (Scrophulariaceae)	Rhizome or underground	Small perennial herb	Kutkin, D- mannitol, vanillic acid, kutkoside	317.0	Western Himalayas
24.	Kalihari	*Glorisa superba* (Liliaceae)	Tubers, leaves, flowers	Tall, stout, climbing herb	Seeds contain colchicines	100.5	S.India
25.	Safed Musli	*Chlorophytum borivilianum* (Liliaceae)	Tuberous roots	Herb	Saponins, alkaloids, carbohydrate	N.A.	Southern Rajasthan, Western M.P and North Gujarat
26.	Gudmar	*Gymnema sylvestre* (Asclepiadaceae)	Leaves and roots	Perennial climber	Tartaric acid, Gymnemic, acid Quercitol etc.	N.A.	Western Ghats, Konkan, Tamilnadu,

Contd.

Table 7

S.No.	Name	Botanical Name (Family)	Parts used	Habit	Constituents	Demand in tonnes (2004-2005)	Habitat (in India)
							Karnataka and Uttar Pradesh.
27.	Kokum	*Garcinia indica* (Clusiaceae)	Ripe Fruit	Tree	Arabin, essential oil, resin, tartaric, citric and phosporic acids	N.A.	Maharashtra, Goa, Karnataka, Kerala, South Gujarat, Assam and West Bengal.
28.	Isabgol	*Plantago ovata* (Plantaginaceae)	Seed	Herb	Mucilage	N.A.	Punjab plains and low hills from Sutlej westwards
29.	Kesar	*Crocus sativus* (Iridaceae)	Stigma	Herb	Crocin, crocetin, safranal and picrocrocin	N.A.	Kashmir

nutrients from components of soil minerals and organic residues to solution, and in nutrient cycling in an ecosystem.

In all types of mycorrhiza, fungal hyphae permeate soil and litter beyond the depletion zones developed around non-mycorrhizal roots. Thus, mycorrhizal roots explore a larger soil volume, and have a greater absorptive area, than non-mycorrhizal roots. The fungal partners in some mycorrhizas may also have chemical mechanisms to liberate fixed inorganic ions or minerals incorporated in organic matter in the soil.

Piriformospora indica is a novel endophytic root colonizing fungus which has great potential for application in agro-forestry, flori-horticulture, arboriculture, viticulture and especially for better establishment of tissue culture raised plants-much needed for the application in plant industry. This would open up numerous opportunities for the optimization of plant productivity in both managed and natural ecosystems, while minimizing risks of environmental damage. This axenically culturable mycorrhiza-like-fungus has been recently described by Varma (JNU, New Delhi) and his collaborators. The fungus was named *Piriformospora indica* based on its characteristic pear-shaped chlamydospores. According to the analysis of 18S rDNA and the ultrastructure of the septal pore, it has phylogenetic relationship within the Hymenomycetes (Basidiomycota), *P. indica* tremendously improves the growth and overall biomass production of diverse hosts, including legumes, medicinal and economically important plants. Pronounced growth promotional effect was also seen with terrestrial orchids. The fungus promises to be a potential orchid mycorrhizal fungus (Fig. 4). The fungus also provides protection when inoculated to the tissue culture raised plantlets by overcoming the 'transient transplant shock' on transfer to the field rendering almost 100% survival (Verma et al. 1998; Varma et al. 1999; Varma et al. 2001; Pham et al. 2004 and Prasad et al. 2005).

14.1 Interaction of *Piriformospora indica* with Some Selected Medicinal Plants

It is scientifically well established that active ingredient(s) present in the medicinal plants, generally, are low. Moreover, synthetic alkaloids (active ingredients) are not as effective as the alkaloids produced in naturally growing plants associated with rhizosphere micro-organisms (bacteria and fungi). Therefore, it is most appropriate and demand of the day to develop an appropriate technology to increase the active ingredients in medicinal plants under investigation by the intervention of symbiotic fungus *P. indica,* an endophyte isolated from desert soil of Rajasthan, is interacted with some selected medicinal plants to assess for its growth promotional activities in them. *P. indica* tremendously improves the

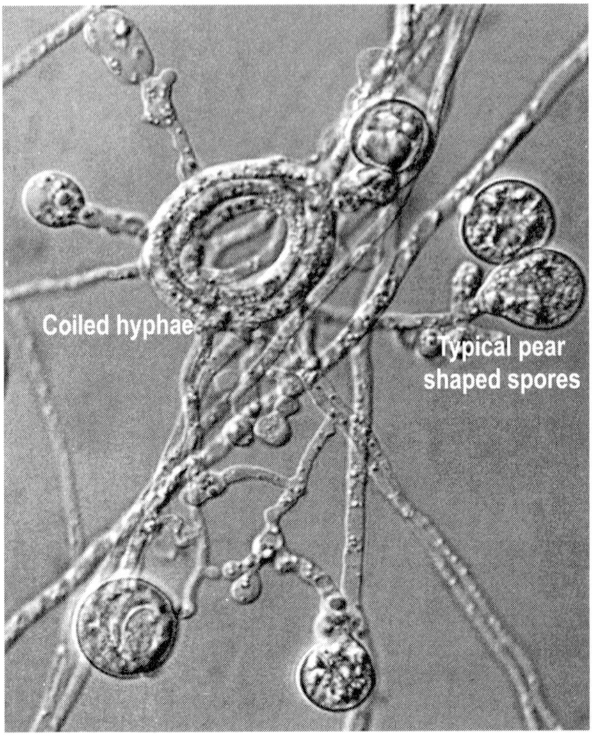

Fig. 4 Coiled hyphae and typical pear shaped spores of *Piriformospora indica*

growth and the synthesis of secondary metabolites (active ingredients) of diverse medicinal and plants of economic importance. *P. indica* colonizes the roots of host plants as diverse group of plants belonging to monocots, dicots including orchids. The fungus could be mass multiplied on cheap and simplified artificial medium.

The medicinal plants tested in the laboratory conditions as well as in the extensive field trial were *Bacopa moniera* (Sahay and Varma 1999, 2000), *Azadirachta indica* (Singh et al. 2002; Singh et al 2003), *Withania somnifera, Spilanthes calva* (Rai et al. 2001) *Tridex procumbans* (Kumari et al. 2004), *Adhatoda vasica* (Rai and Varma 2005), *Abrus precatorius* (Kumari et al. 2004), and *Chlorophytum borivilianum*. Rai et al. (2001) reported growth increase in *Withania somnifera* and *Spilanthes calva* when they were interacted with the fungus *P. indica*. This fungus also enhanced the growth in *A. vasica*.

14.2 Case Study

Bacopa monnieri is a medicinal plant of great economic importance and is known to be used as nerve tonic, adaptogen, antioxidant, antimicrobial, antifungal, sedative, cardio tonic, anticonvulsant and antidepressant and useful for cancer patients experiencing pain. The interaction of the fungus *P. indica* with *Bacopa* plant resulted in an unprecedented increase in the plant biomass, photosynthetic pigments, metabolic regulators and active ingredients like antioxidants and bacosides (Memory plus ingredients) to several fold. Scientists have discovered that boosting the body's natural oxidant level could help humans to live longer life. Man can live 20% longer and have less heart and other age-related diseases. Free radicals are involved in heart disease, cancer and other age-related disease. A patent entitled '*Piriformospora indica* - a symbiotic fungus promotes biomass of *Bacopa monnieri,* enhances the antioxidant activity and bacoside concentration' has been filed to seek the protection of this discovery from European and North American Countries. Thus, studies have showed symbiotic fungus, *P. indica,* enhances the plant biomass, antioxidant activity and bacoside concentration in *Bacopa monnieri.*

Prof. Bisaria and co-workers of Biochemical Engineering Division, IIT New Delhi have got preliminary indication of enhancement of production of podophyllotoxin in *Linum perenne album* (white flax) when it was interacted with mycorrhiza belonging to Sebacinaceae (*Piriformospora indica* and *Sebacina vermifera*). This plant mainly accumulates *podophyllotoxin* and *five methoxypodophyllotoxin* as its secondary metabolites. Podophyllotoxin is a potent anti-cancer agent. Signalling substances when added in small amount to a living cell culture system trigger the formation of specific biomolecules by inducing defense responses, hyper sensitive responses, pathogenesis related protein and lignifications. Interestingly the physical contact of the root with the fungus as well as the fungus culture filtrate enhances the anti-cancer agents in plants.

15. CONCLUSION

Heath for all continues to be a dream for humankind. A major breakthrough occurred when microbiologists discovered that life threatening diseases like plague, tuberculosis, cholera, AIDS etc. were caused by microbes. Surprisingly, many diseases that were previously thought to have only behavioral or genetic components, have been found to involve micro-organisms. The clearest case is that of ulcers, which was long thought to be caused by stress and poor diet; however the causative agent is actually a bacterium, *Helicobacter pylori,* and many ulcers can be cured with appropriate antibiotics. Work on other non-infectious diseases such as heart disease, stroke and some auto-immune diseases also suggest a microbial component that triggers the illness. During the past century, advances in medications have enabled doctors to cure many diseases and save lives. With the increase in life expectancy and the problems of over crowding, air and water pollution, degenerative strata, allergies, diabetes, rheumatic and arthritic conditions, neurological conditions, memory disorders and many more health problems are likely to grow.

Medicinal plants and herbs contain substances known to modern and ancient civilizations for their healing properties. Until the development of Chemistry and, particularly, of the synthesis of organic compounds in the 19th Century, medicinal plants and herbs were the sole source of active principles capable of curing man's ailments. The demand of plant-based therapeutics is increasing, in both developing and developed countries, due to the growing recognition that they are natural products, being non-narcotic, having no side-effects, easily available at affordable prices, and sometimes it is the only source of health care which is available to the poor. The side-effects of medicinal plants seem to be much milder and more infrequent than that of pharmaceutical drugs. Most of the herbs that may have side-effects in high doses are not readily available to buy over the counter at medical shops.

Today, with increase in global population, it is necessary to develop an appropriate technology to increase the active ingredients in medicinal plants by the intervention of symbiotic fungus. In this regard *Piriformospora indica*, which is a symbiotic fungus, can be used as a very promising tool.

16. ACKNOWLEDGEMENTS

The authors acknowledge the support and encouragement received from Dr Ashok K Chauhan, founder president, Ritnand Balved Education Foundation (an umbrella organization of Amity Institutions), Mr Atul Chauhan, Chancellor, Amity University, (UP) and Mr Aseem Chauhan, Trustee and Board Member, Ritnand Balved Education Foundation. The technical support received from Mr Anil Chandra Bahukhandi is highly appreciated.

REFERENCES

Akca E, Claus H, Schultz N, Karbach BS, Debaerdemaeker T, Declercq JP, Konig H (2002) Genes and derived amino acid sequences of S-layer proteins from mesophilic, thermophilic, and extremely thermophilic methanococci. Exremophiles 6: 351-358

Bent S, Ko R (2004) Commonly used herbal medicines in the United States: A review, Am J Med 116: 478-485

Brundrett MC (1991) Mycorrhizae in natural ecosystems. In: Macfayden A, Begon M, Fitter AH (eds) Advances in Ecological Research, Academic Press, London, pp 171-313

Cairns J, Lanza GR, Parker BC (1972) Pollution related structural and functional changes in aquatic communities with emphasis on freshwater algae and protozoa. Proc Natl Acad Sci 124: 79-127

Curds CR (1992) Protozoa and the water industry. Cambridge University Press, MA, pp 122

Dubey NK, Kumar R, Tripathi P (2004) Global Promotion of herbal medicine: India's Opportunity. Curr Med 86: 37-41

Foissner W (1987) Soil protozoa: fundamental problems, ecological significance, adaptations in ciliates and testaceans, bioindicators, and guide to the literature. Progress in Protistology 2: 69-212

Ingraham JL, Ingraham CA (2000) Microbial Biotechnology. In: Ingraham JL, Ingraham CA (eds) Introduction to Microbiology, Second edition, Brooks/Cole, Australia

Kamboj VP (2000) Herbal Medicines. Current Med 78:35-39

Kandler O, Konig H (1985) Cell envelopes of Archaebacteria. In: The Bacteria, Vol VIII. Academic Press, pp 413-457

Kandler O, Konig H (1993) Cell envelopes of archaea: Structure and Chemistry. In: Kates M (ed) The Biochemistry of Archaea (Archaebacteria) Elsevier Science Publishers, Amsterdam, pp 223-259

Kumari R, Pham GH, Sachdev M, Garg AP, Varma A (2004) Symbiotic Fungi for Eco-friendly Environment: A Perspective. Natural Product Radiance 3: 396-400

Morton JB, Benny GL (1990) Revised classification of arbuscular mycorrhizal fungi (Zygomycetes): A new order, Glomales, two new suborders, Glomineae and Gigasporineae, with an emendation of Glomaceae. Mycotaxon 37: 471-491

Niederlehner BR, Pontasch KW, Pratt JR, Cairns J (1990) Field evaluation of predictions of environmental effects from multispecies microcosm toxicity test. Arch Environ Contam Toxicol 19: 62-71

Niemetz R, Karcher U, Kandler O, Tindall BJ, Konig H (1997) The cell-wall polymer of the extremely halophilic archaeon *Natronococcus occultus*. Eur J Biochem 249: 905-911

Pham GH, Singh A, Malla R, Kumari R, Prasad R, Sachdev M, Luis P, Kaldorf M, Tatjana P, Harrmann S, Hehl S, Declerck S, Buscot F, Oelmuller R, Rexer KH, Kost G, Varma A (2004) Interaction of *P. indica* with other Micro-organisms and Plants. In: Varma A, Abbott L, Werner D, Hampp R (eds) Plant Surface Microbiology. Springer-Verlag, Germany, pp 237-265

Pirozynski KA, Dalpe (1989) The geological history of the Glomaceae with particular reference to mycorrhizal symbiosis. Symbiosis 7: 1-36

Prasad R, Pham GH, Kumari R, Singh A, Yadav V, Sachdev M, Peskan T, Hehl S, Oelmuller R, Varma A (2005) Sebacinaceae: Culturable Mycorrhizae-like Endosymbiotic Fungi and their Interaction with Non-transformed and Transformed Roots. In: Declerck S, Strullu DG, Fortin JA (eds) In Vitro Culture of Mycorrhizae. Springer-Verlag, Germany, pp 291-312

Prescott LM, Harley JP, Klein DA (1996) The diversity of the microbial world. Microbiology. WCB Publishers, Dubuque, Iowa

Rai MK, Singh An, Arya D, Varma A (2001) Positive growth responses of the medicinal plants *Withania somnifera* and *Spilanthes calva* to inoculation by *Piriformospora indica* in a field trial. Mycorrhizae 11:123-128

Rai MK, Varma A (2005) Arbuscular mycorrhizae–like biotechnological potential of *Piriformospora indica,* which promotes the growth of *Adhatoda vasica*. Electronic J Biotechnol ISSN 8: 107-112

Report of the Task Force on Conservation & Sustainable Use of Medicinal Plants Government of India, Planning Commission, March – 2000

Sahay NS, Varma A (1999) *Piriformospora indica*: a new biological hardening tool for micropropagated plants. FEMS Microbiol Lett 181: 297-302

Sahay NS, Varma A (2000) Biological approach towards increasing the survival rates of micropropagated plants. Curr Sci 78: 126-129

Singh An, Singh Ar, Kumari M, Rai MK, Varma A (2003) Biotechnology importance of *Piriformospora indica*-A novel symbiotic mycorrhiza-like Fungus: An Overview. Indian J Biotechnol 2: 65-75

Singh Ar, Singh An, Varma A (2002) *Piriformospora indica – in vitro* raised leguminous plants: A new dimension in establishment and phyto-promotion. Indian J Biotechnol 1: 372-376

Varma A, Singh A, Sudha, Sahay N S, Sharma J, Roy A, Kumari M, Rana D, Thakran S, Deka D,Bharti K, Hurek T, Blechert O, Rexer KH, Kost G, Hahn A, Maier W, Walter M, Strack D, Kranner I (2001) In: Hock B (ed) *Piriformospora indica*: An Axenically culturable Mycorrhizae-like endosymbiotic fungus. The Mycota IX, Springer, Berlin, pp 151-161

Varma A, Verma S, Sudha, Sahay N, Britta B, Franken P (1999) *Piriformospora indica* – a cultivable plant growth promoting root endophyte with similarities to arbuscular mycorrhizal fungi. Applied Environ Microbiol 65: 2741-2744

Verma S, Varma A, Rexer Karl-Heinz, Hassel A, Kost G, Sarbhoy A, Bisen P, Buetehorn P and Franken P (1998). *Piriformuspora indica* gen. nov, a new root colonizing fungus. Mycologia - USA, 90: 895-909.

Gloriosa superba L.: Biology and Biotechnological Strategies for Conservation

R ADE and M RAI*

1. INTRODUCTION

The convention on 'Biological diversity' at Rio de Janeiro, Brazil and Biodiversity Bill of Indian Parliament proposes to safeguard the over exploitation of natural resources and protect the right of indigenous people and also our traditional knowledge. There is a need to develop appropriate strategies to protect the IPR of our bioresources and associated knowledge system of our tribal communities.

In India, there are fiftythree million tribal, belonging to more than five hundred fiftyfive tribal groups or communities, under two hundred and twentyseven linguistic groups living in close proximity to nature. These people have unique knowledge about flora and fauna. This indigenous knowledge is a potential tool in searching for new economic plants for food and medicine. Several plants were originally identified and developed through indigenous knowledge. Examples, where ethno-medicines have played a key role in the development of drugs used in the modern system of medicine, are *atropine, cocaine, colchicine, codeine, caffeine, emetine, ephedrine, guguline, morphine, quinine, resurpine, vinblastin, vincristin* etc. (Gupta 1982).

* Department of Biotechnology, Amravati University, Amravati-444602, Maharashtra, India Tel: 91 721 2662207/8; ext. 267 Fax: 91 721 2660649/2662135
E-mail: mkrai123@rediffmail.com; pmkrai@hotmail.com

Human civilization is always influenced by plants and their products. All indigenous remedies and medicines have their roots in ethno medicinal plants. A large number of these ancient medicines and prescription still exist and are restricted to a particular region or people of the world, though they do not exist merely as knowledge but are also practiced largely in primitive societies. The ethno-botanists are trying to discover new medicines from the forests by the help of tribal people.

Gloriosa superba is one of the important species due to its high medicinal values. It is called as 'Mauve beauty', 'purple prince', 'Modest'. 'Orange gem', 'Salman glow', and 'Orange glow'. Many varieties have been originated to introduce a range of colours, forms and size. Though it has been originated in our country, its planting material is very rare and far to meet the present demand. The demand of its seeds in pharma-industries at home and abroad has increased (Sivakumar 2002). Now, it has been included in the Red Data Book by International Union for Conservation of Nature (IUCN).

2. PROPAGATION

Gloriosa can be propagated by seeds and rhizome. The fleshy roots are 'V'- or 'L'-shaped. The arms develop from the base of the plants. After the completion of dormancy, the new sprout emerges from the tip of the arms but never from the joints of the arms. The rhizomes are planted by splitting into two from the joints of the arms. Thus, from one rhizome, only two plants are obtained. The process of multiplication is very slow. The fruit containing a number of hard-coated seeds matures in October. Seeds are sown in April-June, which germinate six to eight weeks after sowing. The seedling grows slowly. Generally, they come to flowering after two season growth.

In new technique, seeds are sown usually in the seed-pans of enriched potting compost of light texture containing plenty of humus, preferentially leaf moulds. Seeds should be sown in the first week of June in the plains. In a 30 cm pan, about 100 seeds are sown to obtain thirty to fifty seedlings.

In September, when seedling reaches to 4-leaf stage, a dose of liquid manure of decomposes oil-cake of mustard or groundnut with a pinch of urea, in the ratio 10:1, for a dose of liquid manure only 30 gm of oilcake per pan, is applied.

During the first week of North winter (December), the seedling decline when only few leaves of dull and green colour at the top can be seen and others turn yellow; now without watering the shoots are left to dry and the tiny tubers are picked out and stored in plastic office-tray on the shelf. Those micro tubers instead of being shriveled up remain plum and sprout at both the ends of the arms during hot summer months (May-June) as usual. The micro tubers can be marketed from January to July through post parcel to district nursery.

G. superba has various vernacular names:

Sanskrit-Langalika, Hindi-Kalahari, English-Superb lily, Climbing lily, Bengali-Bishalguli, French-Glorious du Masaciear, Unani-Muleen, Persian-Buchnak, Burmease-Simadon.

Habitat : Commonly found in the tropical forests of Bengal, Karnataka (India), Myanamar and Sri Lanka.

Parts used : Leaves and rhizome

G. superba, also known as Malabar glory lily, is a perennial tuberous climbing herb, is widely distributed in the tropical and subtropical parts of India, including the foothills of Himalayas (Anon 1956, Rastogi 1993). Adapted to different soil texture and climatic variations, the plant thrives from the arid Bundelkhand to humid Assam valleys. It is known by different names in India such as 'Kalahari' 'Agnishikha,' 'Languliata,' and 'Nangulika.' There are several allied species of *Gloriosa* including *G. superba*, *G. simplex*, *G. grandiflora*, *G. lutea*, *G. planti*, *G. lipolidii*, *G. longifolia*, *G. rotheschildiana*, *G. virenses*, *G. sudanica,* etc. distributed mainly in Africa, besides many hybrids popular garden cultivars like the purple prince, African chief, orange gem, orange gift, lavender lady and orange ball are grown for a wide range of flowers and colour combination of the perianth, which bloom for long during autumn.

The viny stems bear simple, stalkless, linear lanceolate leaves with circular closed tips, spirally twisted in the upper part to serve as tendrils. The flowers are in shades of crimson tapels. The flower bud is green, yellow on opening, changing to orange red and turning to dark pink or red when in full bloom by late autumn.

The asymmetrical 'V'-shaped tubers are the commercial part containing colchicine (0.15-0.3%) together with benzoic acid, salicycilic acid, sterols, and resinous substances (Bellet and Gaignaults 1985; Dvorakova 1984; Fainne 1999). This is used in Ayurvedic medicines as arbortifacient, antipyretic, antinflammatory, antigout, and antileprotic agent. It also provides relief to the swollen joints and in gout. The tubers have long been used as alternative sources of colchicines in chemical and pharmaceutical industry. The seeds are rich source of colchicines and gloriosine (0.7-0.9%). The world market price of the raw material is US $ 50-60 per kilo. The seeds are used as precursor raw material for the manufacture of the drugs for gout, a disease caused due to deposition of micro crystals of uric acid metabolism. The colchicines intercept new cycle of deposition and provide relief in acute pain.

In Tamilnadu, it is raised as small plantation because its aerial parts do not die in winter and produce commercial quantities of seeds in advance. Therefore, parts of Tamilnadu and Karnataka, having equitable climate, provide favorable conditions. The Malabar glory lily grows in a luxurious growth in warm weather having rainfall of 200 cm distributed evenly throughout the year. It is adapted to the peninsular regions; medium sandy loam soil having pH 6.0-7.0 is better suited for its cultivation. High temperature and relative humidity in early period result in a vigorous growth, but rise in temperature from 15 to 20°C during the day and 10 to 15°C at night is ideal for copious flowering and seed set. Humid and cloudy weather for a long period of flowering stage, results into leaf blight disease, since it is a climber, growing up to 6 meters in length preferably to 1.5 m over supporting stalk or wire frame at 30 to 40 cm stage to get more fruit. It can be raised both from seeds and tubers. The seed-propagated plants take 3 to 4 years to bloom, that is why the tuber is the choice for planting material. The land should be ploughed and harrowed until it comes to a fine tilth. All the grass stubbles and permeating roots are removed. The field is levelled and divided into small plots providing slopes for drainage according. About 15 to 20 tons of farmyard manures or compost in a hectare is mixed in the soil. The tubers are brittle and hence its end must be protected from damage, a 50 to 60 gm apical piece is cut out and treated in 0.08% contact fungicide emission-6 (Methoxy ethyl mercuric chloride) for 3 minutes. The vigour of the growing vine depends upon the tuber weight. Use of smaller pieces does not allow it to flower during the first year. The treated tuber pieces are planted at a 6 cm depth into furrows 45 to 60 cm apart. The row-to-row distance is maintained at 30 to 45 cm. The closer spacing helps better cross-fertilization leading to improved fruit set. The glory lily vines respond very well when fed with fertilizers. A dose of 40 kg nitrogen, 50 kg phosphorous pentoxide (P_2O_5) and 75 kg di-potassium oxide (K_2O) per hectare should be applied at the time of planting and the balance 80 kg of nitrogen 8 weeks after planting. Top dressing coincides with providing of stalking of growing vines. The growing vine needs copious irrigation during dry weather in the initial stages of growth, and up to three irrigation in a month, depending upon the rainfall. The crop is not irrigated after flowering because high soil moisture may cause rotting of the under ground tubers.

Superb lily is a perennial herb and remains in the field years. If planted in June (early monsoon) it grows 55 days after plantation and takes another 105-110 days for maturity. The ripen pods are shrunken in position; to spilt open the pods are, in shade for 7-10 days kept. A hectare plant gives 250-300 kg seeds from throughout the year. Estimated 100 tonnes of seeds are required per year to export. The seeds should be packed in moisture proof containers or bags and stored in cold dry place before extraction of alkaloids.

3. DISEASE OF *G. SUPERBA*

Leaf-blight and tuber-rot are two important fungal diseases causing severe damage to the standing crop. A cloudy weather and continuous humid condition favours blight (*Curvularia lunata*). Small lesions appear on leaves, they turn black in colour and spread all over the foliage, causing leaf fall; during severe incidence the whole vine is affected it can diecan. Spraying of 0.3% Dienane M-45 (0.35%) at an interval of 10-15 days twice or thrice, effectively controls this disease.

Soft-rot is caused by *Sclerotium* species. It attacks underground tubers. The affected vine becomes yellow, and in severe stage the plants die. The infected plants, along with underground tubers, should be removed and burnt. Drenching of soil at root zone with Bavistin (0.2%) or Cuprosol is effective in initial stages of the disease.

Lily caterpillar (*Polytella gloriosae*) and green caterpillar (*Pulsia charcites*) attack the foliage and flower buds. The lily caterpillar have red and black bands on the body and lay eggs on the undersurface of tender leaves and crown of the growing shoots, the hatched young caterpillar voraciously eat away the leaves and other parts. The green caterpillar can even eat the flowers. Met-acid spray (0.25%) at fortnightly interval and dusting with DDT and BHC are advised.

Gloriosa superba is diploid (2n=22) and fails to successfully cross with other allies and cultivars, including the only other native species, *G. rothschildiana*. The later is an octaploid (2n=88), medium tall in height with opposite lanceo-cardate leaves. The tetraploid species of *G. virences*, *G. carsoni* and *G. richmondensis* have shown better ability for crossing successfully. Crosses have been reported between *G. virences* Vs *G. carsanii* as well as with *G. richmondensis*. Considering the extensive range of distribution of superb-lily in the Indo-Malayan region of south-east Asia, natural variability and selection amongst germplasm could be exploited with advantageously improving the present cultivars for growth habit, seed yields and its colchicines contents.

4. CHEMICAL CONSTITUENTS

Young leaves contain chelidonic acid; leaves of Indian plant yield colchicines, and dimethyl colchicine. N-formyl de–acetyl-colchicine, lumi-colchicine and two other colchicines and related alkaloid have been identified in the bulb and seeds.

5. PHARMACOLOGICAL ACTION

Gloriosa superba showed the qualities of tonic, antiperiodic, chologogue, antehelmintic, alternative and purgative. The fresh juice of plant exhibited stimulant action on isolated uteri of guinea pig, rabbits and human being; on isolated rat's uterus it showed papaverin-like action. In high doses, the plant extract initiated labour pain in pregnant rabbits. The tuber extract shows antibiotic activity against *Staphylococcus aureus* (Kapoor 2001).

6. MEDICINAL PROPERTIES AND USE

The leaf juice is used to kill lice in the hair. The tubers contain the bitter principles, Superbine and Gloriosin, which in large doses are poisonous, however, in small doses they are used as tonic, antiperiodic, alternative and purgatives. The white flour prepared from the rhizome is bitter. It is given with honey in Gonorrhea, leprosy, colic and intestinal worms, for promoting labor pains a paste of tubers is applied over the supra-pubic region and vagina; its warm poultice is locally applied in rheumatism and *neuralgic pains*.

Doses: 0.1 to 0.25 gm (as bitter tonic)
0.3 to 0.6 gm (as *abortifacient*)

The conventional method of propagation is through corms, since poor seed germination restricts their use in multiplication (Finnie and van Sadden 1989).

G. superba contains about 0.1-0.8% colchicine in their bulb. It is used in plant breeding work to induce mutation and polyploidy and also can solve an important problem in *Fuchsia* breeding.

G. superba also produces another alkaloid, gloriosin.

Colchicines affect cell membrane structure indirectly by inhibiting the synthesis of membrane constituent. It binds to tubulin preventing its polymerization into microtubules. This antimitotic property disrupts the spindle apparatus that separate chromosome during metaphase; cells with high metabolic rates are most involved by the arrest of mitosis.

Indiscriminate over-exploitation of plant for its diverse medicinal use has endangered its survival. Tissue culture approaches are needed for the rapid propagation of the plant (Finnie and Van Sadden 1989).

7. BIOTECHNOLOGICAL STRATEGIES FOR CONSERVATION

The conventional method of propagation is through rhizome, since poor seed germination restricts their use in multiplication (Finnie and Van

Stadden 1989). Indiscriminate over-exploitation of plant for various medicinal uses has endangered its survival. Recently, various scientists have been engaged, in order to conserve this important plant.

Le Roux and Roberties (1997) studied the seed production development in *Gloriosa superba.* Elsawi and Flores (1994) reported *in vitro* propagation and rhizome formation in colchicines alkaloid-producing plants. A micro propagation system was developed for *G. superba* and *Colchicum cornigerum,* a species native to Egypt producing cornigerin, a potent cytostatic agent. *Gloriosa* seedling cultured on Murashige and Skoog medium with 1mg/l naphthalene acetic acid (NAA) developed multiple shoot and rhizome at the base. Rhizome production was enhanced by sub-culturing the regenerated shoot on medium with 2 mg/l kinetin, in contrast corm production. *C. cornigerin* was promoted by the addition of 2% coconut milk and 5% sucrose to half-strength MS medium. Root culture of *G. superba* was established to study alkaloid production. These cultures were initiated from root tips of *in vitro* grown seedlings and were maintained on MS medium supplemented with 1mg/l NAA.

Custers and Bergervoet (1994) reported micropropagation of *G. superba* by shoot-cuttings and explants from nodes, internodes, leaves, flowers, pedicels and tubers of *G. species* (*G. rothschidiana* duphur vs *G. rothschdiana* new accession and *G. rothschildiana* vs *G.superba* were cultured on MS basal medium with 3% w/v sucrose, 0-10mg/l benzyl adenine (BA) and 0.1mg Indole Acetic Acid (IAA) and maintained for 24 days under 16 hr photoperiod. Addition of low level of Benzyl Adenine (BA) (1mg/l) improved plant growth whereas the high level of BA (10mg/l) caused a proliferation of multiple shoot from rhizome meristem. By applying alternatively high and low BA level, a method of continued propagation was achieved which resulted in a 4-7 fold multiplication of qualitatively good plantlets every 18 week. Resulting shoots were incubated on MS medium with 3% sucrose and 0-1 mg/l IAA or NAA. Transplantation into soil was only possible after the plants had formed tubers.

Narain (1981) studied detailed structure of chromosomes and deletion patterns in *Gloriosa superba.* Clonal propagation of *G. superba* from apical bud and node segment of shoot-tip, cultured on agar solidified (0.8% w/v) Gamborg's B5 medium containing BA, IAA, Kinetin, NAA, IBA or 2-4-D (Samarjeeva et al. 1993). The cultures were maintained under fluorescent light at 25-27°C. Primary culture were initiated in solid B5 medium containing 0.5 to 1 mg/l BA and 0.01-.0.5 mg/l IAA, IBA, NAA, when shoot-tips of primary culture were transferred to shoot multiplication media. Shoot proliferation occurred via adventitious bud formation within 4 to 8 weeks. The number of shoots formed on solid media was 2-3 per explants; this was greatly enhanced (40-50 shoot/explants) in liquid culture containing BA (1-5 mg/l) and IBA (0.5-1mg/l) MS (Murashige and Skoog1962). Liquid media was better than B5 liquid medium as a higher rate of shoot multiplication was observed (50-80 shoot per culture). Root formed in media containing any of the auxin except 2-4-D, IAA at 0.1mg/ l was optimal. The regenerated plantlet could be established successfully 100% in soil.

Somani et al. studied *in vitro* propagation and rhizome formation in *G. superba.* Plant Lilaceous, is valued for colchicines and other tropine alkaloid. Fresh sprouts were excised from corms of *G. superba* and dissected propagule with shoot and root primordials were placed on MS basal medium containing 3% sucrose and 0.6% agar. Explants germinated on the MS medium producing shoot and root, which formed new corm within one month. For shoot regeneration and cormlet regeneration, 1-4 mg/l kinetin was added to the medium. Cultures were maintained at 24 degree in white florescent light (2500 lux) with an 8-hr/day photoperiod. Multiple shoot formation occurred directly on the explants after 2-week incubation on M S with 2-4 mg/l kinetin. Only single shoot developed with 1mg/l kinetin. All kinetin concentration inhibited rooting. Plantlet at the 2-leaf stage was transferred to MS medium for rooting. The rooted plants were transferred to sand-soil and compost (1:1:1) mixture in humid chamber for 1 week. Plantlet were later transferred to field condition, rhizome produced *in vitro* were also transferred directly.

Choochote W et al. (2004) evaluated colchicines and associated products from *Gloriosa superba* against mosquitoes. Suri et al. (2001) found the new glycosides, that is, 3-O-demethylcolchicine-3-O-alpha-d-glucopyranoside in seed extract of *Gloriosa superba.* Pederson et al. (1999) reported different pharmacological properties of seven medicinal plants of *Rubiaceae* family from different regions of Mauritius. Mccutcheon *et al* (1992) studied antibiotic screening of some medicinal plants from different regions including native British Colombian area. Studies have been carried out on the regeneration of *Gloriosa superba* (Jadhav 2001; Sachdev *et al*, 2002; Sivakumar *et al*, 2003).

G. superba is a source of colchicines (Bellet and Gaignalt 1985;. Rajgopalan et al. 1994). Due to interest in the therapeutic use an increase in the demand for supplies of colchicinic substances by the pharmaceuticals industries has been observed, an alternative *Colchicum autumnale* as the sole source of industrially produced colchicines was sought (Nidiry et al. 1993). The ornamental plant *G. superba* was sown to produce a range of colchicinic substances including colchicines (0.9%), dimethyl-3-colchicine (0.19%) and colchicoside (0.82%) These minimum values for the colchicine content were higher than for *C. autumnale,* which were reported as 0.62, 9 and 0.39%, respectively.

Rhizomes of Indian *G. superba* were extracted with methanol, and the extract concentrated, diluted with water and acidified with citric acid. This extract was then extracted with ether i.e. chloroform. (Dvorakova 1984). The two chloroform extracts separated by column chromatography on AL 203 and mother liquors after crystallization, separated by preparative Thin Layer Chromatography on silica gel, tropaline and 3-non tropaline alkaloid were isolated from the extract of which cormegerin, (s)-(t), floramultine, bechuanines, 1,12-dihydroxy-2, 10,11-trimethoxy homomorphine, colchicomide, 2-dimethyl colchicines, 3-demethyl colchicolin and colchicoside are reported for the first name from this plant. Alkaloids isolated and assigned the structure 3 -dimensional by ultra violate spectroscopy, infrared spectroscopy, massobaur spectroscopy, nuclear magnetic resonance spectroscopy, and CMR spectral analysis. This was the first corboli alkaloid isolated from the sub-family wurmbaeoideae.

Siva Kumar et al. (2000) studied induction, maturation and germination of embryoids from leaf-tissues of *Gloriosa superba* which were developed by exploiting solid and liquid culture. Nodular calli were obtained through SH medium supplemented with 2-4-D and 1 isopentyldene. In solid culture, the nodular calli, when transferred to 2-4-D along with glycerol, gave the best response (68.4%) in embryoid induction after 20 days. After two subcultures at 7 days of interval in a medium with thiamine instead of glycerol, the embryoids matured; when mature embryoids were transferred to 6-Benzylamino purine (BAP) and Indole Butyric Acid (IBA) medium, they gave rise to plantlet with single shoot and root. In liquid culture, the medium supplemented with NAA and L-Glutamine with agitation, the embryoidogenic calli produced embryoids (85%) after 21 days. The mature embryoid began to turn green and produced shoot and elongated radicals after 35 days.

8. SECONDARY METABOLITE PRODUCTION

It is conventional drug for gout, obtained from corms of *G. superba* and *C. autmnale*, (Family-Liliaceous). Term 'colchicines' is derived from area known as Colchis near black-sea. *C. autumnale* grow wild in Europe and Africa. Thomson proposed early idea of action of colchicines in gout treatment. Gout and uric acid metabolism is same way linked and colchicines might act on this. Gout is caused by deposition of micro crystals of uric acid in joints and may be due to defective regulatory mechanism for endogenous purine synthesis, but conflicting results for the action of colchicines on synthesis and extraction of urates have been recorded. Colchicines interrupts, the cycle of new deposition which seem to be essential for the continuance of acute gout. Distressing side-effect has been recorded occasionally but colchicine remains the drug for acute gout. Modification of the side chain of rings does not abolish anti-gout activity as long as the configuration of C-ring conforms to that of colchicines. It also acts in the metaphase arrest that means doubling of chromosome number, (polyploidy first by perennial in 1899, 1930). It also acts as anti-mitotic, anti-gout agent.

It was also used in cell division by inhibiting mitosis, the division of cells nucleus. It inhibited the development of spindles as the nuclei are dividing (Spindle are formed by the polymerization of tubulin) from a pool of sub-unit during a discrete phase of cell-cycle and then depolymerized during other phase. It was also used to induce polyploidy induction, and some time also to other mutations like chlorophyll mutations, but frequency was low.

It can solve an important problem of fuchsia breeding; most Fuchsia species are diploid or tetraploid (tetraploid species are for instance *F. magellanica, F. magdalenal* and *F. triphylla*). A crossing between diploid and tetraploid result often in a triploid, which is mostly sterile because the process of meiosis (cell division for reproduction) requires the pairing of similar chromosomes and because there is no mechanism allowing for the alignment of three similar chromosomes, triploid plants are not able to produce fertile reproductive cells, they are therefore sterile and unusable as parents. Other advantage of polyploidy plants is that all its parts are bigger (flowers, leaves); a lot of big double fuchsia's are polyploidy. A special problem of colchicines induced ploidy, in particular vagetatively propagated crops, is the chimerism caused by the simultaneous presence of tissue of different ploidy levels in one plant or plant parts.

Colchicine is mostly applied freshly prepared in aqueous. The range of concentration applied varies considerably, for instance from 0.006-3%. A concentration of about 0.05% is the most common used concentration.

Colchicine can also be applied in the lanolin paste or as a solution, for instance, on a cotton dot, placed in a leaf axil. Colchicine works in dividing cells and those can be found in buds, tops of shoots and seeds.

9. CONCLUSION

Since *Gloriosa superba* has proved its own medicinal importance in diverse field such as pharmaceuticals to Ayurvedic systems, there is need of conservation and preservation by applying all possible methods including tissue culture technique, by the help of which we can develop the protocols for its rapid multiplication in order to meet the increasing demands for seeds, tubers and leaves day by day. In 1990, this was rated at 50-60 US $ per kg; from this we can guess its increasing importance. Therefore as a future prospect, its multiplication and evaluation of bioactive compounds is immensely important aspect especially for developing countries like ours, and it is the major thrust area. We can conclude that as the *Gloriosa superba* is a rare and endangered medicinal herb of Asia and Africa having diverse medicinal applications since the Ayurveda; thus to cope with the demand it should be conserved by *in vitro* methods for use in the pharmacological industries.

ACKNOWLEDGEMENTS

The authors are thankful to Dr Sudhir Patil, Hon'ble Vice Chancellor, Amravati University, Amravati for encouragement.

REFERENCES

Anon The Wealth of India, (1956) A dictionary of raw material and industrial product CSIR New Delhi 4: 139-140

Bellet P, Gaignault JC (1985) *Gloriosa superba* L. as a source of colchicineous substances Ann Pharm Fr 43 4: 345-347

Choochote W, Rongsriyam K, Pitasawat B, Jitpakdi A, Rattanachanpichai E, Junkum A, Tuetun B, Chaiwong P (2004) Evaluation of the colchicine-like activity of *Gloriosa superba*-extracted fractions for mosquito (Diptera: Culicidae) cytogenetic study. J Med Entomol 41: 672-676

Custers JBM, Bergervoet JHW (1994) Micropropagation of *Gloriosa*: towards a practical protocol. J Sci Hortic (Amsterdam) 57: 323-334

Dvorakova S (1984) Alkaloid of *Gloriosa superba* L. collect. Czech. Chem Commun 49: 1536-1542

Elsawi SA, Flores HE (1994) *In vitro* propagation and corm formation in colchicines alkaloid-producing plants. J Plant-physiol 105: 121

Finnie JF, Van Staden J (1989) *In vitro* propagation of sander *sonia* and *Gloriosa*. Plant Cell Tiss Org. 19: 151-158

Finnie JF, Van Staden J (1999) Isolation of colchicine from *Sundersonia auracaceae* and *Gloriosa superba* variation in alkaloid level of plant grown *In vivo*. J Plant Physiol 318: 691-695

Gupta BK (1982) Production of colchicine from *G. superba* tubers in cultivation and utilization of medicinal plant edited by Attal, Kapur Regional Research Laboratory, CSIR Journal pp 270-278

Jadhav H (2001) Somatic embryogenesis and plant regeneration in *Gloriosa superba* L. Indian J Expert Biol 39: 943-946

Kapoor LD (2001) Traditional uses of medicinal plants. Ayurvedic medicinal plants pp 327

Le-roux LG, Robberties PJ (1997) Aspects relating to seed production in *Gloriosa superba* L. South African J Bot 63: 191-197

Mccutcheon AR, Ellis SM, Hancock, Towers GH (1992) Antibiotic screening of medicinal plants of the British Colombian native people. J Ethnopharmacol 37: 212-223

Murashigae TF, Skoog F (1962) A revised medium for rapid growth and bioassays with Tobacco tissue culture. Physiol Plant 15: 473-497

Narain P (1981) A case of terminal chromosome deletion in *Gloriosa superba*. Current Sci 50: 285-286

Nidiry ESJ, Khan RM, Reddy PP (1993) *In vitro* nematicidal activity of *Gloriosa superba* seed extract against *Meloidogyne incognita*. Nematol Medit 21: 127–28

Pederson O, Gurib-Fakim A, Subratty, Anderson (1999) Pharmaceutical properties of seven medicinal plants of Rubiaceae from Mauritius. Pharm Biol 37: 202-207

Rai MK (1987) Ethnomedicinal Studies of Patalkot and Tamia (Chindwara). Plant used as Tonic: Ancient Science of life 3: 119-121

Rajgopalan A, Md. Abdul Khader JBM (1994) A comparison of different method of estimation of colchicine in *Gloriosa superba*. Crop Res 8: 549-551

Rastogi RP, Mehrotra BN (1993) Compendium of Indian Medicinal Plants. Vol I-V CDRI, Lucknow, Publication and information Directorate, New Dehli, India

Sachdev K, Prakash HS, Prasad TG, Sathyanarayana BN (2002) Somatic embryogenesis and plantlet regeneration from node and leaf callus cultures of *Gloriosa superba* L. J Pl Biol 29: 179-89

Samarjeewa PK, Dassanayake MD, Jayawardena SDG (1993) Clonal propagation of *Gloriosa superba* L. Indian J Expt Biol 31: 719-720

Sivakumar G, Krishnamurthy KV (2000) Micropropagation of *Gloriosa superba* L; an endangered species of Asia and Africa. Current Sci 78: 647-659

Sivakumar G, Krishnamurthy KV (2002) *Gloriosa superba* L, A very useful Medicinal Plant. In: Singh VK, Govil JN, Hashmi Shamima and Gurdip (eds) Recent Progress in Medicinal Plants Vol. 7: Ethonomedicine & Pharmacognosy II, Eds Singh. Sci. Tech. Publishing LLC, Houston, Texas, USA pp. 465-481

Sivakumar G, Krishnamurthy KV, Rajendran TD (2003) Embryoidogenesis and plant regeneration from leaf tissue of *Gloriosa superba*. Planta Med 69: 479-81

Suri OP, Gupta BD, Suri KA, Sharma AK, Satti NK (2001) A new glycoside, 3-O-demethylcolchicine-3-O-alpha-d-glucopyranoside from *Gloriosa superba* seeds. Nat Prod Lett 15: 217-219

Antimicrobial Activities of Some Ayurvedic Plant Drugs: An Appraisal of Evidence Based Researches

*GS LAVEKAR **ALKA BABBAR

1. INTRODUCTION

Infectious diseases pervade human existence. Great plagues have shaped our history, literature, plumbing, personal hygiene and societal mores. Just centuries ago, cities were devastated by bubonic plague, population scarred by smallpox and whole armies defeated by *vibrio* and spirochetes. Despite improved living conditions, widespread vaccination and availability of effective anti-biotics, infectious diseases continued to take a heavy toll in the developed country among persons with acquired immunodeficiency syndrome, debilitated with chronic disease or treated with immunosuppressive drug. In developing countries, unsanitary living conditions and malnutrition contribute to a massive burden of infectious diseases that kill more than 100 million persons each year. In spite of decades of dramatic progress in their treatment and prevention infectious diseases remain a major cause of death and debility and are responsible for worsening the living conditions of millions of people around the world. Most of these deaths are among children who suffer respiratory and diarrhoeal infections caused by viruses and bacteria. Infection frequently challenges the Physician's diagnostic skill and must be considered in the different diagnoses of syndromes affecting every system of organs.

* Director, Central Council for Research in Ayurveda and Siddha.

** Senior Research Fellow, Central Council for Research in Ayurveda and Siddha, No. 61-65 Institutional area, Opp. D-block, Janakpuri, N. Delhi-110058.

With the advent of antimicrobial agents, some medical leaders believed that infectious diseases would soon be eliminated and become of historic interest only. Indeed in hundreds of chemotherapeutic agents developed since World War-II, most of which are potent and safe, include drugs effective not only against bacteria but also against viruses, fungi and parasites. Nevertheless, we now realize as we developed antimicrobial agents, microbes developed the ability to elude our best weapons and to counter attack with new survival strategies.

2. CONCEPTS OF MICROBES, INFECTION AND INFESTATION IN AYURVEDA

2.1 Etymology

The history of infection and infectious diseases is as old as mankind. The reference of micro-organisms is available in the oldest manuscripts of the Ayurveda and the Vedas as well. In the Atharvaveda, references are available regarding microbes and infectious diseases in the name of *Krimi* and *Krimi roga.* According to Shabda kalpadruma, the term *krimi* is derived as ***'kraamtiti krimi'*** and ***'bhrameh samprasarnaanch'***. These two terms give the meaning of *krimi* as that which moves or roams about. Yakshacharya has described *krimi* as those micro-organisms, which grow on raw flesh (***kravya Madati***). Various terms such as *raksasa, pishacha, asura, vatudana* and *kimidi* are described as synonymous to *krimi.* It has also been stated that these *krimi* travel in night and kill the persons.

2.2 Concept of Microbiology/Pathology

In Charaka Samhita a detailed description of 20 types of *krimi* is given in seven sections which are known as *'Saptaka gana'* viz, *Nidana* (aetiology), *Sthana* (habitat) *Samsthana* (clinical features) *Varna* (colour/description), *Nama* (nomenclature) *Prabhava* (specific effects) and *Chikitsa* (treatment). In present times the medical microbiology is also described on the above-mentioned headings only.

In the description of *Vishama jwara,* Sushruta has accepted involvement of *Agantuka nidana* for its occurrence, which seems nothing but microbial in nature. Acharya Gananath Sen has given the term ***'bhutabhishanga'*** in reference to the *Vishama jwara,* accepting the role of micro-organisms in their occurrence.

भूताभिषडंग नाम भूतानां सूक्ष्मप्राणिनां जीवाणुनामभिषडंग

The term *bhuta* is taken from "भूताभिषडंग नाम भूतानां सूक्ष्मप्राणिनां जीवाणुनामभिषडंग" which collectively means those organisms which produce toxins. These toxins are supposed to manifest the disease in different ways. While describing *Vishama jwara,* Charaka seems to accept this theory as well.

The mode of spread of infectious diseases has been described clearly by Sushruta in reference to *Kustha* (skin diseases), *Jwara* (pyrexia), *Shotha* (tuberculosis), *Netrabhishyandan* (conjunctivitis) etc., spread from human beings to human beings due to sexual intercourse, touching of the body, due to breath, eating together and even sharing the same bed and sharing clothings, garlands, cosmetics etc.

प्रसंडगाद् गात्र संस्पर्शा न्निश्वासात्सह भोजनात्।
सहशय्याडडसनाश्चापि वस्त्रमाल्यानुलेचनात्॥
कुष्ठं ज्वरश्च शोषश्च नेत्राभिष्यन्द एव च।
औपसर्निक रोगाश्च सङ्क्रामन्ति नरान्नरम्॥

(सु नि 5)

Charaka has given a very good explanation of mode of spread in case of *Raja-yakshma* that seems to be similar to that we are observing today by means of droplet infection.

क्रोघोतिः श्वास रूपेण मूर्तिमान निःसृतो मुखात्।

(च चि ८/5)

Charaka has dedicated a chapter on epidemics named as *Janapadodhvamsa vimanam*. The four etiological factors responsible are *jala, vayu, desha*, and *kala.* When contamination and vitiation of these factors take place, epidemics follow. Today water borne diseases, environmental diseases, epidemiological disorders and the seasonal disorders are due to infections that can be correlated with *Janapado-dhwamsa vyadhies.*

Acharya Charaka has described three main objects of *bhuta-vesha* as *rati* (reproduction), *himsa* (production of disease), and *abhyarchanam* (worship by mankind). Sushruta has emphasized that in case of children *grahas* affect them if the mother or *dhatri* does not have adequate hygiene and also does not offer prayers. It is evident from the above description that the great Indian sages had the knowledge of mode of spread, fate of the micro-organism and how to combat the disease, long back. The *krimis, bhutas, grahas, raksasas* and other *Agantuka nidana* are all micro-organisms–may be virus, bacteria and fungal organisms.

Charaka has given three main processes for treating the *krimi rogas.* These are *Nidana parivarjanam* (to avoid the factors responsible for disease), *apakarshanam* (removal of krimis from the affected site) and *prakriti vighata* (to change the environment, favorable to growth of microbes). The concept seems to be very similar to the modern microbiology and practice of medicine and the microbial agents used are prescribed for one or all-purpose.

The overall literacy survey on *krimi* reveals that wherever the symptomatology consists of *jwara, atisara, puya, shotha, shula* etc, the presence of invasion by krimis (microbes) should be considered and the line of treatment should be planned accordingly. Various groups of drugs prescribed in the classics such as *krimighna, kusthaghna, vrana ropana, vrana shodhana, jwaraghna, atisaaraghna, kasaghna, bhutaghna, phiranga rogahara, upadamsahara* etc, must be having more or less antimicrobial activity. Therefore, the need of hour is to explore the existing field of all available Ayurvedic drugs, so that the antimicrobial activities of other drugs should also be re-evaluated.

2.3 Clinical Microbiology

Apart from the description of *Krimi Roga*, acharyas have considered *Krimis* as the etiological factors of several diseases. Some important references regarding the involvement of *krimis* in various diseases are drawn here, to reveal this fact:

(i) *Rakta krimi* is responsible for *Kustha* (M.N. 7/11).
(ii) *Krimi koshtha* is found in *Mridbhakshana janya pandu.*
(iii) *Agantuka chharadi* is because of *koshthagata krimi* (M.N. 15/13)
(iv) *Krimija hridroga* (M.N. 29/6)
(v) *Arumshika* is due to *krimiprakopa* (M.N. 55/31)
(vi) *Krimi danta* (M.N. 56/14)
(vii) *Krimi karna* (M.N. 57/8)
(viii) *Asadhya pratishyaya* is due to *krimi* (M.N. 58/27)
(ix) *Krimi granthi* (M.N. 59/76)
(x) *Krimija shiroroga* (M.N. 60/7)

(M.N. = Madhava nidanam. It is a Classical text of Ayurveda written in 12th century by Acharya Madhava.This book exclusively deals with diagnosis of diseases, and contains 1,522 verses in 69 chapters.)

3. NEED FOR PLANT BASED ANTI-MICROBIAL AGENTS

3.1 Development of Drug Resistance

In recent years, the mainstream medicine have become increasingly receptive to the use of anti - microbial and other drugs derived from plants as the traditional antibiotics derived from microbial sources have become ineffective to the existing antibiotic-resistant pathogens, and particularly viral diseases remain intractable to this type of drug. Furthermore, strains of pathogens resistant to antibiotics have begun to develop at an alarming rate. Such a situation has directed the attention of the natural product chemists and microbiologists, in general, to make a systematic study of the anti-microbial components of medicinal plants.

The technological advancements in the field of medicine and the invention of newer antibiotics, though useful in many cases, have created other problems like the following:

3.2 Toxicity

Practically all-synthetic anti-microbial agents are local irritants. Gastric irritation, pain and abscess formation at the site of IM injection, thrombophlebitis of the injected vein are the complications. Practically all AMAs produce dose-related and predictable organ toxicities.

3.3 Hyper Sensitivity Reactions

Almost all AMAs are capable of causing hypersensitivity reactions. These are unpredictable and unrelated to dose. The whole range of reactions from rashes to anaphylactic shock can be produced.

4. MEDICINAL PLANTS: A POTENTIAL SOURCE OF ANTIMICROBIAL AGENTS

The idea and the practice of using medicinal plants as remedies for human diseases are as old as the human civilizations. Medicinal plants have been recognized as a valuable source of therapeutic components for centuries, and about 60% of the world's population are known to use the traditional medicines derived from medicinal plants. Though the chemotherapy or antimicrobial agents came into existence in the 19th century, their seeds were laid quite earlier. If we have a look at the history of chemotherapy, it may be divided into three phases where one is the empirical use of 'mouldy curd' by Chinese on boils, '*Chaul moogra*' oil by Hindus in leprosy, '*Chenopodium*' for intestinal worms, 'Cinchona bark' (17th century) for fever. This, in true sense, can be said to have laid down the foundation of modern world AMAs. However, attempt to characterize these properties in the laboratories have only been initiated in the early 1900s.Over the years, only a small proportion of several hundred thousand plant species around the globe have been investigated, both, phyto-chemically and pharmacologically, while many more remain to be explored. In India alone, there are about fortyfive thousand plant species of which some three thousand species have been officially documented to have medicinal potential but the traditional practitioners are reported to use more than six thousand species.

In the last few years, plant extracts and phyto-chemicals with known anti-microbial properties have been investigated by a number of researchers in different countries to understand their properties, efficacy and safety. Important medicinal plants with antimicrobial activity are given in Table 1.

Table 1 Some Plants with Antimicrobial Activity

1.1 Antibacterial

Sl.No.	*Name of the Plant*	*Antimicrobial Activity*	*References*
1.	*Adansonia digitata* Linn. (Bombaceae)	*Staphylococcus aureus, Staphylococcus epidermidis, Sterptococcus mutans, Pseudomonas aeruginosa*	Shukla YN et al. (2003)
2.	*Alangium salvifolium* (L.f.) Wangerin (Alangiaceae)	Gram positive and Gram negative group	Mosaddik MA, Kabir KE and Hassan P (2000)
3.	*Allium cepa* Linn. *Allium sativum* Linn. (Liliaceae)	*E. coli, S. faecalis, L. casei, S. sonnei, S. aureus, M. tuberculosis*	Ahsan M and Islam SN (1996)
4.	*Andrographis paniculata* Nees. (Acanthaceae)	Gram positive and Gram negative	Pundarikakshudu K et al. (2003)
5.	*Areca catechu* Linn. (Palmae)	*S. aureus, Trichophyton rubrum, E. coli*	Lalitha Kumari H et al. (1965)
6.	*Azadirachta indica* (Meliaceae)	*S. aureus, B. subtilis, E. coli, Proteus* sp.	Shrivastava AK and Chouhan CS (1977) Ahmad I, Ahmad F and Hussain F (1995) Rao DPC and Satyanarayana T (1977)
7.	*Berberis aristata* (Berberidaceae)	*Vibrio cholerae, L. donovoni*	Bhide MB and Dutta NK (1968) Dutta NK and Pendse MV (1962) Godbole SH and Pendse GS (1960)
8.	*Carum carvi* Linn. (Apiaceae)	Antibacterial and antifungal	Syed M et al. (1987)
9.	*Curcuma longa* Linn. (Zingiberaceae)	*Staphylococci*	Bhavani Sankar et al. (1979)
10.	*Curcuma zeodaria* (Zingiberacae)	*B. subtilis, E. coli, Kl. aerogenes, S. paratyphi, S. aureus, Erwinia carofovora, P. solanacearum, Xantyomonas citri, X. malavacearum*	Banerjee A and Nigam SS (1977)

Contd.

Table 1

Sl.No.	Name of the Plant	Antimicrobial Activity	References
11.	*Datura alba* Nees. (Solanaceae)	*Staphylococcus, Klebsiella* sp., *E. coli, Streptococcus, Pseudomonas, Salmonella* and *Vibrio* sp.	Shanmuga Priya K et al. (2002)
12.	*Elettaria cardamomum* (Zingiberaceae)	Antibacterial	Kubo I et al. (1991) Jawad AM et al. (1988)
13.	*Evolvulus alsinoides* Linn. (Convoluaceae)	*E. coli, Pseudonomes aeruginosa, Staphylococcus aureus, Bacillus subtilis*	Tharan NT et al. (2003)
14.	*Hedychium spicatum* Ham. (Zingiberaceae)	Antibacterial	Sharma GP, Jain NK and Garg BD (1980)
15.	*Mentha arvensis* Linn. (Labiatae)	*Salmonella typhi*	Sampurna N and Nigum SS (1980)
16.	*Momordica charantia* Linn. (Cucurbitacae)	Gram +ve and Gram-ve group	Anwar Z et al. (2000)
17.	*Moringa oleifera* Lam. (Moringacae)	Bark Extract- *B. subtilis, St. pyogenes, E. coli, S. typhosa, Sh. dysenriae, Myc. pyogenes* Seeds-*B. subtilis Myco. phlei*	Bhatnagar SS (1961)
18.	*Morus alba* Linn. (Urticaceae)	*Streptococus aureus*	Yashak Hnoji (1991)
19.	*Myristica fragrans* Houtt. (Myrsitaceae)	Antibacterial	Baxer R and Holzapfel WH (1982) Bhat JV and Broker R (1953)
20.	*Nigella sativa* Linn. (Ranunculaceae)	*Vibrio cholerae, E. coli, Shigella* sp.	Hassan CM et al. Khan MTH and Jabbar S (1999)
21.	*Ocimum sanctum* Linn. (Labiatae)	*S. aureus, E. coli*	Bhat JV and Broker R (1953) Grover GS and Rao JT (1977) Joshi CG and Nagar NG (1952)
22.	*Picrorhiza kurroa* Royle ex Benth (Scrophulariaceae)	Antibacterial V. Cholera, *Staphylococus aurus, Salmonella typhi*	Vohora SB et al. (1972)
23.	*Plumbago zeylanica* Linn. (Plumbaginacae)	Antibacterial, antifungal	Krishnaswamy M and Purushothaman KK (1980) Van Der Vijver LM and Lotter AP (1971)

Contd.

Table 1

Sl.No.	Name of the Plant	Antimicrobial Activity	References
24.	*Pongamia glabra* Vent. (Papilionaceae)	*M. tuberculosis* and many Gram +ve and –ve Bacteria	Chaurasia SC and Jain PC et al. (1978) Ramaswamy AS and Sirsi M (1960)
25.	*Psoralea corylifolia* Linn. (Papilionaceae)	Antibacterial (*Staphylococci*)	Gaind KN, Chopra BM and Kaul RN (1965) Gaind KN et al. (1964) Gaind KN, Dar RN and Kaul RN (1964)
26.	*Rubia cordifolia* Linn. (Rubiaceae)	*Staph. aureus, E. coli*	Kurup PA et al. (1956)
27.	*Tinospora cordifolia* Miers. (Menispermaceae)	Antibacterial	Singh RH and Chaturvedi GN (1974) Dhar ML et al. (1968) Singh RH and Chaturvedi GN (1974)
28.	*Trachyspermum ammi, Trachyspermum roxburghianum* (DC.) Craib. (Umbelliferae)	*P. solanocearum, S. aureus, B. subtilis, P. multicida, S. typhi, E. coli, Shigella dysentery, V. choleriae*	Gautam MP and Purohit RM (1978) Meena MR et al. (1994)
29.	*Tribulus terrestris* Linn. (Zygophyllaceae)	*E. coli, S. aureus*	Joshi CG and Nagar NG (1952)
30.	*Withania somnifera* (Linn.) Dunal. (Solanaceae)	Gram +ve	Bhatnagar SS (1961)
31.	*Zanthoxylum armatum* Roxb.	Antibacterial	Mehta MB, Kharya MD, Srivastava R and Verma, KC (1981)
32.	*Zingiber officinale* Roscoe. (Zingiberaceae)	Antibacterial	Farooq S and Pathak GK (1998) Gugnani HC and Ezenwanze EC (1985)
1.2 Antifungal			
1.	*Amomum subulatum* Roxb. (Zingiberaceae)	*Aspergillus flavus*	Mishra AK and Dubey NK (1990)
2.	*Azadirachta indica* (Meliaceae)	Antifungal	Govindachari TR (1981) Jain JP and Pathak VN (1970)
3.	*Cassica tora* Linn. (Caesalpiniaceae)	Antifungal	Mukherjee PK et al. (1996)
4.	*Nigella sativa* Linn. (Ranunculaceae)	*Moniezia*	Akhtar MS and Javed I (1991)
5.	*Carum carvi* Linn. (Apiaceae)	Antifungal	Guerin JC and Reveillere HP (1985)

Contd.

Table 1

Sl.No.	Name of the Plant	Antimicrobial Activity	References
6.	*Pongamia pinnata Pierre.* (Papilionaceae)	*Aspergillus niger*	Jain PC and Agarwal SC (1978) Jambotkar DK et al. (1962)
7.	*Zingiber officinale* Roscoe (Zingiberaceae)	*Fusarium*	Guerin JC and Reveillers HP (1984) Haware MP and Joshi LK (1974)
8.	*Alstonia scholaris* (Apocynaceae)	*Aspergillus niger*	Versha P et al. (2003)
9.	*Mentha arvensis* Linn. (Labiatae)	*Phytophthora parasitica, Curvularia lunata*	Chaurasia SC et al. (1976) Chaurasia SC and Kher A (1978) Sanyal A and Varma KC (1969)
10.	*Curcuma longa* Linn. (Zingiberaceae)	*Aspergillus niger, A. flavus, P. javanicum, T. viride, C. oryzae, Helminthosporum, P. lapagaricola*	Banerjee A and Nigam SS (1978)
11	*Allium sativum* Linn. (Liliaceae)	*Alternaria tenuis, Helminthosporium gramineum, Curvalaria lunta, Fusarium nivale*	Misra SB and Dixit SN (1977)
12.	*Butea frondosa, B. monosperma*, Roxb. (Leguminosae)	*Helminthosporium sativum*	Masilamani G et al. (1981)
13.	*Mentha arvensis* Linn. (Labiatae)	*Phytophthora parasitica, Curvularia lunata*	Chaurasia SC and Kher A (1978) Sanyal A and Varma KC (1969)
14.	*Ocimum sanctum* Linn. (Labiatae)	Dermatophytes *Aspergillus niger, R. stolonifer, Pencillium digitatum*	Grover GS and Rao JT (1977) Singh L and Sharma M (1978)
15.	*Crotalaria pallida* (Papilionaceae)	*C. albicans*	Muthuswamy P, Chakraborthy GS and Sridhar SK (2003)
16.	*Achyranthes aspera* Linn. (Amaranthaeace)	Antifungal	Misra TN (1922)
17.	*Allium sativum* Linn. (Liliaceae)	*C. albicans,* Dermatophytes	Alkiewicz J and Lutomski J (1992) Amer M, Taha M and Tosson Z (1980) Fromtling RA and Bulmer GS (1978)

Contd.

Table 1

Sl.No.	Name of the Plant	Antimicrobial Activity	References
1.3 Anti-Virals			
1.	*Azadirachta indica, Melia azadirachta* Linn. (Meliaceae)	*Tacarite Virus*	Babbar OP et al. (1982) Singh R and Singh R (1972)
2.	*Argyreia speciosa* Sweet. (Convolvulaceae)	*Vaccinia virus*	Singh R and Singh R (1972)
3.	*Berberis aristata* DC. (Berberidaceae)	*Trachoma virus*	Verma RL (1933)
4.	*Zingiber officinale* Roscoe. (Zingiberaceae)	*Rhinovirus*	Denyer CV et al. (1994)
5.	*Glycyrrhiza glabra* Linn. (Papilionaceae)	*HIV-1 Herpes Simplex*	Badam L (1997)
6.	*Moringa oleifera* Lam. (Moringacae)	*Vacinia* and *Ranikhet disease virus*	Babbar OP (1970)
7.	*Phyllanthus niruri* Hook.f. (Euphorbiaceae)	*Semliki forest encephalitis virus*	Saigopal DVR et al. (1986)
1.4 Anti-Protozoals			
1.	*Azadirachta indica* (Meliaceae)	Antimalarials	Obaseki AO and Jegede-Fadunsin HA (1986)
2.	*Caesalpinia crista* Linn. (Caesalpiniaceae)	Antimalarials	Goyal H et al. (1981)
3.	*Berberis aristata* (Berberidaceae)	*Leishmania donovani*	Choudhary VP et al. (1972) Dutta NK and Iyer NS (1968)
4.	*Zingiber officinale* Rose. (Zingibereraceae)	*Dirorfilaria imminitis*	Datta A and Sukul NC (1987)
5.	*Swertia chirayita* (Gentianaceae)	Antimalarial *P. berghii*	Goyal H et al. (1981)
6.	*Allium sativum* Linn. (Liliaceae)	Antimalarial	Amminuddin et al. (1993)

5. CONCLUSION

In conclusion, it may be mentioned that there has been a marked expansion of our knowledge on anti-microbial agents from medicinal plants due to renewed interest of scientists from diverse fields. These anti-microbial substances, irrespective of their target organisms, have tremendous therapeutic and commercial potential. Although large number of new compounds have been isolated from medicinal plants only some have reached clinical trials, while others are still undergoing various phases of clinical trials. It is, therefore, essentially needed to explore these valuable natural resources for effective utilization in the chemotherapeutic treatment of infection and also for maintaining human health.

REFERENCES

Atrideva (1975), Kushtha Nidanam In: Sushruta Samhita, Motilal Banarsidass, Delhi Publication, Nidana sthana 5/33-34: 246

Amer M Taha M, Tosson Z (1980) The effect of aqueous garlic extract on the growth of dermatophytes. Int J Dermatol 19: 285-87

Akhtar MS, Javed I (1991) Efficacy of *Nigella sativa* Linn. Seeds against *Moniezia* infection in sheep. Indian Vet J 41: 185-87

Alkiewicz J, Lutomski J (1992) Study on the activity of the chloroform extract of garlic on *Candida albicans.* Herba polonica 38: 79-84

Aminuddin, Girach RD, Subhash Khan A (1993) Treatment of malaria through herbal drugs from Orissa. India Fitoterapia 64: 545-548

Ahmad I, Ahmad F, Hussain F (1995) *In vitro* antimicrobial activity of leaf and bark extracts of *Azadirachta indica* A. Juss. *Indian Veterinary Medical Journal* 19: 204-206

Ahsan M, Islam SN (1996) Garlic: A broad-spectrum antibacterial agent effective against common pathogenic bacteria. Fitoterapia 67: 374-76

Anwar Z, Ayub N, Khan AG (2000) Antibacterial ability of extracts from arbuscular mycorrhizal roots of *Allium sativum* L. and *Momordica charantia.* Hamdard Medicus 43: 29-33

Bhat J V, Broker R (1953) Action of some plant extracts on pathogenic staphylococci. *J Sci ind Res* 12: 540-542

Bhatnagar SS (1961) Biological activity of Indian Medicinal Plant Part-I, Antibacterial, antitubercular and anti-fungal action. Indian J Med Res 49: 799-813

Bhide MB, Dutta NK (1968) The antagonisitic action of berberine hydrochloride against certain biogenic substances. Indian J Physiol Pharmacol 12:19

Babbar OP (1970) Nature of antiviral activity detected in some plants extracts screen in cell cultures infected with vacinia and Ranikhet disease virus. Indian J Expt Biol 8: 304

Banerjee A, Nigam SS (1977) Anti bacterial efficacy of the essential oils derived from the various Sp. of *Curcuma* Linn. J Research Ind Med Yoga and Homoeo 12: 89-96

Banerjee A, Nigam SS (1978) Antifungal efficacy of the essential oils derived from various species of the genus - *Curcuma* Linn. J Res Indian Medicine Yoga and Homoeo 13: 63-70

Bhawani Shankar TN, Srinivasa Murthy V (1979) Effect of Turmeric (*Curcuma longa* Linn.) fractions on the growth of some essential and pathogenic bacteria *in vitro.* Indian Journal of Experimental Biology 17:1363-1366

Babbar OP, Joshi MM, Madan R (1982) Evaluation of plants for antiviral activity. Indian J Med Res 76: 54-65

Babbar OP (1982) Evaluation of plants for antiviral activity. Indian J Med Res 76: 54-55

Baxer R, Holzapfel WH (1982) A microbial investigation of selected spices, herbs and additives in South Africa. J Food Sci 47: 570-574

Badam L (1997) *In vitro* antiviral activity of indigenous *glycyrrhizin licorice and glycyrrhizic* acid (Sigma) on Japanese encephalitis virus. J Commun Dis 29: 91-99

Choudhary VP, Sabir M, Bhide VN (1972) Berberine in *giardiasis.* Indian Pediatrics 9: 143

Chaurasia SC, Kher A (1978) Activity of essential oil of three medicinal plants against various pathogenic and non-pathogenic fungi. Indian J Hosp Pharm 15:139

Chaurasia SC, Jain PC (1978) Antibacterial activity of essential oils of four medicinal plants. Indian J Hosp Pharm 15:166-168

Chaurasia SC, Kher A (1978) Activity of essential oil of three medicinal plants against various pathogenic and non-pathogenic fungi. Indian J Hosp Pharm 15:139

Charaka Samhita (1983) edited Charak Chandrika Hindi Commentary, Brahmananda Tripathi, Chaukhambha Surabharati Publication

Dutta NK, Pendse MV(1962) Usefulness of berberine (an alkaloid from *Berberis aristata*) in the treatment of cholera (experimental). Indian J Med Res 50: 1732-36

Dutta NK, Iyer NS (1968) Anti-amoebic value of *berberine* and *Kurchi* alkaloids. J Indian Med Asson 50: 349

Dutta A, Sukul NC (1987) Anti filarial effect of *Zingiber officinale* on Dirorfilaria imminitis. J Helminthol 61: 268-270

Denyer CV, Jackson P, Loakes DM, Ellis MR, Young DA (1994) Isolation of antirhinoviral sesquiterpenes from ginger (*Zingiber officinale*) J Nat Prod 57: 658-662

Fromtling RA, Bulmer GS (1978) In *vitro* effect of aqueous extract of garlic *Allium sativum* on the growth and viability of *Cryptococcus neoformans*. Mycologia 70: 397-405

Farooq S, Pathak GK (1998) A comparative study of *in vitro* antimicrobial activity of total solvent extracts of some medicinal plants with Asava and Aarishta preparation. J Non-*timber Forest Products* 5: 79-81

Godbole SH, Pendse GS (1960) Antibacterial property of some plants. India J Pharm 22: 39

Gaind KN, Dar RN, Kaul RN (1964) Anti-staphylococcal activity of seeds of *Psoralea corylifolia* Linn. J Pharm Sci 53:1428-1429

Gaind KN, Dar RN, Kaul RN (1964) Isolation of an anti-staphylococcal fraction from the seeds of *Psoralea corylifolia* Linn. Indian J Pharm 26:140-141

Gaind KN, Chopra BM, Kaul RN (1965) Antibacterial principle from *Psoralea corylifolia* Linn. Kinetics of *in vitro* antibacterial activity. Indian J Pharm 27: 262-263

Grover GS, Rao JT (1977) Investigations on the antimicrobial efficiency of essential oils from *Ocimum sanctum* and *Ocimum gratissimum*. Perfum Und Kosmef 58: 326-328

Gautam MP, Purohit RM (1978) *In vitro* antimicrobial activity of oils from Indian Medicinal Plants. J Res Indian Med Yoga and Homoeo13: 117-119

Govindachari TR (1981) Survey of contribution from Indian laboratories to plant chemistry. J Indian Chem Soc 58:105-114

Guerin JC, Reveillers HP (1984) Antifungal activity of plant extracts used in therapy. I: Study of 41 plant extracts against 9 fungi species. Ann Pharm *Rf* 42: 553-559

Guerin JC, Reveillere HP (1985) Antifungal activity of plant extracts used in therapy. II: Study of 40 plant extracts against 9 fungi species Ann Pharm 43: 77-81

Gugnani HC, Ezenwanze EC (1985) Antibacterial activity of extracts of ginger and African oil. J Commun Dis 17: 233-236

Hamsaveni Goyal, Saraswathi Sukumar, Purushothaman KK (1981) Antimalarials from Indian Medicinal Plants. J Res Ayursiddha 2: 286

Hassan C M, Ahsan M, Islam SN (1989) *In vitro* antibacterial screening of the oil of *Nigella sativa* seeds. Bangladesh J Bot 18:171-174

Haware MP, Joshi LK (1974) Efficacy of certain fungicides against seed-borne infection by *Fusarium oxysporum* in ginger. Indian Phytopathol 27: 236-237

Jain JP, Pathak VN (1970) Antifungal activity in leaf extracts of certain plants. Labdev J Sci Technol 8B: 58

Jain PC, Agarwal SC (1978) Notes on the activity of some odoriferous organic compounds against some Keratinophilic fungi. Trans Mycol Soc Japan 19: 197

Jambotkar DK, Kane JG, Khurana ML (1962) The *in vitro* and *in vivo* evaluation of soaps from some Indian edible oils. Indian J Pharm 24: 154

Joshi CG, Nagar NG (1952) Antibiotic activity of some Indian medicinal plants. J Sci Industr Res 11: 261

Jawad AM, Jaffer HJ, Al-Naib A, Saber AAW (1988) Anti-microbial activity of some Iraqi plants. Fitoterapia 59:130-133

Krishnaswamy M, Purushothaman KK (1980) Plumbagin- a study of its anticancer, antibacterial and antifungal properties. Indian J Expt Biol 18: 876-77

Kubo I, Himejima M, Muroi H (1991) Anti-microbial activity of flavor components of cardamom *Elettaria cardomomum* (Zingiberaceae) seed. J Agric Food Chem 39:1984-1986

Khan MTH, Jabbar S (1999) Anti-microbial activity of *Nigella sativa* Linn. and *Semecarpus anacardium* L. against *Escherichia coli in vitro.* Hamdard Medicus 42: 16-18

Lalitha Kumari H, Sirsi M, Govindrajan (1965) Antibacterial and antifungal activities of *Areca catechu* Linn. Indian J Expt Biol 3: 66

Misra TN (1922) Antifungal essential oil and long chain alcohol from *Achyranthes aspera.* Phytochemistry 31:1811-1812

Misra SB, Dixit SN (1977) Antifungal properties of *A. sativum* Linn. Sci and Cult 43: 47-48

Masilamani G, Showkath Ali, Subbulakshmi V (1981) Study on karappan (Eczema). J Res Ayursiddha 2:109-21

Mehta MB, Kharya MD, Srivastava R, Verma KC (1981) Anti-microbial and anti-helminthic activities of the essential oil of *Zanthoxylum armatum* Roxb. Indian perfumer 25:19-21

Mishra AK, Dubey NK (1990) Fungitoxicity of essential oil of *Amomum subulatum* against *Aspergillus* flavors. Economic Botany 44: 530-533

Meena MR, Sethi V (1994) Antimicrobial activity of essential oils from spices. J Food Sci Tech 31: 68-70

Mukherjee PK, Saha K, Saha BP, Pal M, Das J (1996) Antifungal activities of the leaf extract of *Cassia tora* Linn. Phytochemistry Res 10: 521-522

Mosaddik MA, Kabir KE, Hassan P (2000) Antibacterial activity of *Alangium salvifolium* flowers. Fitoterapia 4: 447-49

Muthuswamy P, Chakraborthy GS, Sridhar SK (2003) Antibacerial and antifungal activity of *Crotalaria pallida* dry and var extracts. Indian Drugs 40: 718-19

Obaseki AO, Jegede Fadunsin HA (1986) Antimalarial activity of *Azadirachta indica Fitoterapia* Vol 57: 247-251

Pundarikakshudu K, Patel VP, Raval AJ (2003) Antibacterial activity of various extracts of *Andrographis paniculata.* Indian Drugs 40: 539-541

Ramaswamy AS, Sirsi M (1960) Antitubercular activity of some chemical constituents from higher plants. Indian J Pharm 22: 34

Raja Radha Kanta Deva (1967) Shabada KalpaDruma, The Chowkhamba Sanskrit series work No. 93 Varanasi. Part two: 178

Rao DPC, Satyanarayana T (1977) Antibacterial activity of some medicinal plant extracts. Indian Drugs Pharm. Ind. 12: 21-22

Sanyal A, Varma KC (1969) *In vitro* antibacterial and antifungal activity of *Mentha arvensis Var. Piperascens* oil obtained from different sources (Letters to editor) Indian J Microbiol 9:23

Singh R, Singh R (1972) Screening of some plant extracts for antiviral properties. Technology Sindri 9: 415-16

Singh RH, Chaturvedi GN (1974) On the antibacterial activity of some Ayurvedic drugs. J Res Indian Med 9:65-66

Shrivastava AK, Chauhan CS (1977) Antibacerial activity of unsaponifiable matter obtained from fixed oil of seeds of *Melia azedarach* Linn. Indian Drugs Pharmaceut Ind 12:7

Singh L, Sharma M (1978) Antifungal properties of some plant extracts. Geobios 5: 49

Sampurna N, Nigum SS (1980) Efficacy of Indian Essential Oil in combination against *S.Typhi*. Indian drugs Pharmaceut Ind 15:7

Sharma GP, Jain NK, Garg BD (1980) Antimicrobial activity of the essential oil from *Hedychium spicatum* (Zingiberaceae). Indian J Microbiol 20:17

Singhal GD, Tripathi SN, Sharma KR (1985) Krimi Nidanam In: Ayurvedic Clinical Diagnosis based on Madhava Nidana,Chaukhambha Sanskrit Pratishthan, part I : 141-152

Saigopal DVR, Siva Prasad V, Sreenivasalu P (1986) Antiviral activity in extracts of *Phyllanthus fraternus* Webst. Curr Sci 53: 264-65

Syed M Khalid, M R Chaudhary FM, Bhatty MK (1987) Anti-microbial activity of essential oils of the Umbelliferae family Part V *Carum carvi, Petroselinum crispum* and *Dorema ammoniacdum* oils. Pak J Sci Ind Res 30:106-110

Shanmuga Priya K, Gnanamani A, Radhakrishnan N, Mary Babu (2002) Antibacterial activity of *Datura Alba*. Indian Drugs 39(2): 113-116

Shukla YN, Dubey S, Srivastava A, Jain SP, Kumar S (2003) Antibacterial activity and some chemical constituents of *Adansonia digitata* Linn. Indian Drugs 40:186-87

Tharan NT, Vadivu R, Palanisamy M, Justin V (2003) Antibacterial activity of *Evolulus alsinoides* Linn. Indian Drugs 40: 585-586

Verma RL (1933) *Berberine* sulphate in chronic trachoma. Indian Med Gaz 68: 122

Van Der Vijver LM, Lotter AP (1971) Constituents in the roots of *P. zeylanica* responsible for antibacterial activity. Planta Med 20 (1): 8-13

Vohora SB, Peshawar Kumar, Naqvi SAH, Afaq SH (1972) Pharmacological investigations of *P. Kurroa* (Kutki) roots with special reference to its choleretic and antimicrobial properties. Indian J Pharm 34:17

Yashak Hnoji (1991) Inhibitory Effect of Sanggenon-C from root bark of *Morus alba*. Medicinal and Aromatic Plant 34: 634-638

Versha P, Ghosh B, Anroop B, Ramanjit M (2003) Antimicrobial activity of *Alstonia scholaris* leaf extracts. Indian Drugs 40: 412-413

Cyanobacteria in Soil Health and Sustainable Agriculture

R PRASANNA and BD KAUSHIK[1*]

1. INTRODUCTION

Cyanobacteria represent one of the most successful and widespread groups among the prokaryotes, occupying a diverse range of terrestrial and aquatic environments. Besides free-living forms, cyanobacteria also form symbiotic associations with a variety of organisms including bryophytes, pteridophytes, gymnosperms and angiosperms (Rai and Bergman 2002). They play a significant role as primary producers in several ecosystems, besides being pioneers in several inhospitable habitats of the world. They are also capable of excessive proliferation, leading to bloom formation, which cause a significant threat to human and animal health, besides polluting the hydal environment, which are the essential networks for agriculture.

The major ill effects of intensive agriculture during last three decades are manifest in the erosion of soil fertility, in terms of depletion of soil nutrients and organic matter. Long-term fertility experiments have shown that for sustaining high yields under modern intensive farming requires a large turnover of nutrients which neither organic manures nor chemical fertilizers alone can achieve. Only the integrated use of organic manures, bio-fertilizers and chemical fertilizers has been found to be a promising

Centre for Conservation and Utilization of Blue Green Algae (CCUBGA),

1 Division of Microbiology, Indian Agricultural Research Institute (IARI), New Delhi 110 012, India. E-mail: bdkaushik@hotmail.com; radhapr@lycos.com
Tel: 91 (011)25847649; 25848431

* Corresponding author

option not only for maintaining high productivity but also providing sustained stability to crop productivity. In this context, cyanobacteria, like all living organisms, act as sources and sinks of various compounds by *'bio-geochemical cycling'* and being ubiquitous, can play a significant role in integrated nutrient management and sustenance of soil fertility in agriculture (Roger 1996; Kaushik 2003). *Azolla* is an aquatic fern which is symbiotically associated with a prokaryotic, heterocystous, nitrogen-fixing cyanobiont and other eubionts of unknown function. It has been utilized through several countries in south-east Asia in conjunction with rice, and a single crop of *Azolla* is known to provide 20-30 Kg N ha^{-1}, fulfilling 1/3 of the nitrogen requirements of the rice crop (Wagner 1997).

The significance of these phototrophic prokaryotes in agriculture was first recognized by De (1939), who attributed the self maintenance of the N-structure of tropical rice-field soils to the growth of N_2-fixing BGA. The term *'algalization'* was initially applied to the use of defined mixtures of strains (Venkataraman 1972, 1979, 1981) and a methodology was described for its production which was farmer (rural) oriented. Subsequently, efforts were directed towards its improvement at the Centre for Conservation and Utilization of Blue Green Algae (CCUBGA) in terms of selection of better strains and carriers having greater carrying capacity, besides being light-weight and enhancing shelf life (Kaushik 1998; Prasanna et al. 1998). An alternative production technology has been developed in which soil has been replaced by a cheaper (US $ 0.28 per 1000 litre) formulated medium and the production is done under controlled conditions constructing multiplication units in glass or poly-houses to ensure continuous production of quality inoculum throughout the year. The smallest recommended size for these poly or glass-houses are $12 \times 5 \times 3.5$ m.

Also, increasing production levels by adopting polyhouse technology and growing each of the strains separately (to provide equal opportunity for multiplication and greater inoculum load) and then mixing with carrier has been optimized for year round production (Kaushik and Prasanna 1995). Several researchers have also shown the potential of cyanobacteria to ameliorate the saline, saline-sodic and sodic soil of our country, besides their utilization as a source of fine chemicals, bio-polymers and nutraceuticals. In recent years, attempts have been made to create new nitrogen-fixing symbioses of cyanobacteria with plants, and preliminary results indicate feasibility of artificial colonization of roots, which needs to be extended to field level (Rai and Bergman 2002).

2. ECO-PHYSIOLOGY OF CYANOBACTERIA

Cyanobacteria are known to be the primary colonizers in a wide range of habitats, including bare rocks, ice, snow, deserts, saline marshes/

mangroves and deep sea-vents, thereby growing at extremes of temperature and water potential. Most soil and air-dried terrestrial cyanobacteria can survive prolonged dry periods and the desiccation tolerance of certain *Nostoc* strains is indeed remarkable (Potts 2000). The eco-physiology of cyanobacteria has been studied in a wide diversity of deserts. They are typically able to withstand mean summer ground temperatures of 57°C with peaks in excess of 60°C in hot deserts and tolerant low temperature of -15°C in the cold Antarctic. The elaboration of an abundant polymerized extacellular glycans, secretion of UV-absorbing pigments, synthesis of cytoplasmic membrane rich in unsaturated fatty acids and expression of gene involved in water-stress are known to contribute to the desiccation tolerance of *Nostoc commune* (Potts 1994).

Although infrequent at pH below 6.0, their ability to grow in diverse pH ranges and modify their environment makes them successful in any niche. The biodiversity and exploitation of polar cyanobacteria, has created a lot of interest among researchers in relation to the identification of temperature tolerance genes, proteins and the pigments produced. Also, their genetic affinities with their counterparts, growing in hot climates and PCR based sequencing of genes, can go a long way in understanding the mechanism of adaptation to stress.

In India, on an average, BGA accounts to about 33% (Venkataraman 1975) whereas reports show that up to 50% of the total algae was BGA in some of the southern and eastern states. Thirty-eight soil samples from eleven districts of Dhaka division (Bangladesh) were analyzed for cyanobacterial flora (Khan et al. 1994). Of the 84 species recorded, 50% were heterocystous diazotrophic cyanobacteria, predominantly *Fischerella, Nostoc* and *Calothrix*, occurring in about 53%, 47% and 26% of the soil samples respectively. A number of floristic studies have shown the dominance of heterocystous species (*Anabaena, Nostoc, Calothrix, Cylindrospermum, Gloeotrichia, Scytonema*) especially akinetes formers in many rice-fields. These species positively correlated with pH and available P content of the soils (Roger et al. 1983). Among the physical and chemical factors influencing the growth and establishment of these organisms, light exerts the most significant effects. This is manifested in terms of periodicity with respect to season and the cultivation cycle of the crop. Algal succession in rice-fields is manifested in terms of differing populations of unicellular/colonial, non-heterocystous, followed by heterocystous - initially unbranched and by late harvest stage, branched heterocystous forms (Singh and Bisoyi 1989). Nitrogen-fixers do not dominate either in the beginning or late stages of crop growth and the phase between tillering and panicle development leads to production of maximum biomass (Roger and Kulasooriya 1980). Various micro-organisms such as protozoas, fungi and grazers such as copepods, ostracods, snails and larvae significantly diminish cyanobacterial populations (Venkataraman 1972). Management practices such as tillage, transplantation, weeding or water management also influence the proliferation of these organisms in the field. Application of insecticides or fungicides at recommended doses also do not significantly affect the growth of BGA (Venkataraman 1972), as a wide range of tolerance is exhibited by these organisms.

2.1 Agronomic Benefits

Cyanobacteria are most relevant in wetland rice-fields, which supply 86% of the world's requirement for rice, wherein their importance as nitrogen-fixers is well documented (Kulasooriya 1998). It is well known that besides bringing about an improvement in yield of rice (ranging from 5 to 25%), they also, produce indirect or direct beneficial changes in the physical, chemical and biological properties of soil and soil-water interface in rice-fields (Figure 1), which are of agronomic importance (Mandal et al. 1998; Kaushik 2004). Cyanobacterial growth in flooded rice-soils have also been reported to influence the availability of P, Zn, Mn, Fe and this has been indirectly related to the presence of gelatinous sheath in the inoculated species (Das et al. 1991,1995). Cyanobacteria, among other groups of algae, are known to take up P in excess of their immediate needs which may subsequently be released in the form of available P. Cyanobacteria are also known to mobilize insoluble rock phosphate fertilizers and aid in efficient utilization of low cost supplements (Roychoudhury and Kaushik 1989). Algal inoculation is known to result in a build-up of organic matter, however, this has been a controversial area as there are few researchers who strongly claim that organic C is enhanced, ranging from 0.5 – 41.6 $t ha^{-1}$, while others claim that the easy decomposability of algal biomass leads to losses in the fixed carbon (Mandal et al. 1998). The differing susceptibilities of algae to decomposition, which, in turn, is dependent on the algal cell-wall compounds, is another debatable issue. However, *Azolla* biomass is known to be decomposed (thus enhancing organic carbon) completely within 30 days and its incorporation into soil is commonly practiced as a green manuring practice (Singh and Singh 1987).

The photosynthetic liberation of O_2 by cyanobacteria creates an oxygenic environment in the rice-fields, especially in standstill water which is highly beneficial to the paddy ecosystem, because it prevents the accumulation of high amounts of harmful oxidisable organic matter and toxic iron and sulphide compounds. Aiyer et al. (1972) reported a considerable reduction in the oxidisable organic matter, total S^{2-} and Fe^{2+}

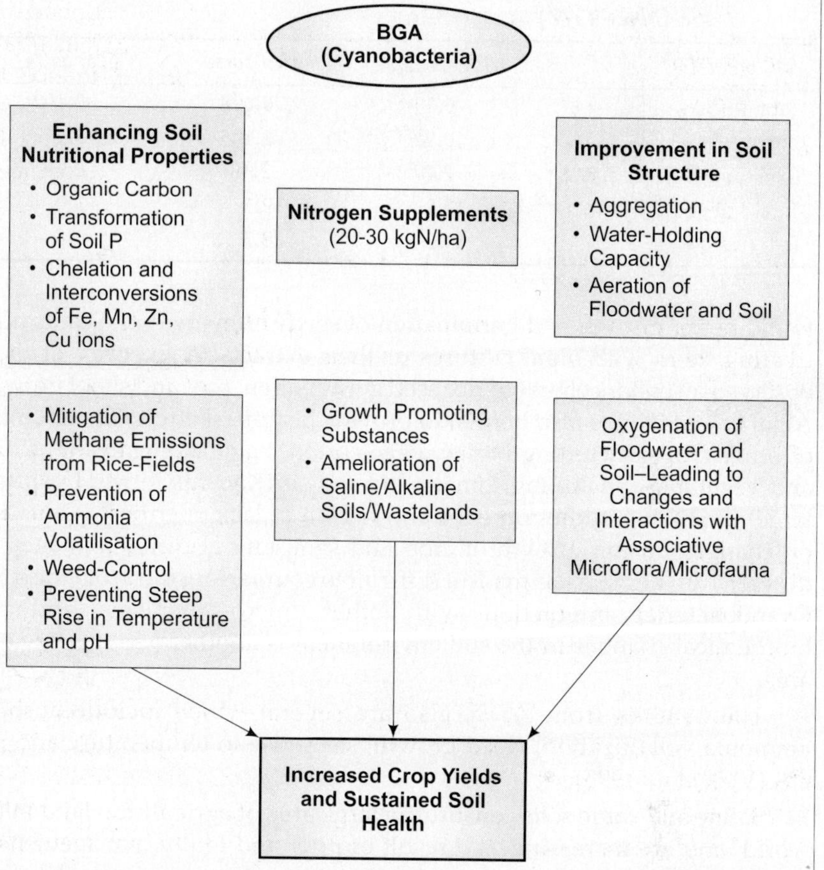

Fig. 1 BGA and its role in agriculture

content of soil after successive rice cropping along with BGA inoculation (Table 1). Similar reports on significant reduction in the water-soluble and exchangeable Fe and Mn content have also been reported (Das et al. 1991). The mitigation of methane emission from rice-fields by the growth of BGA and *Azolla* is also documented (Prasanna et al. 2002).

The stimulatory role of BGA in improving crop-growth and vigour has also been ascribed to the presence of growth regulating substances such as hormones and vitamins excreted by these organisms (Mishra and Kaushik 1989 a,b; Metting and Pyne 1986). A large number of researchers have

Table 1 Effect of algal inoculation on soil properties related to redox system in soil (Aiyer 1972)

Soil properties	*Without algae*	*With algae*	*Change (±)*
Total N (%)	0.1	0.098	−0.002
Organic C (%)	0.98	1.125	+0.145
Oxidisable organic matter	2.97	2.48	−0.49
Total supine (μg/g)	12.2	9.2	−3.0
Fe^{2+} (μg/g)	34.3	28.7	−5.6

found better growth and germination of seeds of many crop-plants after treating them with algal cultures or their extracts. A majority of them observed an enhancement of rice seed germination, root and shoot growth. Algal inoculation is also known to provide beneficial effects on a number of other crops, including barley, oats, cotton, banana, sugarcane, maize and vegetables, including tomato and radish (Kaushik 1998). Despite a large number of studies on BGA and rice-crop, lack of critical evaluation on changes during growth of crop and sampling at different stages by different researchers has made it difficult to compare results from the sites. Cyanobacterial interaction with other micro-organisms and the biochemical changes in the soil environment is another less investigated area.

The benefits from *Azolla* also are several which include curbing ammonia volatilization, weed growth, steep rise in temperature and pH etc. (Vlek et al. 1995).

Saline and sodic soils constitute a large area of agricultural land in the world, and are increasing as a result of poor and faulty management of irrigation practices. Primarily, the reclamation of sodic soils requires the replacement of exchangeable Na with Ca, which is normally done by the application of suitable soil amendments, like gypsum, followed by leaching (Kaushik 1991, 1994). The improvement of saline soils, on the other hand, requires leaching of excess soluble salts from the Rhizosphere by good quality water. Reports of biological reclamation of these soils through the use of BGA are available (Singh 1950; Kaushik 1989). These methods of reclamation were possibly based on the observations of extensive growth of BGA on alkali or '*usar*' soils of India (Singh 1950) and on the salted '*takyr*' soils of the USSR (Gollerbach et al. 1956). Singh (1961) reported that the first alga to appear in the loose of salt-affected soils of Uttar Pradesh was *Microcoleus* followed with *Scytonema*. On the other hand, on compact surface *Porphrosiphon* appeared first followed by several others. The distribution pattern of cyanobacteria in soils of Andhra Pradesh, Haryana, Delhi, Rajasthan, Uttar Pradesh and Punjab revealed that although recurrent combination of forms were discernable, there appeared to be a localized distribution of cyanobacteria depending upon the soil pH, electrical conductivity and exchangeable sodium. The predominant forms recorded were species of *Nostoc, Calothrix, Scytonema, Hapalosiphon,* and *Wetiellopsis* was the only form observed in soils off all the locations and was found to be tolerant to salt fluctuations (Subhashini and Kaushik 1981; Kaushik 1989). In salt-affected soils of Maharashtra the species of *Nostoc* and *Calothrix* were predominant, although the pH of the soil varied from 6.0 to 7.2. Mucilage producing cyanobacterial species of *Scytonema, Lyngbya* and *Tolypothrix* were also common. On analyzing the total cyanobacterial flora, it was observed that out of the total 37 species, 50% were nitrogen-fixing strains, including the non-heterocystous nitrogen-fixers. Unicellular and colonial forms like *Aphanocapsa, Aphanothece, Chroococcus, Gloeocapsa* and *Gloeothece,* rich in mucilage, were also very common in Maharashtara soils. The influence of cyanobacteria on aggregation of rice and semi-arid soils resulting from natural blooms or algalization has been reported (Kaushik and Krishna Murti 1981; Subhashini and Kaushik 1981; Kaushik 1985). The extent of aggregation varies from as low as 51.78% to as high as 292.3%. Such improvements in soil aggregation status results in better hydraulic conductivity. This also reflects in increased air and water movement in the soil and, thus, better root penetration and increased uptake of desired nutrients from soil by plants which are otherwise limiting in sodic and saline-sodic soils. This biological system is capable to remove the sodium from soil complex and binds to its own polysaccharides which are secreted in bulk. The net result of this is a temporary removal of sodium from soil and rendering in reduction in soil pH, electrical conductivity and exchangeable sodium. The physical properties of soils improve like soil aggregation and hydraulic conductivity. Qualitatively the polysaccharide is composed of glucose, galactose, arabinose, xylose, rhamnose, raffinose and two unidentified sugars with Rf values of 0.04 and 0.08 and is identical with the polysaccharides produced without Na^+ stress (Roychoudhury et al. 1983). Additionally, the soils are enriched with carbon and available phosphorus, and suitable crops like paddy and sorghum can be grown.

Increase in the percentage of soil carbon through the cultivation with cyanobacteria varies from one soil type to the other soil type. For example, the increase varied from 22.1 to 28.5% in Andhra Pradesh saline soils (Subhashini and Kaushik 1984), 18.75% due to native flora in pots (Kaushik 1983), 32.15% in saline soil of Delhi (Kaushik and Subhashini 1985). Application of cyanobacteria to the salt affected soils has led to the enrichment of soils with nitrogen content (Subhashini and Kaushik 1981; 1984; Kaushik 1983; Kaushik and Subhashini 1985). The increase in soil nitrogen varied from 17.9 to 28.5% over the initial soil nitrogen (Kaushik

1983, 1985).The availability of the phosphorus is from 68-100% in soils of Andhra Pradesh (Subhashini and Kaushik 1984), and about 11% increase in available phosphorus in saline-sodic soils of Delhi (Kaushik and Subhashini 1985).

A significant reduction in soil salinity (12-35%) due to repeated cultivation of *Anabaena torulosa* in soils rendered saline owing to bad farm management has also been reported (Thomas 1997). The rice yield in saline soils is also affected when N is given in the form of algal inocula vis-à-vis urea (Antarikanonda and Amarit 1991). Successive cultivation of BGA makes the environment more favourable and after a few years it may help to produce a reasonably good yield of crops, as observed by Singh (1961) for sugarcane after 3 years of reclamation with BGA. Although such biological soil amelioration is a time consuming process, it is considered to be a sustainable approach as compared to reclamation by chemical amendments (Oikarinen 1996).

According to Jha et al. (1987) most of the sodium ions removed from the growth medium remains adsorbed externally to the polysaccharides produced by the cyanobacteria. Cyanobacteria also reduce sodium ion content of the soil by making calcium ions available through solubilisation of calcium carbonate nodules, possibly by releasing various organic acids like oxalic, oxaloacetic, lactic and succinic acids (Bhatnagar and Roychoudhury 1992). The protection against alkaline environment is also provided by the synthesis of certain fatty acids (Senthil 1990) and sucrose (Venkataraman and Venkataraman 1991) and osmotic stress induced proteins (Goel et al. 1997)

2.2 Crop Response to Algalization

A large number of field trials have been conducted in diverse agro climatic regions in India and elsewhere. The salient results include:

- Algal inoculation enhances crop yields (ranging from 4 – 32.8%), in the absence of application of chemical fertilizers.
- Increased yields of 8.85 – 12.28% are obtained in the presence of chemical fertilizers, depending on the dose/level and agro climatic region.
- Comparison of yield of rice with the fully recommended dose of chemical fertilizers *vis-a-vis* reduced levels + BGA, leads to a net saving of 20 to 30 kg N/ha/season.
- Residual effect of superimposed inoculum over a period of 3 to 5 years has also been observed.

A comparison of different times of fertilizer N application (basal or 10 days after transplanting, at tillering and panicle initiation) showed that grain yield was better with algalization, irrespective of the method of fertilizer application. As BGA inoculation was generally done one week after fertilizer N application in clay or clay-loam soils, a decrease in mineral nitrogen concentration in floodwater can be expected. It was reported that nitrogenase activity was not depressed in soil-rice-algae system in the presence of less than 40 ppm ammonium-N (Venkataraman 1979). He pointed out the importance of critical evaluation of the relative contribution by algae of N or other substances, or both at high levels of N. Based on 118 field applications of cyanobacteria in Tamil Nadu, Venkataraman (1992) reported an average increase in rice yield by 7.29% when 100 kg N ha^{-1} was applied along with the algae as compared to yields obtained with 100 kg N ha^{-1} fertilizer alone. In our recent report, algal nitrogen fixation was not inhibited at 30 ppm of urea nitrogen (Mekonnen et al. 2002). Algal biofertilizer is recommended only as a supplement to nitrogenous fertilizers and the supplementation effects remain perceptible even in the presence of high levels of fertilizer nitrogen (Venkataraman 1979). A significantly higher increase in grain yield due to algalization under pot culture was reported, both in Boro and Aman crops of rice, with 45 kg N ha^{-1} or without nitrogen in Bangladesh. Kaushik (1998) reported about 10-15% increase in rice yield in the presence of fertilizer nitrogen up to 150kg ha^{-1} is obtained in Haryana. Thus, the response to algalization was generally positive at any level of nitrogen applied in the field, though the response being lower at higher levels (Table 2). Inoculation of rice-fields with cyanobacteria reduces the nitrogen losses through metabolization of the applied combined nitrogen forms. The metabolized combined nitrogen as well as the biologically fixed nitrogen becomes available gradually through exudation and decomposition of these algae.

This clearly illustrates the importance of these organisms as useful supplements, which can lead to net savings of N. Cyanobacteria release the fixed nitrogen mainly in the form of polypeptides, besides free amino acids, vitamins, and auxin-like substances (Venkataraman 1992), either by exudation or by microbial degradation after cell death (Singh et al. 1981).

The transfer of fixed nitrogen from cyanobacteria to the plant has been investigated using the ^{15}N tracer technique. Approximately 40% of the algal nitrogen is known to be recovered by the rice crop (Ladha et al. 2000). The relative availability of cyanobacterial nitrogen to rice depends to a great extent on the susceptibility to decomposition of the biomass, which varies with strain as well as the physiological state. Quantitative estimates of nitrogen from different countries are Philippines 18-33 kg ha^{-1}, Senegal 0-30 kg ha^{-1}, Mali 50-80 kg ha^{-1}, and Japan-11-23 kg ha^{-1}. Algalization seems to be most effective, where native strains are few and allow the establishment of inoculated strains. Therefore, there is a definite need to

Table 2 Effect of algal inoculation at reduced levels of nitrogen fertilizer on the grain yield of rice (figures in parentheses indicate number of field trails).

Treatment[$]	*Grain yield (tonnes ha^{-1})*							
	Orissa (1)	*Bihar* (1)	*MP* (56)	*Maharastra* (1)	*Tamilnadu* (111)	*Kerala* (4)	*UP* (2)	*AP* (5)
0 N	2.98	2.30	2.42	2.07			3.52	3.64
0 N+BGA	3.71	3.06	2.82	2.55			4.36	4.43
60 N+BGA			3.50					
40 N+BGA			3.63					
75 N				3.44	5.24			
50 N+BGA				3.44	5.11			
90 N						3.56		
60 N+BGA						3.84		
100 N					4.70			
75 N+BGA				3.73	5.21			
100 N+BGA				3.66	5.48			
120 N							5.83	
60 N+BGA							5.76	
150 N								5.84
100 N+BGA								6.04

evaluate the competitiveness of the inoculants strains (present in the composite biofertilizer) in soil microcosm studies, before allowing for their mass scale utilization in fields.

Genetic improvement of cyanobacterial strains has mainly focused towards developing ammonia-derepressible, pesticide resistant cyanobacterial mutants, as a viable alternative to the routinely used strains (Venkataraman 1992). However, such strains need to be tested in pot culture, followed by field level experiments before advocating them for bioinoculant production (Vaishampayan et al. 2001). Construction of artificial plant-*cyanobacterial symbioses* is a new area of research which is promising as cyanobacteria known to form associations with a wide range of organisms, including fungi, gymnosperms, pteridophytes, bryophytes and a few angiosperms; however, to date none have been successful. Co-cultivation of cyanobacteria with seedlings of plant species, including rice, wheat, tobacco have shown potential in terms of growth and nitrogen fixation (Rai et al. 2000). *Nostoc* sp. having the widest range of habitats, hosts and locations in host tissues has been the favourite workhorse. Experiments on cyanobacterial-rice associations have shown interesting results and need to be further strengthened with in-depth analyses (Rai and Bergman 2002).

3. CONCLUSION

Cyanobacteria are known for their remarkable ability to flourish in environments exhibiting widely fluctuating chemical and physical parameters, and contribute significantly to the nutrient budget of several ecosystems. Free-living cyanobacteria and *Azolla* (a pteridophyte harboring cyanobacteria as symbionts) represent two important components of integrated nutrient management practices for rice crop. Besides their well documented use as biofertilizer in conjunction with rice crop, they have also been exploited for the production of valuable compounds such as pigments, pharmaceuticals and as biological agents in bioremediation and reclamation of saline-alkali soils. Their independence for C and N makes them ideal inoculants, which not only augment the organic carbon of soils but also improve its physical, chemical and biological structure and functioning. As non-polluting, eco-friendly inputs, they have tremendous biological significance in agriculture and environment.

BGA and *Azolla* are natural components of rice-fields, contributing significantly towards maintaining and improving the productivity of the rice crop. The benefits accrued from organic carbon addition, improvement in soil physical properties, retardation of ammonia volatilization, mobilization of fixed phosphates, regulation of micronutrients far outweigh the benefits of N-increment. There is a definite need to extend the utilization of cyanobacteria, beyond just nitrogen fixation, into the areas where their biomass contributes to the maintenance of long term fertility and sustenance of this unique soil-water ecology; not found elsewhere in agriculture. Basic studies need to be initiated to study the effect of gradual changes in the chemical and electrochemical properties of soil and soil-water interfaces of rice-fields in the presence of BGA and *Azolla*, in order to evaluate the viability and effectiveness of their interactions in long term sustenance and nutrient budgeting of the rice ecosystem.

REFERENCES

Aiyer RS, Salahuddin S, Venkataraman GS (1972) Long-term algalization field trial with high yielding varieties of rice (*Oryza sativa* L.). Indian J Agric Sci 42:380-383

Antarikanonda P, Amarit P (1991) Influence of blue-green algae and nitrogen fertilizer on rice yield in saline soils. Kasctsart J Nat Sci 25:18-25

Bhatnagar A, Roychoudhury P (1992) Dissolution of limestone by cyanobacteria. In: Proc. Natl. Symp. Cyanobacterial Nitrogen fixation Pub. National Facility for Blue-Green Algal Collections, IARI, New Delhi, p 331

Das DK, Santra GH, Mandal LN (1995) Influence of blue-green algae in the availability of micronutrients in soils growing rice. J Indian Soc Soil Sci 43:145-146

Das SC, Mandal B, Mandal LN (1991) Effect of growth and subsequent decomposition of blue-green algae on the transformation of iron and manganese in submerged soils. Plant Soil 138:75-84

De PK (1939) The role of blue-green algae in nitrogen fixation in rice fields. Proc. R. Soc. London, Ser B 127:121-139

Goel S, Gautam M, Kaushik BD (1997) Nitrogen fixation and protein profiles of halotolerant *Nostoc muscorum*-R strain isolated from rice fields and ARM-221 strain. Indian J Expt Biol 35:746-750

Gollerbach MM, Novichkova LA, Sdubrikova NV (1956) The algae of takyrs In: Takyrs of western Turkmenia and routes of their agricultural conquest. Nauk, Moscow, pp 22-29

Gupta AB, Agarwal V, Kushwaha AS (1967) Effect of *Phormidium* extract on growth and yield of *Vigna catjang* (cowpea) T 5269. Proc Natl Acad Sci India 37:349-355

Jha MN, Venkataraman GS, Kaushik BD (1987) Response of *Westiellopsis prolofica* and *Anabaena* sp. to salt stress. J Appl Microbiol Biotechnol 3:307-317

Kaushik BD (1983) Amelioration of salt affected soils with blue-green algae. Spl Lecture. Proc all India applied Phycol Congr. Kanpur pp 60-66

Kaushik BD (1985) Effect of native algal flora on nutritional and physico-chemical properties of sodic soils. Acta Bot Indica 13: 143-147

Kaushik BD (1989) Reclamative potential of cyanobacteria in salt-affected soils. Phykos 28:101-109

Kaushik BD (1991) Cyanobacterial response of crops in saline irrigated with saline ground water In: Shastree NK (ed) Current Trends in Limnology. Vol. 1. Narendra Pub. House, p 201

Kaushik BD (1994) Algalization of rice in salt-affected soils. Ann Agril Res 14: 105-106

Kaushik BD (1998) Use of cyanobacterial biofertilizer in rice cultivation: A Technology Improvement In: Subramanian G, Kaushik BD, Venkataraman GS (eds) Cyanobacterial Biotechnology. Science Publishers. Inc. USA, pp 211-222

Kaushik BD (2004) In Biotechnology in Sustainable and Organic Farming Yadav AK, Chaudhary SR, Talukdar NC (eds) Shree Publishers and Distributors, New Delhi, India, pp 152-168

Kaushik BD, Krishna Murti GSR (1981) Effect of blue-green algae and gypsum application on physico-chemical properties of alkali soils. Phykos 20: 91-94

Kaushik BD, Prasanna R (1995) Improved cyanobacterial biofertilizer production and N-saving in rice cultivation In: Sahoo DB, Qasim SZ (eds) Sustainable Aquaculture. APH Publishing Corporation, New Delhi, India. pp 145-155

Kaushik BD, Subhashini D (1985) Amelioration of salt affected soils with blue-green algae. II. Improvement in soil properties. Proc. Indian Natl. Sci. Acad. Part B 51:386-389

Kaushik BD, Venkataraman GS (1979) Effect of algal inoculation on the yield of vitamin C content of two varieties of tomato. Plant Soil 52: 135-137

Kaushik BD (2003) In Biotechnology in sustainable biodiversity and food security Prasad BN (ed) Science Publishers, Inc Enfield, USA, pp 79-99

Khan ZUM, Tahmida Begum ZN, Mandal R, Hossain MZ (1994) Cyanobacteria in rice soils. World J Microbiol Biotechnol 10: 296-298

Kulasooriya SA (1998) Cyanobacteria and *Azolla* as biofertilizer for rice In: Subramanian GS, Kaushik BD, Venkataraman GS (eds) Cyanobacterial Biotechnology. Oxford & IBH Publishing Co. Pvt. Ltd. New Delhi, pp 201-209

Ladha JK, Dawe D, Ventura T S, Singh U, Ventura W and Watanabe I (2000) Long-term effect of urea and green manure on rice yield and nitrogen balance under long-term green manure and mineral N application. Soil Sci. Soc America J 64: 1993-2001

Mandal B, Vlek PLG, Mandal LN (1998) Beneficial effect of blue green algae and *Azolla* excluding supplying nitrogen, on wetland rice fields: a review. Biol Fertil Soils 27: 329-342

Mekonnen AE, Prasanna R, Kaushik BD (2002) Response of *Anabaena* to different nitrogen sources. Acta Biol Hungarica 53: 367-380

Metting B, Pyne JW (1986) Biologically-active compounds from micro algae. Enzyme Microbial Technol 8: 386-394

Misra S, Kaushik BD (1989a) Growth promoting substances of cyanobacteria. I. Vitamins and their influence on rice plant. Proc. Indian Natn Sci Acad, B55: 295-300

Misra S, Kaushik BD (1989b) Growth promoting substances of cyanobacteria. II. Detection of amino acids, sugars and auxins. Proc. Indian Nat Sci Acad, B55: 499-504

Olkarinen M (1996) Growth promoting substances of cyanobacteria. II. Detection of amino acids, sugars and auxins. Biol Fertil Soils 22: 342-344

Potts M (1994) Desiccation tolerance of prokaryotes. Microbial Rev 58: 755-805

Potts M (2000) *Nostoc* In: The Ecology of Cyanobacteria Whitton BA, Potts M (eds) Kluwer Academic Publishers, Dordrecht. pp 465-504

Prasanna R, Kumar V, Kumar S, Yadav AK, Tripathi U, Singh AK, Jain MC, Gupta P, Singh PK, Sethunathan N (2002) Methane production in rice soils is inhibited by cyanobacteria. Microbial Res 157: 1-6

Prasanna R, Mohammadi SA, Prasanna BM, Singh PK (2002) Inter- and intra-specific variation for nitrogen-fixing potential in *Tolypothrix* germplasm. Acta Bot Hungarica 44: 383-392

Prasanna R, Sharma BK, Sharma RK, Kaushik BD (1998) Standardization of growth parameters and formulation of medium for cyanobacterial biofertilizer strains. Indian J Microbiol 38: 211-215

Rai AN, Bergman B (2002) Creation of new nitrogen fixing cyanobacteria associations. Biol. Environ.: Proc. Royal Irish Acad. 102B 65-68

Rai AN, Söderbäck E, Bergman B (2000) Cyanobacterium-Plant symbioses. New Phytol 147: 449-481

Roger PA (1996) Biology and management of the floodwater ecosystem in rice-fields. IRRI, Manila

Roger PA, Kulasooriya SA (1980) Blue-green algae and rice. IRRI, Manila, pp 112

Roger PA, Zimmerman WJ, Lumpkin TA (1983) Microbiological management of wetland rice-fields. In Soil microbial ecology: application in agricultural and environmental management Meeting B (ed), Dekker, New York pp 417-455

Roychoudhury P, Kaushik BD (1989) Solubilization of Mussorie rock phosphates by cyanobacteria. Curr Sci 58: 569-570

Roychoudhury P, Pillai GR, Pandey SL, Krishna Murti GSR, Saha KC, Mandal LN (1979) Effect of algal growth on the availability of P, Fe and Mn in rice soils. Plant Soil 52: 139-149

Senthil C (1990) Cyanobacterial (*Calothrix* sp.) response to salt stress. M. Sc. Thesis, Indian Agricultural Research Institute, New Delhi

Singh AL, Singh PK (1987) Influence of *Azolla* management on the growth, yield of rice and soil fertility. II, N and P contents of plants and soil. Plant Soil 102: 49-54

Singh PK, Bisoyi RN (1989) Blue green algae in rice-fields. Phykos 28: 181-195

Singh PK, Panigrahi BC, Satapathy KB (1981) Comparative efficiency of *Azolla*, blue-green algae and other organic manures in relation to N and P availability in a flooded rice soil. Plant Soil 62: 35-44

Singh RN (1950) Reclamation of 'usar' lands in India through blue-green algae. Nature 165: 325-326

Singh RN (1961) Role of blue-green algae in nitrogen economy of Indian agriculture. ICAR, New Delhi

Singh VP, Trehan T (1973) Effect of extacellular products of *Aulosira fertilissima* on the growth of rice seedlings. Plant Soil 38: 457-464

Subhashini D, Kaushik BD (1981) Amelioration of sodic soils with blue-green algae Aust. J. Soil Res 19: 361-367

Subhashini D, Kaushik BD (1984) Amelioration of salt affected soils with blue-green algae. I. Influence of algalization on the properties of saline alkali soils. Phykos 23: 273-277

Thomas (1977) J Biological nitrogen fixation. Nucl India 15: 2-8

Vaishampayan A, Sinha RP, Hader DP, Dey T, Gupta AK, Bhan U, Rao AL (2001) Cyanobacterial biofertilizers in rice agriculture. Bot Rev 67: 453-516

Venkataraman GS (1972) Algal Biofertilizers and Rice Cultivation. Today and Tomorrow Publ., New Delhi p 81

Venkataraman GS (1975) The role of blue green algae in tropical rice cultivation. In: Stewart WDP (ed) Nitrogen fixation by free-living microorganisms. Cambridge University Press, London. pp 207-268

Venkataraman GS (1979) Algal inoculation of rice-fields. In: Nitrogen and Rice. International Rice Res. Institute. Los Banos, Philippines. pp 311-321

Venkataraman GS (1981) Blue-green algae for rice production – a manual for its promotion. FAO Soils bulletin no. 46. Rome p 102

Venkataraman GS (1983) Effect of blue-green algae on aggregate stability and rice yield under different irrigation and nitrogen levels. Soil Till Res 3: 61-66

Venkataraman GS (1992) Algal Biofertilizer Technology for Rice-Sankar Printers. Madurai

Venkataraman GS, Neelakantan S (1967) Effect of cellular constituents of nitrogen-fixing blue-green alga *Cylindrospermum* on root growth of rice plants. J Gen Appl Microbiol 13: 53-62

Venkataraman S, Venkataraman GS (1991) Response of *Anabaena* to salt stress I. Structural and metabolic response. Indian J Microbial 31: 131-138

Vlek PLG, Diakite MY, Mueller H (1992) Ammonia volatilization from flooded. Soils Fert Res 42: 165-174

Wagner GM (1997) *Azolla*: A review on its biology and utilization. Bot Rev 63: 1-26

Cyanobacterial Secondary Metabolites: Emerging Trends and Prospects

R PRASANNA[1], S NAYAK[1], A SURESH[2], BD KAUSHIK[2] and DB SAHOO[3*]

1. INTRODUCTION

The large-scale cultivation of microalgae and the practical use of its biomass as a source of diverse valuable products is a relatively young industry. As biological starting points in the energy flow of aquatic and terrestrial food chains, the significance of these micro-organisms is undisputed. Cyanobacteria comprise a versatile assemblage of organisms – heterogeneous in their structure, size and physiology, but united by the presence of a diverse array of photosynthetic pigments, which have wide ranging uses in food, cosmetic and pharmaceutical industries (Borowitzka 1994). In agriculture, their impact as biofertilizers/soil conditioners, especially as nitrogen supplements in rice based agro ecologies is well recognized (Venkataraman 1972; Metting 1988). However, the ubiquity of these organisms is also a source of concern to human health and sanitation. Toxic cyanobacteria waterblooms are found worldwide in eutrophic lakes, ponds, drinking water reservoirs and coastal waters, where they cause animal poisonings and pose risks to human health (Carmichael 1994). Several genera of cyanobacteria form these toxic waterblooms, with *Microcystis* being the most common (Carmichael 1992; Carmichael 1994). However, in recent years, they are recognized as a primary source of

1 Centre for Conservation and Utilization of Blue Green Algae (CCUBGA),

2 Division of Microbiology, Indian Agricultural Research Institute (IARI), New Delhi 110 012, India

3 Department of Botany, Delhi University, Delhi – 110007, India

* E-mail: dbsahoo@hotmail.com; radhapr@lycos.com

exciting novel molecules, exhibiting bioregulatory and therapeutic properties which emphasize the need for in-depth exploration into the structure and function of these secondary metabolites and their significance in health and environment.

2. CYANOBACTERIAL COLOURS

The impact of the physical world on our lives is quite literally, coloured by our perceptions, as humans are decidedly visual creatures. Food colours have become an essential ingredient in food products, aimed at creating wider consumer acceptability and enhancing the aesthetic appeal of products. Until the discovery of the first synthetic dye in 1856 by Sir William Henry Perkins, mankind had been relying on pigments extracted from plants, animals and minerals as natural colourants. However, due to their easy availability, and superior properties of synthetic dyes with respect to tinctorial strength, hue, and stability and low cost, they have been the choice for colouring a wide range of products. But, toxicological studies (Table 1) have shown that many of these synthetic colours are harmful (Branen et al. 2002). Therefore, a perceptible change from synthetic to natural colours has been observed, especially in food and cosmetics in the past decade (Wisgott and Borthlik 1996).

2.1 Pigment Diversity

The vivid colours of blue, green, orange-red or yellow-brown floating masses in water bodies, irrigation channels adjoining fields or cess-pools on the roadside, illustrate their rich and varied pigmentation of these omnipresent organisms. Among algae, Cyanobacteria or Blue Green algae

Table 1 Effects of synthetic food colouring agents on health

S.No.	*Food Colours as per FDA Nomenclature*	*Health Effects*
1.	Red No. 3 (Erythrosine)	Thyroid tumours, chromosomal damage, hyperactivity may cross-react with salicylates.
2.	Red No. 40 (Allura Red)	Lymphatic tumours, hyperactivity
3.	Blue No. 1 (Brilliant Blue)	Chromosomal damage
4.	Blue No. 2 (Indigotine)	Brain tumours
5.	Green No. 3 (Fast green)	Bladder tumours
6.	Yellow No. 5 (Tartrazine)	Thyroid and lymphatic tumours, allergy, hyper activity
7.	Yellow No. 6 (Sun set Yellow)	Kidney tumours, chromosomal damage allergy

(as they are commonly known) and Red Algae are unique in containing coloured protein assemblies called phycobilisomes. These light absorbing antennae comprise a family of highly soluble and reasonably stable fluorescent proteins – phycobilins, which harvest light at wavelengths not efficiently absorbed by chlorophyll. Three major classes of phycobiliproteins—phycoerythrin (red pigment), phycocyanin (blue pigment) and allophycocyanin (bluish green pigment) exist within these two algal groups - which exhibit qualitative and quantitative variation at inter and intrageneric level, and modulate them as a response to environmental parameters (Kaushik 2000; Prasanna et al. 2003; Prasanna et al. 2004 a,b). A number of cyanobacteria have the ability to vary their phycobiliproteins ratio, which allows the regulation of the balance of wavelengths of light absorbed by them, a phenomenon known as chromatic adaptation. The first observation of this kind dates back to 1903 when Gaidukov noticed that *Oscillatoria santa* was red in colour after grown under green light, but assumed blue-green tint when grown under orange light. The colour taken on by the algae was complementary to the incident radiation. This characteristic change in the light-harvesting complex in response to different wavelengths offers the organisms an adaptive advantage, since phycocyanin can efficiently absorb red light and phycoerythrin green light, but not the reverse. These vividly coloured molecules are soluble in aqueous media and constitute upto 50% of the soluble protein and about 20% of the dry weight of the cell (Grossman et al. 1993). The other group of accessory pigments *viz.* carotenoids, which are orange-red to yellow coloured in appearance, also have immense commercial value. The most common carotenoids in cyanobacteria are β-carotene or the zeaxanthin, echinenone and the myxoxanthophyll. Changes in carotenoid content and composition that occur in response to light intensity is also an adaptive mechanism in acclimatized cyanobacteria. In *Oscillatoria terebriformis*, a thermophilic red brown cyanophyte, the ratio of the total carotenoids to chlorophyll is greatly increased in exponentially growing cells by high light intensity mainly by the reduction of chlorophyll and the maintenance of previous carotenoids levels, which indicates the protective role of carotenoids (Kellar and Paerl 1980). Acclimation to high-light, which reduces susceptibility to photoinhibition in *Microcystis aeruginosa* (Zavenboom and Mur 1984) is associated with a decrease in cell-chlorophyll to carotenoid ratio (Raps et al. 1983), in addition to a decline in both, chlorophyll and phycobiliprotein content.

2.2 Use of Algal Colours

A blue colourant extracted from *Spirulina plantensis* known as the Japanese company "Dainippon Inc." and "Chemicals Inc." was among the first commercial ventures utilizing cyanobacteria, and their product 'Lina blue' has been utilized in a range of products. With its increasing popularity, Dainippon Ink has carried out studies on the use of this colourant in chewing gum, soft drinks, alcoholic drinks and fermented milk products such as yoghurt, and patented them in Japan. Other applications of the biliproteins include- confectionaries, candied ices and sherbets (Branen et al. 2002) and toiletries - shampoo, bath foam, coloured powder, make up formulations including lipstick in German laboratories/industries. Phycobiliproteins are commonly used as fluorescent indicators; therefore are a valuable candidate in the design and characterization of light sensing elements in biosensors (Ayyagari et al. 1995). The property that phycobiliproteins retain their colour during electrophoretic movement can be an added advantage for their use as interval protein markers and it can be useful in the field of proteomics. The possible use of phycoerythrin as a time-temperature integrator to predict the destruction of micro-organisms during cooking of food products has also been indicated, by manipulation of chemical environment; the z value of phycoerythrin might be adjusted to approximate the z values of several pathogenic microbes (Ramirez et al. 2001).

The most impressive use of phycobiliproteins has been as 'phycoflours'. These are conjugates of intensely fluorescent algal phycobiliproteins with molecules that confer biological specificity. Their high quantum yields, long extraction and emission-spectra, combined with their solubility in water, permits its binding with a range of compounds, such as immunoglobins and avidins. The prozyme USA based company is producing various phycobiliproteins for commercial use.

PhycoPro™ Phycocyanin from *Spirulina*, SP
PhycoPro ™ Allophycocyanin from *Spirulina platensis*
PhycoPro ™ Allophycocyanin GT5 ™
PhycoPro ™ Allophycocyanin (cross linked)
PhycoPro ™ Y-Phycoerythrin (red algae)
(http://www.prozyme.com) 2004

'Cyanotech' markets the phycobiliprotein conjugated fluorescent probes (http://www.phycobiliproteins.com).

Phycoflours have also been employed in immunoassays, instead of radiolabel led agents, which have several problems such as exposure to high levels of radiation, limited shelf life and disposal dangers. Techniques have also been developed for chemical conjugation of phycobiliproteins to antibodies and other proteins eg. Zenon immunolabeling technology, developed by Molecular Probes, which increases the possibility of detection of diverse combinations of wavelengths in multicolour experiments. Such procedures can also be combined with routine immunoassay/enzyme linked assays using horseradish peroxidase and alkaline phosphatase. The Zenon antibody labelling kits provide numerous advantage, especially when preparing phycobiliprotein-labelled antibodies, as the process is quick (labelling and purification of the complex tubes only minutes), irreversible and can be done with multiple antibodies using sub-microgram quantities.

In last few years, β-carotene commanded 26% of the market share, being applied to a variety of food and beverage products. Apart from being a mere food colourant, β-carotene provides vitamin A nutrition to human body. Aquacarotene, an Australia based firm produces β-carotene from the green alga *Dunaliella* on a commercial scale (http://www.aquacarotene.com).

Recently, Romay et al. (2003) reported the antioxidant, anti-inflammatory, neuroprotective and hepatoprotective effects of C-phycocyanin, when it was evaluated as an antioxidant *in vitro*. It was able to scavenge alkoxyl, hydroxyl and peroxy radicals and inhibited microsomal lipids peroxidation *in vitro*. Carotenoids, although not vitamins per se, serve as a precursor of vitamin A. Approximately 60 carotenoids possess varying levels of provitamin activity. In the IU system 1 μg retinol = 2 μg betacarotene. Carotenoids act as antioxidants, hence protect cells from damage by unstable oxygen molecules. These pigments can boost the immune system and possibly lower the risk of heart disease, prevent onset of cancer and protect against age related diseases such as cataracts and molecular degradation, multiple sclerosis (Rissanen et al. 2002), as shown by clinical trails by National Cancer Institute in which supplements of β carotene alone or together with other micro nutrients were given (http://www.cancer.gov). β-carotene is approved by FDA as colour additive for use in food and drugs and cosmetics. It is also Generally Recognized as Safe (GRAS) as a dietary supplement and as a nutrient. In powder form, it is used as a feed for poultry and fish, colouring salmon fish, egg-yolk and as a nutrient supplement. In cosmetic industries, it is being used in sunscreen lotions, nail polishes, lipsticks and anti-wrinkle creams.

2.3 Extraction and Purification and Stability of Pigments

A number of methods are available for the extraction of biliproteins from algal cells, and the selection of particular procedure is mainly based on the ease of cell breakage. The easiest method involves placing the algae in water and allowing the proteins to leach out for several days. This can be further refined through the use of a mortar and pestle with sand as abrasive or the use of a blender for easily fractured cells. Chauhan et al. (1994) examined different methods for extraction of phycocyanin from

Spirulina sp. In their work, biomass was harvested by filtering through polyester-cotton cloth, washed with demineralized water and suspended in phosphate buffer, which was given various treatments; and 1,800 units lysozyme/ml and 100 ppm linear alkyl benzene sulfonate afforded good phycocyanin level, with high specific content. Approximately, 500+ different naturally occurring carotenoids have now been characterized. Carotenoids need to be extracted from intact and preferably fresh material, so as to avoid oxidative or enzymatic degradation. As carotenoids are not water-soluble, they must be extracted with water-soluble polar organic solvents, usually acetone, methanol or ethanol. A distinct qualitative difference was found in the carotenoids extracted from fresh or desiccated samples of *Nostoc commune* (Olie and Potts 1986). The technique of column chromatography remains extremely valuable especially for preliminary separation and large-scale work, while for smaller samples and delicate separations, thin layer chromatography is widely used. The choice of the adsorbents for carotenoid chromatography is vast-sucrose, cellulose, starch, $CaCO_3$, $Ca_3 (PO_4)_2$, CaO, $MgCO_3$, $ZnCO_3$ or Al_2O_3. Purification of β-carotene from *Chlorella pyrenoidosa* with lipid or oil or by super critical extraction is patented (EP: 586255).

Phycobilisomes (PBs) require a high concentration (usually 0.75 M) of phosphate to be isolated in entire and energetically coupled state. The stability of isolated PBs in a diluted solution can easily be followed by the changes in the fluorescence emission spectra and light scattering technique over wild range of conditions. Pro-enzyme USA based company product phycobiliprotein is supplied as a 60% Ammonium sulphate suspension in 50mM phosphate buffer. It is stable for at least 12 months when stored (4°C) properly (www.proenzyme.com). Phycocyanin of *Anabaena variabilis* extracted under 1 kilo lux white light and with 10 ml air/s/l was stable between pH 6-8, while phycoerythrin of *Nostoc muscorum* under 1 kilo lux green light with 10ml air/s/l was stable between pH 5-9 (Ranjitha 2004).

Beta-carotenes are available as red crystals or crystalline powder (CAS: 7236-40-7). Carotenoids are highly sensitive to loss by oxidation and need to be protected with appropriate packaging materials and storage conditions, but are relatively stable over a wide range of pH and can be stored under an inert gas environment.

3. SELECTION AND MULTIPLICATION OF SUITABLE CYANOBACTERIA

Finding suitable sources of natural colours or bioactive compounds is a serious and major problem, especially when it is necessary to supply large amounts of their secondary metabolites on a commercial scale. The approach is to grow sufficient amounts of native rich sources from which these compounds can be economically isolated. Mass cultivation is akin to agriculture, in that it involves inputs naturally and freely available – sunlight, air, simple nutrients and algal. Biotechnology can be considered as a form of modern agriculture, which involves easier regulation of interacting factors, and on a much smaller scale. Biotechnological application of any organism involves exploring the desirable properties of the organism and attempt at overproducing a product of industrial value. The commercial utilization of microalgae (including cyanobacteria) involves the availability of suitable, cost effective large scale culture systems, which employ preferably strategies for maximum absorption of solar or artificial energy sources. The open systems in use presently are of three major types - large unstirred shallow ponds, circular ponds, and central pivot driven raceway ponds or paddle wheel driven raceway ponds. However, the major problems of contaminants and fluctuations in environmental conditions make 'closed' culture systems more desirable. Closed reactors' designs vary from tubular reactor of wide range of configurations - plate reactor, helical reactor, hanging bags of various dimensions including thin film reactors and fermentors with internal and/ or external lighting. Some of the latest additions to hybrid models of bioreactors include - enclosed Vertical Alveolar Panel (VAP) and Light Diffusing Optical Fibre (LDDF) bioreactors. *Photobioreactors* that may be located indoors-outdoors, but outdoor location is more economical, as it can make use of free sunlight and at the same time, avoid contamination. The helical tubular bioreactor-the Biocoil, is considered as a very efficient and economical design which can be scaled up for large scale production (Borowitzka 1998).

3.1 Bioactive Molecules from Cyanobacteria

The global distribution of cyanobacteria attests to the ecological success of these organisms, which, at times, may cause problems to mankind. As these organisms are more prevalent in water bodies, their 'blooms' produce odorous compounds which bring about unpleasant taste, besides being toxic. Anthropogenic *eutrophication* can exacerbate the risks, allowing toxic cyanobacteria to grow unchecked, leading to harmful blooms with potentially serious economic and health related impacts. These blooms, generally consisting of more than one species, are also known to deplete dissolved oxygen in water, resulting in fish-kills, besides increasing the viscosity of water and hindering gas exchange. In recent years, detection of toxic cyanobacteria has become fundamental for sound water management.

The structural diversity of the known cyanotoxins includes many variants of alkaloids and cyclic peptides (Table 2). The two most common types are microcystins and nodularins, besides a number of non ribosomal peptides and polyketides and lipopolysaccharides (LPS). LPS are known to be potent mediators in the human immune system. The two major types of toxins, hepatotoxins and neurotoxins, have been well characterized but hepatotoxicosis occurs more often than neurotoxicosis (Carmichael 1994). About 50% of the *Microsystis* waterblooms show hepatotoxicity to mammals and other animals. The toxins responsible for hepatotoxicity are the microcystins (Carmichael et al. 1988), which are obtained not only from *Microcystis*, but also from *Anabaena, Nostoc,* and *Oscillatoria* (Rinehart et al. 1994) which also form waterblooms. The microcystins are cyclic heptapeptides like the representative microcystin-LR. More than fifty structural variations in microcystins have been found from the four genera of cyanobacteria (Rinehart et al. 1994). Nodularins are cyclic pentapeptides and have the Adda unit or its derivatives. Microcystins and nodularins show hepatotoxicity through inhibitory activity to protein phosphatases 1 and 2A (MacKintosh et al. 1990) and are potent tumour promoters (Ohta et al. 1994). The cyclic structures of these toxins are essential for the toxicity, since linear compounds which have the same amino acid components as the cyclic peptides, did not show apparent toxicity to mice (Namikoshi et al. 1993). Extensive efforts have been devoted to studies on cyanobacterial toxins resulting in understanding of the toxins and toxin producing organisms.

Table 2 Cyanotoxins and the genera associated as producers

Type of toxin	*Genera associated*
Hepatotoxins	
Microcystins	*Microcystis, Planktothrix, Nostoc, Anabaena, Anabaenopsis*
Nodularins	*Nodularia*
Cylindrospermopsin	*Cylindrospermopsis, Aphanizomenon, Umezakia, Raphidiopsis*
Neurotoxins	
Anatoxin-a	*Anabaena, Planktothrix, Aphanizomenon*
Anatoxin-a(S)	*Anabaena*
Saxitoxins	*Anabaena, Planktothrix, Aphanizomenon, Cylindrospermopsis, Lyngbya*
Dermatoxins	
Lyngbyatoxin-a	*Lyngbya,*
Aplysiatoxins	*Lyngbya, Planktothrix, Schizothrix*

Microcystins are most common causative agent of the cyanobacterial waterblooms and toxicosis, show toxicity to mice at concentrations as low as 50 μg Kg^{-1} (LD_{50}, intraperitoneal injection). The netpen liver disease of salmon observed on the Pacific Canadian coast is thought to be caused by microcystins (Andersen et al. 1993). A structurally unrelated cyanobacterial hepatotoxin, cylindrospermopsin, has been isolated from *Cylindrospermum raciborskii* (Ohtani et al. 1994) and *Umezakia natans* (Harada et al. 1991) and has an acute (24h) LD_{50} of 2.1 mg Kg^{-1} (IP). Neurotoxins are the other group of cyanobacterial toxins (anatoxin-a from *Anabaena* and *Oscillatoria,* ana-toxin-a(s) from *Anabaena flos-aquae,* homoanatoxin-a from *Oscillatoria rubescens*, saxitoxin and neosaxitoxin from *Aphanizomenon* and *Anabaena*; Carmichael, 1992). The molecular systems, implicated in toxin and antibiotic production – non ribosomal peptide synthetases (NRPSs) and Type-I polyketide synthases (PKSs) are known to be present in a number of cyanobacteria (Neilan et al. 1999)

In recent years, there has been a significant increase in the identification of bioactive compounds from cyanobacteria, because of the potential therapeutic or pharmaceutical properties of these metabolites (Shimizu 1996). A number of novel compounds have been isolated, which are similar to those found in marine invertebrates and show immunomodulatory, biomodulatory and therapeutic properties. These include compounds showing antiviral, anticancer, anti-inflammatory and antioxidant properties (Patterson 1996). Several studies on the use of cyanobacterial cells in humans, mice, rats, cats and chicken have demonstrated their effects on phagocytosis, inflammation and NK cell function (Kushik et al. 2000; Jensen and Ginsberg 2000).

Blue-green algae, particularly the marine forms, are the richest source of novel bioactive compounds including toxins having wide pharmaceutical applications (Becker 1994; Patterson 1996). Boyd (1997) has isolated and sequenced an 11kD virucidal protein, christened as cyanovirin-N (CV-N), from *Nostoc ellipsosporum* which irreversibly inactivated diverse T-lymphocyte-tropic (T-tropic), laboratory adapted strains of HIV type-1, HIV type-2 and simian immunodeficiency virus (SIV) as well as T-tropic, macrophage-tropic and T and M tropic primary clinical isolates of HIV-1. Water soluble extract of *Spirulina platensis* was found to have a sulphated polysaccharide calcium spirulinan (Ca-SP), which is an anti-viral agent. This compound selectively inhibits the penetration of enveloped viruses (Herpes simplex, human cytomegalovirus, measles virus, mumps virus, influenza-A virus and HIV-1) into host cells, thereby preventing replication.

Water based extract of *Aphanizomenon flos-aquae* containing high concentrations of phycocyanin inhibited the *in vitro* growth of one out of four tumour cell lines, indicating that at least some tumour cell types may be directly sensitive to phycocyanin. *Phormodium tenue*, contained several diacyl-glycerol compounds which effectively inhibited chemically-induced skin tumours in mice (Tokuda and Nishino 1996). C-phycocyanin is free radical scavenger (Bhat and Madyastha 2000) and has significant hepatoprotective effect. Phycocyanin was shown to inhibit inflammation in mouse ears and prevent acetic acid induced colitis in rats. Several reports have shown that some blue-green algae have cholesterol lowering effect in animal and human models. Increase in total cholesterol, LDL and VLDL-cholesterol in rats, kept on cholesterol feed, was reduced when their diet was supplemented with *Spirulina* (Hori and Ishibashi 1994). This was found due to significant increase in the activity of lipoprotein lipase - a key enzyme in the metabolism of triglyceride rich lipoproteins (Nakaya and Honma 1988).

4. CONCLUSION

The past few decades have witnessed great strides in the production and utilization of algae as food/feed through the efforts of various research groups all over the world. However, with problems related to high cost, acceptability and strict evaluation criteria, there was a cautious approach adopted. But with researchers demonstrating that algal biomass can be used for other applications, such as animal feed, soil conditions and the potentiality of algae as a source of a variety of compounds such as polysaccharides, lipids, proteins, pigments, vitamins, sterols, enzymes, pharmaceuticals and other fine chemicals, the demand is on an increasing trend. Algal biomass has also been utilized for production of biofuels (hydrogen, methane, alcohols), hydrocarbons, labelled amino acids and sugars and as bioassay agents, as microalgae with their short generation time, capability of being easily handled and cultured under controlled conditions, and metabolic flexibility are an excellent bio-resource. The major obstacle is the economics of production of these valuable compounds. Much work is still needed, especially in increasing the product yield, before these processes and products are economically viable – as there exists a wide gap between the well recognized commercial potential of many microalgal species and the actual technical know-how of industrial process. Although many impressive calculations have been published based on extrapolations of algal yields obtained in small ponds, large plants of several hectares - most of these designs/calculations are yet to be fully or partially realized. Therefore, investigations need to be directed towards:

- Building effective and long term linkages between laboratory researchers and industrial technologists/engineers for identifying 'gaps' and evaluating essential criteria in scale up and production technologies.
- Exploiting extreme and novel environments for identifying new strains and novel products.

The time is now ripe to exploit microalgae as a rich source of pigments and bioactive compounds; and with their simple requirements for growth, commercial exploitation holds definite promise. Concerted efforts also need to be made to utilize the tools of genetic engineering for providing a new dimension to the utilization of algae in diverse spheres of agriculture, environmental management and health.

ACKNOWLEDGEMENTS

The authors are grateful to Indian Council of Agricultural Research, New Delhi for the AP Cess fund project (F.No. 13 (37)/2002-SW&DF) for providing financial assistance.

REFERENCES

Andersen RJ, Luu HA, Chen DZX, Holmes CFB, Kent ML, Blanc M, Talyor FJR, Williams DE (1993) Chemical and biological evidence links microcystins to salmon "netpen liver disease". Toxicon 31: 1315-1323

Ayyagari M, Pande R, Kamtekar S, Gao H, Marx K, Kumar J, Tripathy S, Akkara J, Kaplan D (1995) Molecular assembly of proteins and conjugated polymers towards development of biosensors. Biotechnol. Bioengg 45: 116-121

Becker EW (1994) Microalgae: Biotechnology and Microbiology, Cambridge University Press, Cambridge, USA. 301p

Bhat VB, Madyastha KM (2000) C-phycocyanin: A potent peroxyl radical scavenger *in vivo* and *in vitro*. Biochem Biophys Res Commun 275: 20-25

Borowitzka LJ (1994) Commercial pigment production from algae In: Phang CJ (ed) Algal Biotechnology in the Asia Pacific Region University of Malaya, Kuala Lumpur, Malaysia, pp 82-84

Borowitzka MA (1998) Tubular photobioreactor for large-scale algal culture In: Subramanian G, Kaushik BD, Venkataraman GS (eds) Cyanobacterial Biotechnology. Oxford and IBH Publishing Co Ltd, New Delhi, pp 249-258

Boyd MR (1997) Discovery of Cyanovrin-N a novel human immunodeficiency virus inactivating protein that binds viral surface envelope glycoprotein gp 120: Potential applications to microbicide development. Anti Microb Agents Chemother 41: 1521-1530

Branen LA, Davidson MP, Salmine NS, Thorngate III HJ (2002) Food Additives. Marcel Dekker, New York

Carmichael WW (1992) Cyanobacteria secondary metabolites - the cyanotoxins. J Appl Bacteriol 72: 445-459

Carmichael WW (1994) The toxins of cyanobacteria. Sci Amer 270: 78-86

Carmichael WW, Beasley VR, Bunner DL, Eloff JN, Falconer IR, Harada PR Gorham KI, Krishnamurthy T, Yu MJ, Moore RE, Rinehart KL, Runnegar MTC (1988) Naming of cyclic heptapeptide toxins of cyanobacteria (blue-green algae). Toxicon 26: 971-973

Chauhan VS, Kothari RM, Ramamurthy V (1994) Methods of efficient extraction of phycocyanin from *Spirulina*. Biotechnol. Techniq 8: 525-528

Grossman AR, Schaefer MR, Chiang GG, Collier JL (1993) Environmental effects on the light-harvesting complex of cyanobacteria. J Bacteriol 175: 575-582

Harada K-I, Ogawa K, Kimura Y, Murata H, Suzuki M, Thorn PM, Evans WR, Carmichael WW (1991) Microcystins from *Anabaena flos-aquae* NRC-525-17. Chem Res Toxicol 4: 535-540

Hori KG, Ishibashi G (1994) Hypocholesterolemic effect of blue green-alga, *Nostoc commune* in rats fed atherogenic diet. Plant Foods Hum Nutr 45: 63-70

Jensen GS, Ginsberg DI (2000) Consumption of *Aphanizomenon flos-aquae* has rapid effects on the circulation of the circulation and function of immune cells in humans. J Amer Med Assn 2: 50-58

Kaushik BD (2000) Screening of cyanobacterial strains for natural colours. Indian Hydrobiol 3: 81-84

Kellar PE, Paerl HW (1980) Physiological adaptations in response to environmental stress during an N2-fixing *Anabaena* bloom. Appl Environ Microbiol 40: 587-597

Kushak RI, Drapeau C, Van Cott EM (2000) Favourable effects of blue-green alga *Aphanizomenon flos-aquae* on rat plasma lipids. J Amer Med Assn 2: 59-65

MacKintosh C, Beattie KA, Klumpp S, Cohen P, Codd GA (1990) Cyanobacterial microcystin-LR is a potent and specific inhibitor of protein phosphatases 1 and 2A from both, mammals and higher plants. FEBS Lett 264: 187-192

Metting B (1988) Microalgae in agriculture In: Borowitzka MA, Borowitzka LJ (eds) Microalgal Biotechnology. Cambridge University Press, Cambridge, USA, pp 288-304

Nakaya N, Honma Y (1988) Cholestero lowering effect of *Spirulina*. Nutr Reports Int 37: 1329-1337

Namikoshi M, Chori BW, Sun F, Rinehart KL, Evans WR, Carmichael WW (1993) Chemical characterization and toxicity of dihydro derivatives of nodularin and microcystin-LR, potent cyanobacterial cyclic peptide hepatotoxins. Chem Res Toxicol 6: 151-158

NAS/NRC (National Academy of Sciences/National Research Council) (1971) Food colours. National Academy Press, Washington, D.C

Neilan BA, Dittmann E, Rouhiainen L, Bass RA, Schaub, V, Sivonen K, Borner T (1999)

Nonribosomal peptide synthesis and toxigenecity of cyanobacteria. J Bacteriol 181: 4089-4097

Ohta T, Sueoka E, Iida N, Komori A, Suganuma M, Nishiwaki R, Tatematus R, Kim S-J, Carmichael WW, Fujiki H (1994) Nodularin, a potent inhibitor of protein phosphatases 1 and 2A, is a new environmental carcinogen in male F344 rat liver. Cancer Res 54: 6402-6406

Ohtani I, Moore RI, Runnegar MTC (1992) Cylindrospermopsin:a potent hepatotoxin from the blue-green *Cylindrospermopsis raciborskii.* J Am Chem Soc 114: 7941-7942

Olie J, Potts M (1986) Purification and biochemical analysis of the cytoplasmic membrane from the desiccation-tolerant cyanobacterium *Nostoc commune* UTEX 584. Appl Environ Microbiol 52: 706-710

Patterson GML (1996) Biotechnological applications of Cyanobacteria. J Sci Ind Res 55: 669-684

Prasanna R, Pabby A, Saxena S, Singh PK (2004a) Modulation of pigment profiles of *Calothrix elenkenii* in response to environmental stresses. J Plant Physiol 161: 1125-1132

Prasanna R, Pabby A, Singh PK (2004 b) Effect of glucose and light/dark environment on pigmentation profiles in *Calothrix elenkenii*. Folia Microbiol 49: 26-30

Prasanna R, Prasanna BM, Mohammadi SA, Singh PK (2003) Analysis of phycobiliprotein content in *Tolypothrix* germplasm. Folia Microbiol 48: 59-64

Ramirez AO, Merrill JE, Smith DE (2001) Sucrose sodium dodecyl sulphate, Urea and 2-mercaptoethanol affect the thermal inactivation of R-Phycoerythrin. J Food Protection 64: 1806-1811

Ranjitha K (2004) Potential of Cyanobacteria as a Source of Natural Colours, Ph.D. thesis, Indian Agricultural Research Institute, New Delhi

Raps S, Wyman K, Siegelman HW, Falkowski PG (1983) Adaptation of the cyanobacterium *Microcystis aeruginosa* to light intensity. Plant Physiol 72: 829-832

Rinehart KL, Namikoshi M, Choi BW (1994) Structure and biosynthesis of toxins from blue-green algae (Cyanobacteria) J Appl Phycol 6: 159-176

Rissanen T, Voutilainen S, Nyyssonen K, Salonen JT (2002) Lycopene, artherosclerosis and coronary heart disease. Exp Biol Med 227: 900-907

Romay CP, Gonazelz R, Ledon N, Ramirez D, Vimbare V (2003) C-Phycocyanin: A biliprotein with antioxidant, anti-inflammatory and neuroprotective effects. Curr Protein Peptide Sci 4: 207-216

Shimizu Y (1996) Microalgal metabolites: A new perspective. Annu Rev Microbiol 50: 431-465

Tokuda H, Nishino H (1996) Inhibition of 12-O-tetrade-canoylphorbol-13-acetate promoted mouse skin papilloma by digalactosyl diacylgycerols from fresh water cyanobacterium *Phormidium tenue*. Cancer Lett 104: 91-95

Venkataraman GS (1972) Algal Biofertilizers and Rice cultivation, Today and Tomorrow Printers and Publishers, New Delhi. 75p

Wissgott U, Bortlik K (1996) Prospects for new natural food colourants; Trends Food Sci. Technol 7: 298-302

Zavenboom W, Mur RL (1984) Growth and photosynthetic response of the cyanobacterium *Microcystis aeruginosa* in relation to photoperiodicity and irradiance. Arch Microbiol 139: 232-239

Inter-Relationships of Physical and Biological Aspects of Soil Health in Sandy Soil

DJAJADI[1] and LK ABBOTT[1]

1. INTRODUCTION

Agricultural soil management practices have traditionally emphasized high plant production. However, soil degradation is a serious problem in many regions of the world as indicated by declines in various soil health indicators (Arshad and Martin 2002; Wienhold et al. 2004). For example, intensive tillage can decrease aggregate stability (Pagliai et al. 2004), increase soil erosion (Basic et al. 2004), increase gas emission (Lal 2004) and decrease soil organic matter content (Diekow et al. 2005; Sainju et al. 2005). Soil degradation may decrease productivity and lead to issues of environment health such as global warming (Paustian et al. 2000; Rees et al. 2005; Schulze and Freibauer 2005) and presence of residual chemicals in the subsoil and ground water (Prunty and Greenland 1997).

There is an urgent need to widely implement more sustainable soil management practices to improve and maintain soil quality (Carter 2002). However, it has been claimed that strategies of soil management only focus on environmental issues might endanger productivity of food and fibre (Wander et al. 2002). Therefore, the concept of soil management practices needs to be based on an understanding among ecologists, socio-economists, environmentalists and land managers to ensure that a balance

1. School of Earth and Geographical Sciences, Faculty of Natural and Agricultural Sciences, The University of Western Australia, 35 Stirling Highway, Crawley, 6009, WA, AUSTRALIA E-mail: jay@segs.uwa.edu.au

is developed that includes consideration of the impacts of soil management practices on productivity, the environment, economic returns and societal issues. There is a challenge to develop soil management practices that balance the requirements for production and environmental health (Doran and Safley 1997).

Soil health has been defined as 'the continued capacity of soil to function as a vital living system, within ecosystem and land-use boundaries, to sustain biological productivity, promote the quality of air and water environments, and maintain plant, animal and human health' (Doran and Safley 1997). To maintain sustainability of agriculture, establishing ongoing assessment of the condition and health of the soil is very important (Doran and Safley 1997; Arshad and Martin 2002). The health or quality of soil is considered to be the most important elements of sustainable agriculture (Acton and Gregorich 1995; Warkentin 1995) and it depends on a balance among physical, chemical and biological components of soil fertility (Abbott and Murphy 2003).

Soil structure is an important factor regarding the capacity of soil to support agricultural production, soil carbon sequestration and water quality (Bronick and Lal 2005). An important measure of soil structure is aggregate stability (Six et al. 2000). Soil aggregation is the result of soil particle arrangement, flocculation and cementation influenced by soil properties, biota and environment. Aggregate stability is mediated by soil organic carbon, soil organisms, ionic bridging, clay and carbonates (Bronick and Lal 2005). Aggregate stability may be the most important physical indicator of the health of sandy soil because it has a major influence on soil physical (e.g. hydraulic characteristics, soil strength, and erosion), chemical (e.g. nutrient cycling), and biological properties (e.g. microbial activity). Sandy soils are light in texture, have low capacity to retain water and applied nutrients, and are prone to erosion. They also have less capacity to form aggregates than do soils with lower levels of sand. Hence, increasing aggregate stability is important to improving biological and chemical aspects of soil fertility, increasing agricultural productivity, enhancing porosity and minimizing erodibility (Bronick and Lal 2005).

Dynamics of management factors associated with soil health have been extensively reviewed (Guérif et al. 2001; Dani and Ghezzehei 2002; Kay and VandenBygaart 2002; Mrabet 2002; Sauerbeck 2001; Zentner 2002). However, these reviews focus mainly on the effect of soil tillage on soil's physical and chemical properties. Whilst the reviews provided evidence about the effect of tillage on soil properties for a broad range of soil types, there is little information about their effects on soil biological properties. Monitoring changes in biological soil properties may provide valuable information about the health of soil because biological properties of soil are highly sensitive to soil management practices (Pankhust et al. 1997). There is relatively little information about the effect of soil management practices on the health of sandy soil.

This review focuses on the effect of soil management practices on the state of sandy soil, especially the effects of clay, organic matter, liming, temperature, particle size distribution and plant roots. First, an overview is given of the general properties that might indicate the health of sandy soils used for agricultural production. Subsequently, evidence is evaluated concerning the effect of soil management practices on sandy soil, including the interactive roles of the soil physical and biological environment.

1.1 Properties of Sandy Soil

Sandy soils characteristically consist of loose soil particles because the cohesion between them is weak. This natural property of sandy soil can cause problems in agricultural land use. For example, in the Western Australia wheat belt, the soils are often uniform in texture and contain more than 85% sand (Farrington and Campbell 1970). The soils are inherently low in all aspects of soil fertility and have a low capacity to retain water and nutrients (Farrington and Campbell 1970). Many sandy soils in Western Australia contain low proportions of macro-aggregates (McFarlane and Carter 1990; Select Committee into Land Conservation, 1990). Consequently, the soils are prone to erosion and loss of applied nutrients (such as phosphorus) is high (Weaver et al. 1988, Pathan et al. 2002). In contrast, soils dominated by clay form fine granular aggregates because the clay particles are electrically charged and the oppositely charged surfaces provide the basis of a greater aggregation (Shepherd et al. 2001). For a range of soil analysis, the properties of sandy soils are lower than those of clay soils (Table 1, Webster et al. 2001).

Deleterious impacts of management practices of sandy agricultural soils have been reported (Table 2). For example, cultivation of sandy soils more than once and up to three times prior to sowing, increased run off and decreased organic C and aggregate stability (Packer et al. 1992). Long-term continuous cultivation in Western Australian soils is associated with decreased soil pH and increased hard-setting (Gazey and O'Conell 2001). It might be important to establish guidelines for soil management practices in agricultural sandy soils with the objective of reducing erosion, preserving organic matter and optimizing water use. The role of agricultural management that takes into account soil biological processes has potential to increase the sustainable use of these sandy soils.

Table 1 Some soil properties related to soil texture (Webster et al. 2001)

No	*Texture*	*Total C (g C/kg soil)*	*Total N (g N/kg soil)*	*Biomass C (g C/kg soil)*
1	**Sand**	5.6	1.2	0.02
2	Sand	63.2	3.7	0.35
3	Sand	20.1	1.6	0.01
4	Sand	91.8	4.1	0.01
5	Sand	104.1	4.7	0.11
6	Sandy loam	40.5	4.2	0.08
7	Sandy loam	38.1	1.8	0.20
8	Sandy clay loam	32.3	2.2	0.19
9	Sandy clay loam	51.7	3.7	0.68
10	Silty Loam	22.0	3.2	0.11
11	Clay loam	19.7	2.8	0.32
12	Silty loam	51.9	3.7	0.56
13	Clay loam	29.7	1.9	0.62
14	Silty loam	28.5	2.1	0.62
15	Silty clay loam	71.7	4.9	1.09
16	Silty loam	53.0	3.3	0.39
17	Silty loam	105.3	4.7	0.43
18	Silty loam	249.9	9.0	0.73
19	Clay	473.0	17.2	0.06
20	Clay	479.0	20.9	0.93
21	Silty clay loam	383.0	18.4	2.12
22	Loamy sand	423.0	14.0	5.59
23	Sandy loam	347.0	13.0	3.11
24	Silty clay loam	450.0	22.5	4.11
25	Loamy sand	194.0	9.5	0.11

1.2 Aggregate Stability as a Vital Soil Health Indicator for Agricultural Sandy Soil

Soil aggregation is defined as the clustering or grouping of soil particles in which the forces holding the particles together are much stronger than the forces between adjacent aggregates (Martin et al. 1955). Generally, the forces holding the particles together are expressed by soil aggregate stability and assessed by determining the resistance of the aggregates to dry-sieving or wet-sieving.

There are several methods for quantifying soil aggregate size distribution and aggregate stability (Kemper and Rosenau 1986). The

Table 2 Effect of soil management practices on properties of sandy soils.

Soil management practices	Effect on sandy soil properties			Reference
	Physical	*Chemical*	*Biological*	
1. Conventional cultivation (CC) versus direct drilled (DD)	n.o.	The concentrations of extractable P, extractable K, total N and organic C in the soil were all higher with DD than with CC.	n.o.	White 1990
2. Cultivated versus Directed drilled versus pasture	Pasture and direct drilled had higher stable macroaggregate and porosity than cultivated soils	Organic C was higher in pasture and direct drilled	n.o.	Chan and Mead 1986
3. Conventional (T) versus Conservation tillage (C)	T increased run off and decreased aggregate stability	T decreased organic C	n.o.	Packer et al. 1992
4. Direct drilling stubble retained (DDR) versus stubble burnt (DDB) versus cultivation with stubble burnt (CCB)	Aggregate stability in soil with DDR was higher	Organic C was higher in soil with DDR	Microbial biomass C and N was greater in soil with DDR than those in soil with DDB and CCB	Carter and Mele 1992

n.o. = no observation

suitability of these methods depends on the purpose of the study. The most common approaches are based on the wet-sieving methods (Kemper and Rosenau 1986). In this method, a sequence of submerging and sieving in water imitates the natural stresses involved in the entry of water into soil aggregate (Märquez et al. 2004). However, initial water content of soil aggregate before wet-sieving controls the severity of disruption (Kemper and Rosenau 1986). Another method used to determine aggregate stability is capillary-wetted and slaked pretreatments (Elliott 1986; Cambardella and Elliot 1993). In this method, the soil aggregate is slowly wetted before sieving by capillary-wetted pretreatment. Consequently, this pretreatment causes minimal disruption, because moisten aggregates do not arise air pressure in the pores and the air escapes with minimal aggregate disruption (Märquez et al 2004). In contrast, the slaked pretreatment produces substantial disruption, because the air that is trapped inside the soil pores is rapidly displaced with water when air-dry soil is submerged in water. Therefore, the slaked pretreatment method might not be suitable for determining aggregate stability for sandy soil.

1.2.1 Factors Affecting Aggregate Stability

Soil aggregate stability is the result of complex interactions among soil biological, chemical and physical processes (Tisdall and Oades 1982). Three groups of factors affecting aggregate stability are abiotic (clay, sesquioxides, exchangeable cations and particle size distribution), biotic factors (soil organic matter, micro-organisms, plant roots and soil fauna), and environmental (temperature and moisture) (Bronick and Lal 2005). In sandy soils, the distribution of particle size might also contribute to the stability of aggregates. For example, aggregates of sandy soil containing smaller sand particles (<250 mm) were more stable than aggregates in whole sandy soils containing a wide range of sand particles (Fig. 1).

Different models of the formation and stabilization of aggregates indicate the relative contributions of inorganic and organic materials. Soil aggregations can be mainly due to the cementing of soil particles by mineral substances (Miller and Jastrow 1992). In the presence of plants and in soils where organic matter is the major binding agent, the arrangement of micro-aggregates (<0.25 mm diam.) into macro-aggregates (>0.25 mm diam.) can be facilitated by hyphae of arbuscular mycorrhizal fungi and saprophytic fungi in association with fibrous roots (Tisdall and Oades 1979; Tisdall and Oades 1982; Miller and Jastrow 1990). Furthermore, mucigels and polysaccharides released by micro-organisms and roots are involved in binding soil particles and stabilizing aggregates (Oades 1984). It has been reported that glomalin, an insoluble glycoprotein produced by arbuscular mycorrhizal fungi, is associated with stabilization of soil

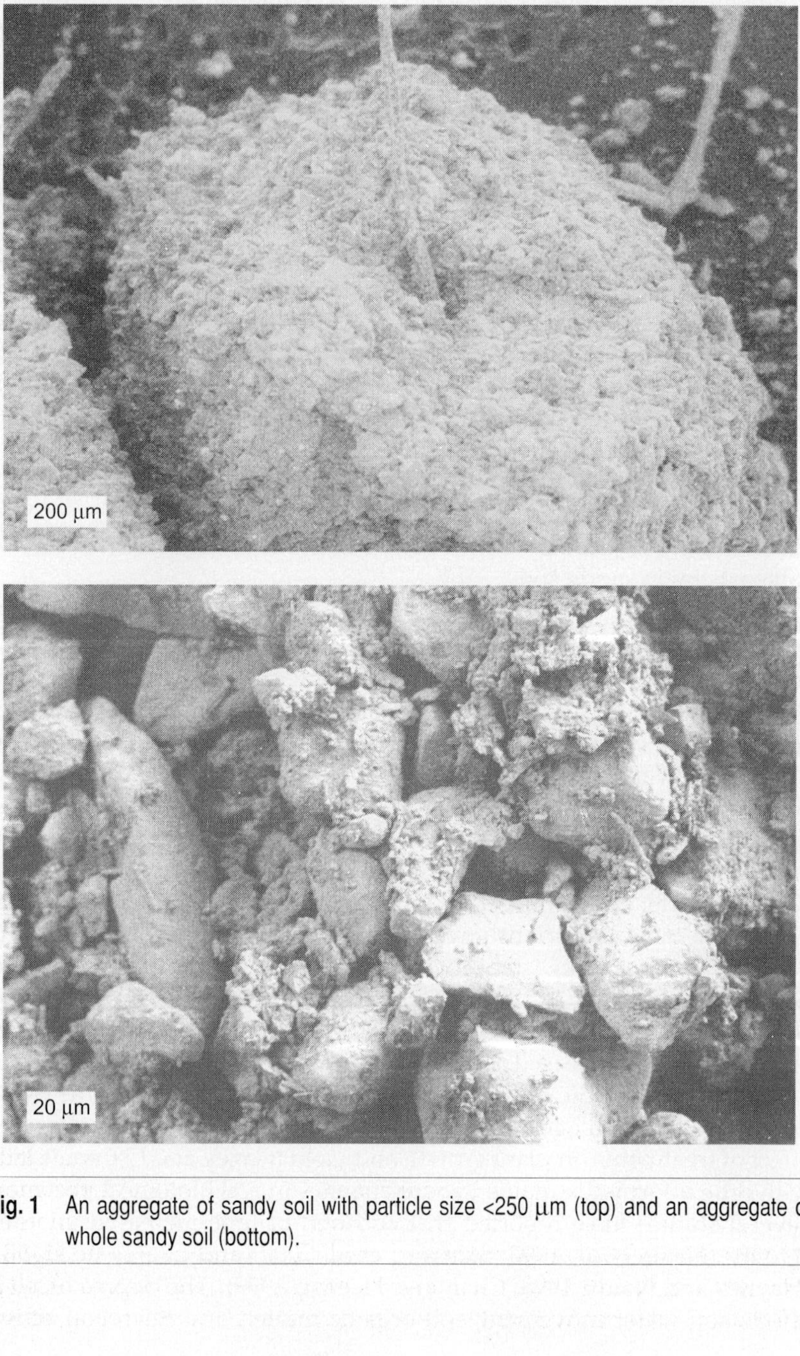

Fig. 1 An aggregate of sandy soil with particle size <250 μm (top) and an aggregate of whole sandy soil (bottom).

aggregates (Wright and Upadyaya 1996; Wright et al. 1996; Franzluebbers et al. 2000). The role of glomalin is to glue soil particles to form soil clusters (Wright and Upadyaya 1996). However, all of these proposed mechanisms have been based on studies conducted in clay and silt loam soils.

Aggregate stability in sandy soils may be the most important aspect of soil health to measure in order to assess the susceptibility of soil to wind erosion. In sandy soils, Degens et al. (1996) suggested that hyphal cross-linkages between sand grains seemed to be a dominant mechanism for the stability of aggregates. Soil amendment with organic materials, such as glucose did not affect water stable aggregates (Degens and Sparling 1996). In addition, ^{14}C microbial biomass and ^{14}C microbial products were poorly correlated with water stable aggregates (Degens and Sparling 1996). In contrast, Kiem and Kandeler (1997) found that microbial biomass had a considerable influence on increasing aggregate stability in sandy soils. Furthermore, de Léon-Gonzáles et al. (2000) reported that the addition of organic material in the form of compost significantly increased the formation of macro-aggregates (>1 mm) that were stable to wind erosion. Clearly, there is no single factor involved in the cohesiveness of primary soil particles in sandy soils.

In sandy soil with different management practices, several factors may be involved in aggregate stability that may have synergistic effects. A conceptual model of inter-relationships between factors is illustrated in Fig. 2. The inter-relationship of some factors is expected to occur because soil management practices alter physical, chemical and biological soil properties (Wang and Gong 1998; Schipper and Sparling 2000; Chan et al. 2001). For example, differences in aggregate stability in a tropical Ultisol (Borneo, Indonesia) were correlated with organic C, clay content and exchangeable sodium percentage (ESP) at sites undergoing erosion (Chappell et al. 1999; Franzluebbers and Arshad 1996). In this soil, organic C was the most important governing factor, accounting for 56% of the variance in aggregate stability. Another demonstration of the inter-relationships among soil characteristics is demonstrated by a long-term continuous cultivation study in Western Australian soils which was associated with decreased soil pH and increased hard-setting (Gazey and O'Conell 2001). Acidic soils in this area have been treated with lime with or without reduced tillage. Unfortunately, the studies have focussed on the effect of treatments on plant growth and yield (Gazey and O'Conell 2001), with little information gained about changes in soil biological properties. Several studies have reported that addition of lime increased microbial activity (Neale et al. 1997; Stenberg et al. 2000) and aggregate stability (Haynes and Naidu 1998; Chan and Heenan 1999). The degree of tillage affects soil water movement, soil organic matter, and microbial activity

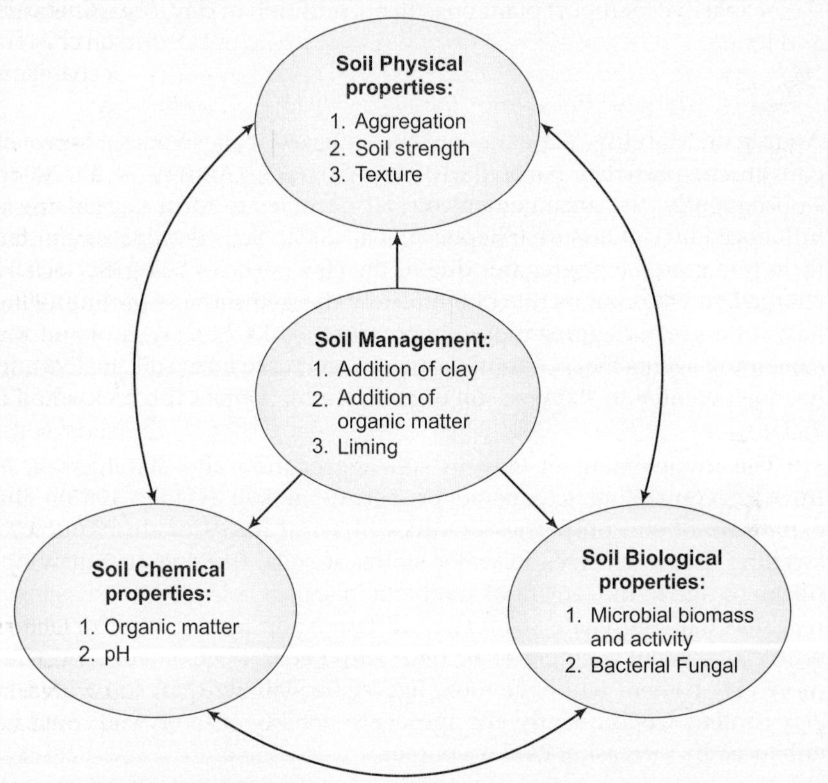

Fig. 2 Conceptual model of inter-relationship of soil characteristics as affected by soil management practices

(Shipitalo et al. 2000; Stenberg et al. 2000), which in turn affect the binding of soil particles.

Many sandy soils in Western Australia contain low proportions of macro-aggregates and are prone to wind erosion (Select Committee into Land Conservation, 1990). Macro-aggregates (binding soil particles >0.25 mm in diam.) in clay and loam soils are sensitive to short-term soil management practices. In sandy soils, aggregate stability may also be sensitive to soil management practices because the binding of sand grains is largely mediated by biological factors (Oades 1993). Consequently, identifying soil biological changes in soil under different soil management practices could be used to determine possible forms of manipulation of soil and crops that enhance soil aggregate stability. The soil management practices that may be applied to agricultural sandy soils to sustain their capacity to support plant growth are addition of clay, organic matter and lime.

1.2.2 The Involvement of Clay in Aggregate Stability

Aggregate stability depends on the internal cohesiveness between constituent particles, particularly clay particles (Andreu et al. 2001). Consequently, the arrangement of soil particles to form aggregates is influenced by soil texture (Shepherd et al. 2002). Soils dominated by clay form fine granular aggregates due to the clay particles being electrically charged and the conjunction of oppositely charged surfaces providing the basis of a greater aggregation (Shepherd et al. 2002). Clay is one of the cementing agents that hold soil particles together to form soil clusters and has the potential to stabilize soil organic matter content (Bronick and Lal 2005).

The involvement of clay in soil aggregation and stabilization is through controlling expansive properties of soil (Oades 1993). The expansion of soil properties involves physical forces of shrinking and swelling due to changes in water status of soils, freezing and thawing, tillage or due to movement of soil biota in soils (Oades 1993). It has been reported that aggregate stability of different soil texture was correlated with clay content (Kemper et al. 1987; Attou et al. 1998). Hence, soil with more clay content will have more aggregate stability than soil with less clay content. Consequently, the aggregate stability of sandy soil could be enhanced by increasing its clay content.

There is some evidence that clay can be used to ameliorate water repellent sandy soil (Carter et al. 1997). Aggregate stability of micro-aggregates was positively correlated with clay content, but the stability of macro-aggregates (>2mm) depended on organic matter content when the organic matter content is greater than 5 to 6% (Boix-Fayos et al. 2001). Amato and Ladd (1992) found a strong correlation between clay content and accumulation of microbial biomass derived from ^{14}C-glucose. Increases in clay content by 1-2% can play an important role in the prevention of water repellency in very sandy soils, even though further increasing the concentration of clay may increase the strength of sandy soil (Harper and Gilkes 1994).

The involvement of clay in aggregation is also through protection of organic matter in the soil from microbial decomposition (Oades 1988). Hence, the process of soil aggregation and stabilization also depends on clay type. Soils dominated by clay minerals with a high specific surface area have a high capacity for absorbing humic substances and consequently for stabilizing aggregates (Parfit et al. 1997). The absorption of organic matter of humin was higher in beidellitic clay soil than in illitic clay soil (Caravaca et al. 2001). The aggregate stability of beidellitic clay soil was significantly correlated with organic matter and humin content of fine silt fraction (Caravaca et al. 2001).

1.2.3 The Involvement of Organic Matter in Aggregate Stability

The involvement of soil organic matter in soil aggregate stability is through the physicochemical interactions of organic compounds with clay and fine silt particles (Caravaca et al. 2001). Hence, the studies of the impact of soil degradation processes on soil properties associated with soil management practices have mainly focused on changes in the physical characteristics and loss in organic matter (Franzluebbers and Arshad 1996; Chappell et al. 1999). However, in soils which are poor in stabilizing media of a physico-chemical nature, soil biological properties could have an important role in stabilizing aggregates (Oades 1993). The total organic C content of soil is considered a poor indicator of organic materials involved in stabilizing macro-aggregates and macro-aggregate stability is sensitive to short-term management (Tisdall and Oades 1982). Consequently, recent studies have concentrated on identifying and understanding labile organic C fractions involved in the short-term (<2 years) stabilization of aggregates. Research in this area has generally focused on the role of microbial biomass C as an indicator of the labile organic C fractions involved in stabilizing macro-aggregates.

The soil microbial biomass can be defined as living organisms with the size smaller than 10 μm (Schloter et al. 2003). Soil microbial biomass content is considered as an integrative indicator of the microbial significance in soil because it is one of the few fractions of soil organic matter that is biologically meaningful, sensitive to soil management or pollution and measurable (Powlson 1994). Soil microbial biomass C has a positive correlation with the degree of soil aggregation (Carter 1992; Edgerton et al. 1995). The microbial biomass has a positive effect on soil aggregation but this is not because the biomass is directly involved as a stabilizing aggregate as it seems likely that the biomass indicates previous microbial turnover of organic C and production of bonding compounds and binding structures (Degens 1997). Hence, soil microbial activity and microbial diversity in the involvement of C turnover and in the production of bonding compounds may have a significant role in aggregate stability of soil under different soil management practices. However, there is still little information about changes in microbial activity and diversity due to the changes in soil management practices in relation to aggregate stability.

1.2.4 The Involvement of Liming in Aggregate Stability

The involvement of liming in soil aggregate stability is through both direct and indirect process (Haynes and Naidu 1998). A direct effect of liming on aggregate stability can be ascribed to the flocculating and cementing actions of $CaCO_3$. Liming of soil will increase the concentration of Ca^{2+} and high ionic strength can result in compression of the double layer and flocculating of clays (Roth 1992). Indirect effect of liming on aggregate stability is associated with increases in microbial biomass, soil respiration, organic matter (Neale et al. 1997; Stenberg et al. 2000) and hyphae of arbuscular mycorrhizal fungi (Abbott and Robson 1985). Chan and Heenan (1999) reported that in soils with low initial aggregate stability, increases in macro-aggregate stability occurred after 1.5 years of addition of lime.

1.3 Implication of Improvement of Soil Health in Sandy Soil

For sandy soils, manipulative techniques to increase aggregate stability might be done by creating a suitable environment for hyphae and roots to grow. Working in clay and loam soils, several authors reported that the length of hyphae and plant roots contributed significantly to soil aggregation (Miller and Jastrow 1990; Boix-Fayos et al. 2001). Hyphal and root enmeshment of soil particles into soil clusters has been suggested to be the main mechanism by which aggregates are stabilised in soils (Tisdall and Oades 1982; Oades 1993; Miller and Jastrow 1992) reported the role of fungi and plant roots in increasing the retention of particulate organic matter (labile organic C) in no-till soil. There is considerable evidence indicating that labile carbohydrate C fractions are important in stabilising macro-aggregates in clay and loam soils (Haynes et al. 1991; Cambardella and Elliot 1993). The labile organic C mainly consists of the organic matter component including plant roots and microbial biomass. Plants that have a root architecture dominated by many fine roots and roots hairs are likely to have greater amount of organic C and greater influence on aggregation than plants with coarse roots systems (Degens 1997). Therefore, as plants have differing root morphologies and differing associations with mycorrhizal fungi, some plants have different effects on binding of soil particles than others (Miller and Jastrow 1990; Oades 1993). The hyphae of arbuscular mycorrhizal fungi produce glomalin that may have an important role in binding soil particles and strains of these fungi differ in their hyphal distribution. Combinations of arbuscular mycorrhizal fungi with dense hyphae and host plants with dense root architecture may have a synergistic effect on the cohesiveness of soil particles of sandy soils in relation to microbial biomass C.

REFERENCES

Abbott LK, Robson AD (1985) The effect of soil pH on the formation of VA mycorrhiza by two species of Glomus. Aust J Soil Res 23(2): 253 – 261

Abbott LK, Murphy DV (2003) What is soil biological fertility? In: Abbott LK, Murphy DV (eds) A Key to Sustainable Land Use in Agriculture: 1-15. Kluwer Academic Publishers, Nedtherland

Acton DF, Gregorich LJ (1995) The health of our soils: Toward Sustainable Agriculture in Canada. Agriculture and Agri-Food Canada, Ottawa

Amato M, Ladd JN (1988) Assay for microbial biomass based on ninhydrin reactive nitrogen in extracts of fumigated soils. Soil Biol Biochem 20: 107-114

Andreu V, Imeson AC, Rubio JL (2001) Temporal changes in soil aggregates and water erosion after a wildfire in a Mediterranean pine forest. Catena 44: 69-84

Arshad MA, Martin S (2002) Identifying critical limits for soil quality indicsators in agro-ecosystems. Agric Ecosyst Environ 88: 153-160

Attou F, Bruand A, Bissonnais Y (1998) Effect of clay content and silt-clay fabric on stability of artificial aggregates. Eur J Soil Sci 49: 569-577

Basic F, Kisic I, Mesic M, Nestroy O, Butorac A (2004) Tillage and crop management effects on soil erosion in central Croatia. Soil Tillage Res 78: 197-206

Boix-Fayos C, Calvo-Cases A, Imerson AC, Soriono-Soto MD (2001) Influence of soil properties on the aggregation of some Mediterranean soils and the use of aggregate size and stability as land degradation indicators. Catena 44: 47-67

Bronick CJ, Lal R (2005) Soil structure and management: a review. Geoderma 124: 3-22

Cambardella CA, Elliott ET (1993) Methods for physical separation and characterization of soil organic matter fractions. Geoderma. 56: 449-457

Caravaca F, Lax A, Albaladejo J (2001) Soil aggregate stability and organic matter in clay and fine silt fractions in urban refuse-amended semi-arid soils. Soil Sci Soc Am J 65: 1235-1238

Carter MR, Mele PM (1992) Changes in microbial biomass and structural stability at the surface of a duplex soil under direct drilling and stubble retention in north-eastern Victoria. Aust J Soil Res 30: 493 – 503

Carter MR, Gregorich EG, Anderson DW, Doran JW, Janzen HH, Pierce FJ (1997) Concept of soil quality and their significance. In: Gregorich EG, Carter MR (eds) Soil Quality for Crop Production and Ecosystem Health. Elsevier, Amsterdam. pp 1-19

Carter MR (2002) Soil quality for sustainable land management: Organic matter and aggregation interactions that maintain soil functions. Agron J 94: 38-47

Chan KY, Mead JA (1988) Surface physical properties of a sandy loam soil under different tillage practices. Aust J Soil Res 26: 549 – 559

Chan KY, Bowman A, Oates A (2001) Oxidizible organic carbon fractions and soil quality changes in an Oxic Paleustalf under different pasture leys. Soil Sci 166: 61-67

Chan KY, Heenan DP (1999) Lime-induced loss of soil organic carbon and effect on aggregate stability. Soil Sci Soc Am 63: 1841-1844

Chappell NA, Ternan JL, Bidin K (1999) Correlation of physicochemical properties and sub-erosional landforms with aggregate stability variations in a tropical Ultisol disturbed by forestry operations. Soil Tillage Res 50: 57-71

Dani Or, Ghezzehei TA (2002) Modelling post-tillage soil structural dynamics: A review. Soil Tillage Res 64: 41-59

Degens BP, Sparling GP, Abbott LK (1996) Increasing the length of hyphae in sand soil increases the amount of water-stable aggregates. Appl Soil Ecol 3: 149-159

Degens BP, Sparling GP (1996) Changes in aggregation do not correspond with changes in labile organic C fractions in soil amended with 14C-glucose. Soil Biol Biochem 28: 453-462

Degens BP (1997) Macro-aggregation of soils by biological bonding and binding mechanisms and the factors affecting these. Aust J Soil Res 35: 431-459

De Leon-Gonzalez F, Hernandez-Serrano MM, Etchevers JD, Payan-Zelaya F, Ordaz-Chaparro V (2000) Short-term compost effect on macro-aggregation in a sandy soil under low rainfall in the valley of Mexico. Soil Tillage Res 56: 213-217

Diekow J, Mielniczuk J, Knicker H, Bayer C. Dick, D.P, Kögel-Knabner I (2005) Soil C and N stocks as affected by cropping systems and nitrogen fertilization in a southern Brazil Acrisol managed under no-tillage for 17 years. Soil Tillage Res 81: 87-95

Doran JW, Safely M (1997) Defining and assessing soil health and sustainable productivity. In: Pankhurst C, Doube BM, Gupta V (eds) Biological Indicators of Soil Health. CAB International, Wallingford, pp 1-28

Edgerton DL, Harris JA, Birch P, Bullock P (1995) Linear relationship between aggregate stability and microbial biomass in three restored soils. Soil Biol Biochem 27: 1499-1501

Elliot ET (1986) Aggregate structure and carbon, nitrogen and phosphorus in native and cultivated soils. Soil Sci Soc Am J 50: 627-633

Farrington P, Campbell NA (1970) Properties of deep sandy soils and the growth of Lovegrass, *Eragrostis curvula* (Schrad.) Nees. Aust J Soil Res 8:123–132

Franzluebbers AJ, Arshad MA (1996) Water-stable aggregation and organic matter in four soils under conventional and zero tillage. Can J Soil Sci 76: 387-393

Franzluebbers AJ, Wright SF, Stuedemann JA (2000) Soil aggregation and glomalin under pastures in the Southern Piedmont USA. Soil Sci Soc Am J 64: 1018-1026

Gazey C, O'Conell M (2001) Soil acidity management pays off. Department of Agriculture, Western Australia. p 4

Guérif J, Richard G, Dürr C, Machet JM, Recous S, Roger-Estrade J (2001) A review of tillage effect on crop residue management, seedbed conditions and seedling establishment. Soil Tillage Res 61: 13-32

Harper RJ, Gilkes RJ (1994) Hardsetting in the surface horizons of sandy soils and its implications for soil classification and management. Aust J Soil Res 32: 603-619

Haynes RJ, Naidu R (1998) Influence of lime, fertilizer and manure applications on soil organic matter content and soil physical conditions. Nutr Cycl Agroecosys 51: 123-137

Kay BD, Vanden Bygaart AJ (2002) Conservation tillage and depth stratification of porosity and soil organic matter. Soil Tillage Res 66: 107-118

Kemper DW, Rosenau RC (1986) Aggregate stability and size distribution. In: Klute A (ed.) Methods of soil analysis, part 1. American Society of Agronomy: Madison. 9: 425-442

Kemper WD, Rosenau RC, Dexter AR (1987) Cohesion development in disrupted soils as affected by clay and organic matter content and temperature. Soil Sci Soc Am J 51: 860-867

Kiem R, Kandeler E (1997) Stabilization of aggregates by the microbial biomass as affected by soil texture and type. Appl Soil Ecol 5: 221-230

Lal R (2004) Agricultural activities and the global carbon cycle. Nutrient cycling in Agro-Ecosyst 70: 103-116

Lehrsch GA, Brown MJ (1995) Furrow erosion and aggregate stability variation in a Portneuf silt loam. Soil Technol 7: 327-341

Marquez CO, Garcia VJ, Cambardella CA, Schultz RC, Isenhart TM (2004) Aggregate-size stability distribution and soil stability. Soil Sci Soc Am J 68: 725-735

Martin JP, Martin WP, Page JB, Ranley WA, De Ment JD (1955) Soil aggregation. Adv Agron 7: 1-37

McFarlane DJ, Carter DJ (1990) The effect of erosion on soil productivity in south-western Australia. In: Working papers-Erosion productivity and erosion prediction workshop. 5th Australian Soil Conservation Conference, Perth, March 1990, pp 3-14

Miller RM, Jastrow JD (1990) Hierarchy of root and mycorrhizal fungi interactions with soil aggregation. Soil Biol Biochem 22: 579-584

Miller RM, Jastrow JD (1992) The role of mycorrhizal fungi in soil conservation. In: Bethlenfalvay GJ, Linderman RG (eds) Mycorrhizae in Sustainable Agriculture, ASA Special Publ. no. 54. Agron Soc Am, Crop Sci Soc Am and Soil Sci Soc Am, Madison, WI, pp 29-94

Mrabet R (2002) Stratification of soil aggregation and organic matter under conservation tillage systems in Africa. Soil Tillage Res 66: 119-128

Neale SP, Shah Z, Adams WA (1997) Changes in microbial biomass and nitrogen turnover in acidic organic soils following liming. Soil Biol Biochem 29: 1463-1474

Oades JM (1984) Soil organic matter and structural stability: Mechanisms and implications for management. Plant Soil 76: 319-337

Oades JM (1993) The role of biology in the formation, stabilization and degradation of soil structure. Geoderma 56: 377-400

Packer IJ, Hamilton GJ, Koen TB (1992) Runoff, soil loss and soil physical property changes of light textured surface soils from long-term tillage treatments. Aust J Soil Res 30: 789-806

Pagliai M, Vignozzi N, Pelligrini S (2004) Soil structure and the effect of management practices. Soil Tillage Res 79: 131-143

Pankhurst CE, Doube BM, Gupta VVSR (1997) Biological indicators of soil health: Synthesis. In: Pankhurst C, Doube BM, Gupta VVSR (eds) Biological Indicators of Soil Health. CAB International, Wallingford, Oxon, UK. pp 419-435

Pathan SM, Aylmore LAG, Colmer TD (2002) Reduced leaching of nitrate, ammonium, and phosphorus in a sandy soil by fly ash amendment. Aust J Soil Res 40: 1201-1211

Parfitt RL, Theng BKG, Whitton JS, Shepherd TG (1997) Effect of clay minerals and land use on organic matter pools. Geoderma 75: 1-12

Paustian K, Six J, Elliott ET, Hunt HW (2000) Management options for reducing CO_2 from agricultural soil. Biogeochemistry 48: 147-163

Powlson DS (1994) The soil microbial biomass: before, beyond and back. In: Ritz K, Dighton J, Giller GE (Eds.), Beyong the Biomass. Wiley, Chichester, UK, pp 3-20

Prunty L, Greenland R (1997) Nitrate leaching using two potato-corn N-fertilizer plans on sandy soil. Agric Ecosyst Environ 65: 1-13

Rees RM, Bingham IJ, Baddeley JA, Watson CA (2005) The role of plants and land management in sequestering soil carbon in temperate arable and grassland ecosystems. Geoderma 128: 130-154

Roth CH (1992) Soil sealing and crusting in tropical South America. In: Sumner ME, Stewart BA (eds) Advances in Soil Science. Soil Crusting-Chemical and Physical Processes. pp 267-300

Sainju UM, Whitehead WF, Singh BP (2005) Carbon accumulation in cotton, sorghum, and underlying soil as influenced by tillage, cover crops, and nitrogen fertilization. Plant Soil 273: 219-234

Sauerbeck DR (2001) CO_2 emissions and C sequestration by agriculture: perspectives and limitations. Nutr Cycl Agroecosyst 60: 253-266

Schulzc ED, Freibauer A (2005) Carbon unclocked from soils. Nature 437:205

Schipper LA, Sparling GP (2000) Performance of soil condition indicators across taxonomic groups and land use. Soil Sci Am J 64: 300-311

Scholter M, Dilly O, Munch JC (2003) Indicators for evaluating soil quality. Agric. Ecosyst Environ 98: 255-262

Select Committee into Land Conservation (1990) Discussion paper no. 2. Agricultural Region of Western Australia. Western Australia Legislative Assembly: Perth, Western Australia

Seybold CA, Herrick JE (2001) Aggregate stability kit for soil assessments. Catena 44: 37-45

Shepherd TG, Saggar S, Newman RH, Ross CW, Dando JL (2001) Tillage-induced changes to soil structure and organic carbon fractions in New Zealand soils. Aust J Soil Res 39: 465-489

Shepherd MA, Harrison R, Webb J (2002) Managing soil organic matter – implications for soil structure on organic farms. Soil Use Manage 18: 284-292

Shipitalo MJ, Dick WA, Edwards WM (2000) Conservation tillage and macropore factors that affect water movement and fate of chemicals. Soil Tillage Res 53:167-183

Six J, Elliot ET, Paustian K (2000) Soil structure and soil organic matter: II. A normalized stability index and the effect of mineralogy. Soil Sci Am J 64: 1042-1049

Stenberg M, Stenberg B, Ridberg T (2000) Effect of reduced tillage on microbial activity and soil properties in a weakly structured soil. Appl Soil Ecol 14:135-145

Tisdall JM, Oades JM (1979) Stabilisation of soil aggregates by the root systems of rye grass. Aust J Soil Res 17: 429-441

Tisdall JM, Oades JM (1982) Organic matter and water-stable aggregates in soils. J Soil Sci. 33: 141-163

Wander MM, Water GL, Nissen TM, Bollero GA, Andrews SS, Cavanaugh-Grant DA (2002) Soil Quality: Science and Process. Agron J 94: 23-32

Wang X, Gong Z (1998) Assessment and analysis of soil quality changes after eleven years of reclamation in subtropical China. Geoderma 81:339-355

Warkentin BP (1995) The changing concept of soil quality. J. Soil and Water Conserv 50: 226-228

Weaver DM, Ritchie GSP, Anderson GC (1988) Phosphorus leaching in sandy soils.II. Laboratory studies of the long-term effects of the phosphorus source. Aust J Soil Res 26: 191 – 200

Webster EA, Hopkins DW, Chudek JA, Haslam SFI, Simek M, Picek T (2001) Relationship between microbial carbon and resource quality of soil carbon. J Environ Qual 30: 147-150

White PF (1990) The influence of alternative tillage systems on the distribution of nutrients and organic-carbon in some common Western Australian wheat-belt soils. Aust J Soil Res 28: 95-116

Wienhold BJ, Andrews SS, Karlen DL (2004) Soil quality: A review of science and the experiences in the USA. Environ. Geochem. Health 26: 89-95

Wright SF, Franke-Snyder M, Morton JB, Upadhyaya A (1996) Time-course study and partial characterization of a protein on hyphae of arbuscular mycorrhizal fungi during active colonization of roots. Plant Soil 181: 193-203

Wright SF, Upadhyaya A (1996) Extraction of an abundant and unusual protein from soil and comparison with hyphal protein of arbuscular mycorrhizal fungi. Soil Sci 161: 575-586

Wright SF (2000) A fluorescent antibody assay for hyphae and glomalin from arbuscular mycorrhizal fungi. Plant Soil 226: 171-177

Zentner RP, Wall DD, Nagy CN, Smith EG, Young DL, Miller PR, Campbell CA, McConkey BG, Brandt SA (2002) Economics of crop diversification and soil tillage opportunities in Canadian prairies. J Agron 94: 216-230

Clostridium botulinum: The Source of Bioterror and Beauty

BR SINGH[1], B LI[1], SK SHARMA[2] and T-WCHANG[1]

1. INTRODUCTION

Botulinum neurotoxins (BoNTs) are a very unique group of proteins, with extreme biological activities as toxins, therapeutics, and cosmetics. There are only about a couple of hundred cases of botulism globally. However, because of the extreme toxicity of the agent (about 100 billion times more toxic than cyanide, based on mouse lethal dose), it is estimated to one of the most expensive food poisoning diseases (Todd 1989).

Currently, there are seven serotypes of BoNTs (A to G) known to be produced by different strains of anaerobic bacteria, *Clostridium botulinum*. Although there is little immuno-cross-reactivity, and there are only less than 50% sequence homologies among various serotypes of BoNTs, their site of action, mode of action, and target of action are remarkably similar, if not identical. Each of the BoNTs binds to the presynaptic region of nerve membrane at nerve-muscle junctions, translocates whole or a part of the toxin inside the nerve cells, and blocks the release of acetylcholine, resulting in a flaccid muscle paralysis (Li and Singh 1999; Arnon et al. 2001; Singh 2000, 2002)

Combination of extreme toxicity, nerve as the site of action and resulting in muscular paralysis, has made botulinum neurotoxin a

1 Department of Chemistry and Biochemistry, and Botulinum Research Center, University of Massachusetts Dartmouth, 285 Old Westport Road, Dartmouth, MA 02747; E-mail - bsingh@umassd.edu

2 Center for Food Safety Applied Nutrition, US Department of Food and Drug Administration, College Park, MD 20740

molecule of elevated anxiety and curiosity. It has been attempted as a bio-terror agent, a fully developed biological weapon for military use, and also as a therapeutic agent against numerous neuro-muscular disorders, such as strabismus, blepherospasm, and torticollis, involving excessive release of neurotransimitter. More curiously, therapeutic botulinum neurotoxin preparations are being used for cosmetic purposes to remove frown lines and facial wrinkles.

Clostridium botulinum, therefore, has become a source of bio-terror and beauty, both being pursued simultaneously for scientific development to counter the former while promoting the latter.

Clostridium botulinum *C. botulinum*, which was first isolated from a contaminated ham and from the spleen of a patient by Van Ermengem in Belgium in 1895 (Foster 1993; Van Ermengem 1897), is a Gram-positive, spore-forming bacterium which grows anaerobically at 37°C or 30°C under pH 6.5-7.0 conditions.

Most of *C. botulinum* as well as *C. butyricum* and *C. baratii* can produce botulinum neurotoxins (BoNTs). Strains of *C. botulinum* are classified into seven types, A to G, according to the antigenic properties of neurotoxins they produce. Generally, one strain of *C. botulinum* can only produce one type of neurotoxin, but several strains that produce more than one type of neurotoxin have been recognized over the years. One type C-strain (C6813) was found to produce the mosaic neurotoxin, of which one-third of the C-terminal region was similar to that of type D neurotoxin (Moriishi et al. 1996). One type A strain, called type AB now, was shown to produce both, type A and type B neurotoxins (Fujinaga et al. 1995). *C. botulinum* type G organism differs phenotypically from other *C. botulinum* types, is now designated as *C. argentinense* (Campbell et al. 1993a). *Clostridium butyricum* and *Clostridium baratii* were found producing type E and type F neurotoxins, respectively (Fujii et al. 1993c; Hutson et al. 1993).

Strains of *C. botulinum* can also be divided into four distinct phenotypic groups (I to IV) based on biochemical properties and nucleic acid hybridization studies. Group-I includes type A, proteolytic strains of types B and F. Group-II includes type E, non-proteolytic strains of types B and F. Group-III is types C and D and Group-IV is type G (Campbell et al. 1993b). Rînner, Stackebrandt (1994) and Campbell et al. (1993b) proved from a very high level of 23S rRNA sequence similarity that 4 Groups I, II, III and IV *C. botulinum* represent a single genetic unit phylogenetically remote from each other and that the marked genotypic variation within the species does not correlate with the neurotoxins produced. *C. baratii* belonged to a new group-group V. The Same conclusions were drawn from 16S rRNA sequence similarities (Hutson et al. 1993). However, the genetic relationship inferred from the BoNT sequences differs markedly from above conclusions and it is clearly established now that all three types of BoNT/F (proteolytic, non-proteolytic and *C. baratii* type F) are genealogically highly related (Elmore et al. 1995).

The spores of proteolytic *C. botulinum* are heat resistant and do not multiply at temperatures below 10°C, but the spores of non-proteolytic *C. botulinum*, which are less heat-resistant, can germinate relatively rapidly at temperatures in the range of 2 to 10°C (Lund and Peck 1994). Type A-*C. botulinum* has 0.39 hour generation time and reaches its exponential growth after five hours of anaerobic incubation of spores (Call et al. 1995).

The bacterial growth curve of type A *C. botulinum* (strain Hall) shows a lag period of four hours, and log phase at 10 hours before reaching the stationary phase (Shukla and Singh 2000).

The studies with a monoclonal antitoxin conjugated with colloidal gold demonstrated that the BoNT was synthesized in the cell cytoplasm at late-exponential phase (seventeen hours) and reached its maximum concentration at stationary phase (24-25 hours). The BoNT was translocated across the cytoplasmic membrane and then exported to the extracellular medium via cell-wall exfoliation. The greatest proportion of BoNT was located within the cell-wall at fortyfive hours (Call et al. 1995).

The spores of *C. botulinum* are widely distributed in soil, mud and surface waters over much of the globe, but different types of *C. botulinum* prevail in different geographical locations. In the western United States, Brazil, Argentina and China, type-A spores predominate, while proteolytic type-B spores tend to predominate in soils of the eastern United States, and non-proteolytic type-B in Britain and Europe. Type E is often associated with freshwater and marine sediments, and northern regions such as northern Canada and Japan (McClure et al. 1994). Initially, the strains of *C. botulinum* type-A were divided into two groups, infant type A and type A, based on the cases of infant botulism in Japan and the classical food-borne botulism (Sakaguchi et al. 1990). But studies of Cordoba et al. (1994) revealed that the strains of *C. botulinum* type A could be divided into two groups, A-1 and A-2, based on different geographical locations isolated and did not correlate with their origins as both are from the cases of infant botulism and classical food-borne botulism. Strains isolated from infant botulism in Japan and several strains isolated from classical food-borne botulism in United Kingdom and in Mauritius fell into group A-2 while all strains examined from the USA and two strains from UK, from both infant and food-borne botulism fell into group A-1. Group A-1 is typical *C. botulinum* type A containing hemagglutinin genes and shows hemagglutinin activity. Several group A-1 strains contain an unexpressed type B neurotoxin gene. Group A-2 lack the hemagglutinin gene and posses no hemagglutinin activity. The type A neurotoxin genes from group A-1 and A-2 are different. Recently, a third isotype of type-A botulinum neurotoxin (A-3) has been identified, which differs significantly with types A-1 and A-2 in its amino-acid sequence (Marks 2004).

3. BOTULISM

Historically, botulism – derived from botulinus meaning sausage, was discovered long before the name appeared in the literature. Earliest reference to possible botulism related disease is found as an edict by Emperor Leo VI of Byzantium (886-911) in which manufacturing of blood sausage was forbidden (Erbguth 2004). However, the first systematic study of 'sausage poisoning' was carried out in 1815 by a health officer in the town of Herrenberg of Wurttemberg (Germany) by the name of J. G. Steinbuch, and later independently by Justinus Kerner, another medical officer in the town of Welzheim in Wurttemberg (Erbguth 2004). Kerner's work was published in journals and monographs in early 1800s. In 1822, Kerner described his observations and experiments with sausage toxin, also referred as fat poison, in a monograph. Kerner wrote, "The nerve conduction is brought by the toxin into a condition in which its influence on the chemical process of life is interrupted. The capacity of nerve conduction is interrupted by the toxin in the same way as in an electrical conductor by rust". Interestingly, Kerner had also hypothesized on the idea of sausage toxin being used as a therapeutic agent (Erbguth 1998).

Botulism is a severe disease characterized by flaccid paralysis and caused by botulism neurotoxins, extremely potent food poisons with a mouse lethal dose of 0.1 ng/kg (Montecucco and Schiavo 1993). Three types of botulism have been observed, so far. Classical food-borne botulism is caused by ingestion of food where the bacteria have produced the neurotoxin. Infant botulism result due to the production of neurotoxin in the intestine after germination and outgrowth of ingested spores. Wound botulism maybe due to the outgrowth of bacteria in the wound or due to unknown origin (Hatheway and Ferreira 1996; Cordoba et al. 1994). Classical food-borne botulism in humans is caused mainly by *C. botulinum* types A, B, E and rarely by type F neurotoxins. Classical food borne botulism in animals is always caused by *C. botulinum* types C-1 and D neurotoxins (Cordoba et al. 1994; Fach et al. 1993). In contrast, the causative agents for infant botulism can be *C. botulinum* types A or B neurotoxins or *Clostridium butyricum* type E and *Clostridium baratii* type F neurotoxins. The wound botulism is rare in humans and the causative agents are either type A or type B from group I (Hatheway 1993), but is increasing significantly in recent years among drug users (Merrison et al. 2002). Neurotoxins can also be used in the therapy of a variety of human muscle disorders such as strabismus, hemifacial spasm and blepherospasm (Schantz and Johnson 1992; Eleopra et al. 2004).

Various animal models are used to examine mechanism of botulism in animals and humans. Different serotypes of BoNT are known to selectively cause the disease in different animals. For example, BoNT/C is mostly associated with avian botulism, BoNT/C and BoNT/D with cattle, sheep and horse, and BoNT/A, BoNT/B and BoNT/E are associated with human, cattle and horse botulism, while BoNT/E is particularly associated with fish botulism (Huss and Eskildsen 1974; Burns and Williams 1975; Ala-Huikku et al. 1977; Fernandez et al. 1989; Baldassi et al. 1991; Haagsma 1991; Jeffrey et al. 1994; Ashie et al. 1996; Ortolani et al. 1997). It is believed that botulism by a selective serotype of BoNT in a given animal is in part related to the presence of a high affinity receptor for that serotype in the host animal system (Fig. 1).

3.1 Botulinum Neurotoxins

Botulism neurotoxins are large proteins (150 kDa, 7S). They remain inactive as a single chain after synthesis and are activated by protease nicking to form a dichain molecule (a 50 kDa light chain and a 100 kDa heavy chain) linked together by a disulphide bond. The proteolytic strains of *C. botulinum* produce endogenous proteases, but non-proteolytic strains of *C. botulinum* require exogenous proteases, such as trypsin in the intestinal tract (Call et al. 1995). The light chain or heavy chain individually are non-toxic and play different roles in the pathway of intoxication. The light chains of neurotoxins are in fact zinc endopeptidases, which catalyze the hydrolysis of synaptic vesicle docking and fusion complex and block the release of acetylcholine (Ahnert-hilger and Bigalke 1995). The heavy chains may fold into a conformation that protects the neurotoxins against the proteolytic cleavage (Schantz and Johnson 1992). The C-terminal part of heavy chains (H_C) is responsible for cell surface binding and the N-terminal part of heavy chains (H_N) is involved in channel formation. The H_C domain is also divided (Fig. 2) into two structural, and possibly functional domains (H_{C1} and H_{C2}) with their specific binding to protein and lipid receptors.

The botulinum neurotoxin is produced in three progenitor toxin forms: M, L and LL forms. The M form consists of neurotoxin (150 kDa) and a non-toxic protein component (120 kDa) which is called neurotoxin binding protein (NBP) (Zhang et al. 1995) or non-toxic non-hemagglutinin component (NTNH) (East and Collins 1994) with 12S molecular size (the molecular size of complex forms is expressed as sedimentation equilibrium values). The L form has molecular weight of about 500 kDa and a molecular size of 16S. The LL form is about 900 kDa and 19S. The

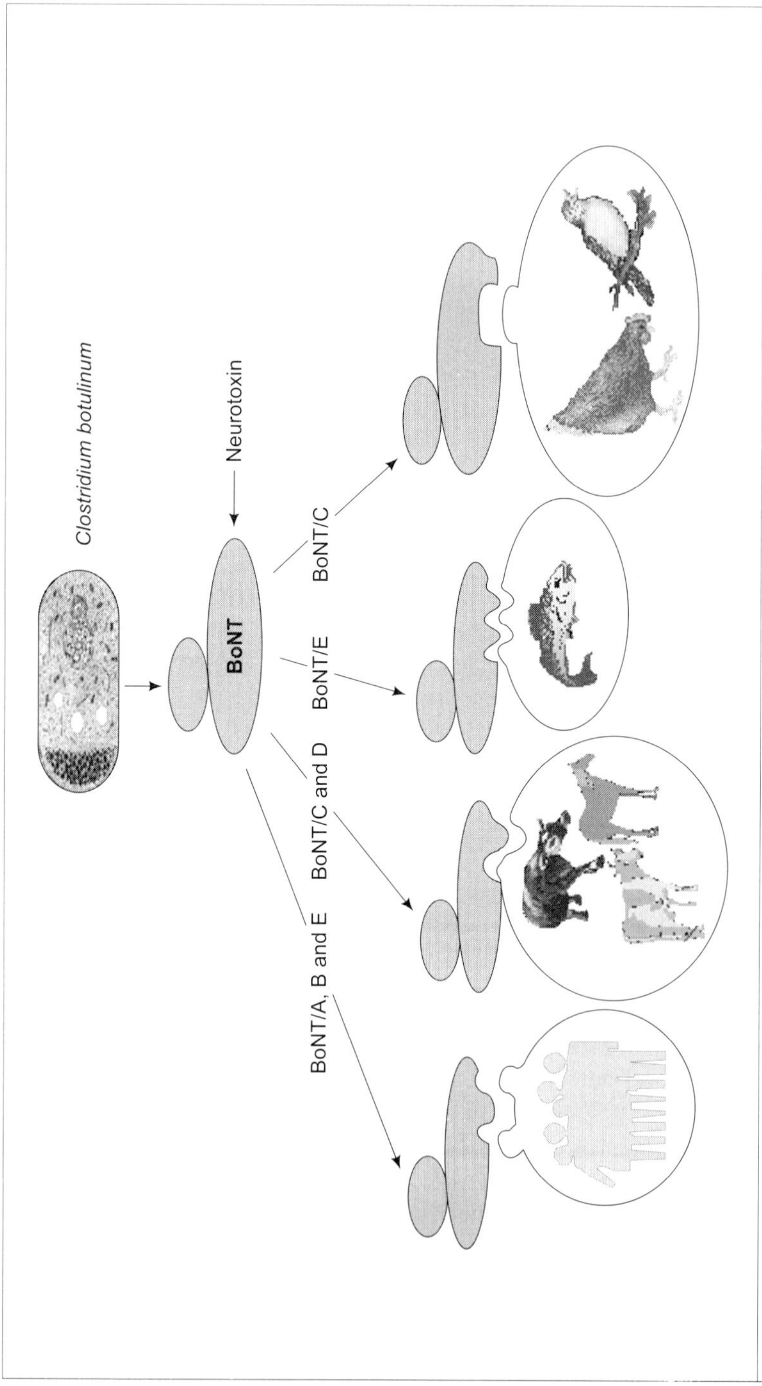

Fig. 1 Schematic representation of different binding topography of various serotypes of BoNT for their interactions with unique protein receptors in different animals.

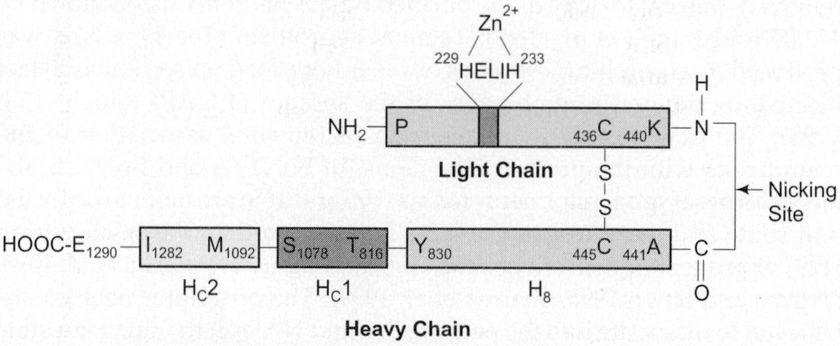

Fig. 2 Schematic diagram of BoNT showing its L and H chains. The two different domains of the H chain shaded with different patterns indicate the N-terminal and C-terminal halves (about 50 kDa each).

L and LL complexes consist of several hemagglutinin components besides the BoNT and NBP, and exhibit hemagglutinin activity (Fujii 1995; Somers and Dasgupta 1991). In 1998, Singh research group named the proteins other than the neurotoxin present in botulinum neurotoxin complex as neurotoxin associated proteins or NAPs (Fu et al. 1998). BoNT/A complex can exist in three forms: M, L or LL. BoNT/B, /C and /D complexes involve in two forms: L and M. BoNT/E and /F complexes are known to exist only in M form, and BoNT/G complex exists only in L form (Fujita et al. 1995). Some of types A and B neurotoxins, which cause the infant botulism, also exist in M form (Cordoba et al. 1994).

The size of the complex formed in BoNT/A and BoNT/B depends on the medium for bacterial growth. The addition of iron or manganese to the growth medium results in a higher concentration of M and L forms of neurotoxin complexes (Schantz and Johnson 1992). In addition, some foods such as vegetables have high botulinogenic properties. *C. botulinum* types A and B are found to produce the stable L and LL forms of neurotoxin complexes in vegetables, whereas they produce the less stable M complex in tuna and pork (Schantz and Johnson 1992).

The non-toxic components of progenitor neurotoxin (NAPs) appear to play a critical role in the toxico-infection by neurotoxin. They are presumed to protect neurotoxins against the digestive proteases and stomach acidity when the progenitor neurotoxins pass through the gastrointestinal tract (Ahnert-Hilger and Bigalke 1995; Schantz and Johnson 1992; Somer and Dasgupta 1991). Such protection is important in the food poisoning activity of the neurotoxin. For example, if NAPs are removed, the oral toxicity of the purified type A neurotoxin goes down by 43,000 fold (Singh et al. 1995). Tetanus neurotoxin (TeNT), which was produced by anaerobic *Clostridium tetani*, is not a food poison and is in fact inactive by the oral route because of the absence of NAPs (Singh et al. 1995). The oral toxicity increases with incremental association of the neurotoxins with the protective proteins. In BoNT/A and BoNT/B, the larger forms of progenitor neurotoxins (19S and 16S) are more toxic by the oral route and more resistant to acid and pepsin than the smaller form (12S) of progenitor neurotoxins (Schantz and Johnson 1992; Fu et al. 1998; Sharma and Singh 1998; Sharma et al. 1999). The progenitor neurotoxins believed to dissociate into the neurotoxins and NAPs in the small intestine or in an alkaline condition and the components of NAPs might also play a role in the adhesion of progenitor neurotoxins to the intestinal tissue before the dissociation of the progenitor neurotoxins (Sakaguchi 1983; Fujinaga et al. 1994, 1997, 2000). Certain carbohydrate groups, which help the NAPs to anchor to the intestinal wall, have been identified (Inoue et al. 2001; Nishikawa et al. 2004).

The neurotoxins and nontoxic components can reassociate spontaneously when the pH is lowered (Hambleton 1992). An ordered interaction between neurotoxins and their NAPs was suggested by the observation that the L and LL forms of type A neurotoxin form crystals (Schantz and Johnson 1992).

3.3 C. *botulinum* Genomic Organisation

C. botulinum (Type A, strain Hall A, ATCC 3502) genomes have an average GC content of about 28.2% (Sanger web 2003), which is lower than that of other bacteria (Hatheway1993). Most *C. botulinum* strains and related nontoxigenic species were believed to carry plasmids. Type A *C. botulinum* (strain Hall A, ATCC3502) contains a 16,344 bp plasmid (Sanger web 2003) and *C. tetani* (strain E88) contains a very large plasmid in the size of 74,082 bp (Holger et al. 2003). All of the proteolytic type F strains tested by Strom et al. (1984) contain a single 11.5 Mdal (17.48Kb, 1Kb of dsDNA = 660KDa) (Brinkmann web 2004) plasmid, but only some of the non-proteolytic type F strains harbour a single 2.2 Mdal plasmid. Codon usage in the botulinum gene was similar to that of the tetanus toxin gene, but it is different from that of *E. coli* genes (Makoff et al. 1989). 90.3% of the degenerated codons from botulinum and tetanus toxin genes end in A or U and AUG, and UAA are translational initiation and termination codons (Schantz and Johnson 1992). A number of codons from neurotoxin genes are rarely used in *E. coli* genes. This is an important factor that will lead to a poor expression of neurotoxin gene in *E. coli* (Clayton et al. 1995).

The genomic organisations of BoNTs and their associated proteins were suggested by researchers (Hauser et al. 1994; East et al. 1994; Fujita et al. 1995), which are summarised in Fig. 3. No characteristic signal peptide sequences are observed in any of the progenitor neurotoxin genes. The genes of progenitor neurotoxins are closely grouped as operons on the chromosome, phage or plasmid. NBP gene is located only 26 bp (type A, strain 667Ab or NCTC2916 or CDC3281) (Santos-Buelga et al. 1998; Hutson et al. 1996; Rodriguez et al. 1998) or 44bp (type A, strain ATCC 3502) (Sanger, 2003) or 15 bp (type C, strain C-6814 or C-Yoichi) (Sagane et al. 2000; 2001) or 15 bp (type D, strain D-4947) (Kouguchi et al. 2002) or 11 bp (type F, Langeland) (East et al. 1998) or 12 bp (type F, strain F202) (East et al. 1994) or 14 bp (type F, *C. baratii*, strain ATCC 43256) (East et al. 1998) or 85 bp (type G, strain ATCC 27322) (Bhandari et al. 1997) upstream of the BoNT gene. There are two promoter regions for neurotoxin genes. One overlaps the C-terminal end of NBP genes and the other is shared with the NBP genes, controlling co-transcription of the two genes. The neurotoxin genes are either transcribed alone or along with NBP genes via a polycistronic mRNA, and thus these two genes form an operon. HA gene clusters form another operon transcribed in the opposite directions from the BoNT and NBP genes. HA gene clusters are located 262 bp (in type C, strain C-6814 or C-Yoichi) (Sagane et al. 2000; 2001) or 261 bp (type D, strain D-4947) (Kouguchi et al. 2002) or 925 bp (in type A, strain Hall A-hyper) (Dineen et al. 2003) or 698 bp (type A, ATCC 3502) or 811 bp (type A(B), NCTC 2916)(Rodriguez et al. 1998) upstream of the NBP gene, respectively. Each HA gene contains its own transcription terminator which is predicted to form a stem-and-loop structure in the mRNA.

3.4 *C. botulinum* Neurotoxin Genes

The genes of all seven types of neurotoxins have been sequenced and the polypeptide chain lengths deduced from the nucleotide sequences are approximately the same, ranging from 1251 (BoNT/E, strain Beluga) to 1315 (TeNT, strain E88 Massachusettes) amino acid residues (Elmore et al. 1995; Hutson et al. 1994; Campbell et al. 1993a; Thompson et al. 1990; East et al. 1992; Whelan et al. 1992; Binz et al. 1990a, 1990b; Fujii et al. 1990). However, the gene localization of different serotypes of BoNT is different. BoNT/A, B and E genes are located in chromosome, BoNT/C1, D in phage and BoNT/G and BuNT/E in plasmids (Hauser et al. 1995; Ahnert-Hilger and Bigalke 1995). The neurotoxin gene (tetX) and its transcription factor (tetR) are also clusterly located in the 74kb plasmid in *C. tetani* (Holger et al. 2003). Whether the BoNT/F genes are located in chromosome or in plasmid is not clear yet (Hauser et al. 1995, Strom et al. 1984). The homology among all types of BoNT genes ranges from 55.2% to 98.2% and

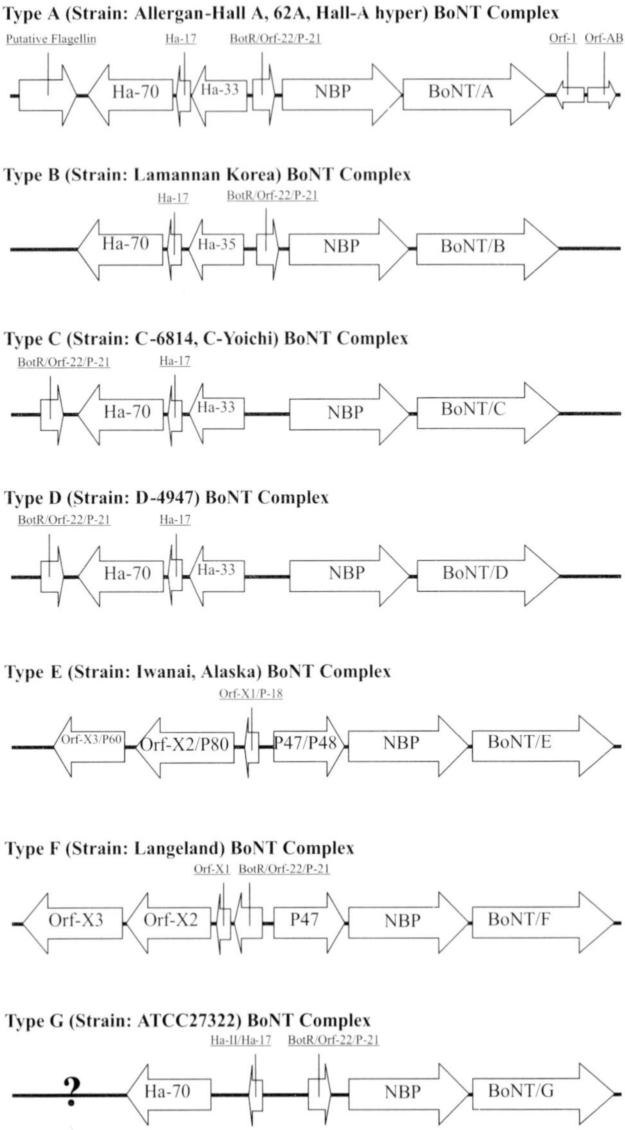

Fig. 3 Genomic organisation of all 7 types of *C. botulinum.* Proteins corresponding to genes labeled as ORF (types E, F and G) are yet to be identified, although tentative assignment has been made for type E genes. The question mark (?) in type G *C. botulinum* reflect unavailability of the sequence data.

is listed in Table 1. The homology of tetanus gene to other BoNT genes ranges from 55.3% to 62.1%, which is lower than that among BoNT genes. In table 1, BoNT/NpB is non-proteolytic type B neurotoxin, BuNT/E is neurotoxin produced by *C. butyricum* type E and BaNT/F is neurotoxin produced by *C. baratii.*

Several strains of *Clostridium botulinum* or *Clostridium butyrium* do not possess BoNT genes (non-toxic *Clostridium* strains) (Zhou et al. 1993). The following evidences from the studies of BoNT and TeTx genes suggest that BoNT and TeTx genes derive from a common ancestor and that the variation of BoNT genes probably result from BoNT gene transfer among *Clostridium* species and subsequent DNA evolution (Elmore et al. 1995; Hauser et al. 1995). The non-toxic *Clostridium* strains may have evolved after loss of the neurotoxin genes (Rînner and Stackebrandt 1994).

- The G+C content of BoNT (26.31%) and TeTx genes (27.83%) is similar, as is that of *C. botulinum* genomes (28.2%) (Fairweather et al. 1986; Holger et al. 2003; Willis 1990).
- The percent identity among BoNTs and TeNT at the amino acid level range from 34.1 to 96.9% (Table 1) and are unrelated to other known protein sequences.

The BoNT genes could localize at chromosome, phage or plasmids.

BoNT/E and BuNT/E are produced by two very different *Clostridium* strains, *C. botulinum* and *C. butyricum*, respectively yet they share 97% identity at the amino acid level, which is much higher than the average identity between different BoNT genes produced by *C. botulinum* (43%). The similar high identity (90%) is observed between BoNT/Bp (proteolytic type B) and BoNT/Bnp (non-proteolytic type B). The identity between BoNT/F and BaNT/F (produced by *C. baratii*) is also high (70.5%) (Table 1).

Nucleic acid sequences of BoNT/A genes from *C. botulinum* type A strains 62 A and NCTC2916 are identical but there are totally unrelated after the ninetyseven nucleotides downstream from the three nucleotide regions of the BoNT/A genes (Binz et al. 1990; Thompson et al. 1990).

The neurotoxin genes of *C. botulinum* type C strains could be transformed into *C. noveyi* type A strains with appropriate vectors (Rînner and Stackebrandt 1994). Evidences show (Zhou et al.1993) that the neurotoxin genes can be transferred from *Clostridium butyricum* to a non-toxigenic *Clostridium botulinum* type E-like strains with a helper strain (non-toxic *C. butyricum*).

The fact that some *C. botulinum* strains contain more than one type of neurotoxin genes (A(B), A(F), or BF) supports the gene transfer hypothesis and suggest that additional genetic events (mutation, deletion, recombination, etc) have occurred. This hypothesis is also proved by the

Table 1 Comparison of clostridial neurotoxins showing per cent identity (lower left) and per cent similarity (upper right) (from Hauser et al. 1995)

	TeTx	*BoNT A*	*BoNT B*	*BoNT NpB*	*BoNT C1*	*BoNT D*	*BoNT E*	*BuNT E*	*BoNT F*	*BaNT F*	*BoNT G*
TeTx		55.3	61.8	62.1	56.2	55.3	57.8	58.0	59.0	57.9	60.8
BoNT/A	35.4		60.0	60.2	55.2	55.2	61.0	60.5	61.8	63.2	58.8
BoNT/B	42.4	44.1		96.0	59.1	57.3	61.6	61.3	61.7	62.5	74.9
BoNT/NpB	42.7	40.7	**92.8**		58.4	56.6	61.9	61.3	61.8	62.8	74.2
BoNT/C1	35.1	33.9	36.0	35.0		69.1	55.9	56.0	56.3	56.4	57.4
BoNT/D	34.1	34.3	36.6	36.4	53.8		57.1	57.1	57.1	56.8	57.6
BoNT/E	37.9	41.3	40.0	40.2	34.3	35.6		98.2	77.3	77.2	60.0
BuNT/E	37.9	41.5	40.0	40.1	34.8	35.4	**96.9**		77.1	76.8	60.0
BoNT/F	38.5	41.4	41.0	41.7	34.6	36.4	62.2	62.1		80.7	58.6
BaNT/F	40.5	44.1	42.8	43.3	35.1	35.5	63.9	63.6	70.5		59.5
BoNT/G	41.6	41.2	58.4	57.7	35.0	37.1	39.5	40.6	39.3	40.7	

results (Hutson et al. 1996) that some of type A strains contain silent type B gene. The type B neurotoxin gene is unexpressed because the deletion and substitution of some nucleotides result in multiple stop signals due to the reading frame shift.

The gene transfers among *Clostridium* strains probably involve a mobile DNA element on the chromosome or the mobilization of a large plasmid harboring the BoNT gene (Hauser et al. 1995).

3.5 C. *Botulinum* Neurotoxin Binding Protein (NBP) Genes

The nucleic acid sequences of *C. botulinum* types A, B, C1, D, E, F and *C. butyricum* type E NBP genes have been determined (Hutson et al. 1996; Fujita et al. 1995; Hauser et al. 1994; East and Collins, 1994; Fujii et al. 1993; 1993; 1993). All of the NBP genes are approximately 3.5kb in length, similar, to BoNT genes. Several experimental results demonstrate that the expression of NBP genes is very important to the BoNTs. First, each NBP gene is located at the N-terminal of BoNT gene with very little space between them (46bp in type A, 14bp in type C, 27bp in type E from both *C. botulinum* and *C. butyricum*, 14bp in type F). Second, the transcription of the NBP gene is always in association with the BoNT gene and only the BoNT gene, not the NBP gene which can be transcribed alone. Third, all types of *C. botulinum* contain a NBP gene.

The homology of NBPs is higher than that of BoNT genes (Table 2), which suggests that the NBP genes are more conserved than the BoNT gene. The close identities between NBP/E and NBP/EBu (98%) (Fujii et al. 1993), and between BoNT/E and BuNT/E (97%) are the strong evidences that the NBP and BoNT genes transfer among the genus *Clostridium*. It is very surprising that the identity of the BoNT/C and BoNT/D genes (53.8%) is much lower than that of the corresponding NBP genes (93.0%).

Table 2 Per cent amino acid identities (lower left-hand triangle) and similarities (upper right-hand triangle) of NBP.

	A	*B*	*C*	*D*	*E*	*F*	*G*
A		90.5	83.0	83.0	79.0	81.5	86.0
B	81.5		81.5	81.5	76.0	78.0	87.0
C	65.4	66.5		95.0	73.0	75.5	82.0
D	65.4	66.5	93.0		72.0	73.5	80.0
E	65.8	59.0	54.0	53.0		77.0	69.0
F	74.0	61.5	56.5	55.5	65.0		73.0
G	72.0	75.0	65.0	64.0	54.0	58.0	

However, this result corresponds to the fact that both types, C and D, are responsible for animal botulism, but cleave the different substrates, Hpc-1/syntaxin and VAMP/synaptobrevin, respectively.

There is a short (14 residues) repeat in the amino acid sequence of the NBPs which could show as L-L/N-S-L-I/M/V-S/T-T/S-A/T-I-P-F-P/L-Y/F-G from 97 to 111 and from 136 to 150. The second repeat may play an important role in distinguishing the M complex from other types of progenitor neurotoxins as evidences from the following observation. First, the amino acid residues from 99 to 149, which include the second repeat from 136-150, were deleted in NBPs from M complex (NBP/E, NBP/F and NBP/EBu). Second, NBPs from M forms of A, C and D progenitor neurotoxins were cleaved in the second repeat region to yield approximately 13 kDa and 106 kDa components (Fujita et al. 1995).

NBP have also sequence homology to both BoNT (all types) and TeNT in light chain area. This area is also the conserved domain named peptidase_M27 area. NBP has not been found any peptidase activity but did contain the protein sequence similarity with a known Zn dependent peptidase.

3.6 C. *Botulinum* Hemagglutinin Genes

The hemagglutinin genes HA33, HA17 and HA70 from type C *C. botulinum* were sequenced by Hauser et al. (1994). The three genes, which are closely linked and form an operon, are transcribed alone or together in the opposite direction to that of NBP and BoNT genes. The HA17 gene encoding 146 amino acids is located between the HA33 and HA70 genes. Homology among the HA33 genes is shown in Table 3.

The high homology between HA/A and HA/B and low homology between HA/A, HA/B, HA/C and HA/D may reflect similarity in specificity and activity of type A and type B, both of which cause human botulism (East et al. 1994).

Table 3 Per cent amino acid identities (lower left-hand triangle) and similarities (upper right-hand triangle) of HA 33

	HA33/A	*HA33/Bnp*	*HA33/Bp*	*HA33/C*	*HA33/D*
HA33/A		93.0	88.5	58.0	58.0
HA33/Bnp*	89.0		89.0	58.0	58.0
HA33/Bp**	83.5	82.0		58.0	57.0
HA33/C	38.5	41.0	39.0		78.0
HA33/D	38.5	40.0	35.0	65.0	

*Bnp: non-proteolytic type B neurotoxin

**Bp: proteolytic type B neurotoxin

The HA70 is cleaved to a predicted 22 kDa protein and a 48 kDa protein after translation, which correspond to the HA20-23 and HA53-57 bands from type A and C on SDS-PAGE (Fujita et al. 1995; Tsuzuki et al. 1992). Homology among the HA70 genes is shown in Table 4.

Table 4 Per cent amino acid identities (lower left-hand triangle) and similarities (upper right-hand triangle) of HA70.

	A	*B*	*C*	*D*	*G*
A		98.5	82.5	82.5	83.0
B	96.0		85.5	85.0	84.0
C	68.5	71.5		95.5	76.0
D	68.5	71.0	93.5		77.0
G	72.0	73.0	65.0	65.0	

The HA70/C has been found to share 27.6% identity and 46.4% similarity with the 259 N-terminal amino acids of *C. perfringens* type A enterotoxin, a protein which binds to a cell membrane receptor and leads to change in plasma membrane permeability. Moreover, a tripeptide cell attachment sequence (Arg-Gly-Asp) was found at amino acid 30-32 of HA22. These data suggest that HA70 might play a role in adhesion of the progenitor neurotoxins to the intestinal tissue before the progenitor toxins dissociate into neurotoxins and nontoxic components in the small intestine (Fujinaga et al. 1994).

The HA33 and HA53/C have been shown to exhibit hemagglutinin activity, but the HA17, HA57/A and HA57/B purified from SDS-PAGE did not show any hemagglutinin activity (Somers and DasGupta 1991). These proteins may only exhibit an hemagglutinin activity when associated with other hemagglutinin components.

Sequence analysis results show that *Clostridium tetani* E88 genome does not contain any one of *C. botulinum* NAPs nucleotide and protein sequences. Therefore, the genetic evidence at the molecular level suggests that *Clostridium tetani* (Massachusettes E88) genotypically lack NAPs genes, and thus pheno-typically lack the protection from NAP-like proteins. This result greatly supports the hypothesis that NAPs might transform the neurotoxin to be food poison and explains the reason why botulinum is food poison but tetanus is not, as suggested by Singh et al. previously (Singh et al. 1995).

4. THE PUTATIVE REGULATION GENE, ORF22

The orf 22 gene encoding 178 amino-acids with a calculated M orf 21.7 kDa, located at downstream of the HA genes in type C and upstream of the

HA genes in types A and B, has the same transcriptional direction as that of the NBP and BoNT genes. Although referred with different names (orf 22/ BotR/P-21) in different types of botulinum serotypes, amino acid sequence homology among different type of orf 22 genes as shown in Table 5 ranges between 58% and 97.5%. The amino acid sequences of type A and type C orf 22 show 52.0% identity in contrast to 98%, 91%, 90% identity between orf 22 of type A and proteolytic type B (Bp), type A and non-proteolytic type B (Bnp), proteolytic and non-proteolytic type B, respectively (East et al. 1994; Hauser et al. 1994). The orf 22 product is postulated to regulate the expression of genes for HA, NBP and BoNT because it displays the characteristics of DNA binding proteins in terms of basic pI (10.4), and helix-turn-helix motifs (Hauser et al. 1994). Moreover, it shows a 29% identity with the *uviA* gene product, a *C. perfringens* regulatory protein (Hauser et al.1995; East et al. 1994).

Table 5 Per cent amino acid identities (lower left-hand triangle) and similarities (upper right-hand triangle) of orf22

	A	*B*	*C*	*D*	*F*	*G*	*TetR*
A		97.5	72.5	72.0	78.5	83.0	84.5
B	95.5		66.5	66.0	71.0	78.0	79.5
C	52.0	48.0		89.0	58.0	60.0	65.0
D	52.0	48.0	86.0		66.0	68.0	71.0
E	60.5	55.0	45.0	53.0		83.0	81.5
F	59.0	54.0	42.0	44.0	60.0		83.5
TetR	66.5	61.5	48.0	52.0	66.5	65.0	

Our BLAST sequence analyses results also showed the botulinum type A, B, C and D are more similar not only because of their NAPs gene loci pattern but also they share more and higher sequence homology with each others. However, the type E and F have different NAPs proteins and interestingly is there is no BotR, which is a transcription regulator, to be found inside the currently discovered gene loci of botulinum type E.

Sequence analyses also suggest that except for Ha-33, most of the NAPs proteins are unique and, generally, have protein sequence similarity with prokaryotic organism only.

4.1 Mode of Action

The mode of action of the BoNT is not well understood at the molecular level. Based on some experimental evidence and analogies with other dichain toxins such as diphtheria, cholera and *Pseudomonas* exotoxin A, a working model involving three steps (Fig. 4) has been proposed (Simpson 1981; 1986; 1989; Singh 1996).

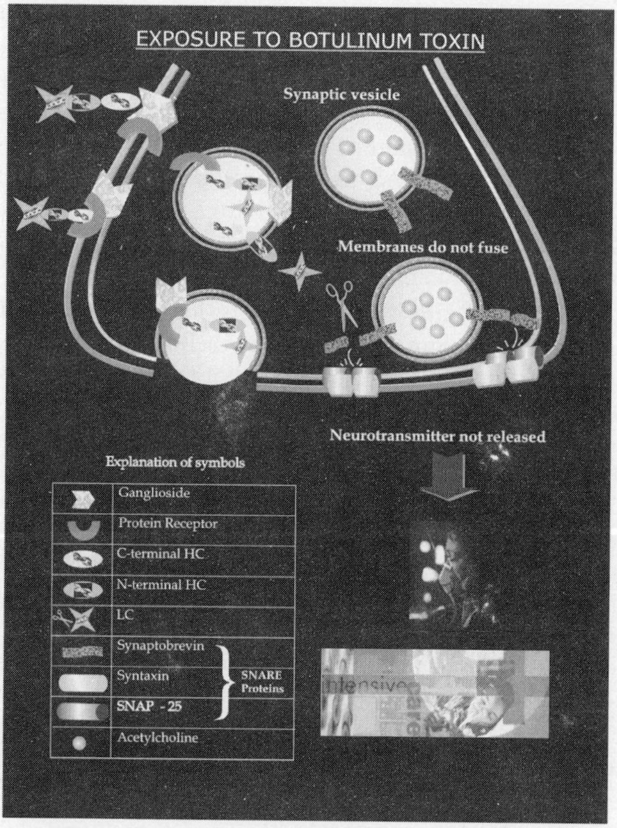

Fig. 4 Schematic representation of the steps involved in the binding, internalization and intracellular activity of BoNTs.

(i) Extracellular Step: It involves binding of the neurotoxin to presynaptic membranes through the C-terminal half of the H chain. The C-terminal half of the H-chain has been suggested to bind to gangliosides on the presynaptic membrane (Simpson 1981; 1986). According to a 'double receptor' model (Montecucco 1986), the C-terminal domain of the neurotoxin binds first with the ganglioside that alters its protein structure and makes it compatible for binding with a protein receptor. Structural changes in botulinum and tetanus neurotoxins upon binding with gangliosides (or detergent) were experimentally observed (Montecucco

1986; Lazarovici et al. 1987; Singh et al. 1991). These changes could also be involved in exposing trans-membrane and surface-seeking peptide domains. Recently, several reports have appeared suggesting existence of different protein receptors for different serotypes of BoNT and for tetanus neurotoxin (Li and Singh 1998; Nishiki et al. 1993; 1994; 1996; Schengrund et al. 1992; Schiavo et al. 1991; 1999; Kozaki 1999; Thilo 1993). Latest results have suggested that the receptor for at least BoNT/B is an isoform of synaptotagmin whose binding is modified by gangliosides (Nishiki et al. 1993; 1994; 1996). Synaptotagmin is involved in the interaction with the synaptic vesicle docking and fusion proteins, and is expected to be exposed on the neuronal surface following exocytotic discharge. It is proposed that gangliosides could prime the structure of the receptor for binding with the neurotoxin.

Critical Analysis of the Role of Gangliosides in BoNT Action: According to the 'double receptor' model of BoNT binding to neuronal cells, gangliosides bind to BoNT H chain that facilitates its binding to the receptor (Montecucco 1986). However, recent studies (Montecucco 1986) and some earlier observations (where gangliosides can be used as antidote against BoNT action; Kitamura et al. 1980; Simpson and Rapport 1971) indicate that binding of gangliosides with BoNT does not actually 'prime' it for binding with the protein receptor. It is becoming increasingly clear that gangliosides are perhaps more important for the activity of the receptor rather than acting as receptor (Nishiki 1993). One observation in favour of this hypothesis is the fact that gangliosides inhibit BoNTs (Kozaki et al. 1984) which will be contrary to their role as a primary receptor that 'primes' BoNT for its eventual binding with the protein receptor.

Two possible modes of ganglioside involvement in BoNT action are as follows:

(a) Gangliosides is important for the binding activity of the protein receptor, most likely by altering its structure. However, the presence of gangliosides in the membrane could also influence the membrane organisation which could change the protein receptor's topography in the membrane that may be relevant for its binding to BoNT.

(b) Gangliosides, present in abundance in nerve tissues, act as low affinity acceptors of BoNT and bind specifically to BoNT binding domain (c-terminal half of H chain). Even though the affinity is low, only a selective group of gangliosides (GT1b) bind with BoNT (Schengrund et al. 1991; 1992), and such binding is very specific, as shown in the crystal structure (Eswaramoorthy, Kumaran and Swaminathan 2000) involving about ten residues in three groups in case of BoNT/B. Although gangliosides do not meet several basic tenets (e.g., high affinity, scarcity, etc.) of a protein receptor (Middlebrook 1989), their binding to specific BoNT segments and their abundance at the nerve membrane can overcome the lack of high affinity.

(c) It is possible that gangliosides play both the functions outlined above.

(ii) Internalization and Translocation Steps: Upon binding, the neurotoxin is internalized through endocytosis (Fig. 4). Inside the cell, pH of the endosome is lowered to 5.5-6.0 (Thilo 1993), which leads to the formation of a membrane channel by the N-terminal half of the H-chain. This channel helps translocate the whole or a part of the neurotoxin into the cytoplasm. At least the 50-kDa BoNT L chain is transported into the cytoplasm from acidic endocytotic vesicles. This transport is dependent upon the 100-kDa H chain (Bandyopadhyay et al. 1987) which has been suggested to form a tetramer in the vesicle membrane as suggested by results of image reconstruction from electron micrographs (Schmid et al. 1993). The H-chain incorporates spontaneously into phospholipid bilayers to form channels that allow ions as well as the L-chain to pass through (Finkelstein 1990; Koriazova and Montal 2003).

Low pH is required for the strong channel formation activity of botulinum and tetanus neurotoxins and their H-chains (Boquet and Duflot 1982; Hoch et al. 1985). A pH of 5.0 or lower induces the channel formation. Two possible effects of the low pH are (i) neutralization of negative charges of the protein and/or conformational changes in the polypeptide folding which allow the integration of the neurotoxin into the membrane bilayer, and (ii) change in the structure of the BoNT receptor which could either release BoNT's H-chain and/or assist in the membrane channel formation. Recent results have suggested that BoNT exists in oligomeric form in aqueous solution (Singh et al. 1993; 1994) as well as perhaps in lipid vesicle (Schmid et al. 1993) that may be relevant to the membrane channel formation by BoNT and its interaction with a receptor.

(iii) Intracellular Step: This step of the BoNT action is relatively better understood. It is known that the L-chain subunit of the neurotoxin, once inside the nerve cells, is sufficient to block the neurotransmitter release (Bittner et al. 1989; Stecher et al. 1989; Mochida et al. 1989) that results into flaccid muscle paralysis. The neurotoxin does not affect either biosynthesis or packaging of the acetylcholine in the nerve cell (Simpson 1989). Recent experimental evidence has suggested that botulinum and tetanus neurotoxins are zinc-proteases, and the substrates for the different serotypes of BoNTs and TeNT are the constitutive components of the secretary machinery (Huttner 1993; Montecucco and Schiavo 1993; 1994). Cleavage of these substrates blocks the docking and fusion of synaptic vesicles (Fig. 4).

Medicinal Use

Even though the crystalline form of type A botulinum neurotoxin (what is now known as BoNT/A complex) was first isolated in 1940s (Lamanna et al. 1946), and its medicinal value was not experimented till 1970s (Scott 1989), the medicinal use of the botulinum neurotoxin, 'sausage poison' or fat poison, as it was referred to in early 1800s, was predicted in a monograph by Justinus Kerner in 1822 (Erbguth 2004). Based on his seven years of studies with sausage poisoning cases and experiments, Kerner concluded that the toxin applied in minimal doses should reduce or block the hyperactivity and hyper excitability of the motor and the autonomic nervous system. Kerner wrote, "The fatty acid or zoonic acid administration in such doses that its action could be restricted to the sphere of the sympathetic nervous system only, could be of benefit in many diseases which originate from hyper excitation of this system", and "as an analogy it can be expected that in outbreaks of sweat, perhaps also in mucous hyper secretion, the fatty acid will be of therapeutic value." Of course, it was just a hypothesis at that time, which was recognized by Dr. Kerner himself, "What is said here about the fatty acid as therapeutic drug belongs to the realm of hypotheses and may be confirmed or disproved by observations in the future" (Erbguth 2004).

Much work has been done in that direction, confirming the predictions of Kerner. Of the seven serotypes of BoNT discovered, so far, two (types A and B) are currently licensed for medicinal uses, and all the serotypes have potential to be used (Eleopra et al. 2004) against many neuromuscular disorders.

Botulinum Neurotoxin A

For about two decades BoNT/A has been successfully used for the treatment of many disorders related to excessive muscle contraction, such as strabismus, blepharospasm, hemifacial spasm and cervical dystonia (Johnson 1999). BoNT/A also significantly reduces pain associated with craniocervical dystonia—an effect that has long been considered secondary to its muscle relaxant action (Brin et al. 2000; Gobel et al. 2001). BoNT/A also has been used successfully to treat several different types of headaches, including tension-type headaches (Wheeler 1998; Schulte-Mattler et al. 1999), cervicogenic headaches (Hobson et al. 1997; Freund et al. 2000) and migraine (Brin et al. 2000; Binder et al. 2000; Silberstein et al. 2000). Botulinum neurotoxin is now widely considered as a pharmaceutical agent with multiple use, and has propelled into the public eye after it was widely reported to act as an anti-wrinkle drug for facial cosmetic enhancement. This has established its new image as a glamour drug. Botulinum neurotoxin is reported to be useful in about a hundred conditions, with indications spanning many specialties (Misra 2002; Jost et al. 2001). In the late 1980s, a group of physicians at Columbia University noticed that patients who received injections for nerve disorders also experienced cosmetic improvement. They pursued this investigation and soon developed the botulinum neurotoxin therapy in common use today. In fact, cosmetic use has become the single most common use of the botulinum neurotoxin-based products.

Clostridium botulinum produces the botulinum neurotoxin in a complex form, consisting of BoNT and NAPs. While there are several laboratories in the world, which produce the BoNT complex for research, the manufacturing of botulinum neurotoxins for therapeutics involves a series of complex and specialized chromatographic protein purification steps. Quality control is the key for the therapeutic products. Two preparations of botulinum toxin A are commercially available, one is BOTOX® from Allergan, Inc. and the other is DYSPORT® from Ipsen, Ltd., now commercially available. These two preparations are widely used for treatment and cosmetic use. They differ from each other on the basis of their preparation and potency. In these two preparations adding either sodium chloride (BOTOX®,Allergan, Inc.) or lactose (DYSPORT® Ipsen, Ltd.) protects the steric conformation of BoNT (Muthane et al. 2003). Human serum albumin is also added to prevent loss from surface adsorption. The toxin is then dried either with freezing (DYSPORT®, Ipsen, Inc.) or without freezing (BOTOX®, Allergan, Inc.) (Muthane et al. 2003). Numerous factors influence the clinical potency of the two preparations and hence, units of each product are not clinically equivalent or interchangeable. However, it is clear from the literature and from clinical experience that the units used to quantify the toxin activity of the two products are not equivalent. This apparent difference in the potency of the two products causes difficulties when comparing the results of studies using different preparations, and when changing from one preparation to the other. It is likely that any difference between the two products is the result of the different assay methods used to quantify the activity of the products (Odergren et al. 1998; Hambleton et al. 1994). Different experimental paradigms have been used to find an appropriate conversion factor in dystonic patients, but the results are conflicting (the ratio Botox:Dysport found being between 1:3 and 1:6) (Ranoux et al. 2002; Durif 1995; Marion et al. 1995; Whurr et al. 1995; Sampaio et al. 1997). Using a 4:1 conversion ratio for Dysport and Botox, similar results were obtained for the two treatments in an appropriately powered study, suggesting that this conversion factor is a good estimate of their comparative clinical potencies (Sampaio, et al. 1997; Sampaio et al. 2004). Pharmacokinetic measurements in terms of compound muscle action potential (CMAPs) with phrenic nerves also provide a similar ratio (4.2:1) for Dysport and Botox (Wohlfarth et al. 2004).

Comparative clinical studies between other botulinum preparations have not yet been published except the toxin preparation produced in china (Tang et al. 2000). In a case study with 785 patients, there were no significant differences found in the clinical effects of two preparations (BOTOX and CBTX-A), including the latency of response, maximal benefit, and duration of improvement. The patients' subjective assessments were similar. But the requested dose of the Chinese preparation, which produced the similar effects, was statistically higher than that of Botox. Side effects included a skin rash, which appeared within a few days after injections in three cases of CBTX-A group, but none from the Botox group. No statistical differences were noted in the other adverse reaction between them. The injections of both kinds of preparation were simple and effective on the patients with cervical dystonia. Chinese preparation is a little less powerful but much cheaper than Botox (Tang et al. 2000).

Injections with botulinum neurotoxin prepared for medicinal use are generally well tolerated. After injection the toxin diffuses into the muscles and adjacent tissues. Its effect diminishes with increasing distance from the injection site, but spread to nearby muscles is enhanced when higher volumes of the toxin are injected (Munchau et al. 2000). Although the use of botulinum toxin is safe, the most frequently adverse reactions are dysphagia, pain, soreness and bruising at the injection site, local weakness, symptomatic general weakness, malaise and nausea. Adverse reactions usually occur within the first week following injection of botulinum toxin and, while generally transient, these reactions may last several months. Localized pain, tenderness and/or bruising may be associated with the injection.

Table 1 Recent medicinal use of botulinum neurotoxin.

	Disorders	*Dysfunction*
1.	Chronic headache	Tension-type headache (Schulte-Mattler and Krack 2004)
2.	Overactive bladder (OAB)	Spastically contraction of detrusor bladder muscles (Wein, 2003)
3.	Laryngeal dystonia	Vocal cord dystonia (Hamano et al. 2004)
4.	Temporomandibular joint dislocation	Dysfunction of the joint, muscles of the jaw (Ricardo et al. 2003)
5.	Dysuria or urinary retention	Non-relaxing urethral sphincter (Leippold et al. 2003)
6.	Tourette's syndrome	Involuntary, rapid, sudden movements of muscles (Porta et al. 2004)
7.	Focal hyperhidrosis	Excessive sweating (Naumann et al. 2004)

Botulinum Neurotoxin B

On December 11, 2000, a botulinum toxin type B product (Myobloc™) was approved by US-FDA as a treatment for patients with cervical dystonia. Myobloc™ is the U.S. trade name for Elan Biopharmaceuticals' botulinum neurotoxin type B product. Since that time, it has been used effectively to reduce facial wrinkles. Myobloc is particularly suggested for relaxing muscles used in frowning and squinting, if for no other reasons then for its name.

Botulinum neurotoxin type B (BTX-B; Myobloc) is approved for general use in the treatment of cervical dystonia (CD). In two large pivotal trials, it was found to be safe and effective in decreasing the movements, pain, and disability associated with CD (Brin et al. 1999; Brashear et al. 1999). Being the newest botulinum toxin based product, it is still being evaluated for various neuromuscular conditions. However, it is being tested with promise against upper and lower-limb spasticity (Bell et al. 2003; Brashear et al. 2003) and piriformis syndrome (Fishman et al. 2004).

Although BTX-B is generally considered safe, recent case reports by Dressler and Benecke (Dressler et al. 2002) indicate that side effects include visual disturbances, dry eyes and dry mouth, which suggest systemic diffusion of physiologically active quantities of toxin from the sites of injection. This interpretation is limited, however, by the small number of cases (Lang 2003). One thing has clearly been observed that there is more antibody response to BTX-B-based drugs because of the requirement of dramatically higher dose (about 100-fold higher compared to BTX-based drug) (Eleopra et al. 2004). Therefore, while BTX-B may be an alternative to BTX-A non-responders; it could be useful for long-term treatment.

The product based on BoNT/B differs from BoNT/A-based products in several ways. It is provided in a liquid form as opposed to a lyophilized powder that requires reconstitution in saline. BoNT/B has shown stability for months when stored appropriately at 2°C to 8°C, whereas BoNT/A must be stored at –5°C as a powder and must be used within hours once reconstituted according to the manufacturer's recommendation (Kim et al. 2003). In practice, BoNT/A may be stable for much longer time. Also, because they are antigenically distinct, BoNT/A non-responders may respond to BoNT/B, and *vice versa* (Setler 2000).

As described earlier, BoNT serotypes have similar structures and basic mechanisms of action. However, there are biochemical differences between them. For example, BoNTs produced in fluid culture or in food are complexes of one or more neurotoxin associated proteins (NAPs), resulting in molecular sizes of 12, 16 and 19S (Schantz et al. 1967; Sakaguchi, 1983; Sugii et al. 1977). BoNT/A, /C, and /E cleave synaptosomal-associated protein of M_r 25,000 (SNAP-25), while synaptobrevin is the target of BoNT/B, /D, /F, and /G. In addition to SNAP-25, BoNT/C also cleaves syntaxin. Therefore, biochemical differences between botulinum toxin serotypes may confer unique *in vivo* biological properties. In some cases, BoNT/B was found to be more effective than BoNT/A. For example, Flynn and Clark (Flynn et al. 2003) compared the rate of diffusion of botulinum neurotoxin types A and B in the forehead and found that BoNT/B had a slightly faster action than BoNT/A. All patients responded to BoNT/B quickly, whereas some had a delayed response to BoNT/A. The study is based on case reports of monitored diffusion of toxin. The biochemical aspect of such faster diffusion is still unknown.

5. CONCLUSION

Generally, neurotoxins are considered lethal to humans when used in high doses either deliberately or accidentally. Botulinum toxin is a rare example of potentially lethal biological agent that can be used as a medicine for several neuromuscular disorders. It has many unique characteristics including exclusive substrate specificity and localized action. Research is underway to use botulinum neurotoxin as a drug delivery vehicle. Despite its extreme toxicity, it has been widely used as a wrinkle remover which is perhaps the single most popular use. While its use as a therapeutic agent is relatively safe, care must be taken as it can interact with other antibiotics, especially those that interfere with neurotransmission. Caution should also be exercised when botulinum toxin type A is utilized for treatment of patients with myasthenia gravis, Eaton Lambert Syndrome, or other disorders that produce a depletion of acetylcholine. Although the most toxic substance known to mankind has been transformed from a killer to cure, safeguards need to be put in place so that the reagents are prepared and used safely. A recent case involving the use of research grade botulinum toxin for therapeutic use, has resulted in severe paralysis of several patients (Wahlberg 2005).

ACKNOWLEDGEMENTS

This work was in part supported by the U.S. Army Medical Research and Material Command under Contract No. DAMD17-02-C-001, and by National Institutes of Health through New England Center of Excellence for Biodefense (AI057159-01).

REFERENCES

Ahnert-Hilger G, Bigalke H (1995) Molecular aspects of tetanus and botulinum neurotoxin poisoning. Progr. in Neurobio 46: 83-96

Ala-Huikku K, Nurmi E, Pajulahti H, Raevuori M (1977) The occurrence of *Clostridium botulinum* type E in Finnish trout farms and the prevention of toxin formation in fresh-salted vacuum-packed trout fillets. Nord Vet Med 29: 386-391

Arnon SS, Schechter R, Inglesby TV, Henderson DA, Bartlett DA, Scher MS, Eitzen, E, Fine AD, Hauer J, Layton M, Lillibridge S, Osterholm MT, O'Toole T, Parker, G, Perl TM, Russell PK, Swerdlow DL, Tonal K (2001) Botulinum Toxin as a biological weapon: Medical and public health management. JAMA 285: 1059-1070

Ashie IN, Smith JP, Simpson BK (1996) Spoilage of shelf-life extension of fresh fish and shellfish. Crit Rev Food Sci Nutr 36:87-121

Baldassi L, Hipolito M, Portugal M A, Calil E M, Moulin AA, Pires D de C (1991) Bovine botulism: laboratory confirmation of clinical diagnosis in 1986-1989. Pev Saude Publica 25:371-374

Bandyopadhyay S, Clark AW, Dasgupta BR, Sathyamoorthy V (1987) Role of the heavy and light chains of botulinum toxin in neuromuscular paralysis. J Biol Chem 262: 2660-2663

Bell KR, Williams, F (2003) Use of botulinum toxin type A and type B for spasticity in upper and lower limbs. Phys Med Rehabil Clin N Am 14:821-835

Bhandari M, Campbell KD, Collins MD, East AK (1997) Molecular characterization of the clusters of genes encoding the botulinum neurotoxin complex in clostridium botulinum (Clostridium argentinense) type G and nonproteolytic Clostridium botulinum type B. Curr Microbiol 35: 207-214

Binder WJ, Brin MF, Blitzer A, Schuenrock LD, Pogoda JM, (2000) Botulinum toxin type A (BOTOX) for treatment of migraine headaches: an open-label study. Otolaryngol Head Neck Surg 123:669–676

Binz T, Kurazono H, Popoff MR, Elkund MW, Sakaguchi G, Kozaki S, Krieglstein K, Henschen A, Gill DM, Niemann H (1990 b) Nucleotide sequence of the gene encoding *Clostridium botulinum* neurotoxin type D. Nucleic Acids Res 18: 5556-5556

Binz T, Kurazono H, Wille M, Frevert J, Wermars K, Niemann H (1990 a) The complete sequence of botulinum neurotoxin type A and comparison with other clostridial neurotoxins. J Bio Chem 265:9153-9158

Bittner MA, Habig WH, Holz RW (1989) Isolated light chain of tetanus toxin inhibits exocytosis: Studies in digitonin permeabilized cells. J Neurochem 53: 966-968

Boquet P, Duflot E (1982) Tetanus toxin fragment forms channels in lipid vesicles at low pH. Proc. Natl. Acad. Sci. USA 79: 7614-7618

Brashear A, Lew M F, Dykstra D D (1999) Safety and efficacy of NeuroBloc (botulinum toxin type B) in type A-responsive cervical dystonia. Neurology 53:1439-1446

Brashear A, McAfee A L, Kuhn E R, Ambrosius W T (2003) Treatment with botulinum toxin type B for upper-limb spasticity. Arch Phys Med Rehabil 84:103-107

Brin MF, Lew M F, Adler C H (1999) Safety and efficacy of NeuroBloc (botulinum toxin type B) in type A-resistant cervical dystonia. Neurology 53 : 1431-1438

Brin MF, Swope D M, O'Brien C et al (2000) Botox for migraine: double-blind, placebo-controlled, region-specific evaluation. Cephalagia 20: 421–422

Brinkmann (2005) Nucleic Acid Conversions (Practical Information for the Molecular Biologist) Eppendorfna.com (http://www.eppendorfna.com/applications/practical-nuc-conv.asp?SX=NF&)

Burns GF, Williams H (1975) *Clostridim botulinum* in Scottish fish farms and farmed trout. J Hyg (London) 74:1-6

Call JE, Cooke P H, Miller AJ (1995) *In situ* characterization of *Clostridium botulinum* neurotoxin synthesis and export. J App Bact 79:257-263

Campbell KD, Collins MD, East AK (1993 a) Nucleotide sequence of the gene coding for *Clostridium Botulinum (Clostridium argentinense)* type G neurotoxin: genealogical comparoson with other clostridial neutoxins. Biochem Biophys Acta 1216: 487-491

Campbell KD, East AK, Thompson DE, Collins MD (1993 b) Studies on the large subunit ribosomal RNA genes and intergenic spacer regions of non-proteolytic *Clostridium Botulinum* types B, E and F. Res Microbio 144:171-180

Clayton MA, Clayton JM, Brown DR, Middlebrook JL (1995) Protective vaccinatin with a recombinant fragment of *Clostridium botulinum* neurotoxin serotype A expressed from a synthetic gene in *Escherichia coli*. Infec Immun 63:2738-2742

Cordoba JJ, Collins MD, East AK (1994) Studies on the genes encoding botulinum neurotoxin type A of *Clostridium botulinum* from a variety of saurces. System Appl Microbio 18:13-22

Dineen SS, Bradshaw M and Johnson EA (2003) Neurotoxin Gene Clusters in Clostridium botulinum Type A Strains: Sequence Comparison and Evolutionary Implications. Curr Microbiol 46: 345-352

Dressler D, Benecke R (2002) Initial experiences with clinical use of botulinum toxin type B[German]. Nervenarzt 73:194-8

Durif F (1995) Clinical bioequivalence of the current commercial preparations of botulinum toxin. Eur Neurol 2: 17–18

East AK, Bhandari M, Hielm S, Collins MD (1998) Analysis of the botulinum neurotoxin type F gene clusters in proteolytic and nonproteolytic Clostridium botulinum and Clostridium barati. Curr Microbiol 37: 262-268

East AK, Collins MD (1994) Conserved structure of genes encoding components of botulinum neurotoxin complex M and the sequence of the gene coding for the non-toxic component in non-proteolytic Clostridium botulinum type F. Curr Microbiol 29: 69-77

East AK, Collins MD (1994) Conserved structure of genes encoding components of the botulinum neurotoxin complex M and the sequence of the gene encoding for the non-toxic component in non-proteolytic *Clostridium botulinum* type F. Curr Microbio 29:69-77

East AK, Richard PT, Allaway D, Collins MD, Thmopson DE (1992) Sequence of the gene encoding type F neurotoxin of *Clostridium botulinum*. FEMS Microbio Lett 96: 225-230

East AK, Stacey JM, Collins MD (1994) Cloning and sequencing of a hemagglutinin component of the botulinum neurotoxin complex encoded by *Clostridium botulinum* types A and B. System. Appl Microbio 17:306-312

Eleopra R, Tugnoli V, Quatrale R, Rossetto O, Montecucco C (2004) Different types of botulinum toxin in humans. Mov Disord 19: S53-S59

Elmore MJ, Hutson RA, Collins, MD, Bodsworth NJ, Whelan S, Minton NP (1995) Nucleotide sequence of the gene coding for proteolytic (group I) *Clostridium botulinum* type F neurotoxin: genealogical comparison with other colstridial neurotoxins. System Appl Microbio 18:23-31

Erbguth FJ (1998) Botulinum toxin, a historical note. Lancet 351: p1280.

Erbguth FJ (2004) Historical notes on botulism, *Clostridim botulinum*, botulinum toxin, and the idea of the therapeutic use of the toxin. Mov Disord 19: S2-S6.

Eswaramoorthy S, Kumaran D, Swaminathan S (2002) A novel mechanism for Clostridium botulinum neurotoxin inhibition. Biochemistry 41: 795-802.

Fach P, Hauser D, Guillou JP, Popoff MR (1993) Polymerase chain reaction for the rapid identification of Clostridium botulinum type A strains and detection in food samples. J App Bact 75: 234-239

Fairweather NF, Lyness VA (1986) The complete nucleotide sequence of tetanus toxin. Nucleic Acids Res 14: 7809-7812

Fernandez RA, Ciccarelli AS, Arenas GN, Gimenez DF(1989) Type D and A *Clostridium botulinum* in necropsy samples from bovines with 'mad de Aguapey'. Rev Argent Microbiol 21:47-53

Finkelstein A (1990) Channels formed in phospholipid bilayer membranes by diphtheria, tetanus, botulinum and anthrax toxin. J Physiol 84:188-190

Fishman LM, Konnoth C, Rozner B (2004) Botulinum neurotoxin type B and physical therapy in the treatment of piriformis syndrome: A dose-finding study. Am J Phys Med Rehabil 83:42-50

Flynn TC, Clark RE (2003) Botulinum toxin type B (MYOBLOC) versus botulinum toxin type A (BOTOX) frontalis study: Rate of onset and radius of diffusion. Dermatol Surg 29:519-522

Foster EM(1993) Reflections on a half-century of foodborne botulism. Botulinum and Tetanus Neurotoxins, Dasgupta BR, Edit. Plenum Press, New York p 505

Freund BJ, Schwartz M (2000) Treatment of chronic cervical-associated headache with botulinum toxin A: a pilot study. Headache 40:231–236

Fu FN, Sharma SK, Singh BR (1998) A protease-resistant novel hemagglutinin purified from type A *Clostridium botulinum*. J Protein Chem 17:53-60

Fujii N (1995) Structure and function of botulinum toxin, Hokkaido igaku zasshi- Hokkaido. J Med Sci 70:19-28

Fujii N, Kimura K, Murakami T, Indoh T, Yashiki T, Tzumuki K, Yokosawa N, Oguma K (1990) The nucleotide and deduced amino acid sequences of EcoRI fragment containing the 5'-terminal region of *Clostridium botulinum* type E toxin gene cloned from Mashike, Iwanai and Otaru strains. Micro Immunol 34:1041

Fujii N, Kimura K, Tsuzuki K, Yokosawa N, Oguma K (1993) Construction and expression of the genes for neurotoxins and non-toxic components in *C. botulinum* types C and E, in Botulinum and Tetanus Neurotoxins. Dasgupta BR, ED., Plenum Press, New York, 405-419

Fujii N, Kimura K, Yokosawa N, Oguma K, Yashiki T, Takeshi K, Ohyama T, Isogai E, Isogai H (1993) Similarity in nucleotide sequence of the encoding nontoxic *Clostridium butyricum* strain BL 6340 and *Clostridium botulinum* type E strain Mashike. Micro Immunol 37: 395-398

Fujii N, Kimura K, Yokosawa N, Yashiki T, Tsuzuki K, Oguma K (1993) The complete nucleotide sequence of the gene encoding the non-toxic component of *Clostridium botulinum* type E progenitor toxin. J Gen Microbio 139: 79-86

Fujinaga Y, Inoue K, Nomura T, Sasaki J, Marvaud JC, Popoff MR, Kozaki S, Oguma K (2000) Identification and characterization of functional subunits of Clostridium botulinum type A progenitor toxin involved in binding to intestinal microvilli and erythrocytes. FEBS Lett 467:179-183

Fujinaga Y, Inoue K, Shimazaki S, Tomochika K, Tsuzuki K, Fijii N, Watanabe T, Ohyama T, Takeshi K, Inoue K, Oguma K (1994) Molecular construction of *Clostridium botulinum* type C progenitor toxin and its gene organization. Biochem and Biophys Res Commun 205:1291-1298

Fujinaga Y, Inoue K, Watanabe S, Yokota K, Hirai Y, Nagamachi E, Oguma K (1997) The haemagglutinin of Clostridium botulinum type C progenitor toxin plays an essential role in binding of toxin to the epithelial cells of guinea pig small intestine, leading to the efficient absorption of the toxin. Microbiology 143:3841-3847

Fujinaga Y, Takeshi K, Inoue K, Fujita R, Ohyama T, Moriishi K, Oguma H (1995) Type A and B neurotoxin genes in a *Clostridium botulinum* type AB strain. Biochem and Biophys Res Commun 213:737-745

Fujita R, Fujinaga K, Inoue H, Nakajima H, Kumon H, Oguma H (2001) Molecular characterization of two forms of non-toxic–non-hemagglutinin components of Clostridium botulinum type A progenitor toxins. FEBS Lett 376: 41–44

Gobel H, Heinze A, Heinze-Kuhn K, Austermann K (2001) Botulinum toxin A in the treatment of headache syndromes and pericranial pain syndromes. Pain 91: 195–199

Haagsma J (1991) Botulism in cattle, a review. Tijdschr Diergerneskd 116: 663-669

Hamano K, Satoko K, Masaharu H, Naito R, Hayachida T, Vchiyama A, Kurata K (2004) Laryngeal dystonia in a case of severe motor and intellectual disabilities due to Japanese encephalitis sequelae. Brain and Development 26:335-338

Hambleton P (1992) *Clostridium botulinum* toxins: a general review of involvement in disease, structure, mode of action and preparation for clinical use. J Neurol 239: 16-20

Hambleton P, Pickett AM (1994) Potency equivalence of botulinum toxin preparations. J R Soc Med 87: 719-724

Hatheway CL (1993) Bacteriology and pathology of neurotoxigenic clostrida. In: Dasgupta BR (ed) Botulinum and Tetanus Neurotoxins. Plenum Press, New York

Hatheway CL, Ferreira J (1996) Detection and identification of Clostridium botulinum neurotoxins. In: Singh BR, Tu A (eds) Natural Toxins II: Structure, Mechanism of Action and Detection. Plenum Press, New York. pp 481-498

Hauser D, Eklund MW, Boqueet P, Popoff MR (1995) Botulinum neurotoxin C1 complex, clostridial neurotoxin homology and genetic transfer in *Clostridium botulinum*, Toxicon 33:515-526

Hauser D, Gibert M, Marvaud JC, Eklund MW, Popoff MR (1994) Organization of the botulinum neurotoxin C1 gene and its associated non-toxic protein genes in *Clostridium botulinum* C 468. Mol Gen Genet 243: 631-640

Hobson DE, Gladish DF (1997) Botulinum toxin injection for cervicogenic headache. Headache 37:253–255

Hoch DH, Romero-Mira M, Ehlrich BE, Finkelstein A, Dasgupta BR,Simpson LL (1985) Channels formed by botulinum, tetanus and diphtheria toxins in planer lipid bilayers: relevance to translocation of proteins across membranes. Proc Nat Acad Sci USA 82:1692-1696

Holger Bruggemann, Sebastian Baumer, Wolfgang Florian Fricke, Arnim Wiezer, Heiko Liesegang, Iwona Decker, Christina Herzberg, Rosa Martinez-Arias, Rainer Merkl, Anke Henne, Gerhard Gottschalk (2003) The genome sequence of *Clostridium tetani*: the causative agent of tetanus disease. Proc Natl Acad Sci USA 100: 1316-1321

Huss HH, Eskildsen U (1974) Botulism in farmed trout caused by *Clostridium botulinum* type E; a preliminary report. Nord Vet Med 26:733-738

Hutson RA, Collins MD, East AK,Thompson DE (1994) Nucleotide sequence of the gene coding for non-proteolytic *Clostridium botulinum* type B neurotoxin: Comparison with other colstridial neurotoxins. Curr Microbio 28: 101-110

Hutson RA, Thompson DE, Lawson PA, Schocken-Itturino RP, Bîtter EC, Collins MD (1993) Genetic interrelationships of proteolytic *Clostridium Botulinum* types A, B, and F and other members of the *Clostridium Botulinum* complex as revealed by small sub-unit rRNA gene sequences. Antonie van Leeuwenhoek. 64: 273

Hutson RA, Zhou Y, Collins MD, Johnson EA, Hatheway CL, Sugiyama H (1996) Genetic characterization of Clostridium botulinum type A containing silent type B neurotoxin gene sequences. J Biol Chem 271: 10786-10792

Huttner WB (1993) Snappy exocytoxins. Nature 365: 104-105

Inoue K, Fujinaga Y, Honke K, Arimitsu H, Mahmut N, Sakaguchi Y, Ohyama T, Watanabe T, Inoue K, Oguma K (2001) Clostridium botulinum type A haemagglutinin-positive progenitor toxin (HA(+)-PTX) binds to oligosaccharides containing Gal beta1-4GlcNAc through one subcomponent of haemagglutinin (HA1). Microbiology 147:811-819

Jeffrey JS, Galey FD, Meteyer CU, Kinde H,Rezvani M (1994) Type C botulism in turkeys: determination of the median toxic dose. J Vet Diagn Invest 6:93-95

Johnson EA (1991) Clostridial Toxins as Therapeutic Agents: Benefits of Nature's Most Toxic Proteins. Annu Rev Microbiol 53:551-575

Jost WH, Kohl A (2001) Botulinum toxin: evidence based medicine criteria in rare indications. J Neurol 248 :39-44

Kim, Eugene JMD, Ramirez Alexander LMD, Reeck Jay BMD, et al (2003) The Role of Botulinum Toxin Type B (Myobloc) in the Treatment of Hyperkinetic Facial Lines Plast Reconstr Surg 112: 88-93

Kitamura M, Iwamori M, Nagai Y (1980) Interaction between *Clostridium botulinum* neurotoxin and gangliosides. Biochim Biophys Acta 628: 328-335

Koriazva LK, Montal M (2003) Translocation of botulinum neurotoxin light chain protease through the heavy chain channel. Nat Struct Biol 10; 13-18

Kouguchi H, Watanabe T, Sagane Y, Sunagawa H, Ohyama T (2002) In vitro reconstitution of the Clostridium botulinum type D progenitor toxin. J Biol Chem 277: 2650-2656

Kozaki S (1999) Botulinum toxin receptors. International Conference 1999: Basic and Therapeutic Aspects of Botulinum and Tetanus Toxins, Orlando, Fl., November 16-18, pp 28

Kozaki S, Sakaguchi G, Nishimura M, Iwamori M, Nagai Y (1984) Inhibitory effect of ganglioside GT1b on the activities of Clostridium botulinum toxins. FEMS Microbiol Lett 21:219-223

Lamanna C, MacElroy OE, Eklund HW (1946) The purification and crystallization of *Clostridium botulinum* type A toxin. Science 103: 613-614

Lang AM (2003) Botulinum Toxin Type A Therapy in Chronic Pain Disorders. Arch Phys Med Rehabil 84: 69-S73

Lazarovici P, Yanai P, Yavin E (1987) Molecular interactions between micellar polysialogangliosides and affinity purified tetanotoxins in aqueous solution. J Biol Chem 262: 2645-2651

Leippold T, Reitz A, Schurch B (2003) Botulinum toxin as a new therapy option for voiding disorders: current state of the art. Eur Urol 44: 165-74

Li L, Singh BR (1998) Isolation of synaptotagmin as a receptor for types A and E botulinum neurotoxin and analysis of their comparative binding using a new microtiter plate assay. J Natural Toxins 7: 215-226

Li L, Singh BR (1999) Structure-function relationship of clostridial neurotoxins. Toxin Reviews 18: 95-112

Lund BM, Peck MW (1994) Heat resistance and recovery of spores of non-proteolytic *Clostridium botulinum* in relation to refrigerated, processed foods with an extended shelf-life. J App Bact Sympo Suppl 76:115-128

Makoff AJ, Oxer MD, Romanos MA, Fairweather NF, Ballantine S (1989) Expression of tetanus toxin fragment C in *E. coli*: high level expression by removing rare codons. Nucleic Acids Res 17:10191-10202

Marion MH, Sheehy M, Sangla S, Soulayrol S (1995) Dose standardization of botulinum toxin. J Neurol Neurosurg Psychiatry 59: 102–103

Marks JD (2004) Development of botulinum neurotoxin immunotherapy. In: Botulinum Neurotoxin and Ricin Investigators Meeting, Bethesda, MD

McClure PJ, Cple MB, Smelt JPP M (1994) Effects of water activity and pH on growth of *Clostridium botulinum*. J App Bact Symp Suppl 76: 105S-114S

Merrison AF, Chidley KE, Dunnett J, Sieradzan KA (2002) Wound botulism associated with subcutaneous drug use. BMJ. 325:1020-1021

Middlebrook JL (1989) Cell surface receptors for protein toxins. In: Simpson LL (Eds.) Botulinum neurotoxin and tetanus toxin. New York: Academic Press, 95–119

Misra VJ (2002) The changed image of botulinum toxin. Bio Med J 325:1188

Mochida S, Poulain B, Weller U, Habermann E, Tauc L (1989) Light chain of tetanus toxin intracellularly inhibits acetylcholine release at neuro-muscular synopses, and its internalization is mediated by heavy chain. FEBS Lett 253: 47-51

Montecucco C (1986) How do tetanus and botulinum toxins bind to neuronal membrane? Trends Biochem Sci 11:314-317

Montecucco C, Schiavo G (1994) Mechanism of action of tetanus and botulinum neurotoxins. Mol Microbiol 13:1-8

Montecucco C, Schiavo G (1993) Tetanus and botulism neurotoxins: a new group of zinc proteases. TIBS 18:324-327

Moriishi K, Koura M, Fujii N, Fujinaga Y, Igoue K, Syuto B,Oguma K (1996): Molecular cloning of the gene encoding the mosaic neurotoxin, composed of parts of botulinum neurotoxin types C1 and D, and PCR detection of this gene from *Clostridium botulinum* type C organisms. App Environ Microbiol 62:662-667

Munchau A, Bhatia KP (2000) Uses of botulinum toxin injection in medicine today (Clinical Review). BMJ 320:161–165

Muthane U, Panikkar D (2003) Botulinum toxins: Pharmacology and its current therapeutic evidence for use. Neurology India 51:455-460

Naumann M, Hamm H (2004) High-dose injection of botulinum toxin to treat focal hyperhidrosis: what's wrong with the concept? J Am Acad Dermatol 50:326-7

Nishikawa A, Uotsu N, Arimitsu H, Lee JC, Miura Y, Fujinaga Y, Nakada H, Watanabe T, Ohyama T, Sakano Y, Oguma K (2004) The receptor and transporter for internalization of Clostridium botulinum type C progenitor toxin into HT-29 cells. Biochem Biophys Res Commun 319: 327-33

Nishiki T, Kamata Y, Nemoto Y, Omori Y, Ito T, Takahashi M, Kozaki S (1994) Identification of protein receptor for *Clostridium botulinum* type B neurotoxin in rat brain synaptosomes. J Biol Chem 269:10498-10503

Nishiki T, Ogasawara K, Kamata Y, Kozaki S (1993) Solubilization and characterization of the acceptor for *Clostridium botulinum* type B neurotoxin from rat brain synaptic membranes. Biochim Biophys Acta 1158: 333-338

Nishiki T, Tokuyama Y, Kamata Y, Nemoto Y, Yoshida A, Sato K, Sekiguchi M, Takahashi M, Kozaki S (1996) The high-affinity binding of Clostridium botulinum type B neurotoxin to synaptotagmin II associated with gangliosides G_{T1b}/G_{D1a}. FEBS Lett 378: 253-257

Odergren T, Hjaltason H, Kaakkola S, Solders G, Hanko J, Fehling C, Marttila RJ, Lundh H, Gedin S, Westergren I, Richadson A, Dott C, Cohen H (1998) A double blind, randomised, parallel group study to investigate the dose equivalence of Dysport® and Botox® in the treatment of cervical dystonia. J Neurol Neurosurg Psychiatry 64: 6-12

Ortolani EL, Brito LA, Mori CS, Schalch U, Pacheco J, Baldacci L (1997) Botulism outbreak associated with poultry litter consumption in three Brazilian cattle herds. Vet Hum Toxicol 39:89-92

Porta M, Maggioni G, Ottaviani F, Schindler A (2004) Treatment of phonic tics in patients with Tourette's syndrome using botulinum toxin type A. Neurol Sci 24: 420-430

Ranoux D, Gury C, Fondarai J, Mas JL, Zuber M (2002) Respective potencies of Botox and Dysport: a double blind, randomised, crossover study in cervical dystonia. J Neurol Neurosurg Psychiatry 72: 459-462

Ricardo GS, Christina MM, Olsson AB, Senno RA, Marciniak CN (2003) Botulinum toxin type A in the treatment of temporomandibular joint dislocation in an adult with anoxic brain injury: A case report. Arch Phys Med Rehabil 84, 9, A8

Rînner SGE, Stackebrandt E (1994) Further evidence for the genetic heterogeneity of *Clostridium botulinum* as determined by 23S rRNA oligonucleotide probing. System Appl Microbiol 17:180-188

Rodriguez Jovita M, Collins MD, East AK (1998) Gene organization and sequence determination of the two botulinum neurotoxin gene clusters in *Clostridium botulinum* type A(B) strain NCTC 2916 Curr Microbiol 36: 226-231

Sagane Y, Kouguchi H, Watanabe T, Sunagawa H, Inoue K, Fujinaga Y, Oguma K, Ohyama T (2001) Role of C-terminal region of HA-33 component of botulinum toxin in hemagglutination. Biochem Biophys Res Commun 288: 650-657

Sagane Y, Watanabe T, Kouguchi H, Yamamoto T, Kawabe T, Murakami F, Nakatsuka M and Ohyama T (2000) Organization of Gene Encoding Components of the Botulinum Progenitor Toxin in *Clostridium botulinum* Type C Strain 6814: Evidence of Chimeric Sequence in the Gene Encoding Each Component. Published Only in DataBase

Sakaguchi G (1983) *Clostridium botulinum* toxins. Pharmac Ther 19: 165–194

Sakaguchi G, Sakaguchi S, Kamata Y, Tabita K, Asao T, Kozaki S (1990) Distinct characters of Clostridiun botulinum type a strains and their toxin associated with infant botulism in Japan. Int J Food Microbiol 11: 231-242

Sampaio C, Costa J, Ferreira JJ (2004) Clinical compatibility of marketed formulations of botulinum toxin. Mov Disord; 19: S129-S136

Sampaio C, Ferreira JJ, Simoes F, Rosas MJ, Magalhaes M, Correia AP, Bastos-Lina A, Martins R, Castro caldas A (1997) DYSBOT: a single-blind, randomised parallel study to determine whether any differences can be detected in the efficacy and tolerability of two formulations of botulinum toxin type A—Dysport and Botox-assuming a ratio of 4:1. Mov Disord 12: 1013–1018

Sanger FTP site for downloading C.botulinum (Hall A ATCC3502) genome data: ftp://ftp.sanger.ac.uk/pub/pathogens/cb/

Sanger web site for C. botulinum (Hall A, ATCC3502) genome data: http://www.sanger.ac.uk/Projects/C_botulinum/

Santos-Buelga JA, Collins MD, East AK (1998) Characterization of the genes encoding the botulinum neurotoxin complex in a strain of Clostridium botulinum producing type B and F neurotoxins. Curr Microbiol 37: 312-318

Schantz EJ, Johnson EA (1992) Properties and use of botulinum toxin and other microbial neurotoxins in medicine. Microbiol Rev 56: 80-99

Schantz EJ, Spero L (1967) Molecular size of *C. botulinum* toxins. Ingram M, Roberts TA (eds). Chapman and Hall, London. pp 296-301

Schengrund CL, DasGupta BR, Ringler NJ (1991) Binding of botulinum and tetanus neurotoxins to ganglioside GT1b and derivatives there of. J Neurochem 57: 1024- S1032

Schengrund CL, Ringler N J, Dasgupta B R (1992) Adherence of botulinum and tetanus neurotoxins to synaptosomal proteins. Brain Res Bull 29: 917-924

Schiavo G (1999) Characterization of tetanus toxin receptors. International Conference 1999: Basic and Therapeutic Aspects of Botulinum and Tetanus Toxins, Orlando, Fl., November 16-18. Abstract page 23.

Schiavo G, Rosetto O, Ferrari G, Montecucco C (1991) Tetanus receptor. Specific cross-linking of tetanus toxin to a protein of NGF-differentiated PC 12 cells. FEBS Lett 290: 227-230

Schmid MF, Robinson JP, Dasgupta BR (1993) Direct visualization of botulinum neurotoxin-induced channels in phospholipid vesicles. Nature 364: 827-830

Schulte-Mattler WJ, Krack P (2004) BoNTTH Study Group: Treatment of chronic tension-type headache with botulinum toxin A: a randomised, double-blind, placebo-controlled multicentre study, Pain 109:110-114

Schulte-Mattler WJ, Wieser T, Zierz S (1999) Treatment of tension-type headache with botulinum toxin: a pilot study. Eur J Med Res 4: 183–186

Scott AB (1989) Clostridial toxins as therapeutic agents. In: Simpson L L(ed) Botulinum Neurotoxin and Tetanus Toxin. Academic Press, San Diego. pp. 399-412

Setler P (2000) The biochemistry of botulinum toxin type B. Neurology, 55: S22-28.

Sharma SK, Fu FN, Singh BR (1999) Molecular properties of a hemagglutinin purified from type A botulinum neurotoxin complex. J Protein Chem 18: 29-38

Sharma SK, Singh BR (1998) Hemagglutinin binding protection of botulinum neurotoxin from proteolysis. J Natural Toxins 7: 239-253

Silberstein S, Mathew N, Saper J, Jenkins S (2000) Botulinum toxin type A as a migraine preventive treatment. For the BOTOX Migraine Clinical Research Group. Headache 40: 445–450

Simpson LL (1986) Molecular pharmacology of botulinum toxin and tetanus toxin. Annu Rev Pharmacol Toxicol 26: 427–453

Simpson LL (1981) The origin, structure and pharmacological properties of botulinum toxin. Pharmacol Rev 33:155-188

Simpson LL (1989) *Botulinum* toxin and Tetanus Toxin. Academic Press, San Diego

Simpson LL, Rapport M M (1971) The binding of *Botulinum* toxin to membrane lipids: sphingolipids, steroids, and fatty acids. J Neurochem 18: 1341-1343

Singh BR (2000) Intimate details of the most poisonous poison. Nature Struc Bio 7: 617-619

Singh BR (2002) Molecular basis of the unique endopeptidase activity of botulinum neurotoxin. In: Scientific and Therapeutic Aspects of Botulinum Toxin. Brin M F, Jankovic J, Hallet M (eds) Lippincott Williams and Wilkins, Philadelphia. pp. 75-88

Singh BR, Barcomb-Caddle L A, Fu F N, Li B (1996) Gene probe-based detection of type E botulinum neurotoxin binding protein using polymerase chain reaction. Toxicon 34: 737-742

Singh BR, Fuller M P, Dasgupta BR (1991) *Botulinum* neurotoxin type A: Structure and interaction with micellar concentration of SDS determined by FT-IR spectroscopy. J Protein Chem 10: 637-649

Singh BR, Li B, Read (1995) *Botulinum* versus tetanus neurotoxins: why is botulinum neurotoxin a food poison but not tetanus? Toxicon 33: 1541–1547

Somers E, Dasgupta B R (1991) *Clostridium botulinum* types A, B, C1, and E produce proteins with or without hemagglutinating activity: Do they share common amino-acid sequences and genes? J Prot Chem 10: 415-425

Stecher B, Weller U, Habermann E, Gratzl M, Ahnert-Hilger G (1989) The light chain but not the heavy chain of botulinum A toxin inhibits exocytosis from permeabilized adrenal chromaffin cells. FEBS Lett 255: 391-394

Strom MS, Elkund M W, Poysky FT (1984) Plasmids in *Clostridium botulinum* and related *Clostridium* species. App Environ Microbio 48: 956-963

Sugii S, Sakaguchi G (1977) Botulogenic properties of vegetables with special reference to the molecular size of the toxin in them. J Food Safety 1: 53–65

Tang X, Wan X (2000) Comparison of botox with a chinese type a botulinum toxin. Chin Med J (Engl) 113: 794-798

Thilo L (1993) Endosome processing: structural, functional and kinetic interrelations. In: BR Dasgupta (ed) Procedings of the International Conference on Botulinum and Tetanus Neurotoxins: Neurotransmission and Biomedical Aspects. Plenum Press. 165-177

Thompson DE, Brehm JK, Oultram JD, Swinfield TJ, Shone CC, Atkinson T, Melling J, Minton N P (1990) The complete amino acid sequence of the *Clostridium botulinum* type A neurotoxin, deduced by nucleotide sequence analysis of the encoding gene. Eur J Biochem 189: 73

Thompson DE, Hutson RA, East AK, Allaway D, Collins MD, Richardson PT (1989) Nucleotide sequence of the gene coding for *Clostridium barati* type F neurotoxin: Comparison with other colstridial neurotoxins. FEMS Microbio Lett 108: 175-182

Todd EC (1989) Costs of acute bacterial foodborne disease in Canada and the United States. Int J Food Microbiol 9: 313-326

Tsuzuki K, Kimura K, Fujii N, Yokoszwa N, Oguma K (1992) The complete nucleotide sequence of the gene coding for the non-toxic–non-hemagglutinin compenent of Clostridium botulinum type C progenitor toxin Biochem Biophy Res Comm 183: 1273-1279

Van Ermengen E (1897) Uber einen neuen anaeroben Bacillus und seine Beziehungen zum Botulisnms. Z Hyg infektionskrankh 26: 1-56

Wahlberg (2005) Fake Botox-injured pair warns others. Palm Beach Post, February 5 issue

Wein AJ (2003) Diagnosis and treatment of the overactive bladder. Urology 62: 20-27

Wheeler AH (1998) Botulinum toxin A, adjunctive therapy for refractory headaches associated with pericranial muscle tension. Headache 38: 468–471

Whelan SM, Elmore MJ, Bodsworth NJ, Brehm JK, Atkinson T, Minton NP (1995) Molecular cloning of the *Clostridium botulinum* structural gene encoding the type B neurotoxin and determination of its entire nucleotide sequence. App Environ Microbio 58: 2345-2354

Whurr R, Brooks G, Barnes C (1995) Comparison of dosage effects between the American and British botulinum toxin A products in the treatment of spasmodic dysphonia. Mov Disord 10: 387

Willis AT(1990) Clostridium The spore-bearing anaerobes. In: Lonton AH, Topley W WC (ed) Topley Wilson's principles of bacteriology, virology and immunity. Edward Arnold, London. 211-246

Wohlfarth K, Kampe K, Bigalke H (2004) Pharmacokinetic properties of different formulations of botulinum neurotoxin type A. Mov Disord 19: S65-S67

Zhou Y, Sugiyama H, Johnson EA (1993) Transfer of neurotoxigenicity from *Clostridium butyricum* to a nontoxigenic *Clostridium botulinum* type E-like strains. App Environ Microbio 59:3825-3831

Forms and Functions of Plant Growth-Promoting Rhizobacteria

CS NAUTIYAL

Where am I
In this maze of life?
A little chain
Of an evolution?
And multitudes of genomic chains
Jumping with their messages?
Or a tiny part of an infinity
Not knowing it is infinity?

–Y.S. Rajan (2002)

1. INTRODUCTION

Soil is one of our most precious non-renewable resources, and the soil biota represents a large portion of the earth's biodiversity. Soil organisms carry out a wide range of ecosystem processes that are essential for crop production, soil resource quality and environmental health in both, natural and managed agricultural soils. Soil is often defined as the earth's surface exploited by roots (Buscot 2005). The soil food-web is extraordinarily complex; its trophic structure and the relationships between its components are still to be understood (Scheu et al. 2005). Although the extent of microbial diversity is not yet known, soil micro-

Microbiology Group, National Botanical Research Institute, Rana Pratap Marg, Lucknow 226 001, India **Tele-fax:** +91-522-2206651 **E-mail:** csnnbri@yahoo.com

organisms probably represent the world's greatest reservoir of biological diversity (Torsvik et al. 1990; Dykhuizen 1998). However, little is known of the forces that drive microbial community structure in soil. The complexity of the soil system is determined by numerous and diverse interactions among its physical, chemical and biological components, as modulated by prevalent environmental conditions (Tiedje 1995; Buscot 2005; Marschner 2005). One of the fundamental characters of soil environment is its heterogeneity, i.e. both, the population level and composition of soil microbiota and the physico-chemical variables, will change considerably over very small distances (e.g. millimetres). In addition, these gradients in space along with the quality of microsites also change over time (seasonal changes). In the majority of dry land cropping regions, moisture availability plays a critical role in determining the activity of both microflora and soil fauna. A coupling of above-ground plant diversity and below-ground microbial diversity has been implied in studies dedicated to assessing the role of macrophyte diversity on the stability, resilience and functioning of ecosystems. Indeed, above-ground plant communities have long been assumed to drive below-ground microbial diversity, but to date very little is known as to how plant species' composition and diversity influence the community composition of micro-organisms in the soil.

A primary goal of ecology is to understand the distribution of organisms. Investigating patterns of biodiversity is a crucial step towards achieving this goal (Lubchenco et al. 1991). While many factors likely affect the biodiversity of a region, primary productivity (the rate of energy capture and carbon fixation by primary producers) is emerging as a key determinant of plant and animal biodiversity, especially species' richness (i.e. the number of species present; Mittelbach et al. 2001). However, it is unknown how, or even if, bacterial diversity varies with primary productivity. Understanding patterns of bacterial diversity is of particular importance because bacteria may well comprise the majority of the earth's biodiversity and they mediate critical ecosystem processes (Torsvik et al. 2002).

The relationship between productivity and diversity has been of long-standing interest to ecologists. Many studies of plants and animals have reported a hump-shaped relationship between productivity and diversity, where diversity peaks at intermediate productivity. Other studies have reported a monotonic increase of diversity with productivity, a decrease, a U-shaped relationship or no discernible pattern (Abrams 1995; Mittelbach et al. 2001). Variation in observed productivity–diversity patterns may result, both, from differences in study design and differential responses of organisms at various spatial and temporal scales (Mittelbach et al. 2001). For example, the geographical scale (e.g. local vs. regional) and ecological scale (e.g. within vs. among communities) of studies often influences, patterns even within the same taxonomic group (Broughton et al.). It is also possible that some studies lump taxa or guilds that differ in their responses to productivity and thus mask patterns at different taxonomic scales (Torsvik et al. 2002). In addition, our understanding of productivity–diversity relationships is influenced strongly by particular well-studied taxonomic groups such as terrestrial plants and, therefore, may be biased by these taxa (Mittelbach et al. 2001). Other taxa (especially micro-organisms) remain relatively unstudied. In particular, the varied genetic and functional activities of the extensive microbial populations have a critical impact on soil functions, based on the fact that micro-organisms are driving forces for fundamental metabolic processes involving specific enzyme activities (Nannipieri et al. 2003).

Loss of biodiversity has thus become a major topic of concern in recent decades, and a significant amount of research has been devoted to understanding the consequences of ecosystem simplification. However, despite the realisation that microbial communities are key to the functioning of terrestrial ecosystems, their response to changes in macrophyte diversity has rarely been investigated directly (Broughton and Gross 2000). The lack of information in this area is at least partly due to the difficulties associated with studying microbial diversity, especially in soil. Microbial diversity has been studied with respect to (i) species' richness, (ii) functional groups and (iii) keystone species (Anderson 2003). Species' richness is frequently used to measure the microbial diversity in soils. This is often studied using a cultivation method. The vast majority of soil microbes (>95%) are not cultivable using currently available techniques; morphological characters are insufficient to allow taxonomy, and the definition of a bacterial species is not at all clear. However, recent use of molecular biological techniques has opened up a new window of observation, which now allows us to view microbial diversity and community structure without the need for laboratory cultivation. To overcome these problems, various methods have been developed to identify and study these micro-organisms, including fatty acid analysis and numerous DNA- and RNA-based methods (Kirk et al. 2004). Functional groups are usually defined with respect to some ecosystem function such as soil respiration and soil enzyme activities (Anderson 2003). However, because the functional groups are aggregated units, the existence of true interlinkage between taxonomic, genetic to functional diversity remains unsolved (Anderson 2003). Keystone species are defined based on the concept that a limited number of organisms and groups of organisms seem to control the critical processes necessary for ecosystem functioning (Walker 1992; Anderson 2003). This method has been used for a wide range of ecosystems. To reveal the consequences of human impacts for ecosystem functioning, microbial biomass carbon was analyzed as keystone in soil faunal community (Bradford et al. 2002). Methanogens are targeted as keystone members in the methane hydrate community (Appenzeller 1991). The keystone method is very useful, because it enables us to estimate the soil fertility from the soil microbiological point of view. Fatty acid methyl ester (FAME) analysis and terminal restriction fragment length polymorphism (T-RFLP) analysis have been used to characterize microbial community structure in soils. FAME analysis method could extract fatty acids from whole cells, not only phospholipids but also neutral lipids and glycolipids. It is known that some unique fatty acids are contained in neutral lipids and glycolipids (Mittelbach et al. 2001). Hence, this method could accumulate more diverse fatty acids, and enable us to classify more sensitively the microbial groups. T-RFLP analysis has been shown to be effective in discriminating between microbial community structures in a range of environments (Kuske et al. 2002; Nikolcheva et al. 2003). This analysis is highly reproducible and high-quality fingerprints consisting of fragments of precise size (Osborn et al. 2000) enable us to analyze many samples, making the analysis useful in field scale studies. Thus, we are now in a position to address more directly this response of soil borne microbial communities in response to changes in macrophyte diversity and species composition of below-ground microbial communities.

As the main input of organic matter in terrestrial ecosystems, plants are thought to have a profound affect in steering soil communities and processes, especially in the rhizosphere (Wardle 1992). However, there exists little data to date to support this assumption. Production, by both, crops and pastures, is supported and enhanced by soil biological processes. There is a two-way relationship between the soil biota and agricultural production. For example, as soil biota play a key role in a number of key nutrient transformation processes, crop residues form the essential supply of carbon (energy source) and nutrients for microbial activity. A diverse, balanced and active soil biota could help provide soil conditions necessary for sustainable crop production with very little negative environmental effects through (i) increased microbial activity, carbon turnover and nutrient supplying potential of soils, (ii) preventing aggressive plant pathogens taking hold and improving plant's ability to withstand disease effects, (iii) supporting the populations of plant growth promoting rhizobacteria (PGPR), (iv) reducing the loss of inorganic fertilizers through erosion and leaching by short-term immobilization, (v) stabilizing soil structure and (vi) reducing the reliance for agrochemicals and reduced persistence of pesticides in soil and thus lessen off-site impacts. The great array of root–microbe interactions results in the development of a dynamic environment known as the rhizosphere where microbial communities also interact (Fig. 1). Broadly, there are three

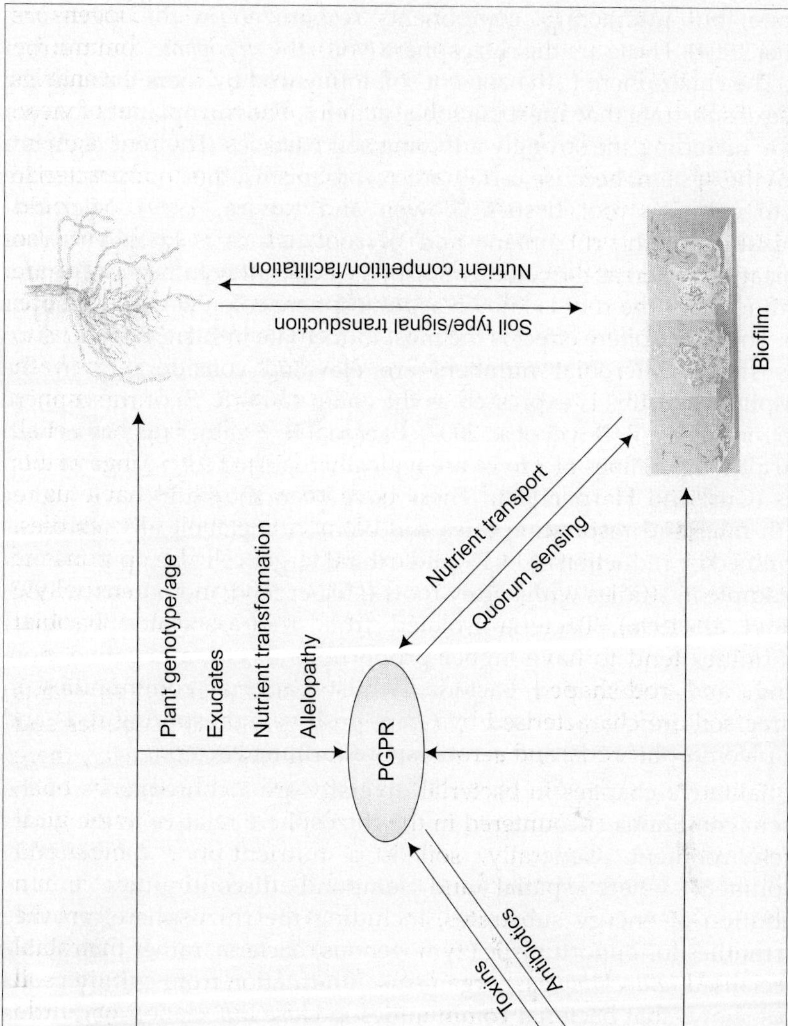

Fig. 1 Plant growth-promoting rhizobacteria (PGPR) forms and functions in soil.

separate, but interacting, components recognized in the *rhizosphere* (Hiltner 1904). These are the rhizosphere (soil), the *rhizoplane*, and the root itself. The rhizosphere is the zone of soil influenced by roots through the release of substrata that affect microbial activity. The rhizoplane is the root surface, including the strongly adhering soil particles. The root itself is a part of the system, because certain micro-organisms, the endophytes, are able to colonize root tissues (Bowen and Rovira, 1999). Microbial colonization of the rhizoplane and/or root tissues is known as root colonization, whereas the colonization of the adjacent volume of soil under the influence of the root is known as rhizosphere colonization (Kloepper 1994). The rhizosphere effect is the most immediate influence of plants on soil systems. Microbial numbers are elevated considerably in the rhizosphere and this is expressed as the count ratio (R/S) of rhizosphere soil to root-free soil (Buyer et al. 2002). Bacterial R/S values may be as high as 100 although values of 3 to 24 are typically reported for a range of crop plants (Curl and Harper1990). These have been shown to have higher growth rates and respiration rates and be more metabolically active, as determined by reduction of INT8, and exhibit larger cell size up to 5.4 mm for example in studies with barley roots (Hojbergand and Sorensen 1993; Ronn et al. 1996). Bacteria isolated from root-associated bacterial communities tend to have higher proportions of Gram-negative, non-sporing, and rod-shaped bacteria; whilst bacterial communities in root-free soil are characterised by Gram-positive, non-sporing rods and cocci, pleomorphic rods, and aerobic spore-forming bacteria.

Qualitative changes in bacterial diversity are a consequence of the different conditions encountered in the rhizosphere relative to the wider soil environment. Generally, soil is a nutrient-poor (*oligotrophic*) environment where spatial and temporal discontinuities in the distribution of energy substrates, including the rhizosphere, provide opportunities for opportunistic (zymogenous) bacteria, rather than stable or specialised (*autochthonous*) organisms. Information from culture based studies shows that bacterial communities in close association with roots have increased proportions of *Pseudomonas, Flavobacterium, Bacillus* and *Streptomyces*, while in bulk soil *Arthrobacter* have been reported to dominate (Williams1985). During development of the plant's root structure from seedling to mature root, the dominance of the zymogenous groups of bacteria over the autochthonous types has been found to decline (Miller 1990; Miller et al. 1990). This reduction probably reflects a transition from so called 'r-selective' conditions (food supply is improved and niche opportunities expand with plant growth) to 'K-selective' conditions (population density approaches the carrying capacity of the environment) (Andrews and Harris 1985). The rhizosphere effect has been found to be strongest generally amongst unicellular bacteria followed by actinomycetes, then fungi, then protozoa and algae, and then, the microfauna (Fig. 2). This means, therefore, that changes in the rhizosphere effect are likely to have a greater and more immediate effect on bacteria rather than on protozoa or algae (Bowen and Rovira 1999; Bonkowski 2004). A variety of microbial forms can be found growing in rhizosphere micro-habitats. It is universally accepted that members of any microbial group can develop important functions in the ecosystem (Giri et al. 2005). Many microbial interactions, which are regulated by specific molecules/ signals (Pace 1997), are responsible for key environmental processes, such as the bio-geochemical cycling of nutrients and matter and the maintenance of plant health and soil quality (Barea et al. 2004; Marschner 2005). This review focuses on the functions of association between plants and PGPR which benefit crops by stimulating plant growth, or by reducing the damage from soil-borne plant pathogens, the biological component of the soil ecosystem, and in particular to review the role of plants within the soil ecosystem and the types of effects that they can confer on both soil organisms and soil processes.

Some examples of the key microbial functions in soil systems are soil biota mediated processes, which can be grouped into two broad categories i.e. single species mediated functions and multiple species/organism mediated functions. For example, symbiotic nitrogen fixation in legumes is carried out by specific partnerships of legume and *Rhizobium* species, whereas a diverse group of bacteria have been shown to perform non-symbiotic nitrogen fixation. Similarly, mineralization of nutrients (e.g. nitrogen, sulphur) and decomposition of soil organic matter or crop residues involves the activity of organisms across different trophic groups. Another important point is that the factors (soil, environment and food and nutrient) that regulate the activity differ for various functional and trophic groups of biota; thus presence of organisms does not necessarily equate to their effective contribution to ecosystem function. The successful functioning of many soil biological processes requires a balance of biota interactions in a complex soil biota community. Thus soil environment is a complex and highly heterogeneous system with its chemical, physical and biological characteristics varying significantly with location and time. The primary role of plants in the soil ecosystem means that changing plants that are cultivated in a soil, or the manner in which they are cultivated, may be expected to have some effect(s) on the ecosystem of that soil. The significance of the impact(s) caused will depend on what has been affected and whether the characteristics of the soil remain altered when the plant (or the causative agent of the change) is removed. Plants are thus a key driver of soil processes, and influence soil systems through a range of interactions in which the activities of the plants (rhizo-deposition and plant litter, water, gas and nutrient exchange) modify the physical,

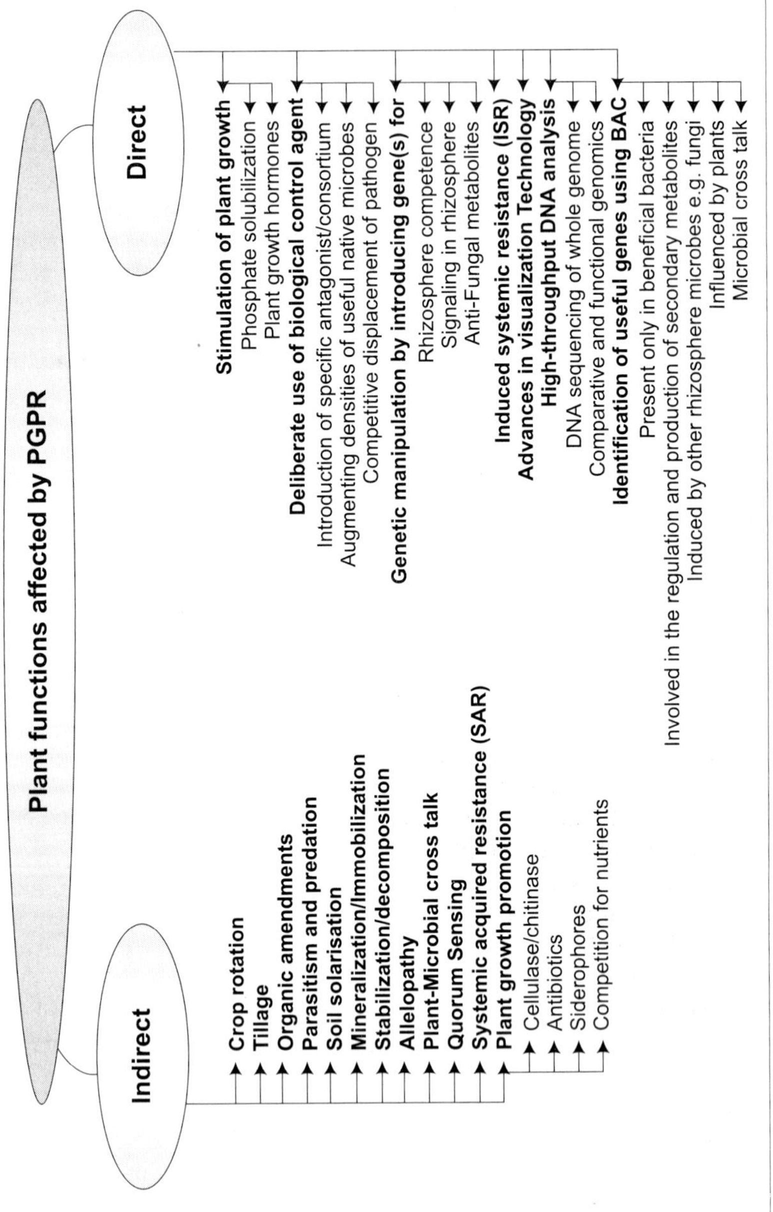

Fig. 2 Indirect and direct functions of plant affected by PGPR and applications thereof

compositional and biological characteristics of the soil (Fig 1). Confining ourselves to the establishment of large numbers of metabolically active populations of beneficial soil microbes is critical for the success of several environmental remediation and agricultural practices (Metting 1992). These micro-organisms are successful in getting established in the soil ecosystem due to their high adaptability in a wide variety of environments, their faster growth rate, and their biochemical versatility to metabolize a variety of natural and xenobiotic chemicals. Majority of the microbial population found in the soil is associated with plant roots, where their numbers can reach up to 10^9 to 10^{12} per gram of soil (Whipps 1990), leading to a biomass equivalent to 500 kg per ha (Metting 1992). This abundance in vegetated soils is due to the availability of nutrients via plant root exudation (Brimecombe 2001), which can stimulate microbial growth in the immediate vicinity of the roots. Soil-borne microbes interact with plant roots and soil constituents at the root–soil interface (Lynch 1990; Glick 1995; Barea et al. 2005). Among rhizobacteria, there is a gradient of root proximity and intimacy as follows: (i) bacteria living in the soil near roots, utilizing metabolites leaked from roots as C and N sources, (ii) bacteria colonizing the rhizoplane (root surface), (iii) bacteria residing in root tissue, inhabiting spaces between cortical cells, and lastly (iv) bacteria living inside cells in specialized root structures or nodules, which generally fall into two groups, the legume associated rhizobia and the woody plant associated *Frankia* sp. These are discussed in order of intimacy with the associated plant, from almost casual to extremely regulated and housed in specialized structures. Within this classification, various mechanisms of plant growth promoting effects have been established with the greatest understanding being of the rhizobia–legume symbiosis. As the quest for definitive knowledge presses on, research into processes underlying plant growth effects of PGPR, at each of the intimacy levels just described, is underway (Gray and Smith 2005).

2. COUPLING OF PLANTS AND PGPR

The increasing emphasis on low-input and 'organic' agriculture requires better understanding of the natural coupling between plant productivity and nutrient cycling in soil. The coupling of plant growth to biological processes in soil has been studied at various levels of complexity. Bardgett et al. (1999), for example, found that biomass production of individual plants is closely linked to that of the microbial biomass associated with roots. However, this correlation does not tell us about the balance of feedback between plants and microbes. Soil micro-organisms have key roles in litter decomposition and nutrient cycling in ecosystems. In addition, their biomass can represent a significant component of the total labile carbon (C), nitrogen (N) and phosphorus (P) in the soil. The activity and biomass of microbial communities can be influenced by several abiotic and biotic factors. Since virtually all soil microbes ultimately depend on autotrophs for their supply of C, the species' composition and activity of the plant community is likely to determine critically both, the biomass and the diversity of microbial species (Curl and Truelove 1986). Much effort has been devoted to characterization of the microbial populations in the rhizosphere of individual plant species, particularly in agricultural monocultures, and evidence is emerging that a given plant supports a distinctive bacterial community (Grayston et al. 1998). However, many such studies have used techniques that depend on culturability of the organisms concerned and so are essentially selective. They target only a small fraction of the total population, often selected preferentially for fast-growing Gram-negative species (e.g. members of the *ã*-proteobacteria). The potential to overcome these limitations has been provided recently by the development of procedures such as phospholipid fatty acid profiling and amplification of 16S rDNA and rRNA, which enable characterization of the whole microbial population. These methods pave the way, in turn, for an evaluation of the relationships between diversity and function in populations of soil micro-organisms. As a result of the past emphasis on agricultural systems we remain largely ignorant of the relationships between plant and microbial diversity in semi-natural plant communities. However, because there are large qualitative and quantitative differences, both in the root exudates from individual plant species and in the nutrient status, e.g. C-N ratio of their tissue residues (Wardle et al. 1997), we can suppose that in permanent grassland, in which plants are typically long-lived, the individual species will sustain distinctive microbial populations. As a consequence, diverse plant communities are hypothesized to sustain greater microbial diversity than monocultures and, in turn, more diversity than bare soil. Specifically, one cannot determine whether the accumulation of microbial biomass contributes positively to plant growth, or is simply a consequence of it. Frederick and Klein (1994) showed the importance of microbial communities in the acquisition of N by individual plants. They found that inoculation of plants with rhizosphere micro-organisms increased the uptake of N, and that this was true for ecotypes from both rich and poor soils, but available N in the rhizosphere was increased with the high-fertility ecotypes only. In soils, mineralization and immobilization occur simultaneously, with the balance shifting according to the availabilities and forms of C and N to microbial communities. In the rhizosphere, the release of C substrata from roots, having a large C-N ratio, most commonly results in an excess of available C and a shortage of N

(Merckx et al. 1987). These conditions promote the microbial immobilization of N, which becomes temporarily unavailable to roots. Where C is available in excess of N, fungal populations can become more prevalent, because they have larger C-N ratio and proportionately smaller requirements for N. The increased availability of C relating to N has led to the conclusion that competition between plants and microbes for N is intense within the rhizosphere, and that root exudation is disadvantageous to the plant as it increases microbial demand for N. The turnover of the microbial biomass in the rhizosphere is rapid (order of hours to days), and is driven by the input of deposits from roots. Consequently roots, which have longer life-spans (order of weeks to months), have repeated opportunity to compete for N as it is cycled through the soil and components of the microbial community. This C–N balance approach provides a useful, but greatly simplified, description of the dynamics of N in the rhizosphere. It is established that microbial communities shift in composition and activity along fertility gradients. However, it is less clear to what extent these differences are a direct consequence of nutrient availabilities in the soil, as distinct from secondary effects related to the prevalent structures of plant communities along these gradients. Bardgett et al. (1999) reported that over a growing season, microbial biomass and activity were positively correlated with changes in plant growth with time for a range of grass ecotypes from soils of intermediate fertility. Further, they showed that this correlation was independent of N fertilization. However, these positive correlations were not apparent for *Lolium perenne*, an ecotype adapted to rich soils. They concluded that there is a stronger coupling of plant growth to biological properties with ecotypes from soils of intermediate fertility, reflecting a greater dependence on this coupling for acquisition of N in their native soils. Short-term interactions between plants, nutrient availability and microbial communities are not necessarily characteristic of these relationships over longer times. For example, Bardgett et al. (1999) found that fertilization with N promoted fungi over bacteria in grassland soil. This is directly opposed to the general finding that microbial communities of rich grassland soils are dominated by bacteria (Bardgett et al. 1999). It is likely that in the longer term, interactions between plants and microbes are increasingly affected by the quality of dead plant inputs (litter and root turnover). In oligotrophic ecosystems, these inputs are generally more recalcitrant and have a larger C-N ratio than inputs from richer ecotypes. Further study is required to determine the extent to which the development and function of the microbial community in the rhizosphere of plants from rich and oligotrophic ecosystems are mediated by root exudation and inputs of dead tissue, respectively.

3. PLANT AND PGPR CROSS TALK

The rhizosphere is a zone of intense competition for resources, and it is not surprising that both, plants and microbes, have evolved strategies to manipulate its functioning. Bacteria have developed efficient systems to perceive their environment through diffusible signals, particularly to sense the microbial population density. Many bacteria produce small signal molecules that are secreted into the local environment and trigger specific behavioural responses in the producing population when they exceed a critical concentration threshold. Under laboratory conditions, this threshold is normally reached when the bacterial culture producing the auto-inducer (AI) signal molecule reaches a critical density. At this point, the population is said to be 'quorate', and a synchronized change in behavior can be triggered. For this reason, the production of and response to such auto-inducers is frequently termed quorum sensing. Among Gram-negative bacteria, the best studied and possibly most common group of auto-inducer signals are *N*-acylhomoserine lactones (AHLs). In plant-associated bacteria, AHLs are found in pathogenic, symbiotic and biological control strains, and they regulate a diverse range of phenotypes including diverse pathogenicity determinants, conjugation, rhizosphere competence and the production of antifungal metabolites (Fig 1). A higher proportion of AHL producing bacteria is found in the immediate vicinity of plant roots (the rhizosphere) than in bulk soil, suggesting a general role in rhizosphere colonization (Elasri et al. 2001) and competence, possibly through regulating mechanisms such as exopolysaccharide production, attachment and biofilms formation (Marketon et al. 2003). Culture-based experiments show that AHL sensing is generally integrated into much larger control networks with many positive and negative inputs. In addition, it is becoming apparent that some plants may be able to interfere with, and possibly respond to, the bacterial AHL signalling system (Teplitski et al. 2000; Mathesius et al. 2003; Marschner 2005). The challenge now is to test the current models in naturally occurring plant–bacterial interactions to determine the key regulators in the AHL signalling network during the plant–microbe interaction. This is important because, under such conditions, it is possible that AI-based signalling systems might be conveying alternative or additional information to population size (Redfield 2002) and, although such signalling mechanisms allow the co-ordination of multicellular behavior, this may not always be the primary function. Newton and Fray (2004) have recently reviewed the importance of plant-derived compounds in contributing to AHL 'quorum-sensing' responses and role of AHL signalling in *Erwinia carotovora* and *Agrobacterium tumefaciens*, a necrotrophic and a biotrophic plant pathogen respectively. It is curious that the most hydrophobic AHL molecules are produced by species of *Rhizobium*, which, during their plant-associated form, are found in multiple small nitrogen-fixing symbiosomes completely surrounded by plant-derived membranes within a host cell. However, it is currently not known whether the differentiated bacteroids within these symbiosomes are producing an AHL signal or whether such communication is reserved for the free-living form. AHL-mediated signalling is clearly important in many plant–microbe associations. The information communicated by such auto-inducers has been questioned but, in most cases, it is likely to include some aspect of population density. However, AHL levels alone are often insufficient to trigger the full range of behavioral changes, and such quorum-sensing systems form part of integrated signaling networks. Inputs from additional auto inducers, the host plant and environmental sources come together to induce the 'quorum-sensing' behaviour (Fig 1).

As discussed above, the composition of organic material released from roots is a strong determinant of the structure of the microbial community. This may function as a broad-scale control by plants of microbial populations, favouring those beneficial to the plant. More specifically, components of the microbial community in the rhizosphere produce plant hormones that affect growth (Pokojska-Burdziej 1981). These hormone producers may benefit from enhanced flow of C from roots through effects on root growth or development (Lippmann et al. 1995). In turn, this may feed back to increased uptake of N by plants as a consequence of increased exploration of soil by roots. Large populations of bacteria feeding micro fauna in the rhizosphere help to cycle microbial N (Clarholm1985). In addition, feeding is selective: some populations are more depleted than others, and so the micro faunal feeders affect the structure of the microbial communities (Griffiths 1994). This may be expected to affect the physiological diversity of the microbial biomass in the rhizosphere, and consequently its mineralization capacity. In addition to micro-organisms' using root exudates as substrata, components of these exudates are thought to act as specific signals to microbes (Grayston et al. 1998). The signal molecules have received much interest in relation to formation of mutualistic associations between host roots and Rhizobia, arbuscular mycorrhizae and ectomycorrhizae (Fries et al. 1987; Le Strange et al. 1990; Dharmatilake and Bauer 1992). Generally, these signal compounds are active at very small concentrations (10^{-6}–10^{-12} M), and effects are independent of the target organism's ability to use the compounds as substrate. Typically, the signal exudates function as specific chemo-attractants, elicitors of spore germination or activators of gene expression required to form the mutualistic symbiosis. The importance of signal exudates for interactions between roots and associated micro-organisms has been studied in much less detail. However, it is likely that with increasing informations about the microbial diversity in the rhizosphere and its dependence on the flow of C from roots, many more examples of signalling between roots and microbes via exudates will be discovered. Bauer and Teplitski (2001) made a discovery with potentially great implications, namely that plants release compounds that have the potential to repress or stimulate microbial signalling in the rhizosphere. A broad range of Gram-negative bacteria detect their population densities through production of diffusive compounds (e.g. N-acetyl homoserine lactones), which, when in excess of a threshold concentration in the environment, induce transcription of specific genes in the population (Faqua et al. 1996). Genes expressed in response to these signals include many involved in interactions between plants and microbes. Teplitski et al. (2000) showed that analogues of bacterial signal molecules are synthesized in plants and released in root exudates. Analogue compounds that repress transduction of bacterial signals may be important in preventing expression of virulence factors such as proteases and cellulase, for which regulation depends on cell density (Pierson et al. 1998). Therefore, exudation of bacterial signal analogues can be considered as a form of defense by the plants against soil-borne pathogens. Intriguingly, analogue compounds that stimulate bacterial signalling have also been detected in root exudates (Teplitski et al. 2000; Bauer and Teplitski 2001). This suggests that plants can actively stimulate specific microbial populations in the rhizosphere. If such signalling were quantitatively significant in nature then plants might stimulate microbial production of exoenzymes to promote mineralization of organic matter around roots (Fig 1).

AHLs accumulate as a function of cell density, and at some threshold level, are described as a bacterial quorum, activate expression of target genes. For instance in *P. aureofaciens*, such a system controls the antibiotic production as these compounds are critical in the competition with other microbes when substratum availability decreases (Pierson et al. 1998). Among the many examples of lactones signalling in bacterial cross-talk are: the stimulation of both sporulation and competence of *Bacillus subtilis*, the induction of fruiting body formation of *Myxococcus xanthus* (Persello-Cartieaux et al. 2003). These auto-inducers allow the cell to avoid constitutive expression of genes that are required only in peculiar environmental conditions. Bacterial cells often engage in elaborate chemical conversations with higher organisms because: (1) sensory transduction system homologous to those involved in quorum sensing have been identified in symbiotic and pathogenic Rhizobacteria–plant interactions (Fuqua et al. 1994); and (2) exudates from pea seedlings were found to contain several separable activities that mimicked AHL signals (Teplitski et al. 2000). Molecular signals are also certainly exchanged between plant and non-pathogenic and non-symbiotic Rhizobacteria.

Indeed, most of bacterial traits required for competitive colonization of root systems were found to be involved in environment perception and more precisely in plant exudates (e.g. an exudates-inducible sugar transporter; Bayliss et al. 1997), which also illustrated their critical role in successful Rhizobacterial colonization. The identification of a bacterial sensor-regulator two-component system and of a type III secretion system, both induced in the rhizosphere (Preston et al. 1998), and the isolation of tomato genes associated with ISR by *B. cereus*, constitute an indirect evidence for the existence of this communication. The need of a threshold initial bacterial Inoculum density (about 10^6-10^7 CFU mL^{-1}) to significantly promote plant growth suggests the role of a quorum sensing system in plant–Rhizobacteria interactions, whereas the perception of eubacterial flagellin peptides allows the plant to sense the presence of a broad range of microbes (Felix et al. 1999). As bacterial plant growth promotion can be mediated by additive mechanisms (e.g. siderophores production and ISR), it is tempting to speculate that plants have also developed many strategies to perceive and select their microbial partner.

Recent work demonstrated that the tomato rhizosphere isolate *P. putida* IsoF produces a wide spectrum of AHLs including 3-oxo-dodecanoyl-homoserine lactone (3-oxo-C12-HSL), 3-oxo-decanoyl-homoserine lactones (3-oxo-C10-HSL) and as minor products, 3-oxooctanoyl-homoserine lactones (3-oxo-C8-HSL), and 3-oxo-hexanoyl-homoserine lactones (3-oxo-C6-HSL). The QS system of this strain consists of PpuI, which directs the synthesis of AHL signal molecules and PpuR, which binds to the AHLs and regulates the PpuI expression in a positive feedback loop. While the wild type *P. putida* IsoF formed very homogenous unstructured biofilms that uniformly cover the surface, a PpuI mutant formed structured biofilms with characteristic microcolonies and water filled channels. When the medium was supplemented with AHL signal molecules, the mutant biofilm lost its structure and converted into an unstructured biofilm similar to the one formed by the wild type IsoF. These results suggest that the QS system influences biofilm's structural development (Steidle et al. 2001). Mature biofilms can be described as complex three dimensional structures where cells are embedded in a thick matrix of extracellular polymeric substances (EPS). These structures are crossed by fluid-filled channels that enable nutrient transport to the interior parts of the biofilms and the elimination of waste products (Hall-Stoodley et al. 2004). Several steps are required for biofilm formation: (I) initial attachment to a surface, (II) formation of microcolonies, (III) maturation of microcolonies into EPS-encased three-dimensional biofilms, and (IV) detachment and dispersion of single cells from the matrix (O'Toole et al. 2000). The dramatic phenotypical changes during these processes must involve a coordinated series of molecular events. Different parameters triggering the transition from plank tonic to sessile life-style have been discussed, including general changes in the genetic program, environmental signals and the interaction between the genetic and environmental responses (Hall-Stoodley et al. 2004). The ability to organize structurally and to distribute metabolic activities between the different bacteria, demands consequently a high degree of coordinated cell-to-cell interaction. Evidences accumulated over the past few years showed that AHL-mediated cell-to-cell signalling is an important regulatory factor that directly controls development of biofilms (Hentzer et al. 2004) in various Gram-negative bacteria, including *Burkholderia cepacia* (Huber et al. 2002), *Aeromonas hydrophila* (Lynch et al. 2002), *P. aeruginosa* (Davies et al. 1998; Yoon et al. 2002; Heydorn et al. 2002) and *Serratia liquefaciens* (Labatte et al. 2004)

While the biochemical mechanisms underlying AHL mediated quorum sensing have been well studied in culture, the functioning of this signalling mechanism under natural biological conditions is more difficult to assess. Recent studies have demonstrated that communication through the use of AHLs is not limited to recognition among cells of the same species, for example, restoration of the AHL-deficient *S. liquefaciens* mutant in a binary swarming colony. The AHLs produced by the co-inoculated bacterium trigger biosurfactant synthesis in the population of AHL-deficient *S. liquefaciens* cells (Andersen et al. 2001). One must always be careful to extrapolate findings on bacteria grown in laboratory conditions to the in vitro situation, where the physiological situation may be different. For example, a study under natural biological conditions revealed anaerobic respiration in *P. aeruginosa* biofilms (Hassett et al. 2002). The latter condition requires the presence of the *rhl* quorum sensing system for bacterial survival. From an applied point of view, influencing the swarming behavior of bacteria may help to control root colonization and containment, and this may have important applications in agriculture. Daniels et al. (2004) have recently reviewed different signal molecules either produced by bacteria (such as other AHLs and diketopiperazines) or excreted by plants (such as furanones, plant signal mimics) might influence the quorum sensing regulated swarming behaviour in bacteria different from the producer. Role and regulation of a surface-associated movement in biofilm formation and how quorum sensing may disperse existing biofilms and control the interaction between bacteria and higher organisms (such as the *Rhizobium*-bean symbiosis) have also been discussed. The traits involved in bacterial rhizosphere competence are still poorly understood; among other factors the ability to form biofilms and QS that enable the bacteria to co-ordinate the expression of special phenotypes in a cell density dependent manner, might play an important role. The use of model systems such as *Arabidopsis thaliana*/*Pseudomonas* spp. opens up the opportunity to apply the deep molecular genetic analysis which is necessary to efficiently understand the molecular ecology of complex inter-kingdom relationships (Fig 1).

4. ALLELOPATHY AMONG PLANT AND PGPR

The term *allelopathic* was first proposed by Molisch (1937) to describe inhibitory or stimulatory biochemical interactions that occurred between members of the plant kingdom. As a class of relationship between organisms, allelopathic is considered to be one where no direct contact occurs; the effect of any interaction being a consequence of some indirect event, controlled by an allelochemical. Since Molisch's time the allelopathic concept has been extended to include any organism-to-organism interaction mediated by the release and subsequent reception of organic compounds (allelochemicals) which result in some beneficial or harmful consequence to the receptor. Recently, allelopathic was redefined again to include "... any process involving secondary metabolites produced by plants, micro-organisms, viruses and fungi that influence the growth and development of biological systems... " (IAS 1998). Thus, while allelopathic events are often reported at the community-species level, allelopathic is more accurately an ecological phenomenon operating at the trophic level, with implications for the regulation of ecosystem health and biodiversity (Malik 2000). By learning how to adapt and manage root zone microbial communities, opportunities arise to produce food crops in a more sustainable manner (Chou 1999). Within the soil environment the free movement of allelochemicals, is now known to influence a wide variety of soil related and crop management processes, including soil fertility, nitrogen transfer, weed control, crop compatibility within rotations, residue management, plant growth, and the development and the maintenance of disease suppressive soils (Narwal 2000). Larger number of allelochemical compounds have been identified from soil microbial sources (Glick et al. 1999). These again involve secondary metabolites comprising lytic agents and enzymes, siderophores, auxins, volatile compounds, and phytotoxic substances (Sturz and Christie 2003).

Plant–microbe interactions extend over time (plant developmental age and season), space (macro and microhabitat) and substrata (energy source and availability). For example, plants appeared are able to influence the composition of the microbial community around their root systems through the selective exudation of specific carbohydrates, carboxylic and amino-acids (Grayston et al. 1998), and these microbial communities can be cultivar-specific (Siciliano et al. 1998). Rhizobacteria can themselves induce root exudation responses in plants (Merharg and Killham 1995), or initiate changes in root biochemistry (Parmar and Dardarwal 1999) prompting the thesis that Rhizobacteria–plant partnerships have a long history of successful co-evolution. As a high proportion of Rhizobacteria are believed capable of producing the plant growth hormone indole acetic acid (IAA) (Glickman et al. 1998), root growth is often stimulated, helping to establish the plant providing more root surface area for microbial habitat. This encourages further exudates' loss and subsequent bacterial colonization. Rhizodermal and root cortical cell-death can be considered to be an autolytic process, attributable to pre-programmed root cell-death (Foster and Bowen 1982); thus early Rhizobacteria colonization can also be initiated by the plant. Similarly, root border cells (sloughed root cap cells) released in advance of the root apical meristem may be used by plants to 'engineer' the microbial ecology of the rhizosphere (Hawes et al. 1998) by loading the rhizosphere with carbon-rich material (Hawes and Brigham1992), thus 'managing' the rate and progress at which root–microbe interactions proceed. In this way, plants can trigger a series of events that result in a set of positive 'allelopathic feedbacks' where the final receptor organism of this allelopathic cascade is also the initiator. In some respects, such mechanisms parallel the process of 'auto toxicity', where photochemical auto-inhibitors—leachates or exudates—collect in the root zone and inhibit alike and unlike species' seed germination and new plant growth, so preventing excessive crowding (Whittaker and Feeny 1971).

Very few studies have quantified the relationship between plant disease and allelopathic. Where it has been reported, the allelochemical event is usually phyto-mediated and triggers or enhances a phytopathogenic outcome (Hartung and Stephens 1983) to the detriment of the host plant. Nevertheless, broadening of the allelopathic concept has enabled the gradual recognition that disease suppression by biological control is, for all intents and purposes, an allelopathic phenomenon. More so, if one accepts the premise that it can be 'plant-directed' through the encouragement and selective development of beneficial microbial communities in the root zone. While Rhizobacteria can influence plant growth directly through the production of plant-hormones such as gibberellins, cytokines and IAA, they can also influence plant growth indirectly through the inhibition of plant pathogens in the root zone soil. In this respect, soil borne phytopathogens encounter antagonism from rhizosphere micro-organisms before, during and after primary infection and secondary spread within the root. Such pathogen antagonism has been collectively termed biological control and was defined by Baker (1987) to be "... a decrease of inoculum or the disease-producing activity of a pathogen accomplished through one or more organisms, including the host plant...". In the root zone, biocontrol is the outcome of multiple allelopathic events, a large proportion of which can be Rhizobacteria in origin (Fujimoto et al. 1995).

Rhizobacterial antagonism can take many forms and is not directed at pathogens specifically, but at any group of organisms 'invading' an established root zone community. Thus, positive or neutral interactions among autochthonous (established) consortia of microflora and micro fauna are more probable, while any invader (colonist or pathogen) is more likely to provoke a negative response (Atlas 1986). Soils with a biological propensity to inhibit or reduce the effect of soil borne phytopathogens have been termed disease suppressive, and several microbial mechanisms involved in regulating disease suppression and pathogen reduction have been described by Sturz and Christie 2003. Niche competition (Stephens et al. 1993) and microbiostasis (Ho and Ko 1986) can develop between pathogens and other microbial populations. In this regard, siderophores-producing bacteria, with high affinities for iron, have been found to inhibit certain phytopathogens, with a requirement for iron, in iron-limited soils (Dowling et al. 1996). Similarly, by establishing partial sinks for nutrients, Rhizobacteria can reduce the amount of carbon and nitrogen available for fungal spore germination and (phytopathogen) pre-infection growth in the root zone (Elad and Baker 1985). Antibiosis through the production of specific or non-specific microbial metabolites, lytic agents, enzymes, volatile compounds or other microbial toxins are often reported as agents of disease suppression (Leyns et al. 1990). Antibiotics synthesized by rhizobacteria can contribute to microbial antagonism and persistence in the root zone soil (Kerry, 2000). Antibacterial, antifungal and anti-nematode activity has been identified in the antibiotic producing strains of a wide range of bacterial genera, but most notably from *Agrobacterium* sp. (agrocin 84), *Pseudomonas* sp. (2,4-*diacetyl phloroglucinol*, *phenazine* derivatives, *pyoleutorin* and *pyrrolnitrin*), *Erwinia* sp. (*herbicolin* A) and *Bacillus* sp. (iturin A, surfactin) (Fravel 1988; Levy and Carmelli, 1995; Sayre and Starr 1988; Thomashow et al. 1997). Suppression of *Meloidogyne incognita* by entomopathogenic nematodes has recently been proposed to be an allelopathic event mediated by symbiotic bacteria occurring within the latter (Grewal et al. 1999).

5. PGPR FUNCTIONS IN SOIL

Major examples of the key microbial functions in soil systems are symbiotic nitrogen fixation in legumes carried out by specific partnerships of legume and *Rhizobium* species, whereas a diverse group of bacteria have been shown to perform non-symbiotic nitrogen fixation. Similarly, mineralisation of nutrients (e.g. nitrogen, sulfur) and decomposition of soil organic matter or crop residues involves the activity of organisms across different trophic groups. However, it must be taken into consideration that factors (soil, environment and food and nutrient) that regulate the activity differ for various functional and trophic groups of biota, thus presence of organisms does not necessarily equate to their effective contribution to ecosystem function. The successful functioning of many soil biological processes requires a balance of biota interactions in a complex soil biota community (Fig 1). Thus, for example, while a variety of bacteria and fungi have been found to be effective inoculants either as biocontrol agents against different crop diseases or through plant growth promotion based on controlled environment experiments, no single microbial inoculants has yet been universally successful under agriculture systems. The maintenance of threshold levels of populations of introduced inoculants is a significant factor in their ability to perform intended function, e.g. effective disease control, plant growth promotion. For example, for an introduced biocontrol agent to be effective it must first survive, establish, acclimatize and grow in field soils and interact with the pathogenic organisms alone or in the presence of plant. Unlike the *Rhizobium* inoculants, which live within the protected environment of a nodule, the soil and environmental conditions are generally harsh and not optimal for introduced microbes in cropping systems, i.e. carbon-poor soils, short-periods of warm and moist soil interjected with long dry and hot periods. Research on the field based ecological aspects of inoculants has been very limited. Some of the key factors important for an introduced micro-organism to be effective include:

1. Availability of source of energy (carbon) or a host plant.
2. Suitable habitat–all functional groups of microbes require specific habitat conditions to perform their function e.g. water, oxygen and nutrient concentration etc.
3. Protection from predators, competition from general soil microbial community.

To complicate the matter further, various management practices that are involved in grain and pasture crop production have an impact on either the populations of different groups of beneficial and deleterious biota and/or their activities in all soil types and cropping regions. The effects on soil biota are through (i) direct effects on the populations, (ii) the changes in the soil habitat (e.g. physical and chemical properties), microclimate and carbon (energy) sources and (iii) influencing on above ground productivity and community composition (Fig 1). However, successful cases, where benefits from adding microbial inoculants were observed, have been reported. Some of the key microbial functions in soil systems, where PGPR have played an important role as microbial inoculants or beneficial products in broad acre agriculture based on reliable scientific evidence are as follows:

5.1 Adding Nutrients to Soil

Organic matter in soil is the most important fraction that supports microbial populations, especially the biologically available portion of soil organic matter. Microbial biomass (MB), the living component of soil organic matter, constitutes 2-5% of the organic carbon in soils. MB acts as the engine for organic matter (OM) turnover and nutrient release. The size of MB in the surface soil may range from 250 mg C per kg in sandy soil to 1100 mg C per kg in OM rich clay soil. Microbial biomass carbon may only represent a small portion of soil organic matter (2-7%) but is dynamic and living and thus is more sensitive to management practices than total soil OM. MB is a store-house of plant essential nutrients, for example nitrogen levels in MB range from 15 mg to 150 kg N/ha. MB also hold 5-15 kg of sulphur and 10-45 kg phosphorus per ha. Nutrients held in MB are, not prone to leaching, only tied up temporarily and are released for plant uptake as a result of predation by micro fauna and the death of microbes during soil drying. It is the interactions between micro-organisms and organic matter in the soil that largely determine the fertility and overall quality of the soil. Therefore it is extremely important to use farm management practices that maintain organic matter levels, especially biologically available organic matter in our soils.

Biological function in soil is mainly regulated by the amount of available carbon. Soil microbes require this carbon as a source of energy, particularly the heterotrophic organisms which constitute the majority of soil micro biota. Plants are the major source of available carbon for biological activity, hence, soil biodiversity and biological activity are more dependant on the quality and quantity of carbon inputs from plants (through root exudation and above & below ground plant residues) and plant-induced changes in soil physical and chemical properties. Pastures are composed of mixtures of plant types (legumes, grasses, C3, C4) and hence considered as having a greater potential to influence on diverse biological processes. However, the availability of carbon in grazed systems is mediated strongly by grazing management through above and belowground plant growth in response to grazing.

Thus, when considering the nutrient transformations and availability in field situations, it is important to account the implications of spatial scales of biota distribution, seasonal patterns of biological activity and landscape position for any ecosystem function. These interactions not only influence our perception of biological functions in an ecosystem but also affect our ability to manage them for maximum benefit. In undisturbed natural ecosystems there is generally a high degree of synchronization of the availability of nutrients and with the need/uptake by plants which results in low levels of nutrients in soil solution at any one time. However, in most of the agricultural systems not only do greater amounts of nutrients flow in and out, but also synchronization of supply with plant requirement is not always optimum (Fig 1).

Nitrogen is a key requisite of life and is used in agriculture as a common fertilizer supplement necessary to maintain high levels of soil fertility. In addition to animal waste, plant residues and other organic inputs, nitrogen enters the soil ecosystem when atmospheric nitrogen (N_2) is fixed as ammonia (NH_3) by specific bacterial populations. Nitrogen fixation is a reducible energy intensive process and nitrogen fixing bacteria are often associated with plants that can provide energy and fixed carbon. Further, ammonia may be oxidized by nitrifying bacteria to nitrite (NO^{2-}) and on to nitrate (NO^{3-}). This nitrification of ammonia means that the soluble nitrate is more readily available to plants and microbes but is also more likely to be lost from soil by leaching, thus decreasing the available fixed nitrogen. Although agricultural supplements and the fixation of new nitrogen are important, a key aspect of soil fertility is the recycling of fixed nitrogen from wastes (plant and animal) to forms which are available to plants. In this mineralisation process nitrogen present in organic wastes is liberated as ammonium by a diverse community of microbes and animals. In soil, ammonia and nitrate may be taken up and utilized by plants or microbes. Bacterial assimilation of NH^{4+} or NO^{3-} is called immobilization. Alternatively, denitrifying bacteria may use the nitrate as an electron acceptor in anaerobic respiration. This involves the reduction of nitrate to nitric oxide (NO), to nitrous oxide (N_2O) and on to N_2. The release of these gases depletes the fixed nitrogen of the soil system. This denitrification happens when soils or parts of soil systems become anoxic (low oxygen availability). The carbon to nitrogen (C:N) ratio of plant rhizodeposition is an influential factor in N-cycling as low ratio values result in N-limited microbial growth and increased microbial immobilization of N. Plants, through rhizo-deposition and other plant-soil exchanges, also have a significant effect on the diversity of the microbial community and its behaviour. Paterson (2003) reviewed the coupling of plant productivity and nutrient cycling and identified a number of mechanisms by which plants can influence nutrient mineralisation by soil microbes, and by which microbes can influence plant productivity.

Biological nitrogen fixation is estimated to contribute 180×10^6 metric tons per year globally (Postgate 1998), of which eighty per cent comes from symbiotic associations and the rest from free-living or associative systems (Graham 1998). The ability to reduce and siphon out such appreciable amounts of nitrogen from the atmospheric reservoir and enrich the soil is confined to bacteria and Archaea (Young 1992). These include, (a) symbiotic nitrogen fixing (N_2-fixing) forms, viz. *Rhizobium*, the obligate symbionts in leguminous plants and *Frankia* in non-leguminous trees, and (b) Non-symbiotic (free-living, associative or endophytic) N_2-fixing forms such as cyanobacteria, *Azospirillum*, *Azotobacter*, *Acetobacter diazotrophicus*, and *Azoarcus*, etc.

As they share common microhabitats in the root–soil interface, Rhizobia and PGPR must interact during their processes of root colonization. Some PGPRs can improve nodulation and N_2-fixation in legume plants (Lucas-Garcia et al. 2004). Studies carried out under field conditions (Bai et al. 2002, 2003), particularly those using ^{15}N-based techniques (Dashti et al. 1998) reinforce such beneficial co-operative effects between microbes. Research on the mechanisms, by which PGPR enhance nodule formation, implicates their production of plant hormones among the co-inoculation benefits. For example, Chebotar et al. (2001) demonstrated that some *Pseudomonas* strains, but not all, increased nodule number and acetylene reduction in soybean plants inoculated with *B. japonicum*. The use of gus-A marked Rhizobacteria allowed the authors to demonstrate that the bacteria colonized the root. Azco´n-Aguilar and Barea (1978), using both cell-free supernatants of PGPR cultures and pure chemicals, first demonstrated that plant-growth-regulating substances produced by PGPR affected nodulation and nitrogen fixation. Recently, Man˜ero et al. (2003) extended these observations. The possibility that metabolites other than phytohormones, such as siderophores, phytoalexins, and flavonoids, might enhance nodule formation has also been proposed (Lucas-Garcia et al. 2004), but this hypothesis has not been verified.

Many of the PGPR described to date are free-living diazotrophs that can convert molecular nitrogen into ammonia in a free state by virtue of the nitrogenase enzyme complex (Postgate 1982). Another feature that has been reported for PGPR is the production of phytohormones which could affect root development directly. Since nutritional capacity and developmental control are very much dependent on each other and because they both affect the growth rate of the plant, one can ask whether the PGPR primarily act on one or the other. It was attractive to explain the positive effect of PGPR on plant growth by the provision of nitrogen fixed by the bacteria to the host plant. This 'biofertilization' hypothesis was all the more attractive since N-availability is the main yield-limiting factor in many agricultural situations and the leaching of N-fertilizers into groundwater causes environmental problems. Experiments using acetylene reduction measurements and the ^{15}N-isotope dilution technique provided conflicting results. For instance, large contributions to the plant's N-budget from plant-associated bacterial N_2-fixation have been reported with sugar cane (Mirza et al. 2001) and mangrove (Bashan et al. 1998). Furthermore, gene reporter fusions demonstrated that the *nif* genes of *Azospirillum* and *Azoarcus* Rhizobacteria strains are expressed (enhanced?) when associated with the roots of wheat and rice, respectively (Vande Broek et al. 1993; Egener et al. 1998, 1999). However the expression of *nif* genes or active N_2-fixation by the rhizobacteria do not imply that there is a large transfer of newly fixed nitrogen to the plant. On the contrary, evidence that growth promotion by PGPR does not rely on the N_2-fixation process have been obtained for tomato seedlings associated with an *Azospirillum brasilense* mutant strain totally deficient in N_2-fixation capacity (Bashan et al. 1989). Overall, most of the inoculation experiments reported in the literature failed to show a significant contribution of N_2-fixation by PGPR to the plant's N status (Bremner et al. 1995). This is in complete contrast to symbiotic associations where relatively large amounts of atmospheric N reach the plant as ammonia released by the bacteroids. By contrast, most of the ammonia produced in PGPR by the nitrogenase catalysed N_2 fixation would be assimilated by the Rhizobacteria through the glutamine synthetase/glutamate synthase (GS/GOGAT) pathway. Considering the high cost of the N_2-fixation reaction (Phillips 1980), the bacteria tend to limit the loss of fixed N. The leak of ammonia out of the cells of bacteria may be minimized by virtue of the GS/GOGAT pathway operating at a high rate (Steenhoudt and Vanderleyden 2000). In addition, ammonium transporters found in several PGPR strains are thought to be involved in the reabsorption of NH^+_4 released as a consequence of NH_3 diffusion through the bacterial membrane (Van Dommelen et al. 1997). The inoculation of tomato roots with a wild-type strain, but not with *nif* mutant strains, of *Azospirillum brasilense* induced the tomato LeAmt1.2 gene coding for an ammonium transporter (Becker et al. 2002). This suggests that due to its N_2-fixation activity the bacteria excrete NH^+_4 in quantities consistent with the induction of the LeAmt1.2 gene, i.e. in the micro molar range (higher concentrations reduces LeAmt1.2 mRNA levels). Quantification of N-transfer would be necessary to assess whether the ammonium released by the bacteria is used as a source of N by the plant. Alternatively, the authors proposed that NH^+_4 ions play a signalling role in the interactions between PGPR and plants (Becker et al. 2002).

Despite their ability to fix atmospheric nitrogen, PGPR are unlikely to provide large amounts of this nitrogen to the plants. However, they have a great impact on nitrogen nutrition by increasing NO^-_3 uptake capacity, indirectly as a consequence of stimulated lateral root development and possibly directly by stimulating NO^-_3 transport systems. The question of the ability of PGPR to stimulate NO^-_3 uptake, however, remains to be addressed directly. Although NO^-_3 transporters are likely to be post-translationally regulated, the results of numerous expression studies suggest that NO^-_3 uptake is primarily regulated at the transcriptional level (Forde 2000; Nazoa et al. 2003). The molecular tools available in Arabidopsis should, therefore, help to determine whether PGPR have an effect on NO^-_3 transporters per se, directly or indirectly, or if the increased N efficiency is only due to the increase of root surface area elicited by the PGPR. The effect of PGPR on root morphogenesis does not appear to be antagonistic to the effect exerted on root architecture by NO^-_3. To investigate whether the two underlying regulatory pathways are totally independent or if they share some common elements will require more detailed knowledge of the individual signalling pathways. In addition, the rapid progress of knowledge on the hormonal transduction pathways in plants will provide tools to determine which steps of these transduction pathways are targets of the PGPR. Finally, the response processes of root development and mineral uptake to NO^-_3 availability and PGPR inoculation are probably independent of each other. If this is true, the effects of these abiotic and biotic factors must be additive, i.e. the total root length would be highest in inoculated plants grown with low N fertilization. This conclusion is consistent with the observation that the effects of inoculation are the highest in fields with low N fertilizer supply (Dobbelaere et al. 2002; Mantelin and Touraine 2004).

5.2 Transferring Nutrients into Plant Available forms or Facilitate their Uptake by Plants

There are abundant micro-organisms thriving in soil, especially in the rhizosphere of plants. It is well known that a considerable number of bacteria possess a functional relationship and constitute a holistic system with plants. They are able to exert beneficial effects on plant growth (Vessey 2003). Application of beneficial microbes in agricultural practices started 60 years ago and there is now increasing evidence that these beneficial microbial populations can also enhance plant's resistance to adverse environmental stresses, e.g. water and nutrient deficiency and heavy metal contamination. PGPR participate in many key ecosystem processes such as those involved in the biological control of plant pathogens, nutrient cycling and seedling establishment, and therefore deserve particular attention for agricultural or forestry purposes (Elo et al. 2000). PGPR may colonize the rhizosphere, the surface of the root, or even superficial intercellular spaces of plants (McCully 2001). Phosphate (P)$^-$ and potassium (K)$^-$solubilizing bacteria may enhance mineral uptake by plants through solubilizing insoluble P and releasing K from silicate in soil (Goldstein and Liu 1987). Some successful examples of inoculation with PGPR have been achieved, both, in laboratory and field trials. For example, strains of *P. putida* and *P. fluorescens* could increase root and shoot elongation in canola, lettuce and tomato (Glick et al. 1997). It has also been reported that wheat yield increased up to 30% with *Azotobacter* inoculation and up to 43% with *Bacillus* inoculation (Kloepper et al. 1991). Soil micro-organisms are important components in the natural soil sub-ecosystem because not only can they contribute to nutrient availability in the soil, but also bind soil particles into stable aggregates, which improve soil structure and reduce erosion (Shetty et al. 1994).

As with nitrogen, the soil system recycles phosphorus (P). This compound is essential for life and taken up by plants (and microbes) from soil as phosphate (PO_4^{3-}). Although mineral phosphorus enters the soil system as phosphates from geological sources, the recycling of phosphorous by decomposition of plant material, animals and wastes is important for soil fertility. Even with the addition of phosphate-based fertilizers, the majority of phosphorus used by a crop (70-90 percent) will be derived from soil reserves. P in soils is immobilized or becomes less soluble either by absorption, chemical precipitation, or both. A survey of Indian soils revealed that 98% of these need phosphorus fertilization either in the form of chemical or biological fertilizer. Although P-content in an average soil is 0.05%, only 0.1% of the total P present is available to the plants because of its chemical fixation and low solubility. Application of chemical phosphatic fertilizers is practiced, though, a majority of the soil P reaction products are only sparingly soluble. Under such conditions, micro-organisms offer a biological rescue system capable of solubilizing the insoluble inorganic P of soil and make it available to the plants (Deubel and Merbach 2005). The availability of phosphates may be limited or stimulated by a variety of factors including microbial immobilization, plant uptake, immobilization on plant residues and release from organic wastes, temperature and weathering of mineral sources. The bioavailability of P is greatest when soil pH is just below neutral and declines with increasing or decreasing pH. Plant access to phosphates may be limited by their poor solubility. Mycorrhizal plants benefit from a symbiotic relationship with a root-infecting fungus which can scavenge phosphates that are too far from the roots and otherwise unavailable. This activity is especially important in drought conditions where low water availability limits the movement of phosphates through the soil. Differences between plants will affect the phosphorus cycle by stimulating different levels of microbial activity by promoting specific mycorrhizal associations and by root-specific scavenging of phosphorus. Sulphur, like nitrogen and phosphorus, is required for life. It is available in soil to plants and microbes mostly as sulphates (SO_4^{2-}). Sulphates arrive in soil through soil minerals, atmospheric deposition, fertilizers and pesticides. As pollution has declined, sulphur inputs too have declined, and sulphur deficiency has emerged as an issue. In soil, the various reduced forms of inorganic sulphur are oxidized to sulphate by a variety of microbial populations including heterotrophic bacteria, fungi, actinomycetes and chemoautotrophs (notably the thiobacilli). This variety probably accounts for the soil to soil variability in factors affecting the availability of sulphate (Killham 1994). Whilst inorganic sulphur is readily oxidized, the mineralisation of organic sulphur from plant and other wastes is more typically limiting. Many microbial populations participate in the mineralisation of organic sulphur. The rate of mineralisation is therefore particularly dependent on the conditions for their growth which, as has been discussed, will be influenced strongly by plant's type and activities. Sulphate may be lost from the system through anaerobic respiration and reduction to hydrogen sulphide. This is limited to anaerobic and therefore to wet soils. The bacterial populations involved are heterotrophs (notably the genera *Desulfobacteriaceae*, *Desulfovibrionaceae* and *Desulfovibrionaceae*). Plants, through rhizodeposition, will directly influence the activity of these Gram-negative sulphate reducers which are dependant on the supply of organic carbon for energy. Phosphate solubilizing micro-organisms (PSM) include largely bacteria and fungi, which can grow in media containing tri-calcium, iron and aluminium phosphate, hydroxyapatite, bone meal, rock phosphate and similar insoluble phosphate compounds as the sole phosphate source. Such microbes not only assimilate P but a large portion of soluble phosphate is released in quantities in excess of their own requirement (Fig 2). The most efficient PSMs belong to genera *Bacillus* and *Pseudomonas* amongst bacteria and *Aspergillus* and *Penicillium* amongst fungi. The reported bacilli include, *B. brevis*, *B. cereus*, *B. circulans*, *B. firmus*, *B. licheniformis*, *B. megaterium*, *B. mesentricus*, *B. mycoides*, *B. polymyxa*, *B. pumilis*, *B. pulvifaciens* and *B. subtilis* from the rhizosphere of legumes, cereals (rice and maize), areca nut palm, oat, jute and chilli. *Pseudomonas striata*, *P. cissicola*, *P. fluorescens*, *P. pinophillum*, *P. putida*, *P. syringae*, *P. aeruginosa*, *P. putrefaciens* and *P. stutzeri* have been isolated from rhizosphere of *Brassica*, chick-pea, maize, soyabean and other crops, desert soils and Antarctica lake. In addition, *Escherichia freundii*, *E. intermedia*, *Serratia phosphaticum* and species of *Achromobacter*, *Brevibacterium*, *Corynebacterium*, *Erwinia*, *Micrococus*, *Sarcina* and *Xanthomonas* are active in solubilizing insoluble phosphates. Cyanobacteria, viz. *Anabaena* sp., *Calothrix brauni*, *Nostoc* sp., *Scytonema* sp. and *Tolypothrix ceylonica* can also solubilize phosphate (Tilak et al. 2005). Goldstein et al. (1999) demonstrated that an efficient mineral phosphate solubilizing phenotype in Gram-negative bacteria resulted from extracellular oxidation of glucose to gluconic acid via the quinoprotein glucose dehydrogenase. A unique bacterial population isolated from the roots of *Helianthus annus jaegeri*, growing at the edge of an alkaline dry lake in the Mojave Desert in Israel, showed no mineral phosphate solubilizing activity and no gluconic acid production. Addition of a concentrated solution containing material washed from the roots to these bacteria in culture however resulted in production of high levels of gluconic acid. This suggested that signalling between bacteria and plant root regulated expression of direct oxidation pathway in this bacterium. The resultant acidification of the rhizosphere played a key role in nutrient availability and/or other ecophysiological parameters essential for the survival of this desert plant. The establishment and performance of PSM is however affected severely under stressed conditions such as high salt, pH and temperature prevalent in degraded ecosystems represented by alkaline soils with tendency to fix phosphorus (Gaind and Gaur 1991). In a screening of 4800 bacterial isolates from the root-free soil, rhizosphere and rhizoplane of *P. juliflora* growing in alkaline soils, 857 morphotypes solubilized phosphate in agar. The incidence of PSB was highest in the rhizoplane, followed by rhizosphere and root-free soil. Phosphate solubilizing ability of strain NBRI4 was higher than control in the presence of salts (NaCl, $CaCl_2$ and KCl) at 30°C and it further increased at 37°C (Johri et al. 1999). Strain NBRI2601 (Nautiyal et al. 2000) isolated from the rhizosphere of chick-pea and alkaline soils could solubilize phosphorus in presence of 10% salt, pH 12, at 45°C suggesting that extensive diversity searches in appropriate habitats may lead to recovery of effective bacteria.

5.3 PGPR Involved in Plant Growth Promotion

PGPR can affect plant growth either indirectly or directly; indirect promotion of plant growth occurs when PGPR lessen or prevent the deleterious effects of one or more phytopathogenic organisms; while direct promotion of plant growth by PGPR involves either providing plants with a compound synthesized by the bacterium or facilitating the uptake of certain nutrients from the environment (Glick 1995). Thus, in the broadest sense, PGPR include the N_2 fixing Rhizobacteria that colonize the rhizosphere, providing N to plants, including the Rhizobia of the well-characterized legume–Rhizobia symbiosis. Regardless of the mechanisms of plant growth promotion, PGPR must colonize the rhizosphere around the roots, the rhizoplane (root surface) or the root itself (within root tissues) (Glick 1995). PGPR are associated with plant roots, and either directly or indirectly stimulates plant growth. Among Rhizobacteria there is a gradient of root proximity and intimacy as follows: (i) bacteria living in the soil near roots, utilizing metabolites leaked from roots as C and N sources, (ii) bacteria colonizing the rhizoplane, (iii) bacteria residing in root-tissue, inhabiting spaces between cortical cells and lastly (iv) bacteria living inside cells in specialized root structures, or nodules, which generally fall into two groups, the legume associated Rhizobia and the woody plant associated *Frankia* species (Fig 2). In a recent review article Gray and Smith (2005) have discussed in order of intimacy with the associated plant, from almost casual, to extremely regulated and housed in specialized structures. Most rhizosphere organisms occur within 50 mm of root surface and populations within 10 mm of root surface may reach $1.2x10^8$ cells $cm^{-}3$ or 10^9–10^{12} microbial cells/g soil. Despite large numbers of bacteria in the rhizosphere, only 7–15% of the total root surface is generally occupied by microbial cells (Foster et al. 1983; Pinton et al. 2001). Rhizobacteria that establish inside plant roots, forming more intimate associations, are entophytes. These include a wide range of soil bacteria forming less formal associations than the Rhizobia–legume symbiosis; endophytes may stimulate plant growth, directly or indirectly (Kobayashi et al. 1995) and include the Rhizobia. Given the semantic overlap, the following definition for endophytic bacteria has been proposed: 'those bacteria that can be isolated from surface-disinfected plant-tissue or extracted from within the plant, and that do not visibly harm the plant' (Hallmann et al. 1997). In general, a greater proportion of endophytes are PGPR than is the case for bacteria inhabiting the rhizoplane or rhizosphere (Nowak 1998). Nodulating (Rhizobia) and other N_2-fixing Rhizobacteria are also endophytes, living in specially developed root organs; given their ability to promote plant growth through N-fixation these bacteria [primarily Rhizobia and the woody plant associated *Frankia* although the cyanobacterial N_2-fixing symbionts of the cycads could also be included] are also PGPR (Lodewyckx et al. 2002).

The list of PGPR is increasing every day as more research groups are engaged in screening Rhizobacteria for growth promotion. Since associative interactions of plants and microorganisms must have come into existence as a result of co-evolution, the use of latter group as bio-noculants must be pre-adapted, so that it fits into a long-term sustainable agricultural system. A number of bacterial species associated with the plant rhizosphere belonging to genera *Azospirillum*, *Alcaligenes*, *Arthrobacter*, *Acinetobacter*, *Bacillus*, *Burkholderia*, *Enterobacter*, *Erwinia*, *Flavobacterium*, *Pseudomonas*, *Rhizobium* and *Serratia* are able to exert a beneficial effect on plant growth. PGPR have one or more specific associations with plants through which they influence plant growth. PGPR communities are generally metabolically highly active and distinct to specific plant types. Among the many mechanisms associated with plant-

PGPR interactions, the production of biologically active metabolites is one of the most important modes of action through which PGPR influence plant growth, either directly on the plant or by modifying the rhizosphere environment (Fig 2). In recent years, the use of PGPR to promote plant growth has increased dramatically in various parts of the world. Several authors have reported that inoculation with PGPR can result in increased germination, seedling emergence and can modify growth and yield of various cereal and non-cereal crops (Van et al. 2000). It has been reported that these growth responses to microbial inoculation involves strain to crop and even variety and site specificity. Similarly, Nowak (1998) found that inoculation benefits of certain strains varied with plant species, cultivar, and growth conditions. Zahir et al. (2004) have recently reviewed screening approaches and practical applications of PGPR in agriculture. In their excellent review on PGPR Gray and Smith (2005) have postulated that during last two decades, we have achieved a remarkable understanding of the subtleties of signalling between rhizobia and their legume hosts. While there are still so many things to learn about this, it is clear that the signalling process in this relationship is extremely sophisticated. It is also clear that there are less intimate plant-PGPR associations, providing a wide range of growth enhancing materials to plants. Will we find signalling systems spanning the gradient from the Rhizobia–legume system to a mere chance association? This seems likely. Plants growing in field soil cannot be viewed as single organisms. They are a source of solar-derived reduced carbon and, as such, are colonized, for good or ill, by a wide range of microbes and other organisms; these plants are communities of organisms and we do not understand the nature of the communities to any great extent. We can expect many more discoveries and many more communication systems. The road ahead will be frustrating at times, but exciting at each milestone achieved.

5.4 PGPR Involved in Control of Plant Diseases

Disease suppressiveness of soil is the ability of a soil to suppress disease severity even in the presence of a pathogen, host plant and favourable climatic conditions. The different types of disease suppression mechanisms are related to the establishment of the pathogen, reduced parasitic activity of the pathogen and the level of disease incidence or severity (Fig 1). For disease suppression known as 'general suppression', the inhibition of pathogenic populations is related to either the activity of the total microflora or diverse microbial-faunal interactions. The 'specific suppression phenomenon' has been attributed to the activity of specific microbial groups (antagonists). Some abiotic factors of soil such as pH and clay content have also been attributed to certain types of disease suppressiveness e.g. *Fusarium* wilts. The increase in disease suppression against a range of cereal root diseases was related to increased carbon inputs (stubble, roots) to the soil from higher yielding crops and greater cropping frequency. Increased C inputs result in changes in the composition and activity of the soil microbial community over time. These changes result in greater competition for soil resources that, along with predation and inhibition of pathogens, lead to increased suppression of many soil-borne fungal diseases. All soils have the ability to suppress soil-borne root diseases to some extent through the activity of soil microbes and thus, disease suppression is not an absolute characteristic but a continuum from highly suppressive soils to poorly suppressive (i.e. conducive) soils. However, the opportunity to improve suppressive activity to an effective level may be limited by the time required for changes in microbial diversity to occur which is dependant on the management practices that impact microbial growth, composition and metabolic status specific to different soil and environmental conditions (Fig 1).

While a variety of bacteria and fungi have been found to be effective biocontrol agents against different crop diseases based on controlled environmental experiments, no single microbial inoculants has yet been successful under broad acre agriculture systems. Briefly, for an introduced biocontrol agent to be effective it must first survive, establish, acclimatize and grow in field soils and interact with the pathogenic organisms alone or in the presence of plant. Soil and environmental conditions are generally harsh and not optimal for introduced microbes in cropping systems, i.e. carbon poor soils, short-periods of warm and moist soil interjected with long dry and hot periods. Unlike the rhizosphere-based inoculants, endophytes escape problems associated with survival in the harsh and carbon poor soil. Research on the field based ecological aspects of inoculants has been very limited. Important research areas include (1) the effect of serial amendment and long-term soil building on soil properties and general suppression; (2) the impact of serial amendment and long-term soil building on soil properties and specific suppression; (3) the impact of reduced tillage on soil properties and disease severity in the short and long term; (4) screening of cover and rotation crops, plant residues, and other organic wastes for specific suppressive qualities; (5) breeding of crops, cover crops, and rotation crops for enhanced support of plant associated beneficial microbes; (6) the relationship between plant nutrient status and plant health; (7) the impact of faunal predators of plant pathogens on disease suppression; and (8) biocontrol agents (single and consortia) with consistent field efficacy.

In the early 1970's several researchers identified microbial populations in the rhizosphere as constituting the first barrier to pathogen infection.

Nowadays, it is well known that some soils are naturally suppressive to some soil-borne plant pathogens including *Fusarium, Gaeumannomyces, Rhizoctonia, Pythium* and *Phytophthora*. Although this suppression relates to both physicochemical and microbiological features of the soil, in most systems the biological elements are the primary factors in disease suppression and the topic of 'biological control of plant pathogens' gained feasibility in the context of sustainable issues (Weller et al. 2002). The groups of micro-organisms with antagonistic properties towards plant pathogens are diverse, including plant-associated prokaryotes and eukaryotes. A detailed overview of mechanisms involved in microbial antagonism, and a compilation of organisms with demonstrated antagonistic properties used in the biocontrol of pathogens, appears in Whipps (1997, 2001). Among the prokaryotes, a wide range of bacteria such as *Agrobacterium, Bacillus* spp. (e.g. *B. cereus, B. pumilis,* and *B. subtilis*), *Streptomyces,* and *Burkholderia* have been shown to be effective antagonists of soil-borne pathogens. The most widely studied bacteria by far in relation to biocontrol are *Pseudomonas* sp., such as *P. aeruginosa* and *P. fluorescens*, which are probably amongst the most effective root colonizing bacteria. Pathogen suppression by antagonistic micro-organisms can result from one or more mechanisms depending on the antagonist involved. Direct effects on the pathogen include competition for colonization or infection sites, competition for carbon and nitrogen sources as nutrients and signals, competition for iron through the production of iron-chelating compounds or siderophores, inhibition of the pathogen by antimicrobial compounds such as antibiotics and HCN, degradation of pathogen germination factors or pathogenicity factors, and parasitism (Fig 2). These effects can be accompanied by indirect mechanisms, including improvement of plant nutrition and damage compensation, changes in root-system anatomy, microbial changes in the rhizosphere, and activation of plant defense mechanisms, leading to enhanced plant resistance. An effective biocontrol agent often acts through the combination of several different mechanisms (Whipps 2001). Rhizobacteria from the genus *Pseudomonas* provide an excellent example of a combination of multiple mechanisms for effective biocontrol including direct antagonism and induction of plant resistance. *Pseudomonas* sp. produce several metabolites with antimicrobial activity towards other bacteria and fungi (Haas and Keel 2003). Indeed, the first clear-cut experimental demonstration that a bacteria-produced antibiotic could suppress plant disease in an ecosystem was made by Tomashow and Weller (1988). Using an elegant genetic approach, they demonstrated the direct correlation between the production of a phenazine antibiotic by a fluorescent *Pseudomonas* sp. and its biocontrol activity against take-all disease of wheat. Competition is another key factor in the antagonistic properties of *Pseudomonas* sp. In addition to competition for substrates research on the siderophores produced by *Pseudomonas* species (pyoverdine, pyochelin) has shown the involvement of siderophores-mediated competition for iron in the control of *Fusarium* and *Pythium* in soils (Duijff et al. 1994; Raaijmakers et al. 1995). Direct evidence for the role of cell-wall degrading enzymes in biocontrol in vitro comes from studies utilizing mutant strains over-expressing or lacking a particular enzyme, or transgenic plants expressing these enzymes.

Over the past decade, specific strains of PGPR have been shown to induce systemic resistance against a broad spectrum of pathogens such as fungi (Van Peer et al. 1991; Wei et al. 1991), bacteria (Alstrom 1991; Press et al. 1997), and viruses (Murphy et al. 2000). PGPR-elicited induced systemic resistance (ISR) is phenotypically similar to pathogen-induced systemic acquired resistance (SAR) (Sticher et al. 1997; van Loon et al. 1998). Both SAR and ISR elicited by PGPR render non-infected parts of previously induced plants more resistant to infection by pathogens and are effective against a broad spectrum of root and foliar pathogens (Zhang et al. 2002). Both pathogen-induced SAR and Rhizobacteria-mediated ISR have been demonstrated in several plant species and are effective against a broad spectrum of root and foliar pathogens including fungi, bacteria, and viruses (Sticher et al. 1997; Van Loon et al. 1998). For the establishment of systemically induced resistance, signal(s) must be transported from the site of induction, which is the primary infection site in the case of SAR, and the root colonization site in the case of ISR (Fig 1). The signal(s) are systemically translocated to trigger the induced state in distant plant parts. The phenomenon of induced resistance offers great opportunities to control plant diseases in a biological way as part of integrated pest management strategies. It may serve as an alternative for conventional chemical control and *R*-gene breeding. Many chemicals have been developed to protect plants against diseases. Most of them are inexpensive and easy to obtain, but both their production and their persistence in the soil after use are potentially harmful to the environment. This is particularly true for chemicals employed in the control of soil-borne fungal pathogens, because often they must be applied repeatedly in large, toxic amounts. The introduction of *R*-genes into plants is attractive because it can render plants completely resistant to a pathogen. However, resistance breeding is dependent on the availability of an *R*-gene, which is not always the case. Moreover, resistance based on a gene-to-gene relationship offers protection against only a single pathogen, which can overcome resistance by mutation, leading to a limited durability of disease resistance in the fields. Induced resistance is an attractive alternative form of plant protection as it is based on the activation of extant resistance mechanisms of the plant. It may, therefore, be considered natural and safe as it offers resistance against a wide range of pathogens (Sticher et al. 1997; Van Loon et al. 1998). Both SAR and ISR confer resistance for lifetime on the plant (Raaijmakers et al. 1995). Both, SAR and ISR, have been shown to be effective under field conditions (Wei et al. 1996). Commercial product Bion, which is based on the active compound benzothiadiazole (BTH) that activates the plant to express induced resistance (Friedrich et al. 1996), has been released to the market. In this age, where the importance of environment-friendly and sustainable agriculture is highly recognized, the contribution of induced resistance to control plant diseases can be of great value. Understanding of the molecular mechanisms underlying PGPR-mediated ISR may contribute to exploitation of the potential of ISR in the control of plant diseases. Initiatives are thus required on the mechanisms involved in induction, signalling and expression of PGPR-mediated induced disease resistance (Fig 2). Several reports show the potential of combining different biocontrol agents with different disease-suppressive mechanisms in the field (de Boer et al. 2003). The development of appropriate combinations should provide a higher level of plant protection, a wider range of effectiveness and a reduction of variability in the results. Thus, the optimal use of the antagonistic properties of the micro biota will result in a more effective and more reliable biocontrol of plant pathogens, as it constitutes a very promising research area.

6. CONCLUSION

The loss of biodiversity has become a major topic of concern in recent decades, and a significant amount of research has been devoted to understanding the consequences of ecosystem simplification. As the main input of organic matter in terrestrial ecosystems, plants are thought to have a profound effect on steering soil communities and processes, especially in the rhizosphere. A variety of microbial forms can be found growing in rhizosphere micro-habitats. Many microbial interactions, which are regulated by specific molecules/signals, are responsible for key environmental processes, such as the bio-geochemical cycling of nutrients, organic matter, maintenance of plant health and soil quality. The successful functioning of many soil biological processes requires a balance of biota interactions in a complex soil biota community. Inputs from the host plant and environmental sources come together to induce the 'quorum-sensing' behaviour. If such signalling were quantitatively significant in nature then plants might stimulate microbial production of exoenzymes to promote mineralization of organic matter around roots. While allelopathic events are often reported at the community-species level, allelopathy is more accurately an ecological phenomenon operating at the trophic level with implications for the regulation of ecosystem health and biodiversity. By learning how to adapt and manage root zone microbial plant growth promoting rhizobacteria (PGPR) communities, opportunities arise to produce food crops in a more sustainable manner. The traits involved in bacterial rhizosphere competence, mechanisms involved in induction, signalling, expression of PGPR-mediated induced plant growth promotion and disease resistance are still to be understood. Among other factors, the ability to form biofilms and quorum-sensing that enable the bacteria to co-ordinate the expression of special phenotypes in a cell density dependent manner, might play an important role. This information will help us further in the development of futuristic agricultural biotechnology products by ecological and/or genetic manipulation of PGPR for the purpose of modifying the soil or microbial flora surrounding the root to achieve desirable environment to improve plant growth and soil health. The use of model systems such as *Arabidopsis thaliana*/*Pseudomonas* sp. opens up the opportunity to apply the deep molecular genetic analysis which is necessary to efficiently understand the molecular ecology of complex inter-kingdom relationships. Future developments in functional genomics (including proteomics and metabolomics) will be useful to identify the genes expressed in the rhizosphere, while the use of promoters to drive gene expression specifically at the root–soil interfaces will allow the engineering of PGPR for beneficial purposes. This review focuses on the functions of association between plants and PGPR which benefit crops by stimulating plant growth, or by reducing the damage from soil-borne plant pathogens, the biological component of the soil ecosystem, and in particular the role of plants within the soil ecosystem and the types of effects that they can confer on both PGPR and soil processes.

PGPR functions are involved in fundamental activities that ensure the stability and productivity of both, agricultural systems and natural ecosystems (Fig 1). Strategic and applied research has demonstrated that certain co-operative microbial activities can be exploited, to help sustainable, environment-friendly agro-technological practices. Since the interaction is so complex it is not surprising therefore to have very few success stories at commercial scale of the use of PGPR (Nautiyal 2000). Thus, at times, it is very frustrating to work in the area of 'Plant-Microbial Association' in general and PGPR in particular. However, in spite of these bottlenecks we must find ways, means and vision to successes. As Abdul Kalam and Rajan (2002) stated not so long ago, "If we tie ourselves into knots over problems and project that attitude over 365 days that can not be the vision. A vision has to cut across the ordinary and aim at bigger things, but just take care that it is not impossible. At the time of articulating the vision, however, it should appear nearly impossible!"

Improvement of PGPR functions by ecological or genetic means is an important approach to enhancing their performance (Fig 2). This strategy is a likely prerequisite if these microbes are to be exploited commercially and routinely for plant growth promotion. The advantages would include better yield, lower costs and more liberty for farmer in the choice of crop rotation, and reduce dependence on chemical fungicides. Developing predictive models for PGPR is necessarily a complex endeavour because of the multi component nature of the system. We must develop a thorough understanding of the environmental and host factors that affect the microbial community and the efficacy of a particular mechanism of PGPR in the plant environment. A massive research effort on population biology and mechanisms of interactions of PGPR is required to accumulate and integrate the information that will supply the basis for predictive models. Although population biology of PGPR has been studied in both the laboratory and the field, research directed towards elucidating mechanisms of interactions has been primarily laboratory-based. In addition to its importance for developing models, an understanding of the mechanisms underlying these interactions may allow us to manipulate the soil environment to create conditions conducive to successful PGPR functions. In addition, an understanding of these mechanisms may provide a logical basis for selection and construction of more effective PGPR strains (Fig 2). Ultimately, however, better strains will have to be constructed by genetic engineering and a better understanding of the ecological factors that interfere with PGPR activity. Despite the fact that these efforts are still at a very early stage, this approach should have the effect of accelerating progress in this field so that it may not be unreasonable to expect to see improved genetically engineered PGPR strains being used within next 10 years (Fig 2). Recent advances in our understanding of the ecology and molecular biology of the systems responsible for PGPR are opening the ways to strain improvement. Substantial advances in elucidating the genetic basis of the beneficial effects of PGPR have been made, some from whole-genome sequencing projects.

Developments in high throughput DNA sequencing have resulted in elucidation of the whole-genome sequences. Data as of August 2005 on BLAST with microbial genomes (387 bacterial/26 archaeal genomes tree). For future updates and further details for work being done on various PGPRs please refer to the URL http://www.ncbi.nlm.nih.gov/sutils/genom_table.cgi data base and references quoted therein. *P. fluorescens* SBW25 (PfSBW25) is a Gram-negative PGPR that grows in close association with plants. In common with a broad range of functionally similar bacteria, it plays an important role in the turnover of organic matter and certain isolates can promote plant growth. Despite its environmental significance, the causes of its ecological success are not well understood is building a genomic encyclopedia of the PGPR strain PfSBW25 on the basis of short-run non-contiguous sequence data. It is anticipated that the obtained sequence data will, by comparative and functional genomics, facilitate the identification of genes that are specifically present in plant beneficial rhizosphere bacteria, that are specifically expressed on the seed or in the rhizosphere, that are involved in regulating the production of secondary metabolites or whose expression is influenced by other rhizosphere microbes. Recently development and application of a simple promoter trapping strategy (IVET) to identify PfSBW25 genes showing elevated levels of expression in the sugar beet rhizosphere has been described. A total of twenty-five rhizosphere-induced (*rhi*) fusions are reported with predicted roles in nutrient acquisition, stress responses, biosynthesis of phytohormones and antibiotics. One *rhi* fusion is to *wss*, an operon encoding an acetylated cellulose polymer. A mutant carrying a defective *wss* locus was competitively compromised (relative to the wild type) in the rhizosphere and in the phyllosphere, but not in bulk soil. The rhizosphere-induced *wss* locus therefore contributes to the ecological performance of PfSBW25 in the plant environment and supports our conjecture that genes inactive in the laboratory environment, but active in the wild, are likely to be determinants of fitness in natural environments. It is anticipated that these methods, used in combination with existing methods, may provide shortcuts to the discovery of new genes and give a holistic perspective to plant beneficial bacteria (Fig 2). This progress will lead to a more efficient use of these strains and possibly to their improvement by genetic modification. This information will help us further in the development of futuristic agricultural biotechnology products, by ecological and/or, genetic manipulation of plant beneficial bacteria, engineered with rhizosphere competence gene(s), for the purpose of modifying the soil or microbial flora surrounding the root to achieve desirable environment to improve plant growth. Thus, future research in rhizosphere biology will rely on the development of molecular and biotechnological approaches to increase our knowledge of rhizosphere biology and to achieve an integrated management of soil microbial populations. From the agricultural and ecological viewpoints, the aims will be to increase food quality and to improve sustainable plant productivity maintaining environmental quality. However, to achieve this, basic and strategic studies must be undertaken to improve our understanding of microbial interactions in the rhizosphere. Only then can the corresponding agro-biotechnology be applied successfully. Hence, future investigation in the field of microbial co-operation in the rhizosphere will include: (i) advances in visualization technology; (ii) analysis of the molecular basis of root colonization; (iii) signalling in the rhizosphere; (iv) functional genomics; (v) mechanisms involved in beneficial co-operative microbial activities; (vi) engineering of micro-organisms for beneficial purposes; and (vii) biotechnological developments for integrated management (Fig 2). Many traits of root colonization by PGPR have already been identified, but novel molecular approaches are being used to screen for new traits. These are important to decipher the genes encoding proteins involved in transport or signal transduction pathways involved in colonization. An increase in current knowledge on quorum sensing systems, such as those based on N-acyl-homoserine lactones, will be important for understanding the ecodynamics of microbial populations in the rhizosphere, and the cellular and molecular aspects of signalling processes in microbe to microbe interactions. Future developments in functional genomics (including proteomics and metabolomics) will be useful to identify the genes expressed in the rhizosphere, while the use of promoters to drive gene expression specifically at the root–soil interfaces will allow the engineering of micro-organisms for beneficial purposes. The new tools of recombinant DNA technology, mathematical modelling, and computer technology combined with a continuation of the more classical approaches such as crop rotation, various tilling strategies, addition of organic amendments such as compost, mulch or manures, should quickly move PGPR research and technology into a new era. All in all, the availability of new and powerful technologies for studying co-operative microbial interactions in the rhizosphere guarantees a greater understanding of useful PGPR functions, which will facilitate their successful applications in agricultural biotechnology.

ACKNOWLEDGEMENTS

Thanks are due to Dr. P. Pushpangadan, Director, National Botanical Research Institute, Lucknow for his valuable encouragement and providing necessary support. Author is highly indebted to Dr. H. R. Bhojwani, Adviser to Minister of Science & Technology, Government of India; Professor Y. S. Rajan, Principal Adviser, Confederation of Indian Industry, New Delhi, and Professor R. P. Sharma, Secretary, National Academy of Agricultural Sciences, New Delhi, for useful discussions. The work was supported by Mission Mode Task Force Project Exploration and Exploitation of Microbial wealth of India, Council of Scientific & Industrial Research (CSIR), New Delhi.

REFERENCES

Abrams PA (1995) Monotonic or unimodal diversity-productivity gradients: what does competition theory predict? Ecol 76: 2019–2027

Alstrom S (1991) Induction of disease resistance in common bean susceptible to halo blight bacterial pathogen after seed bacterization with rhizosphere pseudomonads. J Gen Appl Microbiol 37: 495–501

Andersen JB, Heydorn A, Hentzer M, Eberl L, Geisenberger O, Christensen BB, Molin S, Givskov M (2001) gfp-based N-acyl homoserine–lactone sensor systems for detection of bacterial communication. Appl Environ Microbiol 67: 575–585

Anderson TH (2003) Microbial eco-physiological indicators to assess soil quality Agriculture. Ecosys Environ 98: 285–293

Andrews JH, Harris RF (1985) r- and K- Selection and microbial ecology. In: Marshall KC (eds) Advances in Microbial Ecology, Plenum Press: New York

Appenzeller T (1991) Fire and ice under the deep sea floor. Sci 252: 1790–1792

Atlas RM (1986) Applicability of general ecological principles to microbial ecology. In: Poindexter JS, Leadbetter ER (eds) Bacteria in Nature vol.2 Plenum Press, New York pp. 339–370

Azco´n-Aguilar C, Barea JM (1978) Effect of interactions between different culture fractions of phosphobacteria and Rhizobium on mycorrhizal infection, growth and nodulation of *Medicago sativa.* Can J Microbiol 24: 520–524

Bai YM, Pan B, Charles TC, Smith DL (2002) Co-inoculation dose and root zone temperature for plant growth promoting rhizobacteria on soybean (*Glycine max* (L.) Merr) grown in soil-less media. Soil Biol Biochem 34: 1953–1957

Bai YM, Zhou XM Smith DL (2003) Enhanced soybean plant growth resulting from co-inoculation of *Bacillus* strains with *Bradyrhizobium japonicum*. Crop Sci 43: 1774–1781

Baker KF (1987) Evolving concepts of biological control of plant pathogens. Annu Rev Phytopathol 25: 67–85

Bardgett RD, Mawdsley JL, Edwards S, Hobbs PJ, Rodwell JS, Davis WJ (1999) Plant species and nitrogen effects on soil biological properties of temperate upland grasslands. Functional Ecol 13: 650–660

Barea JM, Azco´n R, Azco´n-Aguilar C (2004) Mycorrhizal fungi and plant growth promoting rhizobacteria. In: Varma A, Abbott L, Werner D, Hampp R (eds.) Plant surface microbiology. Springer-Verlag, Germany 351–371

Barea JM, Marý´a Jose´ Pozo, Rosario Azco´n, Concepcio´n Azco´n-Aguilar (2005) Microbial co-operation in the rhizosphere. J Exp Bot 56(417): 1761–1778

Bashan Y, Holguin G (1998) Proposal for the division of plant growth-promoting rhizobacteria into two classifications: biocontrol-PGPB (plant growth-promoting bacteria) and PGPB. Soil Biol Biochem 30: 1225-1228

Bauer WD, Teplitski M (2001) Can plants manipulate bacterial quorum sensing? Aust J Plant Physiol 28: 913–921

Bayliss C, Bent E, Culham DE, MacLellan S, Clarke AJ, Brown GL, Wood JM (1997) Bacterial genetic loci implicated in the *Pseudomonas putida* GR12–2R3 – canola mutualism: identification of an exudate-inducible sugar transporter. Can J Microbiol 43: 809–818

Becker D, Stanke R, Fendrik I, Frommer WB, Vanderleyden J, Kaiser WM, Hedrich R (2002) Expression of the NH+4-transporter gene LEAMT1;2 is induced in tomato roots upon association with N_2-Fixing bacteria. Planta 215:424-429

Benhamou N, Kloepper JW, Quadt-Hallman A, Tuzun S (1996) Induction of defense-related ultrastructural modifications in pea root-tissues inoculated with endophytic bacteria. Plant Physiol 112: 919–929

Boer M de, Bom P, Kindt F, Keurentjer JB, van der Sluis I, van Loon LC, Bakker PAHM (2003) Control of *Fusarium* wilt of radish by combining *Pseudomonas putida* strains that have different disease-suppressive mechanisms. Phytopathol 93: 626–632

Bonkowski M (2004) Protozoa and plant growth: the microbial loop in soil revisited. New Phytol 162: 617–631

Bowen GD, Rovira AD (1999) The rhizosphere and its management to improve plant growth. Adv Agron 66: 1–102

Bradford MA, Jones TH, Bardgett RD, Black HIJ, Boag B, Bonkowski M, Cook R, Eggers T (2002) Impacts of soil faunal community composition on model grassland ecosystems. Sci 298: 615–618

Bremner E, Jenzen H, Gilbertson C (1995) Evidence against associative N_2 fixation as a significant source of N in long-term wheat plots. Plant Soil 175: 13-19

Brimecombe MJ, De Leij FA, Lynch JM (2001) The effect of root exudates on rhizosphere microbial populations. Pinton R, Varanini Z, Nannipieri P (eds) The Rhizosphere. Marcel Dekker, New York pp 95–140

Broughton LC, Gross KL (2000) Patterns of diversity in plant and soil microbial communities along a productivity gradient in a Michigan old-field. Oecologia 125: 420–427

Buscot F (2005) What are soils? Microorganisms in soils: Roles in genesis and functions. In: Buscot F, Varma S (eds) Springer-Verlag, Berlin Heidelberg, Germany, pp 1-17

Buyer JS, Roberts DP, Russek-Cohen E (2002) Soil and plant effects on microbial community structure. Can J Microbiol 48: 955–964

Chebotar VK, Asis CA, Akao S (2001) Production of growth promoting substances and high colonization ability of rhizobacteria enhance the nitrogen fixation of soybean when inoculated with *Bradyrhizobium japonicum*. Biol Ferti Soils 34: 427–432

Chou CH (1999) Roles of allelopathy in plant biodiversity and sustainable agriculture. CRC Crit Rev Plant Sci 18: 609–636

Clarholm M (1985) Interactions of bacteria, protozoa and plants leading to mineralisation of soil nitrogen. Soil Biol Biochem 17: 181–187

Cordier C, Pozo MJ, Barea JM, Gianinazzi S, Gianinazzi-Pearson V (1998) Cell defense responses associated with localized and systemic resistance to Phytophthora parasitica induced in tomato by an arbuscular-mycorrhizal fungus. Mol Plant–Microbe Interactions 11: 1017–1028

Curl EA, Truelove B (1986) The Rhizosphere, Springer-Verlag, Berlin

Daniels R, Jos Vanderleyden, Jan Michiels (2004) Quorum sensing and swarming migration in bacteria. FEMS Microbiol Rev 28: 261–289

Dashti N, Zhang F, Hynes R, Smith DL (1998) Plant growth promoting rhizobacteria accelerate nodulation and increase nitrogen fixation activity by field grown soybean [*Glycine max* (L.) Merr.] under short season conditions. Plant Soil 2: 205–213

Davis DG, Parsek MR, Pearson JP, Iglewski BH, Costerton JW, Greenberg EP (1998) The involvement of cell to cell signals in the development of a bacterial biofilm. Sci 280: 295–298

Deubel A, Merbach W (2005) Influence of micro-organisms on phosphorus bio-availability in soils In: Buscot F, Varma A (eds) Springer-Verlag, Germany, pp 177-191

Dharmatilake AJ, Bauer WD (1992) Chemotaxis of Rhizobium meliloti towards nodulation gene-inducing compounds from alfalfa roots. Appl Environ Microbiol 58: 1153–1158

Dobbelaere S, Croonenborghs A, Thys A, Ptacek D, Okon Y, Vanderleyden J (2002) Effect of inoculation with wild type *Azospirillum brasilense* and *A. irakense* strains on development and nitrogen uptake of spring wheat and grain maize. Biol Fert Soil 36: 284-297

Dowling DN, Sexton R, Fenton A, Delany I, Fedi S, McHugh B, Callanan M, Moënne-Loccoz Y, O'Gara F (1996) Iron regulation in plant-associated *Pseudomonas fluorescens* M114. In Molecular Biology of Pseudomonads. In: Nakazawa K, Furukawa K, Haas D, Silver S (eds) Implications for biological control ASM Press, Washington, DC, pp 502–511

Duijff BJ, Bakker PAHM, Schippers B (1994) Suppression of *Fusarium* wilt of carnation by *Pseudomonas putida* WCS358 at different levels of disease incidence and iron availability. Biocontrol Science and Technology 4: 279–288

Dykhuizen DE (1998) Santa Rosalia revisited: Why are there so many species of bacteria? Antonie van Leeuwenhoek 73: 25–33

Egener T, Hurek T, Reinhold-Hurek B (1998) Use of green Fluorescent protein to detect expression of nif genes of Azoarcus sp. BH72, a grass-associated diazotroph, on rice roots. Mol Plant Microbe Interactions 11: 71-75

Egener T, Hurek T, Reinhold-Hurek B (1999) Endophytic expression of nif genes of Azoarcus sp. strain BH72 in rice roots. Mol Plant Microbe Interactions 12: 813-819

Elad Y, Baker R (1985) Possible role of competition for iron and carbon in suppression of chlamydospore germination of *Fusarium* spp. by *Pseudomonas* spp. Phytopathol 75: 1053–1059

Elasri M, Delorme S, LeManceau P, Stewart G, Laue B, Glickmann E (2001) Acyl-homoserine lactone production is more common among plant-associated *Pseudomonas* spp. than among soilborne *Pseudomonas* spp. Appl Environ Microbiol 67: 1198–1209

Elo S, Maunuksela L, Salkinoja-Salonen M. Smolander A, Haahtela K (2000) Humus bacteria of Norway spruce stands: plant growth promoting properties and birch, red fescue and alder colonizing capacity. FEMS Microbiol Ecol 31: 143–152

Faqua C, Winans SC, Greenberg EP (1996) Census and consensus in bacterial ecosystems: lux R–lux I family of quorum-sensing transcriptional regulators. Ann Rev Microbiol 50: 727–751

Felix G, Duran JD, Volko S, Boller T (1999) Plants have a sensitive perception system for the most conserved domain of bacterial flagellin. Plant Journal18: 265–276

Forde BG (2000) Nitrate transporters in plants: structure, function and regulation. Biochemica Biophysica Acta 1465: 219-235

Foster RC, Bowen GD (1982) Plant surfaces and bacterial growth: the rhizosphere and rhizoplane. In: Mount MS, Lacy GH (eds.) Phytopathogenic Prokaryotes, Marcel Dekker, New York, USA pp.159–185

Foster RC, Rovira AD, Cock TW (1983) Ultrastructure of the Root– Soil Interface The American Phytopathological Society, St Paul, MN p 157

Fravel DR (1988) Role of antibiosis in the biocontrol of plant diseases. Annu Rev Phytopathol 26: 75–79

Frederick BA, Klein DA (1994) Nitrogen effects on rhizosphere processes of range grasses from different successional seres. Plant Soil 161: 241–250

Friedrich L, Lawton K, Ruess W, Masner P, Specker N, Gut Rella M, Meier B, Dincher S, Staub T, Métraux JP, Kessmann H, Ryals J (1996) A benzothiadiazole derivate induces systemic acquired resistance in tobacco. Plant J 10:61-70

Fries N, Serck-Hanssen K, Dimberg LH, Theander O (1987) Abietic acid, an activator of basidiospore germination in ectomycorrhizal species of the genus Suillus (Boletacaea). Exp Mycol 11: 360–363

Fujimoto DK, Weller DM, Thomashow LS (1995) Role of secondary metabolites in root disease suppression. In: Inderjit, Dakshini KMM, Einhellig FA (eds) Allelopathy: Organisms, Processes and Applications, ACS Symposium Series, Washington, DC pp 330–347

Fuqua WC, Winans SC, Greenberg EP (1994) Quorum sensing in Bacteria: the LuxR-LuxI family of cell density-responsive transcriptional regulators. J Bacteriol 176: 269–275

Gaind S, Gaur AC (1991) Thermotolerant phosphate solubilizing micro-organisms and their interaction with mungbean. Plant Soil 133: 141–149

Giri B, Giang PH, Kumari R, Prasad R, Varma A (2005). Microbial diversity in soils. In: Buscot F, Varma A (eds) Micro-organisms in soils: Roles in genesis and functions. Springer-Verlag, Berlin Heidelberg, Germany, pp19-58

Giri B, Sachdev M, Giang PH, Kumari R, Prasad R, Garg A.P, Oelmueller R, Varma A (2005). Mycorrhizosphere: Strategies and Functions. In: Buscot F, Varma A (eds) Micro-organisms in soils: Roles in genesis and functions. Springer-Verlag, Berlin Heidelberg, Germany, pp 213-252

Glick BR (1995) The enhancement of plant growth by free-living bacteria. Can J Microbiol 41: 109–117

Glick BR, Changping L, Sibdas G, Dumbroff EB (1997) Early development of canola seedlings in the presence of the plant growth-promoting rhizobacterium *Pseudomonas putida* GR12-2. Soil Biol Biochem 29: 1233–1239

Glick BR, Patten CL, Holguin G, Penrose DM (1999) Biochemical and Genetic Mechanisms Used by Plant Growth Promoting Bacteria. Imperial College Press, London, UK

Glickman E, Gardan L, Jaquet S, Hussain S, Elasri M, Petit A, Dessaux Y (1998) Auxin production is a common feature of most pathovars of *Pseudomonas syringae.* Mol Plant–Microbe Interact 11: 156–162

Goldstein AH, Liu ST (1987) Molecular cloning and regulation of a mineral phosphate solubilizing gene from *Erwinia herbicola.* Biotechnol 5: 72–74

Goldstein AH, Rogers RD (June 15 1999) Biomediated continuous release phosphate fertilizer. (Lockheed Idaho Technologies Co. USA) US 5912398 A, p.19

Graham AH (1988) Principles and Application of Soil Microbiology. 322–345

Gray EJ, Smith DL (2005) Intracellular and extacellular PGPR: commonalities and distinctions in the plant–bacterium signaling processes. Soil Biol Biochem 37: 395–412

Grayston SJ, Wang S, Campbell CD, Edwards AC (1998) Selective influence of plant species on microbial diversity in the rhizosphere. Soil Biol Biochem 30: 369–378

Grewal PS, Lewis EE, Ventkatachari S (1999) Allelopathy: a possible mechanism of suppression of plant-parasitic nematodes by entomopathogenic nematodes Nematol 1: 735–743

Griffiths BS (1994) Soil nutrient flow. In: Darbyshire JF (ed) Soil Protozoa CAB International, Wallingford pp 65–91

Hallmann J, Quadt-Hallmann A, Mahaffee WF, Kloepper W (1997) Bacterial endophytes in agricultural crops Can J Microbiol 43: 895–914

Hall-Stoodley L, Costerton JW, Stoodley P (2004) Bacterial Biofilms: from the natural environment to infectious diseases Nature Rev 2: 95–108

Hartung AC, Stephens CT (1983) Effects of allelopathic substances produced by asparagus on incidence and severity of asparagus decline due to *Fusarium* crown rot. J Chem Ecol 8: 1163–1174

Hass D, Keel C (2003) Regulation of antibiotic production in root colonizing *Pseudomonas* spp. and relevance for biological control of plant disease. A Rev Phytopathol 41: 117–153

Hassett DJ, Cuppoletti J, Trapnell B, Lymar SV, Rowe JJ, Sun YS, Hilliard GM, Parvatiyar K, Kamani MC, Wozniak DJ, Hwang SH, McDermott TR, Ochsner UA (2002) Anaerobic metabolism and quorum-sensing by *Pseudomonas aeruginosa* biofilms in chronically infected cystic fibrosis airways: rethinking antibiotic treatment strategies and drug targets. Adv Drug Deliv Rev 54:1425–1443

Hawes MC, Brigham LA (1992) Impacts of root border cells on microbial populations in the rhizosphere. Adv Plant Pathol 8: 119–148

Hawes MC, Brigham LA, Wen F, Woo HH, Zhu Y (1998) Function of root border cells in plant health: pioneers in the rhizosphere. Annu Rev Phytopathol 36: 311–327

Hentzer M, Eberl L, Givskov M (2004) Quorum-sensing in biofilm: gossip in the slime city? In: O'Toole GA (ed) Microbial Biofilms. American Society for Microbiology Press, Washington pp 118–140

Heydorn A, Ersbøll B, Kato J, Hentzer M, Parsek MR, Tolker-Nielsen T, Givskov M, Molin S (2002). A statistical analysis of Pseudomonas aeruginosa biofilm development: impact of mutations in genes involved in twitching motility, cell-to-cell signalling and stationary phase gene expression. Appl Environ Microbiol 68: 2008–2017

Hiltner L (1904) ber neuere Erfahrungen und Probleme auf dem Gebiet der Bodenbackteriologie und unter besonderer Beru»cksichtigung der Gru»ndu»ngung und Brache. Arbeiten Deutscher Landwirtschafts Gesellschaft 98: 59-78

Ho WC, Ko WH (1986) Microbiostasis by nutrient deficiency shown in natural and synthetic soils. J Gen Microbiol 132: 2807–2815

Hojbergand O, Sorensen J (1993) Microgradients of Microbial Oxygen-Consumption in a Barley Rhizosphere Model System. App Environ Microbiol 59(2): 431-437

Huber B, Riedel K, Ko¨the M, Givskov M, Molin S, Eberl L (2002) Genetic analysis of functions involved in the late stages of biofilm development in *Burkholderia cepacia* H111. Mol Microbiol 46: 411–426

International Allelopathy Society (IAS) (1998) A rticle 2, IAS Constitution (draft), SecondNewsletter1998,http://www2.uca.es/dept/quimica_organica/ias/newslett2.htm#draft, International Allelopathy Society. Department of Biochemistry, Oklahoma State University, Stillwater, Oklahoma, USA

Johri JK, Surange S, Nautiyal CS (1999) Occurrence of salt, pH and temperature-tolerant phosphate solubilizing bacteria in alkaline soils. Curr Microbiol 39: 89-93

Kalam Abdul APJ, Rajan YS (2002) India 2020: A vision for the new Millennium, Penguin Books, London

Kerry BR (2000) Rhizosphere interactions and the exploitation of microbial agents for the biological control of plant-parasitic nematodes. Annu Rev Phytopathol 38: 423–441

Killham K (1994) Soil ecology Cambridge University Press, London

Kirk JL, Beaudette LA, Hart M, Moutoglis P, Klironomos, Lee H, Trevors JT (2004) Methods of studying soil microbial diversity. J Microbiological Methods 58: 169–188

Kloepper JW (1994) Plant growth-promoting rhizobacteria (other systems) In: Okon Y, Boca Raton FL (eds.), *Azospirillum*/plant associations, USA: CRC Press pp111–118

Kloepper JW, Liftshitz K, Zablotowicz RM (1989) Free-living bacterial inocula for enhancing crop productivity. Trends Biotechnol 7: 39– 43

Kobayashi M, Suzuki T, Fujita T, Masuda M, Shimizu S (1995) Occurrence of enzymes involved in biosynthesis of indole-3-acetic acid from indole-3-acetonitrile in plant-associated bacteria, *Agrobacterium* and *Rhizobium*. PNAS 92: 714–718

Kuske CR, Ticknor LO, Miller ME, Dunbar JM, Davis JA, Barns SM, Belnap J (2002) Comparison of soil bacterial communities in rhizospheres of three plant species and the interspaces in an arid grassland. Appl Environ Microbiol 68: 1854–1863

Labatte M, Queck SY, Koh KS, Rice SA, Givskov M, Kjelleberg S (2004) Quorum-sensing-controlled biofilm development in *Serratia liquefaciens* MG1. J Bacteriol 186: 692–698

Le Strange KK, Bender GL, Djordjevic MA, Rolfe BG, Redmond JW (1990) The Rhizobium strain NGR 234 nodD1 gene product responds to activation by the simple phenolic compounds vanillin and isovanillin present in wheat seedling extracts. Mol Plant Microbe Interaction 4: 214–220

Levy E, Carmelli S (1995) Biological control of plant pathogens by antibiotic-producing bacteria. In: Inderjit, Dakshini KMM, Einhellig FA (eds) Allelopathy: Organisms, Processes and Applications, ACS Symposium Series, Washington, DC pp 300–309

Leyns F, Lambert H, JoosSwings J (1990) Antifungal bacteria from different crops. In: Hornby (ed) Biological Control of Soil-borne Plant Pathogens, CAB International, Wallingford, Oxfordshire, UK pp 437–444

Lippmann B, Leinhos V, Bergmann H (1995) Influence of auxin producing rhizobacteria on root morphology and nutrient accumulation of crops. 1. Changes in root morphology and nutrient accumulation in maize (*Zea mays* L.) caused by inoculation with indole-3-acetic acid producing pseudomonas and Acinetobacter strains or IAA applied exogenously. Angewandte. Botanik 69: 31–36

Lö honis F (1926) Nitrogen availability of green manures. Soil Science 36:253–290

Lodewyckx C, Vangronsveld J, Porteous F, Moore ERB, Taghavi S, Mezgeay M, Van der Lelie D (2002) Endophytic bacteria and their potential applications. Crit Rev Plant Sci 21: 583–606

Lubchenco J, Olson AM, Brubaker LB, Carpenter SR, Holland MM, Hubbell SP (1991) The Sustainable Biosphere Initiative: an ecological research agenda: a report from the Ecological-Society-of-America. Ecol 72: 371–412

Lucas-Garcia JA, Probanza A, Ramos B, Colo´n-Flores JJ, Gutierrez-Man˜ero FJ (2004) Effects of plant growth-promoting rhizobateria (PGPRs) on the biological nitrogen fixation, nodulation and growth of *Lupinus albus* I. cv. Multolupa Engineering Life Sciences 4: 71–77

Lynch JM (1990) The rhizosphere. John Wiley New York

Malik AU (2000) Challenges and opportunities in allelopathy research: a brief overview. J Chem Ecol 26: 2007–2009

Man˜ero FJ, Probanza A, Ramos B, Flores JJ, Garcý´a-Lucas JA (2003) Effects of culture filtrates of rhizobacteria isolated from wild lupin on germination, growth, and biological nitrogen fixation of lupin seedlings. J Plant Nutrition 26: 1101–1115

Mantelin S, Bruno Touraine (2004) Plant growth-promoting bacteria and nitrate availability: impacts on root development and nitrate uptake. J Expt Bot 55 394: 27-34

Marketon MM, Gronquist MR, Eberhard A, González JE (2002) Characterization of the *Sinorhizobium meliloti sinR/sinI* locus and the production of novel *N* acyl homoserine lactones. J Bacteriol 184: 5686–5695

Marschner F (2005) Microbial community structure and function in the rhizosphere. In: Varma A, Podile A, IK International and Thiema Press, (eds) Biotechnological applications of microbes, India & Germany pp 43–65

Mathesius M, Mukders S, Gao M, Teplittski M, Caetano-Anolles G, Rolfe BG Bauer W (2003) Extensive and specific responses of a eukaryote to bacterial quorum-sensing Proc Natl Acad Sci USA 100: 1444–1449

McCully ME (2001) Niches for bacterial endophytes in crop plants: a plant biologist's review Aust J Plant Physiol 28: 983–990

Merckx R, Dijkstra A, Denhartog A, van Veen JA (1987) Production of root-derived material and associated microbial growth in soil at different nutrient levels. Biol Fert Soil 5: 126–132

Merharg AA, Killham K (1995) Loss of exudates from roots of perennial rye-grass inoculated with a range of micro-organisms. Plant Soil 170: 345–349

Metting Jr FB (1992) Structure and physiological ecology of soil microbial communities. In: Metting Jr FB, Dekker Marcel (eds), Soil Microbial Ecol, New York, pp 3–25

Miller HJ Symbiosis (1990) Notes on the behaviour of fluorescent pseudomonas in rhizosphere studies 9: 377-381

Miller HJ, Liljeroth E, Henken G, van Veen JA (1990) Fluctuations in the fluorescent pseudomonas and actinomycete populations of rhizosphere and rhizoplane during the growth of spring wheat. Can J Microbiol 36: 254-258

Mirza MS, Ahmad W, Latif F, Haurat J, Bally R, Normand P, Malik KA (2001) Isolation, partial characterization, and the effect of plant growth-promoting bacteria (PGPB) on micro-propagated sugarcane *in vitro*. Plant and Soil 237: 47-54

Mittelbach GG, Steiner CF, Scheiner SM, Gross KL, Reynolds HL, Waide RB (2001) What is the observed relationship between species richness and productivity? Ecol 82: 2381–2396

Murphy JF, Zehnder GW, Schuster DJ, Sikora EJ, Polston JE, Kloepper JW, (2000) Plant growth-promoting rhizobacterial mediated protection in tomato against Tomato mottle virus. Plant Dis 84: 779–784

Nannipieri P, Ascher J, Ceccherini MT, Landi L, Pietramellara G, Renella G (2003) Microbial diversity and soil functions. European J Soil Science 54: 655–670

Narwal SS, Hoagland RE, Dilday RH, Reigosa MJ (2000) Proceedings of the III International Congress on Allelopathy in Ecological Agriculture and Forestry, Dharwad, India (August 18–21, 1998). In: Allelopathy in ecological agriculture and forestry, Kluwer Academic Publications, London, UK p 267

Nautiyal CS (2000) Biocontrol of plant diseases for agricultural sustainability. In: Upadhyay RK, Mukherji KG, Chamola BP (eds) Biocontrol potential and its exploration in sustainable agriculture. Kluwer Academic/Plenum Publishers, USA, pp 9-23

Nautiyal CS, Bhaduria S, Kumar P, Lal H, Mondal R, Verma D (2000) An efficient microbiological growth medium for screening phosphate solubilizing micro-organisms. FEMS Microbiol Lett 182: 291–296

Nazoa P, Vidmar JJ, Tranbarger TJ, Mouline K, Damiani I, Tillard P, Zhuo D, Glass ADM, Touraine B (2003) Regulation of the nitrate transporter gene AtNRT2.1 in *Arabidopsis thaliana*: responses to nitrate, amino acids and developmental stage. Plant Mol Biol 52: 689-703

Newton JA, Fray RG (2004) Integration of environmental and host-derived signals with quorum-sensing during plant–microbe interactions. Cellular Microbiol 6: 213–224

Nikolcheva LG, Cockshutt AM, Barlocher F (2003) Determining diversity of freshwater fungi on decaying leaves: comparison of traditional and molecular approaches. Appl Environ Microbiol 69: 2548–2554

Nowak J (1998) Benefits of *in vitro* Biotization of plant tissue cultures with microbial inoculants. *In Vitro* Cell Dev Biol Plant 34: 122–130

O'Toole GA, Kaplan HB, Kolter R (2000) Biofilm formation as microbial development. Ann Rev Microbiol 54: 49–79

Osborn AM, Moore ERB, Timmis KN (2000) An evaluation of terminal-restriction fragment length polymorphism (T-RFLP) analysis for the study of microbial community structure and dynamics. Environ Microbiol 2: 39–50

Pace NR (1997) A molecular view of microbial diversity in the biosphere. Science 276: 734–740

Parmar N, Dardarwal KR (1999) Stimulation of nitrogen fixation and induction of flavonoid like compounds by rhizobacteria. J Appl Microbiol 86: 36–44

Paterson E (2003) Importance of rhizodeposition in the coupling of plant and microbial productivity. European J Soil Science 54: 741-750

Phillips DA (1980) Efficiency of symbiotic nitrogen fixation in legumes. Annual Rev Plant Physiol 31: 29-49

Pierson EA, Wood DW, Cannon JA, Blachere FM, Pierson LSI (1998) Interpopulation signalling via N-acyl homoserine lactones among bacteria in the wheat rhizosphere. Mol Plant Microbe Interactions 11: 1078–1084

Pinton R, Varanini Z, Nannipieri P (2000) The rhizosphere as a site of biochemical interactions among soil components, plants, and micro-organisms. In: Pinton R, Varanini Z, Nannipieri P (eds) The Rhizosphere, Mercel Dekker, Inc, New York, USA pp 1–18

Pokojska-Burdziej A (1981) The effect of carbon and nitrogen sources on auxins and gibberellin-like substances synthesis by bacteria isolated from the roots of pine seedlings (*Pinus silvestris* L.). Acta Microbiologia Polonica, 30: 347–354

Postgate J (1998) Nitrogen Fixation. 3rd edn, Cambridge Univ. Press, Cambridge p. 112

Postgate JR (1982) Biological nitrogen fixation: fundamentals. Philosophical Transactions of the Royal Society of London, Series B, 296: 375-385

Press CM, Wilson M, Tuzun S, Kloepper JW (1997) Salicylic acid produced by *Serratia marcescens* 90-166 is not the primary determinant of induced systemic resistance in cucumber or tobacco. Mol Plant–Microbe Interact 10:761–768

Preston GM, Haubold B, Rainey PB (1998) Bacterial genomics and adaptation to life on plants: implications for the evolution of pathogenicity and symbiosis. Curr Opin Microbiol 1: 589–597

Raaijmakers JM, Leeman M, Van Oorschot MMP, Van der Sluis I, Schippers B, Bakker PAHM (1995) Dose–response relationships in biological control of fusarium wilt of radish by *Pseudomonas* spp. Phytopathol 85: 1075–1081

Rajan YS (2002) In: Agony and Harmony, New Century Book House (P) Ltd., Chennai, India pp 2-3

Redfield RJ (2002) Is quorum-sensing a side effect of diffusion-sensing? Trends Microbiol 10: 365–369

Reynolds HL, Waide RB (2001) What is the observed relationship between species richness and productivity? Ecology 82: 2381–2396

Ronn R, Griffiths BS, Ekelund F, Christensen S (1996) Spatial distribution and successional pattern of microbial activity and micro-faunal populations on decomposing barley roots. J Appl Ecol 33: 662-672

Ryals JA, Neuenschwanderm UH, Willits MG, Molina A, Steiner HY, Hunt MD (1996) Systemic acquired resistance. Plant Cell 8: 1809–1819

Sayre RM, Starr MP (1988) Bacterial diseases and antagonisms of nematodes. In: Poinar GO, Jansson HB (eds) Diseases of Nematodes CRC Press, Boca Raton, FL pp 69–101

Scheu S, Ruess L, Bonkowski M (2005) Interactions between micro-organisms and soil micro- and mesofauna. In: Buscot F, Varma A (eds) Microorganisms in soils: Roles in genesis and functions, Springer-Verlag, Berlin Heidelberg, Germany, pp 253-275

Shetty KG, DHetrick BA, Figge DAH, Schwab AP (1994) Effects of mycorrhizae and other soil microbes on revegetation of heavy metal contaminated mine spoil. Environ Pollu 86: 181–188

Siciliano SD, Theoret CM, de Freitas JR, Hucl PJ, Germida JJ (1998) Differences in the microbial communities associated with the roots of different cultivars of canola and wheat. Can J Microbiol 44: 844–851

Steenhoudt O, Vanderleyden (2000) *Azospirillum* a free-living nitrogen-fixing bacterium closely associated with grasses: genetic, biochemical and ecological aspects. J FEMS Microbiol Rev 24: 487-506

Steidle A, Sigl K, Schuhegger R, Ihring A, Schmid M, Gantner S, Toffels M, Riedel K, Givskov M, Hartmann A, Langebartels C, Eberl L (2001) Visualization of N-acylhomoserine lactone-mediated cell-to-cell communication between bacteria colonizing the tomato rhizosphere. Appl Environ Microbiol 67: 5761–5770

Stephens PM, Crowley JJ, Connel CO (1993) Selection of pseudomonad strains inhibiting *Pythium ultimum* on sugar beet seed in soil. Soil Biol Biochem 25: 1283-1288

Sticher L, Mauch-Mani B, Metraux JP (1997) Systemic acquired resistance. Annu Rev Phytopathol 35: 235–270

Sturz AV, Christie BR (2003) Beneficial microbial allelopathies in the root zone: the management of soil quality and plant disease with rhizobacteria. Soil Tillage Res 72: 107–123

Teplitski M, Robinson JB, Bauer WD (2000). Plants secrete substances that mimic bacterial N-acyl homoserine lactone signal activities and affect population density-dependent behaviors in associated bacteria. Mol Plant Microbe Interaction 13: 637–648

Thomashow LS Weller DM (1988) Role of a phenazine antibiotic from Pseudomonas fluorescens in biological control of *Gaeumannomyces graminis* var. *tritici*. J Bacteriol 170: 3499–3508

Thomashow LS, Bonsall RF, Weller DM (1997) Antibiotic production by soil rhizosphere microbes in situ. In: Hurst CJ, Knudsen GR, McInerney MJ, Stetzenbach LD, Walter MV (eds) Manual of Environmental Microbiology. ASM Press, Washington DC pp 305–319

Tiedje JM (1995) Approaches to the comprehensive evaluation of prokaryote diversity of a habitat. In: Allsopp D, Hawksworth DL, Colwell RR (eds) Microbial Diversity and Ecosystem Function CAB International, Wallingford, UK pp 73–97

Tilak KVBR, Ranganayaki N, Pal KK, De R, Saxena AK, Nautiyal CS, Mittal S, Tripathi AK, Johri BN (2005) Diversity of plant growth and soil health supporting bacteria. Curr Sci 89: 136-150

Torsvik V, Goksoyr J, Daae FL (1990) High diversity in DNA of soil bacteria. Appl Environ Microbiol 56: 782–787

Torsvik V, Ovreas, Thingstad LTF (2002) Prokaryotic diversity – magnitude, dynamics and controlling factors. Sci 296: 1064–1065

Van Dommelen A, Van Bastelaere E, Keijers V, Vanderleyden J (1997) Genetics of *Azospirillum brasilense* with respect to ammonium transport, sugar uptake and chemotaxis. Plant Soil 194: 155-160

Van Loon LC, Bakker PAHM, Pieterse CMJ (1998) Systemic resistance induced by rhizosphere bacteria. Annu Rev Phytopathol 36: 453–483

Van Peer R, Niemann GJ, Schippers B (1991) Induced resistance and phytoalexin accumulation in biological control of *Fusarium* wilt of carnation by *Pseudomonas* sp. strain WCS417r. Phytopathol 81: 728–734

Van VT, Berge O, Ngoke S, Balandreau J, Heulin T (2000) Repeated beneficial effect of rice inoculation with a strain of *Burkholderia vietnamiensis* on early and late yield components in low fertility sulphate acid soil of Vietnam. Plant Soil 218: 273–284

Vande Broek A, Michiels J, Van Gool A, Vanderleyden J (1993). Spatial-temporal colonization patterns of *Azospirillum brasilense* on the wheat root surface and expression of the bacterial *nif*H gene during association. Mol Plant Microbe Interactions 6: 592-600

Vessey JK (2003) Plant growth-promoting rhizobacteria as biofertilizers. Plant Soil 255: 571–586

Walker BH (1992) Biodiversity and ecological redundancy. Conservation Biol 6: 18–23

Wardle DA, Bonner KI, Nicholson KS (1997) Biodiversity and plant litter: experimental evidence which does not support the view that enhanced species richness improves ecosystem function. OIKOS 79: 247–258

Wei G, Kloepper JW, Tuzun S (1991) Induction of systemic resistance of cucumber to *Colletotrichum orbiculare* by select strains of plant growth promoting rhizobacteria. Phytopathol 81: 1508–1512

Wei G, Kloepper JW, Tuzun S (1996) Induction of systemic resistance to cucumber disease and increase plant growth by plant growth-promoting rhizobacteria under field conditions. Phytopathol 86: 221–224

Weller DM, Raaijmakers JM, Gardener BBM, Thomashow LS (2002) Microbial populations responsible for specific soil suppressiveness to plant pathogens. Annu Rev Phytopathol 40: 309–348

Whipps JM (1990) Carbon economy. In: Lynch JM, Wiley (ed) In The Rhizosphere, New York pp 59–97

Whipps JM (1997) Developments in the biological control of soil-borne plant pathogens. Adv Botanical Res 26: 1–134

Whipps JM (2001) Microbial interactions and biocontrol in the rhizosphere. J Exper Bot 52: 487–511

Whittaker RH, Feeny PP (1971) Allelochemics: chemical interaction between species. Sci 171: 757–770

Williams ST (1985) Oligotrophy in soil: Fact or fiction? In: (eds) Fletcher M, Floodgate GD Bacteria in their natural environments, Academic Press: London

Yoon S, Hennigan RF, Hilliard GM, Ochsner UA, Parvatiyar K, Kamani MC, Allen H, DeKievit T, Gardner PR, Schwab U, Rowe JJ, Iglewski BH, McDermott TR, Mason RP, Wozniak DJ, Hancock RE, Parsek MR, Noah T, Boucher RC, Hassett DJ, Dev (2002) Development and persistence of anaerobic *Pseudomonas aeruginosa* biofilms: relevance to pathogenesis and therapy of cystic fibrosis lung disease. Cell 3: 593–603

Young JPW (1992) Phylogenetic classification of nitrogen-fixing organisms. In: Stacey G, Burris RH, Evans HJ ((eds)) Biological Nitrogen Fixation. Chapman and Hall, New York pp 43–86

Zahir A, Zahir MA, William T, Frankenberger Jr (2004) Plant growth-promoting rhizobacteria: Applications and perspective in agriculture. In Advances in Agronomy, Academic Press: USA 81: 97-168

Zhang S, Moyne AL, Reddy MS, Kloepper JW (2002) The role of salicylic acid in induced systemic resistance elicited by plant growth-promoting rhizobacteria against blue mold of tobacco. Biol Cont 25: 288–296

Microbial Population and Biomass C and N in the Rhizosphere of *Albizia lebbeck* L. and *Gmelina arborea* Roxb. in a 'jhum' fallow in Northeast India

K SHRIVASTAVA, A ARUNACHALAM and K ARUNACHALAM

1. INTRODUCTION

Cycling of nutrients is crucial to the restoration of degraded ecosystems in the hills (Arunachalam and Pandey 2003). Trees growing on degraded lands in the hill slopes (e.g. abandoned shifting agricultural land, locally called 'jhum' cultivation), particularly in the geologically young eastern Himalayan plateau, holds together the loose sandy–loam soil and helps in slope stability, reducing run-off and soil erosion (Toky and Ramakrishnan 1982; Ramakrishnan 1992). Some of the tree species commonly used in the afforestation and/or land reclamation activities in northeastern India are *Albizia lebbeck, Albizia procera, Albizia lucida, Gmelina arborea, Duabanga grandiflora, Terminalia myriocarpa, Bombax ceiba,* and bamboos (Arunachalam and Arunachalam 2002a). Agroforestry and silvipastoralism have been advocated as alternative land use practices to shifting agriculture and fallow management in the humid environments (Belsky et al. 1993a; Schroth 1998; Arunachalam et al. 2002). We chose *Albizia lebbeck* L. and *Gmelina arborea* Roxb. that rapidly colonize the degraded lands in the region due to their adaptability, faster growth and nutrient conservation role (Shukla 1992) in order to assess their role in succession and reconstruction of degraded ecosystems. While the impact

Department of Forestry, North Eastern Regional Institute of Science and Technology, Nirjuli 791109, Arunachal Pradesh, India (E-mail: karunashrivastava@yahoo.co.in)

of tree growth on the soil may differ at species level (Schroth 1998), it is expected to increase the microbial population and biomass, particularly in the rhizosphere zone, by providing a larger root surface area that would help in enriching soil fertility by acting as a 'sink' and 'source' of plant available nutrients (Singh et al. 1989).

The role of microbial biomass in soil fertility management was evaluated in various terrestrial ecosystems and was found to play crucial role in N and P dynamics in the tropical soils (Hernot and Robertson 1994; Arunachalam et al. 1999). However, its role in the restoration of degraded lands has not received the attention of ecologists, foresters and soil scientists (Arunachalam and Arunachalam 2002a; Arunachalam and Pandey 2003). Nevertheless, data on microbial biomass as influenced by tree growth could prove to be a potential index in soil nutrient restoration during the recovery of degraded ecosystems. Therefore, one N-fixing tree species, *A. lebbeck* and another timber-yielding species *G. arborea* were selected to evaluate their influence on the physico-chemical and biological properties of rhizosphere soil and to determine the contribution of microbial biomass to nutrient pool in the top soil. The study is a part of a major research project that aims to identify potential tree species for rehabilitating the abandoned sloping agricultural lands ('jhum' fallows) at lower elevations of north-east India in general, Arunachal Pradesh in particular.

2. MATERIALS AND METHODS

2.1 Study Area

The study sites are located in the humid tropical forest belt dominated by native tree species like *Mesua ferrea, Chukrasia tabularis, Terminalia myriocarpa, Anthocephalus cadamba,* etc. The understorey has dense growth of ferns, and other species like *Lantana camara, Eupatorium* sp., *Musa sapientum, Oxalis* sp., *Symplocos* sp., etc. Almost all the original vegetation has been cleared in the study area due to various anthropogenic stress events and also to a certain extent by frequent landslides and floods during monsoon (Arunachalam et al. 2000; Arunachalam and Arunachalam 2002b). The main anthropological stress was shifting cultivation on the hill slopes and illegal felling (Arunachalam 2002; Upadhyaya and Arunachalam 2004). Our study sites were (1) jhum fallow (1.27 ha) and (2) a grassland (0.9 ha) which were in close proximity to each other, located at 132 m above sea-level with 6-13% slope facing north-east in the Itanagar capital complex of Arunachal Pradesh (Latitude 26°28′ to 29°30′ N, Longitude 91°31′ to 97°30′ E), north-east India. *Albizia lebbeck* and *Gmelina arborea* plants were growing in the abandoned jhum field, cultivated fifteen years earlier.

The parent rock of the study area is of sub-himalayan type consisting Neogene molassic sediments (Siwaliks). The soils were sandy loam, having about 75% sand content. The study area experiences three distinct seasons namely a warm and dry summer (March to May), monsoon (June to September) and a cool and dry winter (October to February). The average annual rainfall is 2500 mm approximately. The average minimum and maximum air temperatures during the study period were 23°C and 29°C respectively; the relative humidity varied from 64 to 85%. The light intensity varied from 690 to 26200 lux and soil temperature (0-15 cm depth) ranged 25°C to 32°C during the study period.

2.2 Sampling Procedures

Five individuals of two different tree species planted fifteen years ago in a jhum fallow as a rehabilitation measure were selected for detailed sampling. Adjacent naturally revegetated grassland was also selected as control site during October 2003. Understudy vegetation and soil samplings in the case of tree species were restricted to 2 m distance away from the main trunk of the respective species, and well within the plant canopy. Plant height (using Ravi altimeter) and girth (using measuring tape) were measured. The height of the plant averaged 11.8 m and 10.1 m for *A. lebbeck* and *G. arborea* respectively. Girth, tree volume and canopy cover were greater in *A. lebbeck* than in *G. arborea* (Table 1).

Five 1 m × 1 m quadrates were laid for ground vegetation analysis within the canopy of each of the tree species and in the grassland, and all plants within those quadrates were counted. Density and dominance were calculated according to Misra (1968). Nomenclature of plant species followed Hooker (1872-1897).

In all the five quadrates of an individual tree used for ground vegetation analysis, microclimatic variables such as relative humidity and air temperature (using thermo-hygrometer), light intensity (using lux

Table 1 Basal area and canopy cover of *Albizia lebbeck* and *Gmelina arborea*

Species	*Girth (cm)*	*Basal Area (m^2)*	*Height (m)*	*Volume (m^3)*	*Canopy Cover (m^2)*
Albizia lebbeck (15 years old)	129.00 ±12.14	0.33 ±0.02	11.76 ±1.23	3.88 ±0.08	22.79 ±1.02
Gmelina arborea (15 year old)	98.75 ±8.43	0.28 ±0.11	10.12 ±0.94	2.83 ±0.11	19.10 ±1.34

±S.E. (n=5)

meter) and soil temperature (using soil thermometer) on the floor within the canopy of the tree species and in grassland. All measurements were conducted during peak daylight conditions. Below the canopy of each individual tree and in grassland five soil samples in the rhizosphere zone down to a depth of 60 cm (0-15, 15-30, 30-45, 45-60 cm) were collected from those quadrates using a soil corer (5.5 cm inner diameter), mixed thoroughly species-wise and/or site-wise. The composite soil sample of each of the tree species and grassland was divided equally into two parts; one part was immediately (within 24 hours) sieved (2 mm mesh screen) and analysed for pH (digital pH meter) and moisture content (gravimetric method). The other part of the soil was sieved through 2 mm mesh screen, air-dried under laboratory conditions for seven days, and was determined for texture (Boyoucous hydrometric method). The remaining air-dried soil samples were ground and sieved through 0.5 mm mesh screen and used for analysis of soil organic carbon (rapid titration method) and total nitrogen (semi-micro Kjeldahl procedure). All procedures followed are as outlined in Allen et al. (1974) and Anderson and Ingram (1993).

For the estimation of microbial population and biomass, another set of five soil samples (0-15 cm depth) were collected below the tree canopies and in grassland. In this case, the core was wiped with absolute ethanol before every insertion to prevent any external microbial contamination. Soils were used within 24 hours of sampling for determination of all microbial properties. We considered five replications for all analytical determinations. The bacterial and fungal populations were determined using dilution plate techniques on nutrient agar and rose Bengal agar medium, respectively. Soil bacterial population was estimated by Waksman's (1952) method using the nutrient agar medium at 10^5 dilution. Fungal population was estimated by dilution plate method (Johnson and Curl 1972) using Martin Rose Bengal agar medium at 10^3 dilution in water. The inoculated petri-dishes were incubated at 30±1°C for 24 h and 25±1°C for five days for bacteria and fungi, respectively.

As many reports suggest that microbial biomass is active in the top 0-15 cm soil layer, we also considered the top 0-15 cm soil depth for determination of microbial C and N using chloroform fumigation extraction technique (Anderson and Ingram 1993) using two sets of treatment (chloroform fumigated and unfumigated) and extracted in 0.5 N K_2SO_4 and simultaneously digested and titrated against ferrous ammonium sulphate using 1 : 10 phenanthroline monohydrate as the indicator and N/140 HCl using boric acid indicator, respectively. In all cases, the values of unfumigated samples were subtracted from fumigated one to get the values for microbial C and N.

2.3 Statistical Analysis

Tukey's test was used to compare the mean values across the sites. Linear regressions were worked out whenever necessary following Zar (1974).

3. SALIENT OBSERVATIONS

3.1 Ground Vegetation

There were nine herbaceous species under the canopy of *A. lebbeck,* of which *Oplismenus* sp. (a monocot) had the highest dominance value of 43.7 (Table 2). Under the canopy of *G. arborea,* six species were identified of which one was a pteridophyte (*Polypodium sp.*) which constituted 10.4% of the total dominance value (=100); *Achyranthes aspera* had the highest dominance (40.2%). In the grassland, *Axonopus compressus* was the dominant species (32.9%), followed by *Andropogon aciculatus* and *Cynodon dactylon*. The total density of ground vegetation was 38.6, 17.3 and 41.5 m^{-2} below the canopy of *A. lebbeck and G. arborea* and in grassland respectively. The total number of species was also highest (13) in the grassland (Table 3).

3.2 Microclimate and Soil Properties

Air temperature, relative humidity and soil temperature did not show any significant difference between species and in grassland (Table 3). Among the tree species, light intensity was greater under the canopy of *G. arborea* than under *A. lebbeck*. Bulk density of soils ranged 1.19-1.56 g/cm^3. Soil moisture content was greater in grassland as compared to the soils under tree canopy (Table 3).

In general, the soil was slightly acidic (5.99-6.54). Soil organic matter (SOM) was greater in grassland as compared to the two study species. Among themselves, total nitrogen (N) was greater under *A. lebbeck* and SOM was greater under *G. arborea*. Soil C–N ratio was 8 in case of *A. lebbeck* and 20 in *G. arborea* and 41 in the grassland (Table 3). In general, pH, moisture, SOM and total N decreased with increasing soil depth (Fig. 1).

3.3 Microbial Population and Biomass

The soil biological properties were determined in terms of microbial population (bacteria and fungi) and microbial biomass C and N. Over all, microbial population decreased with increasing soil depth (Fig. 2). Both bacterial and fungal populations in soil were greater under *A. lebbeck,* while the grassland soil harbored the least microbial population (Table 4).

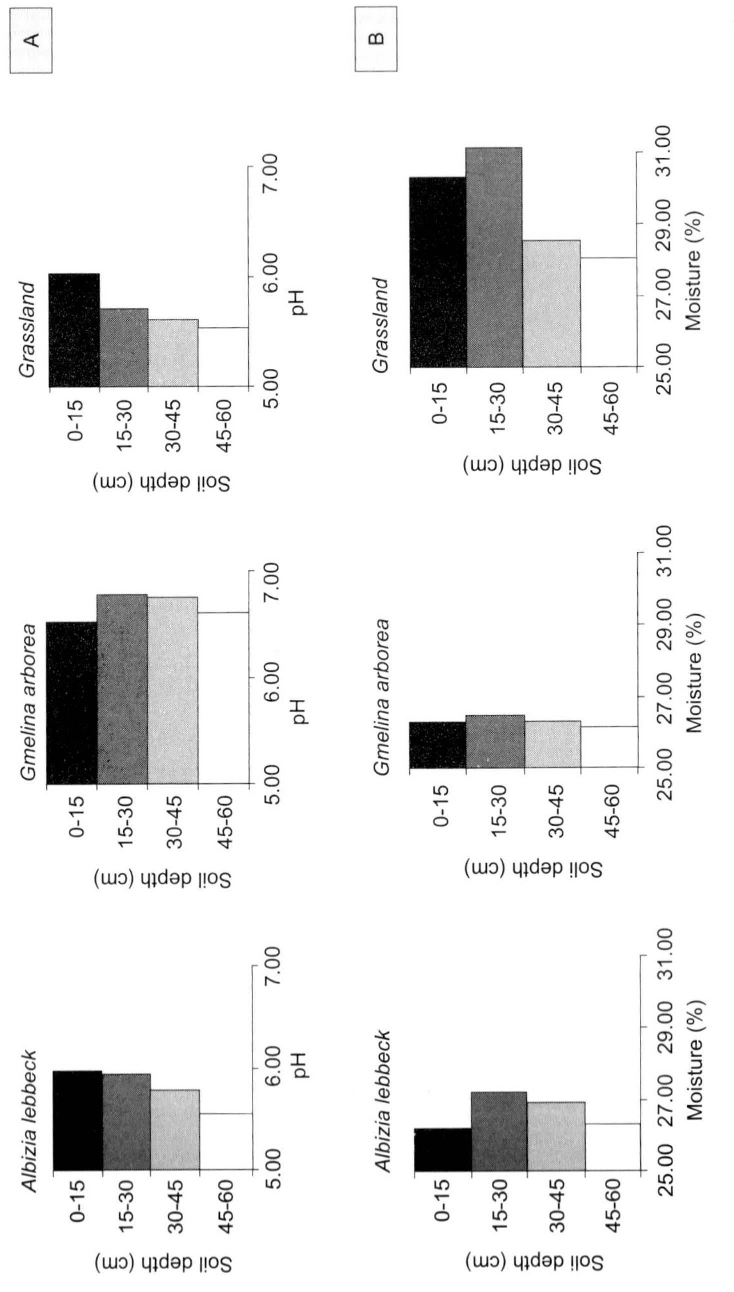

Figure Contd.

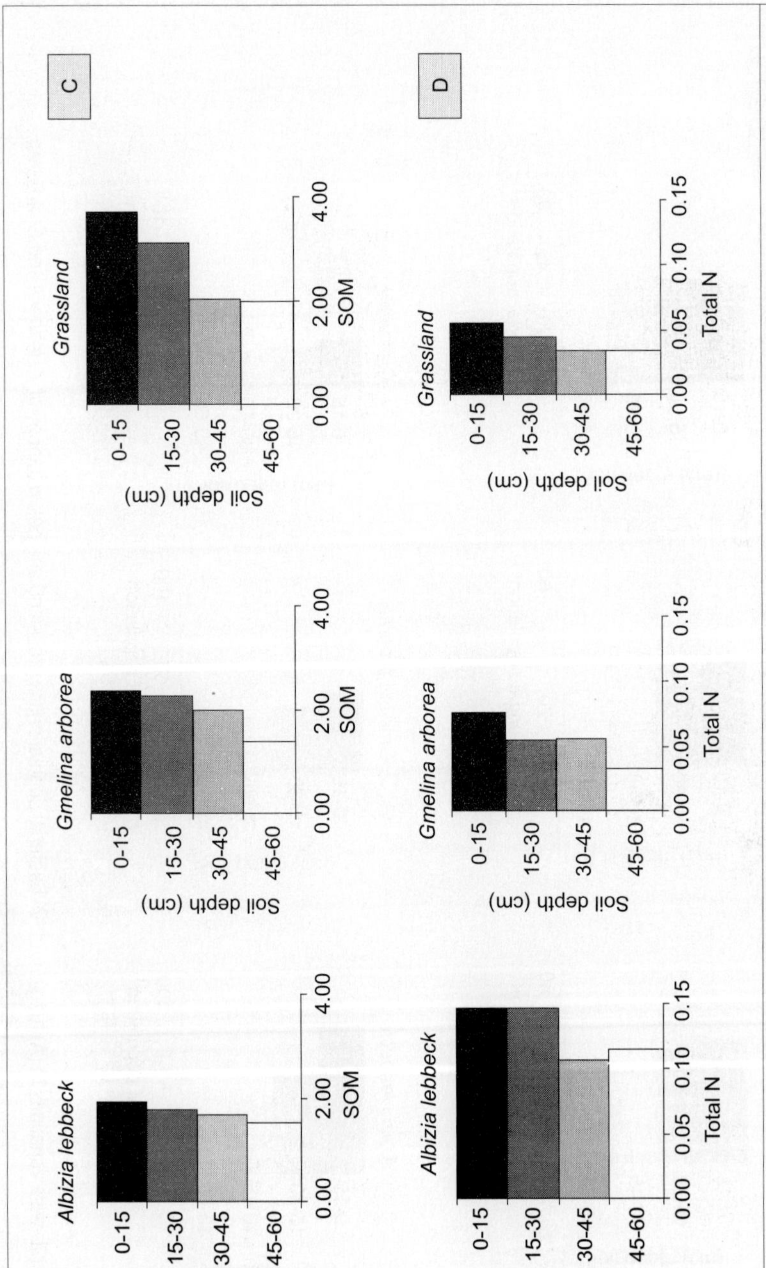

Fig. 1 Depth-wise variation in (A) soil pH, (B) moisture (C) organic C and (D) total N in grassland and below the canopy of *Albizia lebbeck* and *Gmelina arborea*.

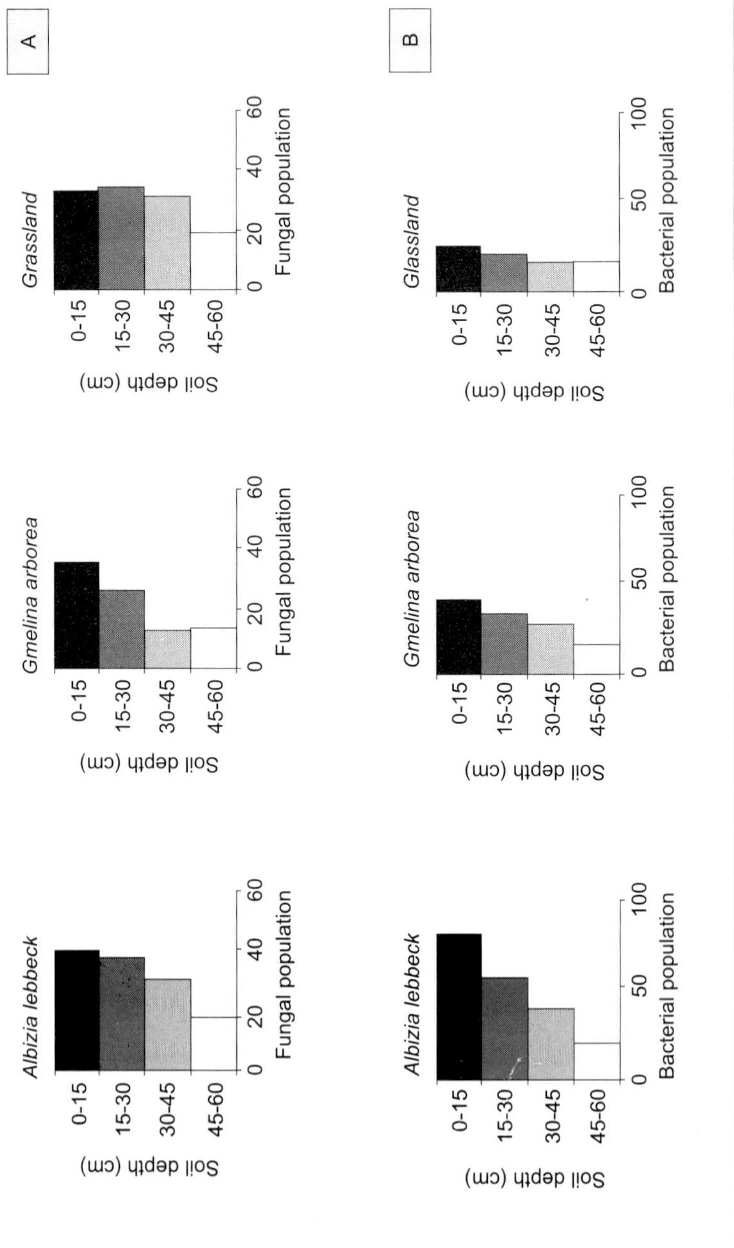

Fig. 2 Depth-wise variations in (A) fungal and (B) bacterial populations in grassland and below canopy of *A. lebbeck* and *G. arborea*.

Table 2 Species composition, density (m^{-2}) and dominance (%) of ground vegetation below tree canopy and in grassland

Species	*A. lebbeck*		*G. arborea*		*Grassland*	
	Density	*Dominance*	*Density*	*Dominance*	*Density*	*Dominance*
Achyranthes aspera L.	9.32	18.11	9.65	40.23	-	-
Ageratum conyzoides L.	3.37	9.72	-	-	1.32	3.94
Andropogon aciculatus. Retz	-	-	-	-	6.31	18.73
Axonopus compressus (Sw.) Beauv	6.63	12.89	2.32	14.59	16.31	32.92
Bonnaya reptans (Roxb.).Spreng	-	-	-	-	2.66	5.24
Borreria articularis (Lf) FN.Williams	1.00	2.92	-	-	3.64	7.2
Cuphea carthagensis. Macbr	-	-	-	-	1.68	3.33
Cynodon dactylon. (L.) *Pers*	-	-	-	-	4.00	7.88
Desmodium sp.	-	-	-	-	0.63	3.94
Drymaria cordata (L.) *Willd.*	1.62	4.86	-	-	-	-
Kyllinga brevifolia Rottb.	-	-	-	-	2.00	3.94
Mikania micrantha Kunth.	0.68	1.94	1.34	5.59	-	-
Mimosa pudica Linn.	-	-	-	-	0.35	1.97
Oplismenus sp.	15.00	43.73	-	-	-	-
Polygonum vulgare L.	0.34	1.94	1.34	16.67	-	-
Polypodium sp.	-	-	1.67	10.42	-	-
Spilanthes acmella Murr.	0.68	3.89	1.00	12.51	1.66	4.94
Sida acuta Burm.	-	-	-	-	0.64	3.94
Urena lobata L.	-	-	-	-	0.33	1.97
Species number	9	-	6	-	13	-
Total density/dominance	38.64	100	17.32	100	41.53	100

–absent; values are the means of 5 replicated $1m^2$ quadrats.

Table 3 Microclimatic variability and soil (0-15 cm depth) physico-chemical properties under the canopy of two different tree species and in grassland.

Parameters	*A. lebbeck*	*G. arborea*	*Grassland*
Microclimate			
Air temperature (°C)	28.1 ± 0.35	28.8 ± 1.18	28.9 ± 1.45
Humidity (%)	85 ± 2	84 ± 3	83 ± 6
Light intensity (lux)	17330 ± 213	29500 ± 339	38070 ± 246
Soil temperature (°C)	25.0 ± 1.05	25.1 ± 2.10	25.2 ± 1.83
Soil physical properties			
Texural class	Sandy loam	Sandy loam	Sandy loam
Bulk density (g cm^{-3})	1.19 ± 0.05	1.37 ± 0.18	1.56 ± 0.23
Moisture (%)	26.20 ± 0.01	26.27 ± 0.07	30.07 ± 0.07
Soil chemical properties			
pH (1:2.5 w/v H_2O)	5.99 ± 0.03	6.54 ± 0.14	6.03 ± 0.08
Organic C (%)	1.16 ± 0.05	1.38 ± 0.57	2.07 ± 0.06
Organic Matter (%)	1.99 ± 0.09	2.37 ± 0.98	3.57 ± 0.10
Total N (%)	0.14 ± 0.02	0.07 ± 0.01	0.05 ± 0.01
C-N	8.29	19.71	41.40

±S.E. (n=5)

Table 4 Soil microbial population and biomass C and N (0-15 cm depth) under the canopy of two different tree species and in grassland.

Parameters	*A. lebbeck*	*G. arborea*	*Grassland*
Microbial population (g^{-1} dry soil)			
Fungi (no. of colonies × 10^3)	39.87 ± 2.33	34.12 ± 2.56	32.07 ± 1.24
Bacteria (no. of colonies × 10^5)	73.80 ± 1.12	40.30 ± 1.09	24.45 ± 1.01
Microbial biomass ($\mu g\ g^{-1}$)			
C	881.90 ± 9.03	671.12 ± 3.14	1024.56 ± 2.08
N	321.11 ± 0.09	189.43 ± 0.41	157.82 ± 0.28
C-N	2.75	3.54	6.49
Contribution of microbial biomass to soil nutrient pool (%)			
Microbial C to Soil organic C	7.60	4.86	4.95
Microbial N to Soil total N	22.94	27.06	31.56

±S.E. (n=5)

On the contrary, soil microbial biomass carbon (C) was greater in grassland (Table 4) and lowest under *G. arborea*. Microbial N was greater in *A. lebbeck* soil (321 μg g^{-1}) and lowest in the grassland. The contribution of microbial C to soil organic carbon (SOC) was significantly ($P<0.05$) lower in the grassland as well as under *G. arborea* as compared to that of *A. lebbeck*. The contribution of microbial N to total soil N was, however, greater in grassland and in *G. arborea* soil (Table 4).

3.4 Fungal Species Composition

Although 40 forms of fungi were isolated from the soils under the canopy of two tree species and grassland. Only five species, such as *Aspergillus flavipes, A. fumigatus, A. vstus, Penicillium funiculosum* and *Scopulariopsis racemosum* were present in all soil samples analyzed (Table 5). In total, there were twenty five, twenty one and fiftheen fungal forms identified in soils under *A. lebbeck, G. arborea* and grassland, respectively. Some species were exclusively present in a particular soil; eight under *A. lebbeck*, ten under *G. arborea* and one in grassland (Table 5).

Table 5 Fungal species composition in the top soil (0-15 cm depth) below tree canopy and in grassland

Fungal species	*A. lebbeck*	*G. arborea*	*Grassland*
Absidia heterospora	-	+	-
Acremonium sp.	-	+	-
Alternaria humicola	+	-	-
Aspergillus cervinus	-	+	+
Aspergillus flavipes	+	+	+
Aspergillus fumigatus	+	+	+
Aspergillus ochraceous	+	-	-
Aspergillus sulphurius	+	-	+
Aspergillus terreus	-	-	+
Aspergillus ustus	+	+	+
Aspergillus versicolar	+	+	-
Chaetomium globosum	+	-	+
Cladosporium cladosporioides	-	+	-
Cladosporium herbarum	+	-	-
Cladosporium sp.	-	+	-
Curvularia lunata	-	+	+
Fusarium oxysporum	-	+	-
Fusarium solani	+	-	+

Contd.

Table 5

Fungal species	*A. lebbeck*	*G. arborea*	*Grassland*
Helminthosporium sativum	-	+	+
Mucor circinelloides	+	-	-
Myrothecium soridum	+	+	-
Mycelia sterila 1	+	-	-
Mycelia sterila 2	-	-	+
Mycelia sterila 3	+	-	-
Nirospora sphaerica	-	+	-
Paecilomyces varioti	+	+	-
Papularia sphaerosperma	-	+	-
Penicillium funiculosum	+	+	+
Penicillum rubrum	+	-	-
Penicillium chrysogenum	-	+	-
Penicillium sp.	+	-	+
Phoma glomerata	+	-	+
Phomopsis sp.	+	-	-
Rhizoctonia solani	+	-	-
Sclerotium rolfsii	-	+	-
Scopulariopsis racemosum	+	+	+
Scopulariopsis brevicaulis	+	-	-
Trichoderma glaucum	-	+	-
Torula convoluta	+	-	-
Verticillium terrestre	+	+	-
Total species number	25	21	15

+ present; - absent

4. INTERPRETATIONS

Although the two tree species were growing contiguously in the same site, we observed spatial differences in the distribution of soil nutrients and microbial population. The root causes of this spatial heterogeneity are not presently understood. Nevertheless, in an environment where rainfall is high (over 2000 mm annually) and *monsoonic*, and the soil is sandy loam and porous, this spatial heterogeneity may have potential to nutrient retention, especially when the system is ecologically fragile and nutrient poor (Pandey and Singh 1985; Belsky et al. 1989). In the grassland, only light demanding and shade intolerant species like *Cynodon dactylon*, *Axonopus compressus* and *Kullinga brevifolia* showed greater dominance. While, beneath the canopy of tree species, much shade loving dicot plants

(*Achyranthes aspera, Polygonum rude, Spilanthes acmella)* were abundant (Table 2). This is further substantiated by the microclimatic variability in the undercanopy environment of the two tree species and in grassland (Table 3) (Belsky et al. 1993b).

Soil pH remained slightly acidic. Differences in soil organic C content below the canopies of two tree species were not significant as they were growing in the same site. However, total N was significantly higher ($P<0.05$) in the rhizosphere soil of *A. lebbeck*, while it was reduced by 50% in *G. arborea* and again half-reduced in the grassland soil. It appears that growth of tree species exerts a greater impact on N turnover than C turnover in the soil. Reduction in N-level below the canopy of *G. arborea* may be due to greater uptake of N from soil by this species and also low N return to soil (Hosur and Dasog 1995). Thus this species would have put the ground flora under severe competition and therefore low ground vegetation below its canopy (Belsky 1992). The heterogeneity in soil nitrogen between the N_2-fixing and non-N_2-fixing tree species in this study may be attributed to their rhizosphere characters that may have differential effect on the decomposer population (Arunachalam et al. 1997). This is confounded by depth wise decrease in soil nutrient concentrations (Fig. 1) and microbial population (Fig. 2).

High counts of bacteria and fungi and greater microbial biomass in *A. lebbeck* soils compared to *G. arborea* may be attributed to dense growth of herbaceous vegetation and to greater availability of nutrients on account of greater accumulation of litter and fine roots (Table 6). Jha et al. (1992) pointed out that for a given community, one or few species are numerically dominant. The results obtained fully corroborate this point, as five species of fungi (*Aspergillus flavipes, A. fumigatus, A. vstus, Penicillium funiculosum* and *Scopulariopsis racemosum*) were dominant in all soil samples studied. These fungi thus reveal their wider ecological amplitude. The genus *Aspergillus* was represented by eight species, *Penicillium* by four species, *Cladosporium* by three species and *Fusarium* by two species (Table 5). The greater species diversity of the genus *Aspergillus* and *Penicilium* could be due in part to their greater spore production and dispersion (Arunachalam 1992). However, there were a few species unique to rhizosphere zone of different tree species studied. Thus the dynamics of fungal species was greatly influenced by the changes in canopy cover and soil nutrient changes (Maithani and Tripathi 1996).

Microbial C (882-1025 $\mu g\ g^{-1}$) values were well within those reported by Vance et al. (1987) for various terrestrial ecosystems (61-1900 $\mu g\ g^{-1}$). The microbial C (801-1432 $\mu g\ g^{-1}$) in *A. lebbeck* soil was comparable to that of a 7-year old jhum fallow in this region (Arunachalam and Pandey 2003). There was a significant positive correlation between soil organic-C and

Table 6 Litter and root biomass (kg ha^{-1}; 0-15 cm soil depth) below tree canopy and in grassland

Detritus	*A. lebbeck*	*G. arborea*	*Grassland*
Aboveground			
Leaf litter	128.31 ± 24.12	98.42 ± 8.32	78.12 ± 7.18
Others	31.19 ± 2.87	14.78 ± 1.91	3.44 ± 0.91
Total	159.50	113.20	81.56
Belowground			
Fine roots (< 2 mm)	632.4 ± 2.1	124.0 ± 1.1	620.0 ± 1.8
Coarse roots (>2 mm)	979.6 ± 2.5	446.4 ± 1.6	-
Nodules	74.4 ± 0.9	-	-
Rhizomes	-	-	131.0 ± 1.1
Total roots	**1686.4**	**570.4**	**620.0**

- absent; ±S.E. (n=5)

microbial C (r=0.503, df.=24, P<0.01). The dynamics of N in the mineral soil is also reportedly linked to C, because most N exists in organic compounds and heterotrophic microbes, which utilize organic-C for energy (Arunachalam et al. 1999). But in this study, microbial N showed negative correlation with microbial C (r=-0.831, df.=24, P<0.01). Joergensen et al. (1995) reported that above soil pH 5.0, microbial C–N ratios vary within a narrow range. Our study does corroborate this as the differences in microbial C–N ratio between sites were low, as the soil pH did not vary significantly (Tables 3, 4). They also suggested that soils with comparatively low C and N availability may result in microbial C–N ratios which are well below the optimum values, i.e. 5-8. In this study, the soils under the tree canopies had microbial C–microbial N ratios below 5 and in grassland the ratio exceeded 6. This again indicates low availability of N in the soils studied (Tripathi and Singh 1994). However, soil-specific differences in population structure and associated functioning of microbial population are also important in regulating the C–N ratio in microbial biomass. Nonetheless, the microbial biomass in the soils under the tree canopy was dormant, because of a very small microbial C–N ratio (2.75-3.54) (Bremner and van Kessel 1992). A low range of microbial C–N ratio (2-6) in this study also indicated that bacteria dominated the microbial biomass of the study sites (Anderson and Domsch 1989) and hence may have tremendous potential in rapid soil nutrient turnover during community redevelopment on abandoned shifting agricultural lands (Arunachalam et al. 1997). Further, abundant fungal forms in the rhizosphere of the tree species would help in nutrient immobilization that is crucial for soil nutrient restoration in rehabilitated sites occurring on slopes where runoff and leaching losses are tremendous (Mohan 1992).

5. CONCLUSION

The influence of *Albizia lebbeck* L. and *Gmelina arborea* Roxb. on the ground vegetation and physico-chemical and microbiological characteristics of rhizosphere soil (up to 60 cm depth), as a measure to the rehabilitation of the abandoned shifting agricultural land in Arunachal Pradesh, north-east India have been characterized. The results were compared with grassland that has developed through the fallow period in adjacent plot. Soil was slightly acidic. Soil total nitrogen was significantly lower below the canopy of *G. arborea* that had less ground flora as compared to *A. lebbeck*. Interestingly, grassland had greater soil organic matter and low nitrogen as compared to the rhizosphere soil of the tree species. Soil microbial population and microbial biomass carbon and nitrogen were greater in the rhizosphere zone of *A. lebbeck* as compared to *G. arborea*. Both, soil nutrients and bacterial-fungal populations decreased with increasing soil depth. The contribution of microbial biomass to soil organic carbon pool was lower (4.8-7.6%) as compared to its contribution to soil total nitrogen (22.9-31.5%). Below the canopy of the N_2-fixing *A. lebbeck*, the microbial biomass contributed more to soil organic carbon, and under the canopy of *G. arborea* it registered greater contribution to the soil nitrogen pool. Based on the morphological and rhizosphere microbiological properties, the study concludes that *A. lebbeck* has greater potentials to restore the soil nitrogen cycling, particularly nitrogen which is vital to the rehabilitation of fallow agricultural lands on the hill slopes at lower elevations.

Studies further indicate that the contribution of microbial biomass to soil organic C was greatest in the soils of *A. lebbeck* due mainly to greater microbial population as compared to *G. arborea* (Table 4). Further, *A. lebbeck* being a N_2-fixing species, a lot of soil microbial and/or metabolic activity is expected in the rhizosphere due to symbiosis. Eventually, the soil N-level is high in the soils under *A. lebbeck* as compared to *G. arborea*. Considering the physiography of the jhum fallow i.e. sloppy, N is more leacheable (Mohan 1992). Thus, growth of N_2-fixing tree species may help in enriching soil N and improve soil metabolism. Plantation using *G. arborea* may not help improving the soil nutrient pool. Interestingly, in such nutrient-poor soil, the contribution of microbial N to total soil N was significantly greater than in the soils under the canopy of the N_2-fixing species (Table 5) indicating a greater role of microbial biomass in N turnover. Over all, tree plantation would help conservation of nutrient elements vis-à-vis support growth of several herbaceous plants under its canopy and also the plant residue or forage of the tree (Belsky 1992; Arunachalam et al. 2003) itself by acting as a 'sink' and 'source' of plant available nutrients. It is concluded that *A. lebbeck* with its fairly a good interaction between the morphological and rhizosphere characteristics as compared to *G. arborea* could prove to be a potential species for rehabilitating the ecologically fragile jhum fallow by agroforestry and/or silvipastoralism. Nevertheless, further extensive studies are required to arrive at any holistic conclusion.

ACKNOWLEDGEMENTS

The authors are grateful to GBPIHED, Almora, Ministry of Environment and Forests, Govt. of India and the Indian Council of Agricultural Research, New Delhi for financial support. Mr. Jadav Saikia helped in field works. Special thanks to Mr. P.C. Nath for identification of plants. Mr. S. Deb assisted soil analysis.

REFERENCES

Allen SE, Grimshaw HM, Parkinson JA, Quarnby C (1974) Chemical Analysis of Ecological Materials. Blackwell Scientific Publications, Oxford p 541

Anderson JM, Ingram JSI (1993) TSBF-Handbook of Methodology, CAB International, Wallingford, UK. p 221

Anderson TH, Domsch KH (1989) Ratios of microbial carbon to soil organic carbon in arable soils. Soil Biol Biochem 21: 211-216

Arunachalam A (1992) Studies on mycoflora and biochemical changes during storage of decaying fruits and vegetables. M.Sc. Thesis, A.J.College, Sivakasi (Affiliated to Madurai Kamraj Univesity) India, 147

Arunachalam A (2002) Dynamics of soil nutrients and microbial biomass during first year cropping in an 8-year jhum cycle. Nutrient Cycling in Agroecosys 64: 283-291

Arunachalam A, Arunachalam K (2002a) Evaluation of bamboos in ecorestoration of 'jhum' fallows in Arunachal Pradesh: ground vegetation, soil and microbial biomass. Forest Ecology and Management 159: 231-239

Arunachalam A, Arunachalam K (2002b) Dynamics of soil microbial biomass as affected by floods in the humid tropics. Indian J Soil Conser 30: 21-28

Arunachalam A, Pandey HN (2003) Ecosystem restoration of jhum fallows in north-east India: Microbial C and N along altitudinal and successional gradients. Restor Ecol 11:168-173

Arunachalam K, Arunachalam A, Tripathi RS, Pandey HN (1997) Dynamics of microbial population during the aggradation phase of a selectively logged subtropical humid forest in north-east India. Trop Ecol 38: 333-341

Arunachalam K, Arunachalam A, Melkania NP (1999) Influence of soil properties on microbial populations, activity and biomass in humid subtropical mountainous ecosystems of India. Biol Fertil Soils 30: 217-223

Arunachalam A, Arunachalam K, Bhattacharjee A, Nag A (2000) Natural revegetation on landslides in humid tropical Arunachal Pradesh: Community dynamics and soil properties. J Tropical Fort Sci 12: 682-696

Arunachalam A, Khan ML, Arunachalam K (2002) Balancing traditional jhum cultivation with modern agroforestry in eastern Himalaya – A biodiversity hot spot. Current Sci 83: 117-118

Arunachalam K, Singh ND, Arunachalam A (2003) Decomposition of leguminous crop residues in a 'jhum' cultivation system in Arunachal Pradesh, India. J Plant Nutrit Soil Sci 166:731-736

Belsky AJ (1992) Effects of trees on nutritional quality of understorey gramineous forage in tropical savannas. Tropical Grassland 26:12-20

Belsky AJ, Amundson RG, Duxbury JM, Riha SJ, Ali AR, Mwonga SM (1989) The savanna in Kenya. J Appl Ecol 26:1005-1024

Belsky AJ, Effects of trees on their physical, chemical and biological environments in a semi-arid Mwonga SM, Amundson RG, Duxbury JM, Ali AR (1993a) Comparative effects of isolated trees on their undercanopy environments in high rainfall and low rainfall savannas. J Appl Ecol 30:143-155

Belsky AJ, Mwonga SM, Duxbury JM (1993b) Comparative effects of isolated trees on their undercanoy environments in high rainfall and low rainfall savannas. Agroforestry Systems 24:1-20

Bremner Evan Kessel C (1992) Seasonal and microbial biomass dynamics after addition of lentil and wheat residues. Soil Sci Soc Am J 56:1141-1146

Hernot J, Robertson GP (1994) Vegetation removal in two soils of the humid tropics: effect on microbial biomass. Soil Biol Biochem 26:111-116

Hooker JD (1872-1879) The Flora of British India. L. Reeve & Co., London 7: 883

Hosur GC, Dasog GS (1995) Effect of tree species on soil properties. J Indian Soc Soil Sci 43: 256-259

Jha DK, Sharma GD, Mishra RR (1992) Ecology of soil microflora and mycorrhizal symbionts in degraded forests at two altitudes. Biol Fertil Soils 12:272-278

Joergensen RG, Anderson TH, Wolters T (1995) Carbon and nitrogen relationships in the microbial biomass of soils in beech (*Fagus sylvatica*) forests. Biol Fertil Soils 19: 1414-147

Johnson LF, Curl EA (1972) Methods for the research on ecology of soil-borne plant pathogens. Burgess, Minneapolis p 247

Maithani K, Tripathi RS (1996) Species diversity of soil microfungi in the humid subtropical forests of north-eastern India. J Swamy Botanic Club 13: 63-66

Misra R (1968) Ecology Work Book. Oxford & IBH, Calcutta p 224

Mohan S (1992) Nutrient losses from soil due to jhumming practices in Arunachal Pradesh. Arunachal Forest News 10:29-31

Pandey AN, Singh JS (1985) Mechanism of ecosystem recovery: A case study from Kumaun Himalaya. Recrea Revege Res 3: 271-292

Ramakrishnan PS (1992) Shifting Agriculture and Sustainable Development, UNESCO-MAB Series, Volume 10, Parthenon Publishing, Paris. p 424

Schroth G (1998) A review of below ground interactions in agroforestry, focusing on mechanisms and management options. Agroforest Syst 43: 5-34

Shukla GP (1992) Status paper on afforestation of wasteland and rehabilitation of 'jhum' fallows in Arunachal Pradesh. Arunachal Forest News 10: 4-10

Singh JS, Raghuvanshi AS, Singh RS, Srivastava SC (1989) Microbial biomass acts as a source of plant nutrients in dry tropical forest and savanna. Nature (London) 399:499-500

Tripathi SK, Singh KP (1994) Productivity and nutrient cycling in recently harvested and mature bamboo savannas in the dry tropics. J Appl Ecol 31: 109-124

Toky OP, Ramakrishnan PS (1982) Role of bamboo (*Dendrocalamus hamiltonii* Nees & Arn.) in conservation of potassium during slash and burn agriculture (jhum) in north-eastern India. J Tree Sci 1:17-26

Upadhyaya K, Arunachalam A (2004) Immediate effect of clear-felling on soil C, N and P in a humid tropical forest in Arunachal Pradesh. J Trop For Sci 16:136-139

Vance ED, Brookes PC, Jenkinson DS (1987) Microbial biomass measurements in forest soils: The use of chloroform fumigation-incubation method for strongly acid soils. Soil Biol Biochem 19: 697-702

Waksman SA (1952) Soil Microbiology. John Wiley & Sons, New York. P 356

Zar JH (1974) Biostatistical Analysis. 2nd edn., Prentice Hall, Englewood Cliffs, NJ p 718

Effect of Co-inoculation of AM fungi and *Bradyrhizobium japonicum* on Nodulation, Nitrogen and Phosphorus Content in Soya Bean

S NEUPANE and BN PRASAD

1. INTRODUCTION

Soya bean [*Glycine max* (L.) Merrill] is one of the leguminous plants grown in tropical to temperate region of an elevation from 500m-3000m in Nepal. Soya bean is considered as a good source of dietary protein, since it contains 38-40% protein and 20% fat.

For vegetarian people, soya bean becomes most valuable proteinaceous food in their diet. And also for the people who can not afford money to buy meat and other proteinaceous product, soya bean becomes cheapest protein supplement. Beside protein and fat, soya bean also contains more of calcium and phosphorus than any cereal. It is also rich in iron, potassium, magnesium, amino acids and vitamins.

Soya bean seeds are consumed as green, dry or sprouted. Unripe seeds are consumed as vegetable; roasted and salted seeds are used in cakes and candies. Soya bean milk is used for infant feeding, and is also used to make curd, butter, milk cheese and other milk products. Soya bean flour used in bakery products and other food stuffs. Soya bean oil is used for cooking purpose. It is used in paints and varnishes and in soaps and other food products. The oil cakes are used as cattle feed.

Central Department of Botany, Tribhuvan University, Kirtipur, Kathmandu, Nepal.
E-mail: prasadbn@tubraj.wlink.com.np

Besides the above uses, soya bean is the largest source of edible oil and accounts for roughly 50% of the total oil seed production of the world. Soya bean, being legume, has the capacity to fix large amount if atmospheric di-nitrogen by symbiotic association with biological nitrogen-fixer (*Bradyrhizobium japonicum*). Thus it is used to improve soil fertility and reduce production cost of sustainable soil fertility.

The leguminous plants can benefit from the symbiotic association with *B. japonicum* as well as AM fungi. Rhizobial symbiosis provides nitrogen to the plant necessary for growth. Likewise, AM symbiosis enhances the plant growth through the ability of extraradial fungal hyphae taking up the low diffusing nutrients such as phosphorus from soil (Varma and Hock 1998). Symbiotic association between plants and AM fungi is ubiquitous and is particularly important in improving plant phosphorus uptake efficiency. The importance of legume plants has been traditionally attributed to high phosphorus requirements of nodulation and nitrogen fixation processes (Barea and Read 1997). The role of AM fungi on the tripartite symbiosis Rhizobium-legume-AM fungus may not be limited due to its nutritional effect (Barea et al. 1983). Phosphorus plays a vital role in plant metabolism and nitrogen fixation; legumes require high P levels for their growth and effective nodulation (Bergersen 1971). The nitrogenase activity is dependent on ATP for reduction of atmospheric dinitrogen to ammonia.

The present paper reports the effect of AM fungi and *B. japonicum* on total dry weight, nodulation, total nitrogen and phosphorus content in soya bean plant.

2. SALIENT OBSERVATIONS AND INTERPRETATIONS

In soya bean cultivar 'Sathiya' the microbial treatments increased the total dry weight, shoot dry weight, nodule number, nodule dry weight, N and P content in plant.

The dry weight of plant inoculated with only AM fungi or *B. japonicum* was found more than uninoculated plant, where dual inoculation of both AM fungi and *B. japonicum* was found highest (Fig. 1 and 2). The increment of dry matter production on co-inoculated plant, may be due to AM fungi, makes more P and other nutrients available to the plants by absorbing them from the soil and higher nitrogen fixation by *B. japonicum* which enhanced the nodulation and plant development. *Glomus mosseae* colonized soya bean plants increased their shoot dry weight when inoculated with *Bradyrhizobium*.

The nodule number as well as nodule dry weight in plant co-inoculated with AM fungi and *B. japonicum* found highest (Fig. 3 and 4),

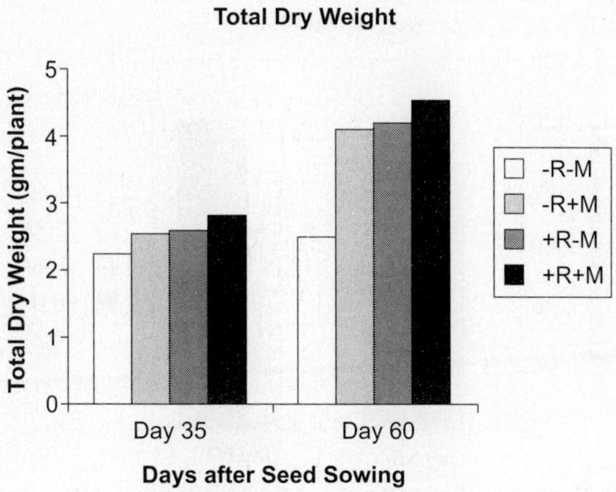

Fig. 1 Effect of microbial treatment on total dry weight of plant

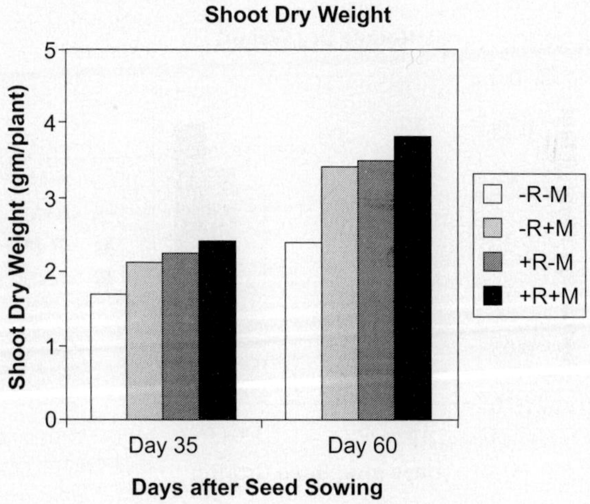

Fig. 2 Effect of microbial treatment on shoot dry weight of plant

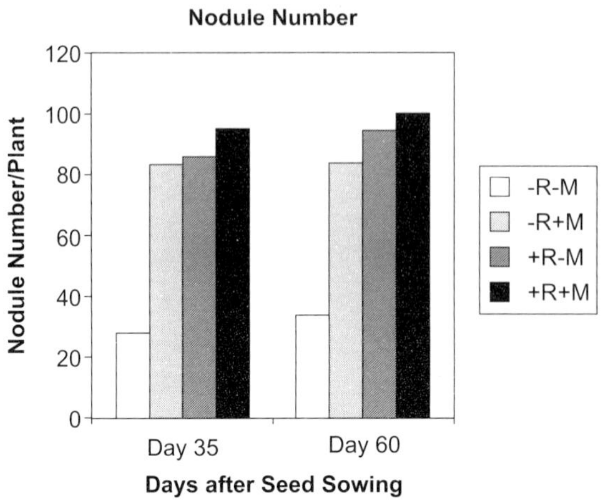

Fig. 3 Effect of microbial treatment on nodule number

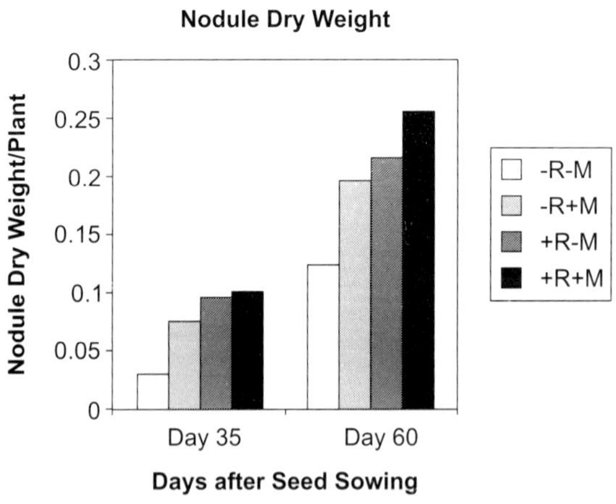

Fig. 4 Effect of microbial treatment on nodule dry weight

where presence of sufficient bradyrhizobial cells in the soil nodulate the soya bean plants. The precise exchange of molecular signals between bradyrhizobia and host plant is essential to the development of an effective nodulation (Varma 1992). Several legumes grow poorly and fail to nodulate effectively in autoclaved soil unless they were microbial. But in the case of uninoculated plant only ineffective nodulation occurs. The number and dry weight of these ineffective nodules are less.

Nitrogen content in nodule as well as plant tissue in co-inoculated plant with AM fungi and *B. japonicum* was found higher than the single inoculation of the AM fungi or *B. japonicum* and control. The highest percentage of N content in nodule was 5.92% and 5.89% was recorded in co-inoculated plant on day 35th and 60th after seed sowing respectively (Fig. 5). Their increments were 35.09% and 39.95% over uninoculated (control) plant. Similarly the increment percent of nitrogen in shoot of co-inoculated plant was found 38.24% and 39.90% on day 35th and 60th after seed sowing respectively (Fig. 6), over the uninoculated plant. This is because of AM fungi increase the effectiveness of *Rhizobium* on soya bean (Ross and Harper 1970) where AM fungi stimulate nitrogen fixation by legume-*Rhizobium* symbiosis. AM fungi produce some growth hormones like auxins, gibberellins, cytokinins. Gibberellins are found to stimulate nodulation and *in vitro* nitrogenase activity (Prasad and Mathur 1992). The additional phosphate uptake through fungal hyphae also stimulated the nitrogen fixation and accumulation of nitrogen content in nodule and plant tissue occurred.

Phosphorus content in plant tissue of co-inoculated plant was found highest over single inoculated and uninoculated plant (Fig. 7). The P content in co-inoculated plant was 3.18% and 3.01% on day 35th and 60th respectively. In these days increment percentage was 70.05% and 69.10% respectively. The improvement of plant's P-status is due to permeability of the root cell membrane under low nutrition. Increased root cell membrane permeability leads to increased loss of metabolites, which is sufficient to sustain the growth of the mycorrhizal fungus. Subsequently, mycorrhizal infection leads to improve plant's P-nutrient and reduce loss of metabolites.

3. PROTOCOL OF THE EXPERIMENTS

Seed of soya bean cultivar 'Sathiya' was collected from Agronomy Division of Nepal Agricultural Research Council (NARC), Kathmandu, Nepal. The inoculum of *B. japonicum* was provided by Soil Science Division of NARC. The mycorrhizal inoculum (resting spores) was isolated from the maize rhizosphere via wet sieving (Gerdmann and Nicolson 1963) and sucrose centrifugation method (Jenkins 1964), and

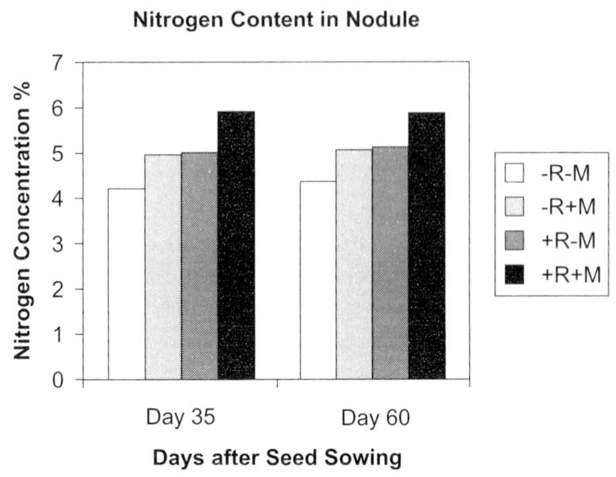

Fig. 5 Effect of microbial treatment on nitrogen content in nodule

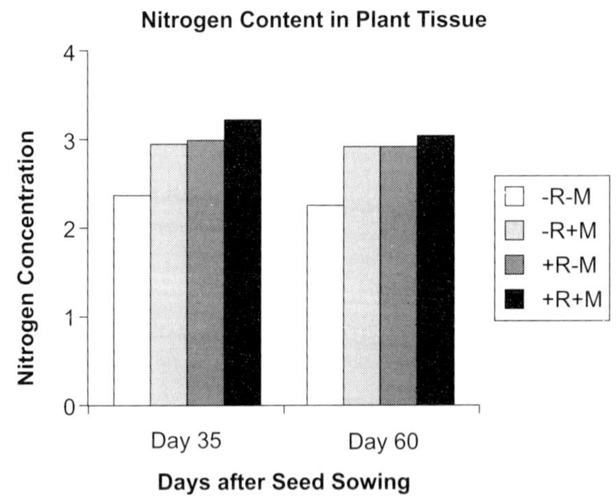

Fig. 6 Effect of microbial treatment on nitrogen content in plant tissue

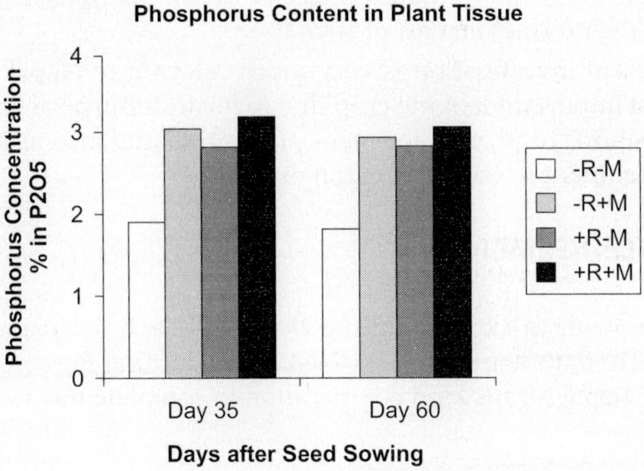

Fig. 7 Effect of microbial treatment on phosphorus content in plant tissue

these isolated spores were surface sterilized by immersing in 2.5% chloramin T for 10 minutes followed by several washing with sterilized water.

The pot culture experiment was conducted during August 2002 to October 2002 with replication to study the response of microbial treatments. There were four inoculant treatments viz., plant inoculated with *B. japonicum* (+R), plants inoculated with AM fungi (+M), plants co-inoculated with *B. japonicum* and AM fungi (+R+M) and control (-R-M). The pots were placed under natural condition of light and temperature. The observations were taken on 35th and 60th day after seed sowing.

The percentage of mycorrhizal infection was determined after cleaning roots in 10% KOH and staining with 0.05% trypan blue (Philips and Hayman 1970).

The dry weights of different parts of the plants were recorded after 24 hours of heating at 70°C in oven. Nitrogen and phosphorus contents in plant tissue were estimated by Micro-Kjeldahl method (PCARR 1980) and Vanadomolybdate method (PCARR 1980) respectively.

4. CONCLUSION

Arbuscular Mycorrhizal Fungi markedly improve the nodulation and nitrogen fixation by interaction with *B. japonicum*, a legume bacterium, mainly by providing high phosphorus requirement for the fixation process. Thus, these micro-organisms can be used to improve soil fertility and reduce the production cost of soya bean.

The present investigation is very much relevant to Nepal since soya bean is most important legume crop due to its multipurpose use in Nepal as a major source of protein for mass population and also as a source of nitrogen-fixer plant in the hilly region of Nepal.

ACKNOWLEDGEMENTS

The authors want to express sincere thanks to Dr B R Khadage, Senior Scientist, Plant Pathology division, Nepal Agricultural Research Council, Khumaltar, Nepal for his kind co-operation to complete this work.

REFERENCES

Barea JM, Azon-Agiilar C (1983) Mycorrhizas and their singnificance in nodulating nitrogen-fixing plants. Adv Agron 36: 1-54

Bergersen FT (1971) Biochemistry of symbiotic nitrogen fixation in legume. Ann Rev Plant Physiol pp121-130

Gerdmann JW, Nicolson TH (1963) Spores of mycorrhizal endogone species extracted from soil by wet sieving and decanting. Trans Bra Mycol Soc p 235

Jenkins WR (1964) A rapid centrifugal-flotation technique for separating nematodes from soil. Plants Dis Rep p 492

Philips JM, Hayman DS (1970) Improved procedure for clearing roots and staining parasitic and vesicular-arbuscular mycorrhizal fungi for rapid assessment of infection. Trans Brit Mycol Soc 55:158-160

Prasad BN, Mathur SN (1992) Effect of GA_3 on nitrogen fixation in forage legumes in Nepal. In: Role of Biotechnology and Agriculture. Prasad, Ghimire and Agrawal (eds) Oxford and IBH Publication. pp 85-90

Ross JP, Harper JA (1970) Effects of endogone mycorrhiza on soya bean yields. Phytopathology 60:1552

Smith NC, Read DJ (1997) Mycorrhizal symbiosis (second ed.) academic press p 605

Varma A, Hock B (1998) Mycorrhiza: structure, function, molecular biology and Biotechnology. Spring-Verlag, Germany

Varma DPS (1992) Signals in root nodule organogenesis and endocytosis of *Rhizobium*. Plant and Soil pp 373-382

Fungus Protoplast: Impediments on Biotechnology

R HAMPP[1], T HUREK[2], AC KHARKWAL[3], H KHARKWAL[3] and A VARMA[3]*

1. INTRODUCTION

Protoplasts are, by definition, all the components of a live cell after experimental removal of cell-wall (Hawksworth et al. 1995). They contain all the intracellular organelles of cells and form a vital link in transfer of micromolecules between cyto-organelles.

Currently, most of the researchers engaged in fungal genetics are using gene manipulation procedures based on protoplast. In addition, fungus breeding by protoplast mutagenesis and fusion has become a useful model for microbial breeding. Although, the main interest in the use of fusion techniques is the production of interspecific and intergeneric hybrids, the success of the hybrid formation mainly depends on the taxonomic proximity of the strains under study.

The protoplast can be obtained in filamentous fungi from the mycelium, germinated or intact conidia, although it is more complicated in the last case. For every fungus, factors effecting protoplast yield must be assayed in order to establish ideal conditions for protoplast preservation without internal material loss (Azevedo 1998).

*Corresponding author

1. Institute for Plant Physiology and Ecology, University of Tuebingen, Auf der Morgenstelle 1, Tubigen-72076, Germany
2. Cooperation Laboratory, Max Planek Institute for Marine Microbiology, University of Bremen FB 2, Leobener Stv. NW 2, Bremen - 28359, Germany
3. Amity Institute of Microbial and Herbal Studies, Amity University, Block A, Amity Campus, Sector 125, Noida, 201303 E-mail: agitvarma@aihmr.amity.edu

Since protoplasts are physiologically normal, they are important for studies of cell-wall biosynthesis, secretive processes and biosynthesis of secondary metabolism products. The isolation of the protoplasts can also be used to understand the mystery of symbiosis between the fungal partner and mycelia protoplast and to address the questions pertaining to metabolic exchange (Singh 2001). Their direct applications in genetics are protoplast fusion, transformation, electrophoretic karyotype analysis and plant-microbe interaction.

2. GENERATION OF PROTOPLAST

2.1 Protoplast Isolation: The Developmental Era

The first report of an enzyme of microbial origin that attacked the chitin component of fungal walls appeared at the start of the last century (Benecke 1905). Although the work of Giaja (1919) identified the lytic activity of gastric juice of snail, *Helix pomatia*, against yeast cell-walls, but it was the work of Weibull (1953) on the isolation of bacterial protoplasts using lysozyme that provided the impetus for large-scale production of protoplasts from fungi. Initially, the protoplasts were isolated from *Saccharomyces cerevisiae*, *S. carlsbergenesis* (Eddy and Williamson 1957) and *Neurospora crassa* (Batchmann and Bonner 1959). Since then the protoplasts have been isolated from all the taxonomic groups of fungi by enzymatic digestion of cell-wall (Table 1).

The process of generation of protoplasts i.e., protoplastation involves both enzymic and non-enzymatic protocols (Peberdy 1979a). The most common and widely used method of protoplast release is lytic enzyme method. The choice of any lytic enzyme depends upon the composition and structure of the fungal cell-wall (Hamlyn et al. 1981; Elbouami 2000).

2.2 Non-Enzymic Methods

2.2.1 Mechanical Method

Intact *Saccharomyces cerevisiae* cells, when grown on quartz sand or subjected to mechanical pressure by squeezing them between slide and coverslip, has produced spherical fragile plasma droplets, some containing the nucleus, which, under some conditions, might give rise to regenerated cells (Necas 1956). Takada and Yamamoto (1963) produced protoplasts by squeezing out the protoplasm from ruptured yeast cell-walls under hypertonic conditions. These protoplasts can regenerate if the cells are inoculated into normal medium.

This method necessitated drastic treatments to produce cell fractions, generally causing loss and damage to cellular components.

Table 1 Protoplast isolation from mycelial fungi: optimal reported yields in recent reports

Species	*Enzyme*	*Osmotic stabilizer*	*Yield (per g fr wt)*	*Reference*
Acremonium diospyri	A[b]	0.4 M $(NH)_2SO_4$	2.4×10^{6}[b]	Deed et al. 1990
Agaricus bisporus[m]	D	0.35 M KCl	$3\text{-}4 \times 10^{7}$	Chen and Hampp 1993
Alternaria kikuchiana	F	1.2 M $MgSO_4$	32.5×10^{6}	Kitamoto et al.1988
Aspergillus niger	F	1.2 M $MgSO_4$	16.5×10^{7}	Kitamoto et al.1988
Aspergillus oryzae	F	1.2 M $MgSO_4$	14.5×10^{8}	Kitamoto et al.1988
Aspergillus sojae	F	1.2 M $MgSO_4$	16.8×10^{8}	Kitamoto et al.1988
Botrytis cinerea	F	1.2 M $MgSO_4$	22.0×10^{8}	Kitamoto et al.1988
2 Cenococcum geophilum[m]	B	**KMPC**	2.1×10^{6}	Barrett et al. 1989
Cladonia aggregata	A	0.6 M $MgSO_4$	3.7×10^{5}	Kinoshita et al. 1991
C. bellidiflora	A	0.6 M $MgSO_4$	9.0×10^{4}	Kinoshita et al. 1991
C. cristatella	A	0.6 M $MgSO_4$	2.3×10^{6}	Kinoshita et al. 1991
C. boryi	A	0.6 M $MgSO_4$	″	Kinoshita et al. 1991
C. pleurota	A	0.6 M $MgSO_4$	6.0×10^{4}	Kinoshita et al. 1991
3 C. stellaris	A	0.6 M $MgSO_4$	5.6×10^{6}	Kinoshita et al. 1991
Cladosporium didymum	F	1.2 M $MgSO_4$	13.7×10^{8}	Kitamoto et al. 1988
Coprinus cinereus	F	1.2 M $MgSO_4$	40.0×10^{8}	Kitamoto et al. 1988
C. macrorhizus	D	0.5 M mannitol	30.0×10^{8}	Yanagi et al.1985
C. phlyctidosporous	F	1.2 M $MgSO_4$	21.0×10^{8}	Kitamoto et al. 1988
Cryponectria parasitica	E	0.5 M mannitol/ 1 mM $CaCl_2$	8.0×10^{4}[b]	Jang et al. 1993
Cylindrocarpon didymum	F	1.2 M $MgSO_4$	13.7×10^{7}	Kitamoto et al. 1988
Emericella nivea	F	1.2 M $MgSO_4$	60.0×10^{7}	Kitamoto et al. 1988

Contd.

Table 1

Species	*Enzyme*	*Osmotic stabilizer*	*Yield (per g fr wt)*	*Reference*
Eurotium chevalieri	F	1.2 M $MgSO_4$	90.0×10^5	Kitamoto et al. 1988
Eurotium repens	F	1.2 M $MgSO_4$	65.0×10^5	Kitamoto et al. 1988
Favolus arcularius	F	1.2 M $MgSO_4$	45.0×10^7	Kitamoto et al. 1988
Flammulina velutipes	F	1.2 M $MgSO_4$	90.0×10^8	Kitamoto et al. 1988
Fusarium culmorum	F	1.2 M $MgSO_4$	10.0×10^7	Kitamoto et al. 1988
Gibberella fujikuroi	F	1.2 M $MgSO_4$	90.0×10^3	Kitamoto et al. 1988
Hebeloma circinans[m]	A	MMC	17.0×10^{6b}	Barrett et al. 1989
H. cylindrosporum[m]	A	MMC	12.6×10^{7b}	Barrett et al. 1989
H. cylindrosporum[m]	J	0.7 M $MgSO_4$	41×10^6	Hebraud and Fevre 1988
H. sinapizans[m]	J	0.7 M $MgSO_4$	5×10^6	Hebraud and Fevre 1988
H. edurum[m]	J	0.7 M $MgSO_4$	0.5×10^6	Hebraud and Fevre 1988
Helminthosporium oryzae	F	1.2 M $MgSO_4$	18.0×10^6	Kitamoto et al. 1988
Laccaria bicolor[m]	A	MMC	8.6×10^{6b}	Barrett et al. 1989
L. bicolor[m]	A	0.6 M mannitol	12.4×10^6	Kropp and Fortin 1986
L. laccata[m]	A	0.6 M mannitol	17.9×10^{7b}	Kropp and Fortin 1986
Malbranchea pulchella	C	0.6 M KCl	18.0×10^7	Virk et al. 1992
Monascus anka	E	0.6 M KCl	11×106	Virk et al. 1992
Neurospora crassa	E	0.6 M KCl	62.5×10^7	Virk et al. 1992
Oidiodendron maius[m]	K	1M sorbitol	3.1×10^8	Bardi et al. 1999
Penicilliun chrysogenum	E	1.2 M $MgSO_4$	22.0×10^7	Kitamoto et al. 1988
P. cyclopium	A[a]	1.2 M $MgSO_4$	1.6×10^7	Roncal et al. 1991
Pholiota nameko	F	1.2 M $MgSO_4$	32.5×10^7	Kitamoto et al. 1988

Contd.

Table 1

Species	*Enzyme*	*Osmotic stabilizer*	*Yield (per g fr wt)*	*Reference*
Pisolithus tinctorius[m]	A	MMC	2.5×10^6	Barrett et al. 1989
Pleurotus ostreatus	A[a]	0.8 M mannitol	3.5×10^7	Peng et al. 1993
Pyricularia oryzae	F	1.2 M $MgSO_4$	22.5×10^7	Kitamoto et al. 1988
Schizophyllum commune[m]	F	1.2 M $MgSO_4$	35.0×10^7	Kitamoto et al. 1988
Sclerotinia rolfsii	A	0.6 M KCl	5.5×10^6	Kelkar et al. 1990
Sporotrichum thermophile	A[b]	0.6 M KCl	1.6×10^{6b}	Sharma et al. 1988
Suillus bellini[m]	J	0.7 M $MgSO_4$	34×10^6	Hebraud and Fevre 1988
Suillus luteus[m]	F	1.2 M $MgSO_4$	25.0×10^6	Kitamoto et al. 1988
Suillus granulatus[m]	A	0.7 M $MgSO_4$	2.7×10^7	Dias et al. 1996
Thelephora terrestris	A	MMC	3.2×10^6	Barrett et al. 1988
Trametes sanguinea	F	1.2 M $MgSO_4$	52.5×10^7	Kitamoto et al. 1988
Trichoderma harzianum	H	0.4 M KCl	6.0×10^6	Tashpulatov et al. 1991
T. reesei	F	0.7 M KCl	25.0×10^9	Kumari and Panda 1992
T. viride	I	0.7 M KCl	25.0×10^9	Tamaova et al. 1993
Ustilago maydis sporidia	A	0.5 M $NH_4\ (SO)_4$	25.0×10^9	Wellmann and Schauz 1993

[a] Lytic enzymes: A Novozym 234; A[a] protease reduced Novozym 234; A[b] Novozym SP 249; B Novozym 234 + chitinase; C Novozyme 234 + b glucuronidase; D Novozym 234 + cellulsae + chitinase; E *Trichoderma* enzyme (Sigma); F preparation from culture filtrate of *Trichoderma harzianum*; G culture filtrate preparation from *Trichoderma reesei*; H culture filtrate preparation from *Streptomyces afghaniensis*; I snail gut juice enzymes; J cellulase Onozuka R 10 and Driselase; K *Trichoderma harzianum* lytic enzyme

[b] Yields expressed on alternative basis, e.g., per g dry wt., per ml or per membrane sheet

[m] Mycorrhizal fungus

2.2.2 Metabolic Disturbances Inhibiting Cell-Wall Synthesis

Some compounds interfere with the biosynthetic reactions involved in cell-wall formation without affecting other reactions connected with the synthesis of protoplasm (McQuillen 1960). This causes the cells to produce an abnormal cell-wall or none at all. The cells should be in actively growing state and in the presence of stabilizing conditions such as hypertonic sucrose or mannitol (Hamlinton and Calvet 1964). Batchmann and Bonner (1959) showed that the hyphae of *Neurospora* became bulgy and irregular when grown in 4% sorbose medium. Results with glucose, sucrose and fructose, which served as osmotic stabilizers as well as carbon sources, were similar to those with sorbose plus 2% sucrose when considered on a molar basis. Berliner (1971) obtained protoplasts from *Schizosaccharomyces octosporus* upon incubation in Sabouraud medium with a high concentration of $MgSO_4$ with 2-deoxy-D-glucose. The phenomenon involved may be the selective cell-wall inhibition by extracellular loss of necessary enzymes or substrates, although an alternative explanation would be the extracellular movement and activation of autolytic enzyme. While adopting such procedures, comparison of properties of protoplast obtained by enzymatic and non-enzymatic methods are required. Foury and Goffeau (1973) demonstrated that 2-deoxy-D-glucose caused a reduction in respiratory activity of *S. pombe* protoplasts, and other metabolic effects are also possible.

2.2.3 Cultivation of Fungi on Thickened Guinea-Pig Serum

Meinecke (1960) obtained protoplasts of *Penicillium glaucum* by inoculating on thickened between two sterilized glass plates fastened with parafilm. After 7-14 days, protoplasts were formed. However, the effectiveness of this technique is doubtful.

Mechanical and non-enzymatic methods for protoplast isolation have not been used extensively. This may be not only because they are specific for a particular organism, but also due to possible fears regarding the physiological state that may be induced in the protoplasts by the treatments used.

2.3 Enzymic Methods

The use of lytic enzymes for protoplast isolation has been employed on a large scale, these being the less drastic and more rapid (Davis 1985; Woestmeyer and Woestmeyer 1998). Protoplastation with lytic enzymes entails following steps are shown in Fig 1. The fungus is grown on a suitable growth medium under optimal growth conditions till an appropriate growth phase best suited for protoplast yield is obtained. The

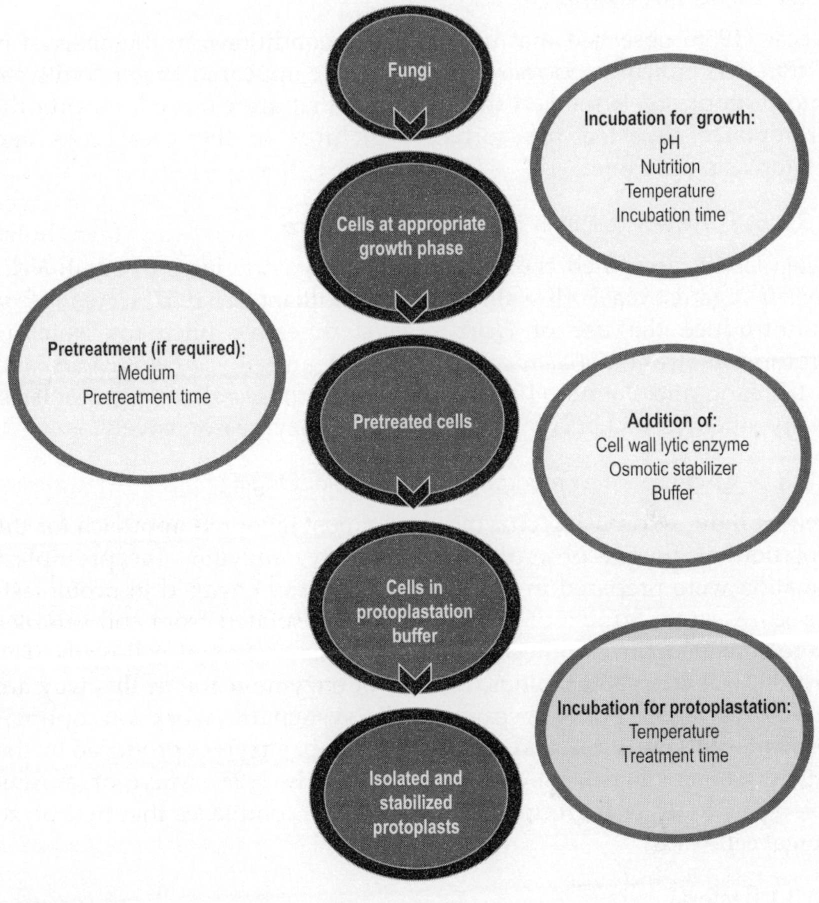

Fig. 1 Protoplastation with lytic enzymes

fungal cells are then separated from the medium and subjected to cell-wall lytic enzymes in the presence of an appropriate osmotic stabilizer under optimal incubation conditions. In some cases, a pretreatment of the cells prior to exposure to lytic enzymes is required in order to release the protoplasts. The lytic enzymes degrade the cell-wall and release the protoplast in the medium, which are stabilized by osmotic stabilizers present in the medium. Subsequently the protoplast yield is monitored microscopically. Different enzymatic processes are as follows.

2.3.1 Controlled Autolytic Process

Necas (1956) observed that under certain conditions, in the absence of extraneous enzymes, *Saccharomyces cereviseae* appeared to get converted into protoplasts. It seemed that enzymes that are closely bound to the protoplasm digested the surface structures of the yeast cells and protoplasts were released.

2.3.2 By Enzymes Present in The Snail Gastric Juice

Giaja (1919) identified the lytic activity of gastric juice of snail, *Helix pomatia*, against yeast cell-walls. Eddy and Williamson (1957) were the first to introduce the use of *Helix pomatia* digestive juice for isolating protoplasts from *Saccharomyces cerevisiae* and *S. carlsbergenesis* and Batchmann and Bonner (1959) used it for *Neurospora crassa* protoplasts. Many other researchers have used the same enzyme extensively.

2.3.3 By Crude Enzyme Preparations of Microbial Origin

Cell-wall digestion using enzymes is the most favoured approach for the isolation of fungal protoplasts. Previously, enzymes for protoplast isolation were prepared in-house by laboratories engaged in protoplast-based research. Strains of micro-organisms isolated from soil samples were screened for colonies that caused lysis of fungal cell-walls. The process was long and tedious. Batches of enzyme made in this way are highly variable, partly because little systematic work on optimal fermentation conditions and on the spectrum of enzymes produced by the lytic organisms had been carried out (Peberdy 1995). Micro-organisms belonging to diverse groups produce enzyme complexes that hydrolyze fungal cell-walls.

2.3.3.1 Bacteria

An *Arthrobacter* species caused lysis of yeast was isolated by Rowley and Bull (1977). Several *Bacillus* species have been shown to produce mycolytic enzymes (Tsujibaka et al 1975). An isolate of *Cytophaga jhonsonii* also caused lytic activity on yeast cell-wall (Bacon et al 1965). Several representatives of *Streptomyces* and related genera are known to be active producers of lytic enzymes (Price and Strock 1975). Fawcett et al (1973) and Hamlyn and Ball (1979) reported the application of the *Cytophaga* lytic enzyme L1. Another commercially available enzyme, popularly used for the isolation of yeast and fungal protoplasts, is Zymolyase obtained from *Arthrobacter leuteus*. Many researchers prefer to use the laboratory prepared lytic enzyme of this organism for the isolation of protoplasts of filamentous fungi and yeasts. Protoplasts of *Saccharomyces cereviseae* and *Kluyveromyces fragilis* (Stewart 1981 a,b), and *Candida tropicalis* and *Candida albicans* were prepared by using laboratory prepared Zymolyase. Fukuda and Kirimura (1991) isolated protoplasts from the yeast *Hansenula jaldinii* also by using Zymolyase.

2.3.3.2 Fungi

The lytic enzymes produced by *Trichoderma* species are effective against a wide range of fungal species (Vries and Wessels 1973 a,b). When the fungus was grown on the hyphal walls of *Schizophyllum commune*, several glucanases and chitinases were produced in the culture broth. A strain of *Rhizopus* that produces a β-1,3-glucanase which is lytic for yeasts-cell' walls (Yamamoto et al. 1974).

Many fungi showing autolytic actions may be the source of their own lytic enzymes. Isaac and Gokhale (1982) reported autolytic activities in cultures of *Aspergillus nidulans*. These lytic activities are quite effective, but further a lot of work has to be done to optimise cell-lysis and to access the specificity of the preparations.

2.3.3.3 Actinomycetes

These widely used lytic enzymes are called Strepzymes. Isaac and Gokhale (1982) used enzyme from *Streptomyces* RA for protoplast formation from *Fusarium culmorum*. It was also very effective against *Aspergillus nidulans* (Peberdy and Gibson 1971). When used in combination with crude cellulase from *Oxysporus*, it produced protoplasts from *Penicillium chrysogenum* (Anne and Peberdy 1976). Strepzyme from *Streptomyces graminopfaciens* was used in *Geotrichium candidum* protoplast formation (Dooijewaard-Kloosterziel et al. 1973) and that of *Streptomyces* S4 was used with conidial spores of *Aspergillus flavus* (Moore and Peberdy 1976). Protoplasts of *Trichoderma viride* were formed by treatment with *Micromonospora chalcea* lytic enzymes (Benitez et al. 1975).

2.3.3.4 Using Commercial Hydrolytic Enzymes

Commercial enzymes like cellulase CP, Chitinase, Driselase, Glusulase, Novozym 234, (Gokhale 1991), Novozym SP 249, β-glucuronidase have been used successfully for protoplast formation in filamentous fungi and yeasts (Peberdy 1995). The gastric juice of the snail, *Helix pomatia* is probably the most used of all mycolytic enzymes. The digestive juice of *Helix pomatia* contains many digestive enzymes, including lipases, more than twenty carbohydrases, and proteinases. The large number of carbohydrases may explain its usefulness for digesting fungal wall while the lipases and proteases are probably important for the breakdown of lipoprotein structures. This enzyme is also called Helicase, Lyticase or Glusulase. Novozym 234 produced by *Streptococcus mutans* induces lysis of several fungal species including yeasts (Dickinson and Isenberg 1982; Peberdy 1985). It is a combination of cellulase, chitinase and protease activities. It is very effective against yeasts as well as filamentous fungi (Eddy and Williamson 1957). Sandhu et al (1989) compared the effects of several lytic enzymes such as Novozym 234 from *Trichoderma harzianum* and *Aspergillus nidulans* lytic enzymes such as β-glucanase, α-glucanase, exo-β-1,4-glucanase, endo-β-1,4-glucanase, β-1,4-glucosidase and protease, and cellulases of *Aspergillus nidulans* on protoplast formation of hyperproducing cellulase mutant *Trichoderma reesei*. Novozym 234 at a concentration of 4 mg/ml gave the best results. Stephen and Nasim (1981) referred to Novozym 234 as Mutanase and used to produce protoplasts from a wide variety of yeasts. As more and more fungi were investigated, it became clear that not all species were susceptible to Novozym 234. Subsequently, several more commercial preparations such as driselase and other cellulases have been found to be useful for protoplast isolation from several fungi (Davis 1985; Peberdy 1985). Screening for novel mycolytic organisms and their enzyme profile, a study was carried out (Kaul et al 1993). One of the isolates was of the genus, *Acremonium* that had not been previously associated with mycolytic activity. Despite these alternate sources, most enzymes have been derived from strains of *Trichoderma harzianum* (Kitamoto et al 1988; Selitrennikoff and Bloomfield 1984).

2.4 Factors Effecting Protoplast Yield by Using Lytic Systems

Growth medium composition and culture conditions are the chief factors responsible for optimal yield of fungus protoplast. In *Aspergillus nidulans* protoplasts yields were higher from mycelium growing on glucose salts medium than from mycelium growing on the same medium plus yeast extract (Peberdy 1976). In *A. niger*, mycelium grown on mineral salts medium supplemented with glucose and asparagine, released significantly more protoplasts than the mycelium grown on the same medium with malt extract or malt extract alone (Musilkova and Fencl 1968). However, in case of the yeast *Aureobasidium pullulans*, yield was significantly increased when the cells were grown under anaerobic conditions (Finkelman et al. 1980)

2.4.1 Growth Stages

In general, protoplast yield is much greater for the mycelium in the exponential phase of growth than cells from stationary or late stationary phase of growth (Peberdy 1976; Elbouami 2000; Schwencke et al. 1977). However, large yields of protoplasts were obtained in *Penicillium chrysogenum* cultures at stationary phase, and it was suggested that endogenous lytic activity might have triggered the protoplast release (Cabib et al. 1979).

2.4.2 Pretreatment of Cells

The function of pretreatment changes the structure of cell-wall by artificial control, which can increase the sensitivity of cell-wall to enzymes and further raise the frequency of protoplasts (Zhou and Ping 1990). Thiol compounds are known to destroy the protective layer of protein outside the cell-wall by breaking the disulfide bond of excretion protein of the mycelium (Peberdy 1979a; Harris 1982). However, Zhou et al. (1984) considered that the pretreatment could lower the frequency of protoplast regeneration.

The pretreatment time differs for different organisms and strains. Usually, the fungal cell-walls containing significant amounts of mannans and proteins seem to require pretreatment. In *dimorphic fungus Mucor rouxii* pretreatment was reported more commonly in yeast-form cells than in mycelial-form cells, which was attributed to higher mannan content in yeast form cells (Wessels 1994).

2.4.3 Lytic Enzymes

Different enzyme mixes have been used singly or in combination for release of fungal protoplasts (Peraza et al. 2003; Zhou et al. 1984). Usually these mixes exhibit activities such as chitinase, glucanase, protease, mannanase etc. Commercial lytic enzyme systems have been used successfully mostly for the fungi belonging to the class Ascomycetes, Basidiomycetes and Deuteromycetes (Hamlyn et al. 1981). In case of Zygomycetes, effective enzyme preparations are not available commercially which could be due to the qualitative difference in the cell-wall composition of higher and lower phycomycetous fungi (Chitinis and Deshpande 2002; Ruiz-Díez 2002; Peberdy 1979a). In case of dimorphic organisms, the two morphological forms require separate lytic enzyme systems in order to yield protoplasts (Chitinis and Deshpande 2002).

2.4.4 Effects of Osmotic Stabilizer

The release of intact fungal protoplast largely depends on the nature and osmolarity of the osmotic stabilizer present in the medium. The osmoticum of the medium may stimulate the release of protoplast from the cells (Rodriguez Aguiree MJ et al. 1964; Thomas and Davis 1980). In *A. niger* it was shown that Ca^{2+} ions stimulated the release of protoplasts in certain strains by stimulation of lytic enzyme activity (Musilkova and Fencl 1966).

A wide range of inorganic and organic compounds such as NH_4Cl, $(NH_4)_2SO_4$, $CaCl_2$, $MgCl_2$, $MgSO_4$, KCl, NaCl, glucose, sucrose, sugar alcohols (sorbitol and mannitol), citric acid and sodium citrate have been used (Tully and Gilbert 1985). Since the cell-wall composition varies according to the species, it is safe to assume that there must be an optimum osmotic concentration for each species (Cheng and Bélanger 2000), although Solís et al. (1996) did not report significant variation at testing KCl, $MgSO_4$ and NH_4Cl (0.7 mol.L^{-1}) for the release of *Aspergillus flavipes* protoplast. However, for a particular fungal cell, there is no reasonable explanation that is going to be more suitable as on osmotic stabilizer than another (Zhao et al. 2004).

2.4.5 Treatment Conditions

Temperature and pH affect the activities of lytic enzymes and the osmotic stabilizer. Temperature higher than optimal may cause agglutination of certain organelles in isolated protoplasts while low temperature effects protoplast membrane stability (Kovac and Subik 1970). The temperature at which fungi lose their cell-wall by enzymolysis varies between 24°C and 35°C (Zhou et al. 1984). pH value is also an effective factor that affects the preparation of protoplast because of its effect on enzyme activity (Balasubramanian et al. 2003; Peraza et al. 2003).

3. MYCORRHIZAL FUNGI AND PROTOPLASTS

Most terrestrial plants distributed worldwide establish at least one of the types of mutualistic associations in their roots (Smith and Read 1997; Varma 1999) called mycorrhiza (Frank 1885; Trappe 1987). Mycorrhiza occur as three types:

Endomycorrhizae colonize root-cells inter and intracellularly; ectomycorrhiza grow only between the root cortical cells and over the root surface, while ericoid mycorrhizae share features of both, endo- and ectomycorrhizae. The most widespread and probably most ancient is arbuscular mycorrhizal (AM) symbiosis (endomycorrhizal) between soil-borne fungi (mycobiont) presently classsified in the phylum Zygomycota, order Glomales (Morton et al 1995) and approximately ninety percent of terrestrial plant species (Varma 1995, 1999). The symbiosis is termed arbuscular because the mycrobiont produces specialized arbuscules in root cortical cells involved in bi-directional exchange of carbon, phosphorus and other physiologically important molecules.

AM fungi play an indispensable role in upgrading plant growth, vigour and survival by a positive impact on nutritional (Smith and Gianinazzi-Pearson 1988) and hydratic status of the plant (Nelson 1987; Davies et al 1992) and on soil aggregation (Tisdall 1994), increasing the reproductive potential, improving root performance and providing a natural defense against invaders including pests and pathogens.

While these fungi have been used to stabilize forests since the very beginning of last century, the novelty in recent years has increased recognition that biological processes can be manipulated genetically, opening numerous opportunities for the optimization of plant productivity especially in man managed ecosystems, while minimizing risks of environmental damage (Bagyaraj and Varma 1995; Varma 1995). However, the growth of arbuscular mycorrhizae in pure culture in the absence of living host roots is a matter of global concern. The obligate biotrophy of AM fungi and the inability of the ectomycorrhizal fungi to sporulate or complete asexual cycle in laboratory is a bottleneck for fundamental and applied research.

In the early 1970s, a few studies for the production of protoplasts were conducted with basidiomycetes (de Vries and Wessels 1973). Only since 1986 reports involving mycorrhizal fungi have been published (Anunciacao et al 1990; Barrett et al 1989; Dias et al 1996; Farquhar and Peterson 1990; Hebraud and Fevre 1988; Kropp and Fortin 1986) (Table 1). The ability to form large numbers of regenerative protoplasts is indispensable for experiments with the ectomycorrhizal fungi involving genetic transformation or mutagenesis. Till date, *Laccaria* and *Hebeloma* are the only genera among several evaluated species with potential for such experimentation (Barrett et al 1989; Marmeisse et al 1992). There is only one report for protoplast isolation from ericoid mycorrhizal fungus, *Oidiodendron maius* (Bardi et al 1999). However, there is no report of protoplast preparation from AM fungi.

4. REGENERATION OF PROTOPLASTS

The sequence of events leading from protoplast to normal cell, capable of growth has been referred to as protoplast regeneration (Necas and Svoboda 1985; Necas 1980; Peberdy 1979b). Cell-wall synthesis is the key event in the process of protoplast regeneration (Peberdy 1979a). The phenomenon of regeneration serves as a model system for the study of various developmental processes. The regeneration of protoplasts is also a prerequisite for all the experiments employing hybridization and genetic manipulations in fungal cell (Zhao et al. 2004; Khedkar et al. 2005).

Wall formation can be followed microscopically by the use of fluorescent dyes and biochemically by the incorporation of radiolabelled sugars into the nascent wall polymers (Peberdy 1979b). Fukui et al (1969) quantitatively studied the detailed regeneration process for *Geotrichum candidum* protoplasts using a thin layer of stabilized agar. Three phases of regeneration were described:

Lag Phase: protoplasts were slightly swollen;

Log Phase: protoplasts rapidly gained osmotic stability and started growing;

Stationary Phase: protoplasts produced germ tubes and microcolonies became visible.

Regeneration of the cell-wall follows the same general pattern in all fungal systems and, hence, for the initial studies, yeast protoplasts were used as the model system (Necas and Svoboda 1974). Protoplasts synthesise and release all the chemical constituents of the cell-wall onto the surface. Some of these are produced in the quantities different from those found in the normal cells (Farkas and Svoboda 1980). In some yeast species, aberrant glucans not present in the normal cell-walls are incorporated in the regenerating wall (Kreger and Kopecka 1976). The fibrillar and amorphous components are synthesized and transported independently irrespective of their differing chemical composition in different fungi (van der Valk and Wessels 1977). The mode of wall material secretion onto the protoplast surface is still unclear. The synthesis of glucan and chitin macromolecules was found to be associated with the plasma membrane (Vermeulen and Wessels 1984). Glycoproteins, the main components of the matrix are discharged via exocytosis (Farkas 1979). First structure assembled on the surface of regenerating protoplasts was reported to be the microfibrillar net composed either of glucan (Eddy and Williamson 1959; Popov et al. 1980), chitin (Gibson et al. 1976) or chitin and glucan (van der Valk and Wessels 1976). For microfibril formation, two possible mechanisms were postulated (Necas and Svoboda 1985). One assumes the self-assembly of the macromolecules secreted on the protoplast surface. The second assumes that microfibrils are organised immediately after polymer synthesis occurs in particular enzyme complexes like chitosomes or gluconosomes (Bartnicki-Garcia 1980; Necas and Svoboda 1981). In the case of normal cell-wall synthesis the existing wall operates as the epigenic information system (Martínez et al. 2004). However, in the case of protoplasts, cell-wall synthesis occurs completely *de novo* (Peberdy 1979a). The only information determining the supramolecular structure of the wall is inherent in the secreted polymers. The self-assembly of these polymers results in the formation of the normal wall and is also controlled by the environmental conditions (Kreger and Kopecka 1976; Necas 1971). The morphology of the protoplast growth and consequently the morphology of reversion depend on the relationship between an increase in cytoplasmic volume and the rate of wall regeneration (Chitnis and Deshpande 2002). If the rate of wall regeneration and the increase in cytoplasmic volume are balanced, protoplasts revert rapidly resuming normal morphogenesis and are usually iso-diametrical. If wall regeneration proceeds at a low rate, protoplasts grow in an unisodiametric fashion; i.e., protoplasts of both yeast and mycelial fungi develop tubular, chainlike or other irregularly shaped formations that revert to cells after completion of wall regeneration. Studies on the assembly of yeast protoplasts during regeneration showed that net structures of normal and protoplast cells were different and the difference could be due to the absence of β-1, 6-glucan synthetase effected by the liquid medium for cultured protoplasts (Kreger and Kopecka 1976).

5. FUNGAL PROTOPLAST: APPLICATIONS

The intact fungal protoplast has been used for a variety of purposes such as protoplast fusion, transformation, electrophoretic karyotype analysis and plant-microbe interactions.

5.1 Protoplast Fusion

Protoplast fusion has proved to be a highly efficient procedure for obtaining heterokaryons and enabling the parasexual cycle of filamentous fungi readily available for genetic studies and industrial strain improvement (Anne and Peberdy 1985; Peberdy 1989).

The process of protoplast fusion is rarely observed in a simultaneous way, but can be easily achieved by using polyethylene glycol and Ca^{2+} (Anne and Peberdy 1976; Pigac et al. 1982; Svoboda 1978; Svoboda and Piedra 1983). Intraspecific protoplast fusion involving strains with the same mating types has been obtained with frequencies of about 1×10^{-3} to 5×10^{-3} in *Saccharomyces cerevisiae* (Ferenczy and Maraz 1977), *Rhodosporidium toruloides* (Sipiczki and Ferenczy 1977), *Candida utilis* (Delgado and Herrera 1981) and *Candida albicans* (Sarachek et al. 1981). In filamentous fungi, protoplast fusion has been successfully used to produce heterokaryons between strains, which are sexually incompatible (Typas 1983). The procedure is especially valuable for *Phytophthora* because of the rare occurrence of hyphal fusion in this group (Judelson and Yang 1998). Lucas et al. (1990) have used protoplast fusion to generate somatic hybrids of *P. capsici*. Double drug-resistant strains were obtained when protoplasts of a metalaxyl resistant mutant of *P. sojai* Kaufmann and Gerdemann were fused with flurotryptophan-resistant protoplasts (Layton and Kuhn 1988). However, evidence that the selective markers represented nuclear genes was lacking (Layton and Kuhn 1988). Subsequently with the availability of the nuclear gene markers (Chang and Ko 1990), Gu and Ko (2000) were able to perform protoplast fusion and the resulting nuclear hybrids also underwent karyogamy and diploidization.

The main objective of fusion techniques is the production of interspecific and intergeneric hybrids, but the success of the hybrid formation mainly depends on the taxonomic proximity of the strains under study. Results of the earliest studies suggested that hybrid formation could be achieved only if the closely related parental species were used (Lewis 1969). However, further experiments suggested that this might not be the case (Peberdy 1979b), since interspecific somatic hybrids between *Penicillium roquefortii* and *P. chrysogenum* (Anne et al. 1976), *Aspergillus nidulans* and *A. rugulosus* (Kevei and Peberdy 1977, 1979), *Saccharomycopsis diastaticus* and *S. rouxii* (Spencer 1985), and between other species have been described. Furthermore, intergeneric protoplast fusion has been reported between *Candida tropicalis* and *Saccharomycopsis fibuligera* (Peberdy 1979a) and *Saccharomycopsis diastaticus* and *Schizosaccharomyces pombe* (Tamaki 1982). In these cases the fusion frequency was very low, about 10^{-6} to 10^{-7} (Tamaki 1982). Many of the hybrids were unstable and readily dissociated into their parental strains (Delgado and Herrera 1981); in others parental nuclei fuse and either gave stable hybrid progeny (Delgado and Herrera 1981), or else the hybrid nuclei undergo random loss of chromosomes to stabilize at various levels of aneuploidy prior to segregation (Peberdy 1979a; Sarachek et al. 1981).

Protoplast fusion has been used for the improvement of enzyme producing strains, such as cellulases (Furlaneto and Pizzirani-Kleiner 1992), β-glycosidases (Hoh et al. 1992), pectinases (Solís et al. 1997), amylases (Rubinder et al. 2000) and lipase (Sawicka-Zukowska et al. 2004), penicillin producing strains (Tahoun 1993), citric acid producers (Kirimura et al. 1988; Martinková et al. 1990) and in fungi of agricultural interest (Viaud et al. 1998; Ogawa et al. 2000).

5.2 Genetic Transformation

Transformation extends the potential for genetic manipulation not only in established genetic systems but also in fungi less amenable for study by conventional genetic analysis. Transformation of a filamentous fungus was originally reported by Mishra and Tatum (1973) who transformed an inositol-requiring mutant to prototrophy by supplying the DNA from wild- type to growing cultures. Fungal transformation typically involves the use of regenerative protoplasts, identification of selectable marker genes, and stable integration of the transforming DNA into the chromosome of the organism (Amsellem et al. 2002; Fincham 1989; Finkelstein 1992; van den Hondel and Punt 1991; Lopes et al. 2004). However, there are the following alternative methods for transformation (Costanzo and Fox 1988; Delmore 1989; Dhawale et al. 1984; Richey et al. 1989; Sanford 1988).

a) Electroporation/Electropermeabilization: Electroporation is non-destructive permeabilization of biological membranes in short-duration, high amplitude electric fields (Delmore 1989; Richey et al 1989)
b) Biolistic/Particle bombardment/Microprojectile Method: Bombarding the intact mycelium with DNA bound to small tungsten or gold particles (Sanford 1988).
c) Intact cells can be treated with high concentrations of alkali metal ions such as Li^+ or Cs^+ to induce permeability before addition of DNA and treatment with PEG (Dhawale et al 1984; Ito et al 1983).
d) Partial cell-breakage by blending with glass beads (Costanzo and Fox 1988). This violent treatment kills 80-90% of the cells.

The low level of homology required for integration in the fungal genome allows the use of heterologous genes that have been employed for molecular studies of genetically uncharacterized but economically important fungi (Goosen et al.1992).

Fungal protoplast transformation can be done by using polyethylene glycol (PEG), but frequencies are considerably lower than those obtained with bacteria and yeast; nevertheless, this approach has found widespread applications in various areas of fungal research and biotechnology (Fincham 1989; Azevedo 1998; Robinson and Sharon 1999; De Guido et al. 2003; Varavallo et al. 2004). An alternative approach to inserting DNA into cells involves permeabilization of cell-membranes via electroporation. In this technique a high-voltage electric pulse is used to create a population of small, aqueous pores in the cell-membrane through which large molecules (e.g. DNA) either diffusely or electrophoretically enter the cell (Weaver 1995). Electroporation has been used to transform a number of fungi (Brown et al. 1998; Richey et al. 1989; Goldman et al. 1990).

Different methods of fungal transformation may involve different DNA transfer mechanisms e.g. when transformed with the similar gene construct (*vgb* and bleomycin resistance genes) PEG-mediated transformant of *P. chrysogenum* showed salt resistance as compared to the *Agrobacterium*-mediated ones which couldn't (Sun et al. 2002).

Successful transformation of fungus requires selective markers like dominant or semi-dominant genes responsible for antibiotic resistance e.g. *Sh ble* or *hph*, conferring resistance to phleomycin or hygromycin B, respectively (Gritz and Davies 1983; Kaster et al. 1983; Jain et al. 1992; Santos et al. 1996), or for fungicide resistance e.g. *Bml*^{r} gene from *Neurospora crassa* which confers resistance to benzimidazoles (Orbach et al. 1986).

The effectiveness of genetic transformation is low (1-25 transformants ug^{-1} plasmid DNA) when hetrologous genes are used (Fincham, 1989; Hynes 1986). Transformation frequency can be enhanced by using non-integrative autonomously replicating plasmids carrying DNA sequences with a replication origin, as the 2 μm plasmid (Beggs 1978) and chromosomal ARSs (Autonomous Replicating Sequences) of *S. cerevisiae* (Stinchcomb et al. 1979). ARS-like sequences have rarely been observed in filamentous fungi (Huang et al. 1989; Santos et al. 1996; Suarez and Eslava, 1988); AMA1 sequence (Autonomous Maintenance in *Aspergillus*) of *A. nidulans* being a prime example (Gems et al. 1991; Aleksenko and Clutterbuck, 1996,1997). Autonomously replicating plasmids carrying the AMA1 sequence have been successfully used in a simple gene-cloning strategy, known as 'Instant Gene Bank', based on co-transformation of linearized plasmids and genomic DNA fragments obtained with an appropriate restriction enzyme (De Guido et al. 2003). Plasmids and useful flanking genomic sequences can be readily recovered from transformants (Gems et al. 1994; Verdoes et al. 1994). For single copy plasmid integration a technique called Restriction Enzyme-Mediated Integration (REMI) is used. The target plasmid is linearized with restriction enzymes by adding the same enzyme to the transformation mixture at different concentrations. It is a useful tool for mutagenesis and gene cloning because single-copy insertions make it easy to rescue transforming plasmid and flanking sequences (Kahmann and Basse, 1999; Maier and Schafer 1999).

Mycorrhizal fungi are highly recalcitrant to transformation because of the difficulties in culturing and obtaining protoplasts. Very few reports of transformation of ectomycorrhizal fungi have been published (Barrett et al 1990; Bills et al 1995,1999; Marmeisse et al 1992; Peng et al 1993). Despite the existence of diverse transformation techniques, gene delivery remains a limiting step in innumerable fields of research.

5.3 Electrophoretic Karyotype Analysis

Fungal cytogenetics has been hampered by the small size of fungal chromosomes, the lack of known sexual stages in many medically and industrially important species, and the occurrence of endomitosis (Chiu 1996). However, the karyotype of several fungal species has been determined by pulse-field gel electrophoresis, a technique requiring large amount of protoplast to prepare the agarose gels for blocks (Mills and McCluskey 1990). This has allowed the electrophoretic karyotype determination of species such as *A. nidulans* (Brody and Carbon 1989), *P. janthinellum* (Kayser and Schulz 1991), *P. notatum*, *P. chrysogenum* (Fierro et al. 1993), *Agaricus bisporus* (Sonnenberg et al. 1996), *P.paxilli* (Young et al.

1998), *Pleurotus ostreatus* (Larraya et al. 1999), *P. nalgiovense* (Färber and Geisen, 2000), *A. nidulans* strains with chromosome duplications (de Queiroz et al. 2000) and *Crinipellis perniciosa* (Rincones et al. 2003). The molecular karyotype of *Coprinus cinereus*, obtained by PFGE, has been correlated with its genetic map by the use of cloned gene probes and genetic studies (Pukkila and Casselton 1991; Pukkila and Skrzynia 1993). Electrophoretic karyotyping of different fungi has shown that chromosome length polymorphisms (CLPs) are a common and prominent feature of these organisms (Zolan, 1995). Two mechanisms have been proposed for the generation of these polymorphisms: increasing the copy number of particular sequences, such as the rDNA (Pukkila and Skrzynia 1993; Sonnenberg et al. 1996) and subtelomeric repeats (Farman and Leong 1995; Louis 1994), and mitotic and meiotic recombination processes (Zolan 1995; Zolan et al. 1994). In many cases these CLPs seems to have minor genetic consequences, since many different karyotypes are found in a given species (Larraya et al. 1999). However, some reduction in spore viability has been observed in outcrosses between *C. cinereus* strains with differences in their chromosomal sizes (Pukkila, 1992) and in crosses between *S. cerevisiae* strains with pronounced CLPs (Zolan 1995). For some species it has been reported that CLPs within a given strain will eventually disappear by chromosome recombination (Zolan et al. 1994).

5.4 Plant-Microbe Interactions

Viable protoplasts can be used to address questions regarding the metabolic or biochemical compartmentation, which are not accessible with intact hyphae, root tissues, or the fungus under functional symbiosis.

Protoplastation is useful in case of endosymbiotic fungi because they can be grown on synthetic media (Rai and Varma 2005; Singh, 2001; Varma et al. 2001) and thus can be manipulated apart from the fungal partner. The isolation of the protoplast can also be used to understand the mystery of symbiosis between the fungal partner and mycelia protoplast and to address the questions pertaining to metabolic exchange.

One of the glaring examples of plant-microbe interaction is *Piriformospora indica*. *P. indica* is a novel endophytic root colonizing fungus, which mimics the capabilities of a typical AM fungus (Verma et al. 1998; Varma et al. 1999; Oelmüller et al. 2005). The fungus colonizes the roots and improves the health, vigour and survival of a wide range of mono- and dicotyledon plants (Rai and Varma 2002, Rai et al. 2001). This fungus mediates uptake of phosphorus from the substratum and its translocation to the host by an energy-dependent active process (Malla et al. 2005). It serves as a strong agent for biological hardening of tissue culture-raised plants, protecting them from 'transplantation shock', rendering almost hundred percent survival rate on the hosts tested (Rai et al. 2001). This fungus is also a potential biological agent against potent root pathogens. Thus, it displays immense potential to be utilized as biological tool for plant promotion, protection from pests, and for relieving stress conditions such as those caused due to acidity, desiccation and heavy metal toxicity (Waller et al. 2005).

6. A CASE STUDY: *PIRIFORMOSPORA INDICA*

Researchers from the School of Life Sciences, Jawaharlal Nehru University, New Delhi, have screened a novel endophytic fungus (Verma et al. 1998), which mimics the capabilities of typical, AM fungus. The fungus was isolated from the rhizosphere of the woody shrubs *Prosopsis julifera* and *Zizyphus nummularia* growing in the western part of Rajasthan, a typical desert region of the Indian subcontinent. The characteristic features of *P. indica* are the following:

- axenically cultivable on synthetic media
- no *clamp connections*
- *anastomosis* occurs frequently
- hypha-hypha aggregation often observed
- no *hyphal knots*
- simple septum with *dolipores* and continuous, straight *parenthosomes*
- spore 8-45 mm in diameter
- 8-25 nuclei per spore.

The fungus promises to serve as the substitute of AM fungi to overcome the long-standing enigma of science. The functional similarities with AMF are the following:

- broad and diverse host spectrum
- hyphae extramatrical, inter- and intracellular
- hyphae never invade the endodermis
- chlamydospores in soil and within cortical tissues
- sexual stages not seen
- positive phytopromotional effects on tested hosts
- phosphorus mobilizer
- phosphorus transporter
- tool for biological hardening of micropropagated plantlets
- potent biological control agent against root pathogens.

6.1 *Piriformospora Indica*: A New Root Symbiont

Based on the 18S and 28S rDNA analysis and the ultrastructure of the septal pore, its phylogenetic relationship is within the Hymenomycetes (Basidiomycota).

P. indica tremendously improves the growth and overall biomass production of a wide host spectrum, like herbaceous mono- and dicots, and trees, including medicinal plants, and several economically important crops (Varma et al 1999, 2001). Pronounced growth promotional effect was also seen with terrestrial orchids (Blechert et al 1999). A recent report indicated the ability of *P. indica* to colonize the rhizoids of a liverwort (bryophyte) and the *thalli* failed to grow under *in situ* conditions in the absence of this fungus (Varma et al 2001).

6.2 The Physiological and Functional Identity

The fungus enters the root cortex and forms inter- and intracellular hyphae. Within the cortical cells, the fungus often forms dense hyphal coils or branched structures, intracellularly. *P. indica* also forms spore- or vesicle-like structures within or between the cortical cells. Like AM fungi, hyphae multiply within the host cortical tissues and never traverse through the endodermis. Likewise, they also do not invade the aerial portion of the plant (stem and leaves).

Interestingly, the host spectrum of *P. indica* is very much like AMF. *P. indica* colonize the roots of host plants as diverse as *Zea mays* L., *Nicotiana tabacum* L., *Petroselinum crispum* L., *Populus tremula* L., *Setaria italica* L., *Oryza sativa* L., *Sorghum vulgare*, *Triticum sativum*, *Glycine max* (L.) Merr., *Cicer arietinum* L., *Solanum melongena* L., *Artemissia annua* L. and *Bacopa monniera* (L.) Wett. (Varma et al 1999, 2001). This phenomenon may be connected with some identical functional aspects as indicated by the serological characterization (Singh, 2001).

6.3 Phosphate Mobilization and Transport

P. indica mediates uptake of phosphorus from the medium and translocates to the host in an energy-dependent process. *P. indica* produces significant amounts of acid phosphatases for the mobilization of broad range of insoluble forms of phosphate, enabling the host plant the accessibility of adequate phosphorus from immobilized reserves in the soil (Varma et al 2001).

6.4 Biological Hardening Agent

P. indica promises to be an excellent candidate for biological hardening of micropropagated plantlets as the fungus rendered more than 90 per cent survival rate of the transferred plantlets of (*Nicotiana tabacum* L., and *Bacopa monniera* L. Wett. (Sahay and Varma 1999, 2000) by excessive root proliferation and induction of secondary rootlets, protecting them from transplantation shock and potent root pathogens (Singh et al 2000; Varma et al 2001).

6.5 Immobilization of the Endosymbiont

P. indica have been successfully immobilized in alginate beads, and retained the germinating capacity even after 90 days storage at low (4°C) and room temperature (30°C), when used as an inoculum in pot-culture experiments using *Sorghum vulgare* as the host (Roy 1999). This finding ascertains that the entrapment of fungal propagules inside alginate beads stabilizes the infective capacity of the fungus and promises its use as a viable inoculum for various biotechnological applications and feasible long distance transportation.

6.6 *P. Indica* Protoplasts: Applied and Fundamental Research

6.6.1 Protoplast Production from Mycelium

The fungal hyphae, used as the starting material for protoplast isolation, after an incubation period of 4 hr. in the *Trichoderma harzianum* Lysing Enzyme (L2265 Sigma, St. Louis), either alone or used in combination with cellulase, chitinase and hemicellulase gave the appearance of beaded chains. The cell-wall residues around the released spherical-to-oval bodies were observed by calcofluor white staining by observing under fluorescent microscope. These spheroplasts were also resistant to osmotic lysis in distilled water.

When the fungal mycelium was subjected to 4 hr. incubation in the *Trichoderma harzianum* lysing enzyme (L1412 Sigma, St. Louis), either alone or in combination with cellulase, spherical protoplasts were released as evident by their non-fluorescence with calcofluor white staining and bursting under hypotonic shock of distilled water. The protoplasts were mostly aggregated and clustered, frequently two to four together. Numerous protoplasts appeared as if undergoing the process of fusion.

6.6.2 Protoplast Regeneration

When appropriately diluted suspensions of purified protoplasts were incubated on Kaefer/MMNC$_{1/2}$ medium, both supplemented with

0.5 M KCl/sorbitol or mannitol, neither visible colonies nor regenerated hyphae was visible as observed till 120 days.

6.6.3 Chlamydospore Production

Circular discs infested with *P. indica* culture on inoculation onto the surface of solidified Kaefer medium in petriplates, produced prominent growth zones. The microscopic analysis of a ten-day-old inoculum revealed highly aggregated, overlapping and intertwined hyphae. The entire surface of culture was covered by the formation of pear-shaped chlamydospores within twenty-eight days. Chlamydospore production was further induced by subjecting the culture to temperature stress by an overnight incubation at 4°C.

6.6.4 Optimization of Chlamydospore Germination

The conditions were optimized such that the spores could be induced to germinate simultaneously. The different modes of spore germination are depicted in Fig. 2. The spores scrapped from Kaefer medium agar plates on incubation in fresh Kaefer medium for 24 hr. gave a high germination frequency of 94.36 per cent. In contrast, a germination frequency of only 77 per cent was achieved after a 24 hr. incubation when the source of inoculum and substrate was PDA medium.

The effect of organic and inorganic nitrogenous sources was assessed. The spore germination in water agar fortified with yeast extract (0.3 per cent) was found to be 91.6 per cent at 24 hours. However, high concentrations of yeast extract were inhibitory to spore germination. Similarly high spore germination was observed with inorganic nitrogenous sources such as NH_4NO_3 (Fig. 2) and $NaNO_3$ at a concentration of 0.5 per cent the frequency of germination being 88.28 per cent and 62 per cent, respectively. A similar pattern of high spore germination at low concentrations of the substrates and their higher inhibitory concentrations was also observed with the non-nitrogenous sources, *viz.*, $CaSO_4$ and K_2SO_4, although their positive effect on spore germination was quite low; the germination frequencies at 0.5 per cent being 42.5 and 52.88 per cent, respectively.

These findings indicate that nitrogen may have a stimulatory effect on spore germination, which becomes inhibitory/toxic at its higher concentrations.

6.6.5 Protoplast Production from Germinated Chlamydospores

6.6.5.1 Effect of Commercial Enzymes

Ranges of commercially available enzyme preparations were screened for their ability to release protoplasts from germinated chlamydospores of

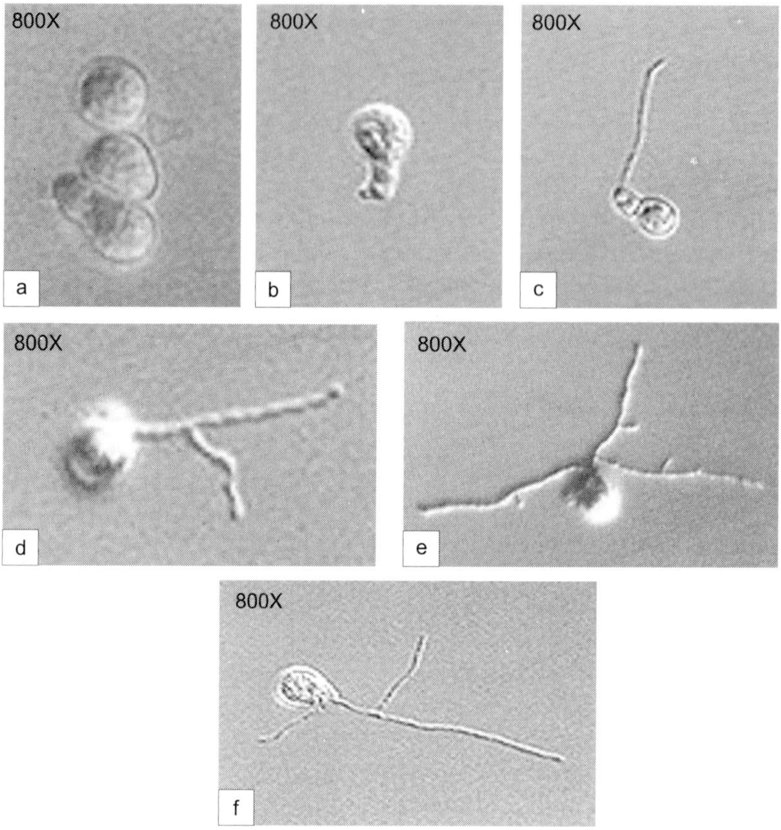

Fig. 2 Germinating Chlamydospores of *P. indica*

P. indica. The yield of protoplasts attained by the *Trichoderma harzianum* lysing enzyme cocktail (Sigma, St. Louis) was of highest magnitude and gave optimal results of 2×10^8 protoplasts per gram (fresh weight) of culture per ml of enzyme mixture. Cellulase Type II (Sigma, St. Louis), *Cellulolysin Cellulase* (Calbiochem) and Cellulase Onozuka R-10 were highly effective, releasing 0.83×10^8, 0.7×10^8 and 0.6×10^8 protoplasts, respectively. *Aspergillus niger* pectinase (Sigma, St. Louis) was inactive. Some lytic activity was observed with mutanase (Merck), glucanase (Merck) and chitinase.

6.6.5.2 Effect of Enzyme Concentration

Different concentrations of *T. harzianum* lysing enzyme (Sigma, St. Louis), dissolved in an iso-osmotic medium with 0.5 M KCl, were tested for protoplast yield at different periods of incubation. In one set of experiments with low enzyme concentrations of 3 mg/ml, 6 mg/ml and 25 mg/ml, the protoplasts yield was the same. However, in another set of experiments, the protoplast yield slightly increased when the enzyme concentration was increased from 25 mg/ml to 50 mg/ml.

6.6.5.3 Effect of *Osmotic Stabilizers*

Various concentrations of sorbitol, using the optimized enzyme mixture (*Trichoderma harzianum* lysing enzyme, Sigma, St. Louis), were tested for their ability to support protoplast release and stability. The highest yield of protoplasts was obtained at 0.5 M solution.

The effect of different osmotic stabilizers on protoplast release was tested using *T. harzianum* lysing enzyme (Sigma, St. Louis), dissolved in different stabilizers, all of which were at the concentration of 0.5 M. Most protoplasts were stable with the use of KCl, sorbitol, mannitol and glucose. $MgSO_4$ was found ineffective as an osmotic stabilizer and the protoplasts lysed on emergence. KCl gave the best results, and to a lesser extent, mannitol and sorbitol were also effective as stabilizers.

6.6.5.4 Effect of Incubation Temperature

The most suitable incubation temperature with the lysing enzyme was 30°C, which produced 0.71×10^8 protoplasts. At 37°C, yields were reduced to less than 49 per cent of this value was released while at 20°C or 25°C, the yield was still lower, 91 per cent of the former value.

6.6.5.5 Effect of Culture Age

The age of *P. indica* culture significantly affected the yield of protoplasts. A maximum yield of 0.73×10^8 protoplasts was obtained with a 24 hr. old culture. The protoplast yields sharply declined to 92 per cent less with a 44 hr. culture, and 47 per cent less protoplasts with an 18 hr. old culture.

6.6.5.6 Morphological Changes

Within ten minutes after incubating with the lytic enzyme mixture, the hyphae swelled at certain points, mostly at tips, presumably the points of greatest sensitivity to the enzyme action. The mycelial contents seemed to aggregate inside the hyphae. Subsequently, the protoplasts emerged as a small, round, bud-like structure at one side or at the end of a broken hypha. Finally, the protoplasmic contents of most hyphae formed spherical protoplasts. After the completion of the lytic action of the enzyme, the mycelial wall was degraded and majority of hyphal cells were converted into protoplasts. However, the chlamydospores were resistant to degradation by the lytic enzyme. Not all the hyphae were equally sensitive to the lytic enzyme attack. While some parts of the mycelia swelled within 10-30 m of the reaction and released the protoplasts, other parts took longer time. However, significantly high yields could be obtained by half hour incubation.

6.6.5.7 Morphology of Protoplasts

The protoplasts were spherical, of variable sizes depending on the cell-wall digesting enzyme, and appeared fragile. The contents of the protoplasts were non-uniform.

6.6.5.8 Sensitivity and Stability of Protoplasts

The protoplasts were sensitive to osmotic shock; when placed in distilled water or hypotonic solutions, they swelled and bursted.

After a 24 hr. storage in the osmotic medium, 99.7 per cent of the protoplasts were stable at –20°C, 93.09 per cent at 4°C and 21.28 per cent at room temperature.

6.6.6 Protoplast Staining with Fluorescent Dyes

Staining with calcofluor white showed that the protoplasts were free of cell-wall material. The percentage of viable protoplasts as determined by FDA staining was 36.11 per cent (Fig. 3a). Staining the protoplasts for DNA with ethidium bromide revealed the presence of one to four nuclei per protoplast (Fig. 3b,c,d,e).

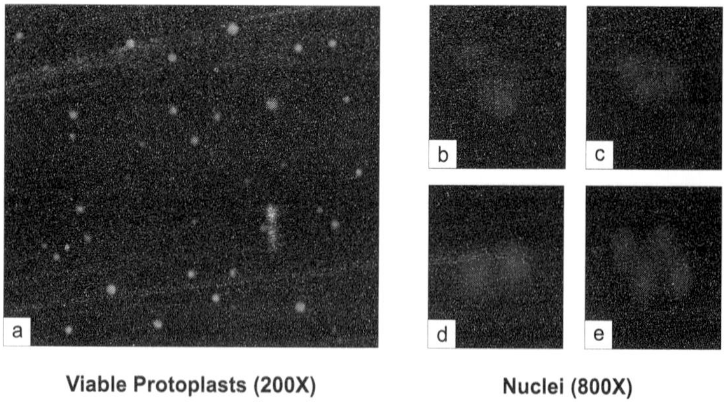

Fig. 3 Viable Protoplasts and Nuclei observed under fluorescence microscope

6.6.7 Protoplast Regeneration

6.6.7.1 Effect of Regeneration Media

When appropriately diluted suspensions of purified protoplasts were incubated on Kaefer medium supplemented with 0.5 M KCl/sorbitol or mannitol, no protoplast regeneration was visible as observed for sixty days. Protoplasts were regenerated on $MMNC_{1/2}$ regeneration media made isotonic with 0.5 M sorbitol and 0.5 M KCl.

Neither visible colonies nor regenerated hyphae were observed in the medium without osmotic stabilizers.

6.6.7.2 Effect of Osmotic Stabilizers

Regeneration frequencies of protoplasts cultured on $MMNC_{1/2}$ regeneration media fortified with 0.5 M sorbitol and 0.5 M KCl were different. Visible colonies appeared after nine days of culture on sorbitol containing medium. However, colonies appeared on KCl containing medium within 3-4 weeks. The regeneration frequency on sorbitol containing medium was higher than on KCl supplemented medium.

6.6.7.3 Effect of Enzyme Concentration

Although the protoplast yields with low enzyme concentration of 3 mg/ml and 6 mg/ml were almost the same, their regeneration frequency was reduced three folds with enzyme concentration of 6 mg/ml. At higher enzyme concentration of 50 mg/ml, the regeneration frequency drastically decreased on the corresponding medium.

6.6.7.4 Effect of Protoplast Density

The optimal protoplast density was between 10^4 and 10^6 protoplasts per ml. The protoplasts did not regenerate at low densities.

6.6.7.5 Microscopic Analysis

Microscopic examination revealed that reversion of protoplasts started within 2-3 days. Initially, the protoplasts, mostly clustered together, swelled and increased in size (Fig. 4a). On third day of incubation, when the aliquots of liquid protoplast culture was stained with calcoflour white, a faint staining of the newly generated wall material on some protoplasts was visible (Fig. 4b). On fourth day, the intensity and frequency of protoplast staining increased (Fig. 4c,d). The fluorescence was more intense and germination of one to two hyphae in a cluster was visible on the fifth day (Fig. 4e,f). On the sixth day, mycelium with a bright fluorescence were visible (Fig. 4g,h).

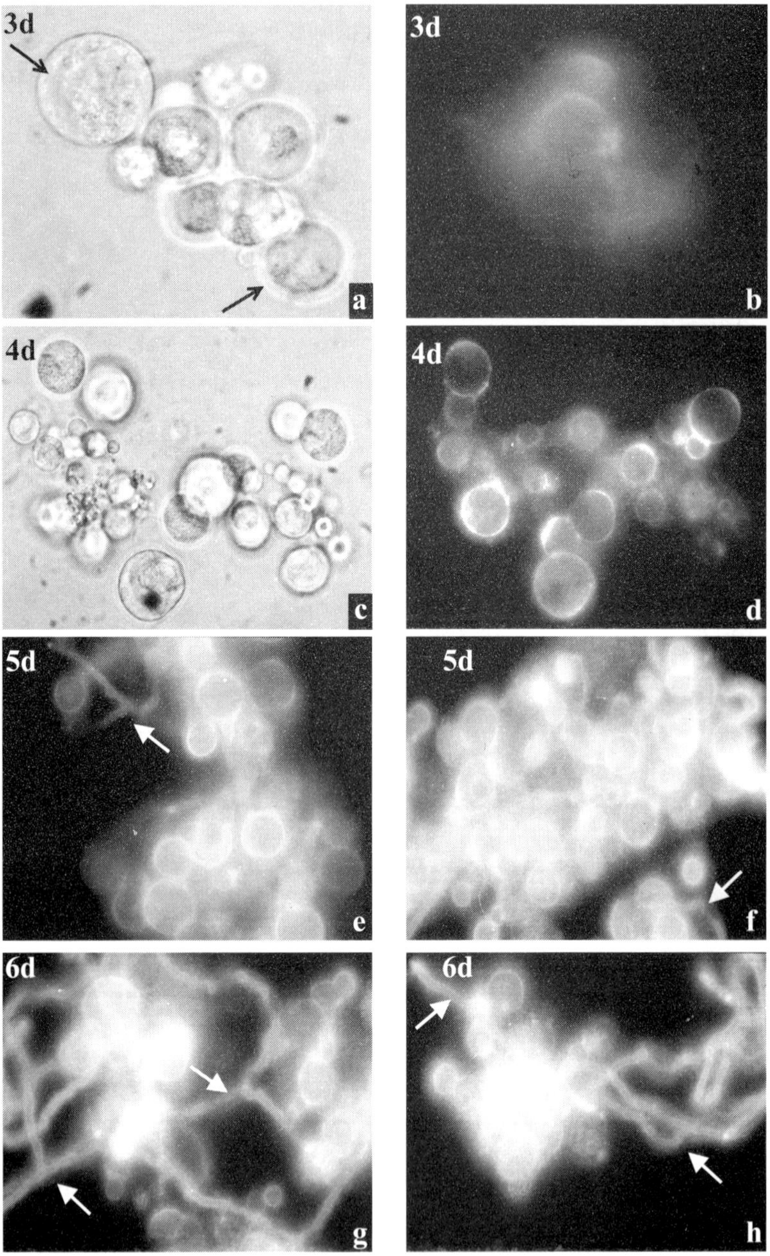

Fig. 4 Regenerating protoplasts as observed under light and florescence microscope (800 X)

The protoplasts produced short irregular protuberances developing into a germ-tube. Analysis under a phase contrast microscope chains (Fig. 5) and light microscope (Fig. 6) at high magnification revealed that the newly formed hyphae were extremely undulating giving the appearance of beaded. Various stages of protoplast regeneration are depicted in Fig. 7a,b,c and Fig. 8a,b,c.

6.6.8 Growth on Non-isotonic Medium

After two weeks of incubation in isotonic (0.5 M sorbitol) $MMNC_{1/2}$ regeneration medium, the regenerated protoplasts spread plated on non-osmotically adjusted Kaefer agar medium rapidly produced normal colonies indicating the reversion to normal cellular functions.

6.6.9 Myco-photobiont Interaction

6.6.9.1 Photosymbiont Promotional Features

Inoculation of *Zea mays* seedlings with regenerated *P. indica* colonies resulted in a significant increase in the shoot length, number of leaves and overall plant biomass as compared to the uninoculated control. An extensive root proliferation was prominently visible in the inoculated plants with the induction of numerous enlarged secondary rootlets.

6.6.9.2 Cytochemical and Histochemical Analysis

On microscopic analysis of the stained root segments of *Zea mays* inoculated with regenerated *P. indica*, differentiated fungal structures, *viz.*, hyphae, and chlamydospores were prominently visible in the cortical tissues. The fungal hyphae often adhered together, and gave the appearance of intertwined cords (Fig. 9a,b). The chlamydospores appeared singly (Fig. 9b,c) or in clusters (Fig. 9d,e), and were distinctive due to their pear-shaped and double-walled structures. The fungus did not invade the endodermis. Control plant did not contain any fungal structures.

These findings indicated that the host phytopromotional and root colonizing potential of *P. indica* remained unaltered subsequent to protoplast regeneration.

6.6.10 Effect of Antimycotics

To identify a selection marker to develop a transformation system with *P. indica*, among the different antimycotics tested at various concentrations, *P. indica* was susceptible to hygromycin (Sigma, St. Louis) atrazine (Fluka) and cycloheximide (Sigma, St. Louis). The minimum inhibitory concentration for hygromycin was 100 mg/ml, and for atrazine was 10^{-3} M. The colonies developed on the medium without antimycotics

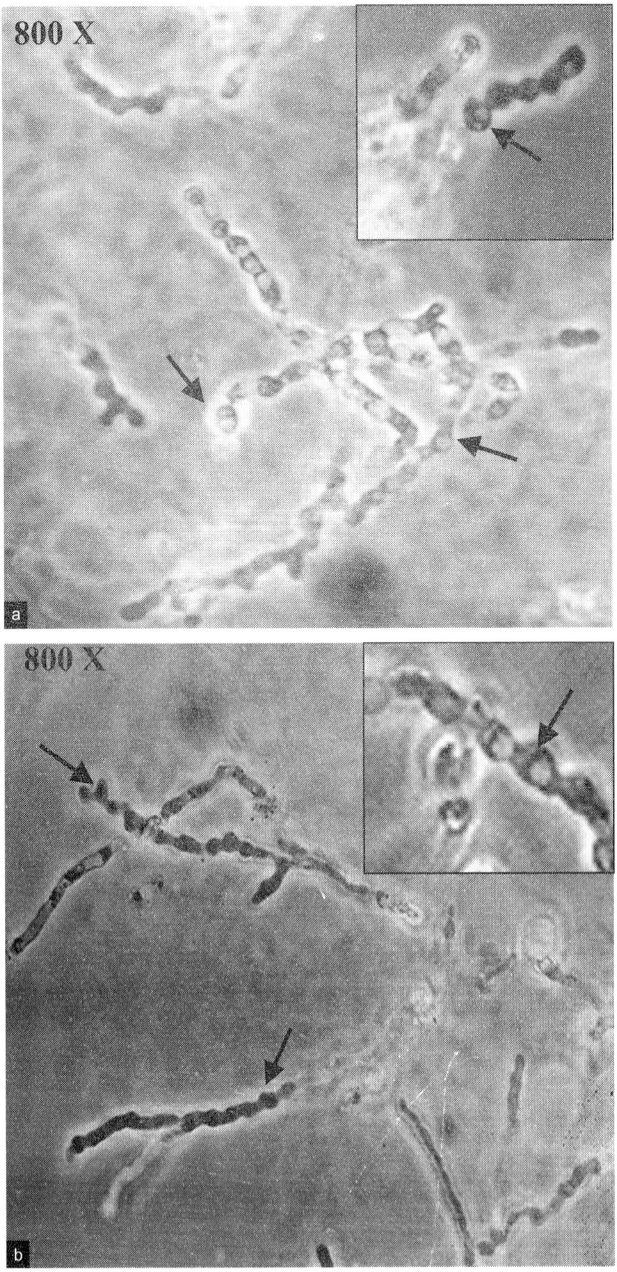

Fig. 5 Regenerating protoplasts as observed under phase contrast microscope

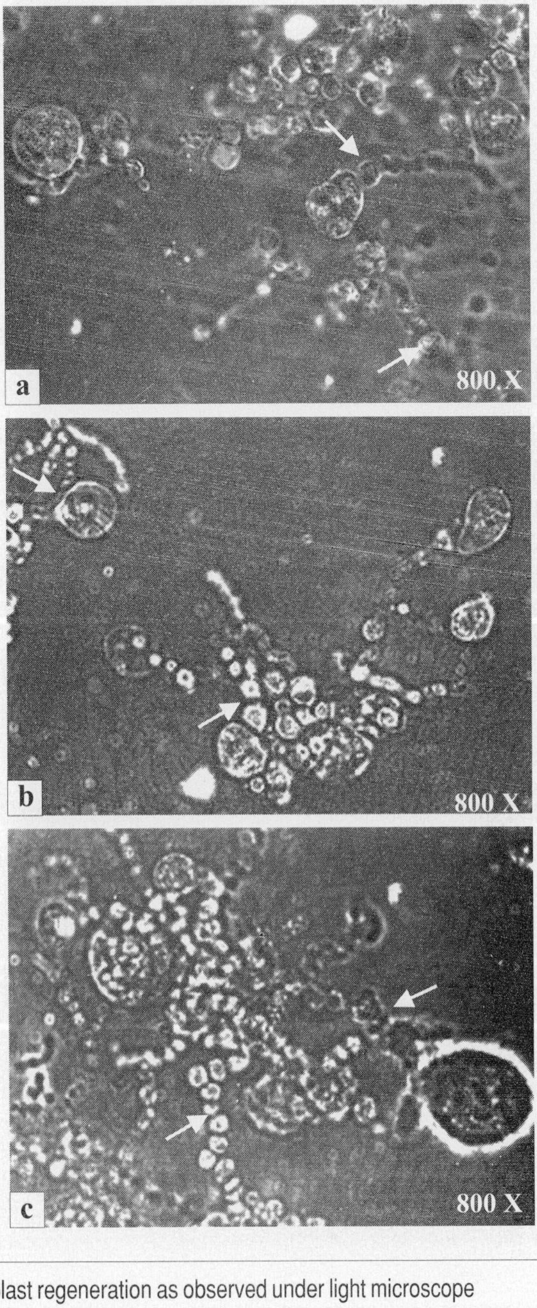

Fig. 6 Protoplast regeneration as observed under light microscope

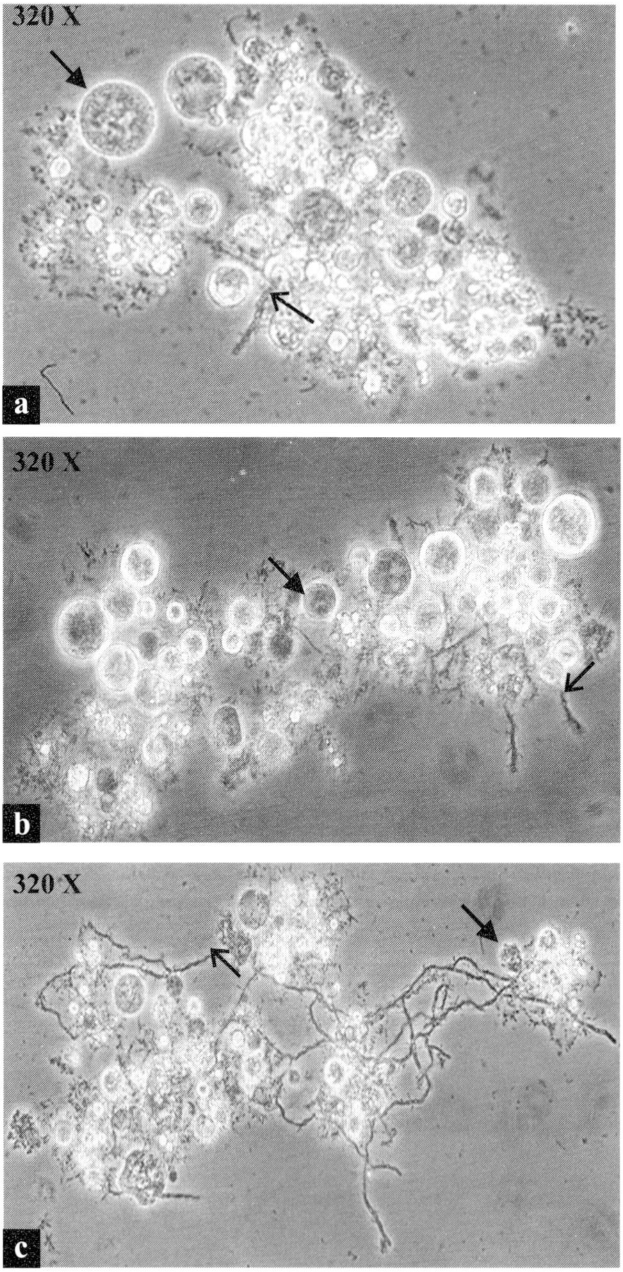

Fig. 7 Protoplast regeneration as observed under phase contrast microscope

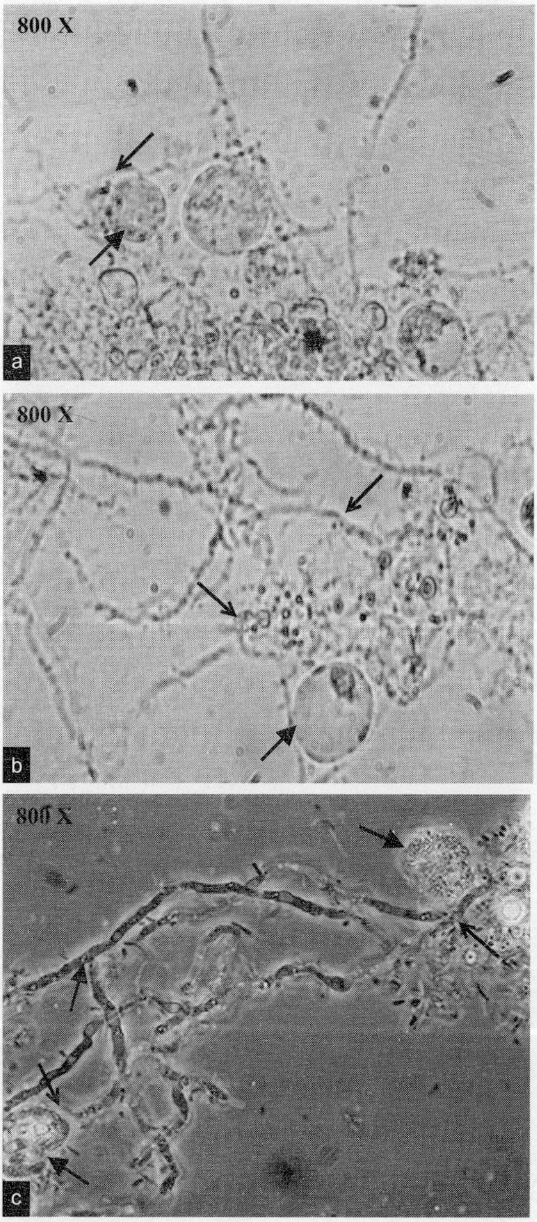

Fig. 8 a, b. Regenerated protoplasts as observed under light microscope; c. Regenerated protoplasts as observed under phase contrast microscope

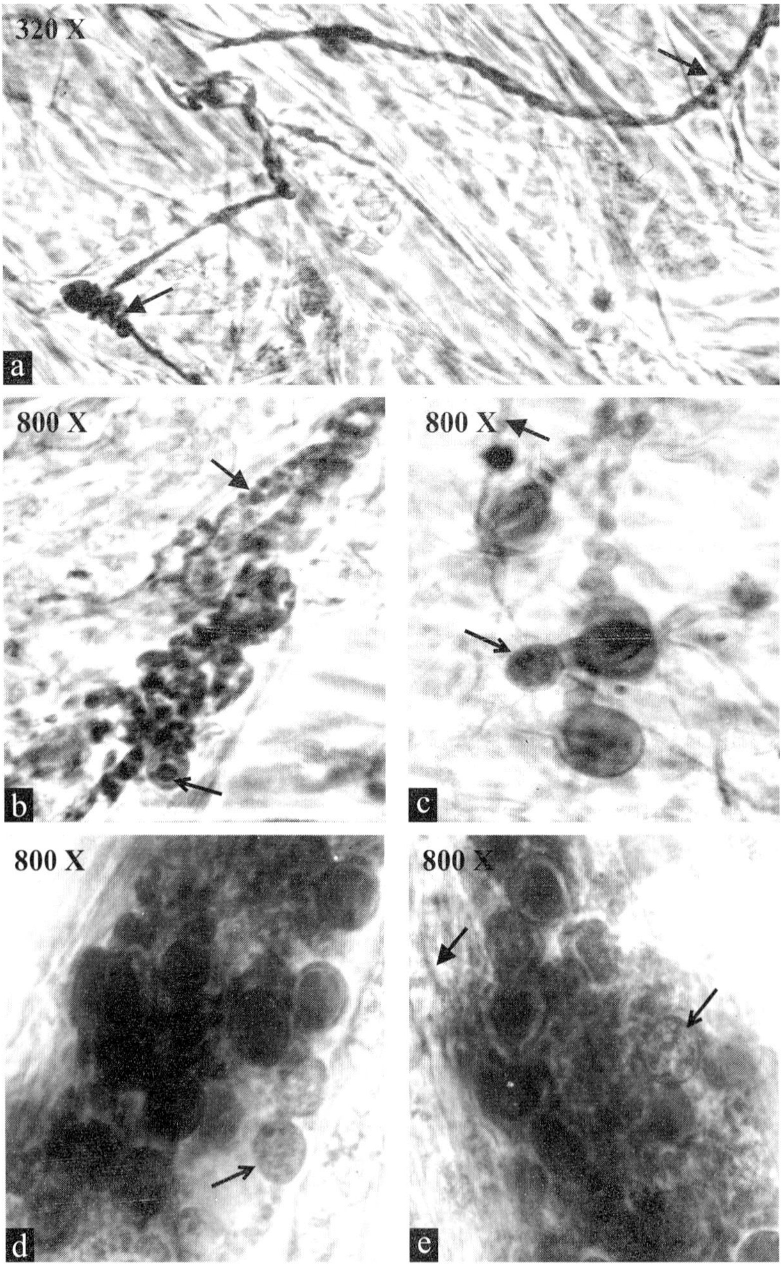

Fig. 9 Root colonization potential of regenerated protoplasts

showed normal growth. However, it was resistant to Baasta even at high doses of 1000 mg/ml.

6.6.11 Transformation of P. indica

Subsequent to protoplast transformation with pCSN43, selection for hygromycin resistance on plates containing $MMNC_{1/2}$ medium supplemented with 100mg/ml as an indicator of putative transformants, resulted in seven colonies per 10mg of pCSN43 per 10^7 protoplasts. However, the growth of the colonies stopped after 20-25 days of transfer, indicative of an unstable DNA integration.

7. CONCLUSION

Fungus protoplasts serve as a potent tool for fungal biotechnology research. The protocol for protoplast isolation needs to be refined more so as to have a window for developing standardized isolation procedures. Regeneration of protoplast is one of the important steps towards improving the economically important fungal traits and for further manipulation. The startling aspect of fungal protoplast is its wide applications in development of novel genetic clones by protoplast fusion and genetic transformation, karyotyping and in understanding of plant-microbe interactions. The adaptability of fungi in general to undergo interspecific and intergeneric protoplast fusion has obliterated the need of parasexual stage in all the groups of fungi. The somatic hybrids have shown stable regeneration with incorporation of selective gene markers from both of the parents. The usage of protoplasts in karyotyping makes better characterization of fungus feasible and also provides a window of opportunity for chromosome breeding and manipulation. Lastly, fungus protoplasts can become an important tool in understanding plant-microbe interactions especially in case of axenically cultivable non-AM fungi *P. indica*.

ACKNOWLEDGEMENTS

This chapter is dedicated to late Dr Archana Singh who left for heavenly abode at a very young age, while at peak of career.

REFERENCES

Aleksenko AY, Clutterbuck AJ (1996) The AMA1 plasmid replicator in *Aspergillus nidulans* is an inverted duplication of a low-copy-number dispersed genomic repeat. Mol Microbiol 19: 565-574

Aleksenko AY, Clutterbuck AJ (1997) Autonomous plasmid replication in *Aspergillus nidulans*: AMA1 and MATE elements. Fungal Genet Biol 21: 373-387

Amsellem Z, Cohen BA, Gressel J (2002) Engineering hypervirulence in a mycoherbicidal fungus for efficient weed control. Nature Biotechnol 20: 1035-1039

Anne J, Peberdy JF (1976) Induced fusion of fungal protoplasts following treatment with polyethylene glycol. Arch Microbiol 105: 201-205

Anne J, Eyssen H, Somer de P (1976) Somatic hybridization of *Penicillium roquefortii* with *P. chrysogenum* after protoplast fusion. Nature 62: 719-721

Anne J, Peberdy JF (1976) Induced fusion of fungal protoplasts following treatment with polyethylene glycol. J Gen Microbiol 92: 413-417

Anne J, Peberdy JF (1985) Protoplast fusion and interspecies hybridization in *Penicillium*. In: Peberdy JF, Ferenczy L (eds) Fungal Protoplasts, Marcel Dekker, New York, pp 259-277

Anunciacao CE, Guimaraes, Araujo EF, Muchovej RMC, Souza (1990) Production and regeneration of protoplasts of *Pisolithus tinctorius*. Biotechnol Tech 4: 215-220

Azevedo JL (1998) Genética de microrganismos. Goiânia: Editora UFG

Bacon JSD, Milne BD, Taylor IF, Webley DM (1965) Features of the cell-wall of yeast revealed by the action of enzymes from a non-fruiting myxobacterium (*Cytophage jhonsonii*). Biochem J 95: 25-30

Bagyaraj DJ, Varma A (1995) Interaction between arbuscular mycorrhizal fungi and plants and their importance in sustainable agriculture in arid and semi-arid tropics. Advances in Microbial Ecology 14: 119-142

Balasubramanian N, Annie Juliet G, Srikalaivani P, Lalithakumari D (2003) Release and regeneration of protoplasts from the fungus *Trichothecium roseum*. Can J Microbiol 49: 263-268

Bardi L, Perotto S, Bonfante P (1999) Isolation and regeneration of protoplasts from two strains of the ericoid mycorrhizal fungus *Oididendron maius*: Sensitivity to chemicals and heavy metals. Microbiol Res 154: 105-111

Barrett V, Lemke PA, Dixon RK (1989) Protoplast formation from selected species of ectomycorrhiza fungi. Appl Microbiol Biotechnol 30: 381-387

Barrett V, Lemke PA, Dixon RK (1990) Genetic transformation of a mycorrhizal fungus. Appl Microbiol Biotech 33: 313-316

Bartnicki-Garcia S (1980) In: Ferenczy L, Farkas GL (eds) Advances in protoplast research. Akademiai kiado, Budapest, Pergamon Press, Oxford, pp 475-484

Batchmann BJ, Bonner DM (1959) Protoplasts from *Neurospora crassa*. J Bact 78:150-156

Beggs JD (1978) Transformation of yeast by a replicating hybrid plasmid. Nature 275: 104-109

Benecke W (1905) Uber *Bacillus chitinovororus*, einen chitin zersetzenden spaltpilz. Bot Ztg 63: 227

Benitez T, Ramos S, Acha IG (1975) Protoplasts of *Trichoderma viride*. Arch Microbiol 103: 199-203

Berliner MD (1971) Induction of protoplasts of *Schizosaccharomyces octosporus* by magnesium sulphate and 2-deoxy-D-glucose. Mycologia 63: 819-825

Bills S, Podila GK, Hiremath S (1999) Genetic engineering of an ectomycorrhizal fungus *Laccaria laccata* for use as a biological control agent. Mycologia 91: 237-242

Bills S, Richter DL, Podila GK (1995) Genetic transformation of the ectomycorrhizal fungus *Paxillus involutus* by particle bombardment. Mycol Res 99:557-561

Blechert O, Kost G, Hassel A, Rexer R-H, Varma A (1999) First remarks on the symbiotic interactions between *Piriformospora indica* and terrestrial orchids. In: Varma A, Hock B (eds) Mycorrhizae 2nd Edition, Springer-Verlag, Germany, pp 683-688

Brody H, Carbon J (1989) Electrophoretic karyotype of *Aspergillus nidulans*. Proc Natl Acad Sci 86: 6260-6263

Brown JS, Aufauvre-Brown A, Holden DW (1998) Insertional mutagenesis of *Aspergillus fumigatus*. Mol Gen Genet 259: 327-335

Cabib E, Roberts R, Bowers B (1979) Synthesis of the Yeast cell-wall and its regulation. Ann Rev Microbiol 33:21-39

Chang TT, Ko WH (1990) Resistance to fungicides and antibiotics in *Phytophthora parasitica*: Genetic nature and use in hybrid determination. Phytopathology 80: 1414-1421

Cheng Y, Bélanger R R (2000) Protoplast preparation and regeneration from spores of the biocontrol fungus *Pseudozyma flocculosa*. FEMS Microbiol Lett 190:287-291

Chitinis AMV, Deshpande MV (2002) Isolation and regeneration of protoplasts from the yeast and mycelial form of the dimorphic zygomycetes *Benjaminiella poitrasii*: Role of chitin metabolism for morphogenesis during regeneration. Microbiol Res 157: 29-37

Chiu SW (1996) Nuclear changes during fungal development. In: Chiu SW, Moore D (eds) Patterns in fungal development. Cambridge University Press, Cambridge, United Kingdom, pp 105-125

Costanzo MC, Fox TD (1988) Transformation of yeast by agitation by glass beads. Genetics 120: 667-670

Davies JFT, Potter JR, Linderman RG (1992) Mycorrhiza and repeated drought exposure exposure affect drought resistance and extraradical hyphae development of pepper plants independent of plant size and nutrient content. J Plant Physiol 139: 289-294

Davis B (1985) Factors influencing protoplast isolation. In: Peberdy JF, Ferenczy L (eds) Fungal Protoplasts, Dekker, New York, pp 45-71

De Guido MA, Pollastro S, Carlucci A, De Miccolis Angelini RM, Faretra F (2003) *Phomopsis viticola* is easily transformed with hph and Bmlr genes. J Plant Pathol 85:43-52

de Queiroz MV, Pizzirani-Kleiner AA, Azevedo JL (2000) Electrophoretic characterization of *Aspergillus Nidulans* strains with chromosomal duplications Genet Mol Biol 23: 293-297

de Vries OM, Wessels JG (1973) Release of protoplasts from *Schizophyllum commune* by combined action of purified 1,3-glucanase and chitinase derived from *Trichoderma viride*. J Gen Microbiol 76:316-330

Delgado JM, Herrera LS (1981) Protoplast fusion in the yeast *Candida utilis*. Acta Microbiol Acad Sci 28: 339-345

Delmore E (1989) Transformation of *Saccharomyces cerevisiae* by electroporation. Appl Environ Microbiol 55: 2242-2246

Dhawale SS, Paietta JV, Marzluf GA (1984) A new, rapid and efficient transformation procedure for *Neurospora*. Curr Genet 14: 241-246

Dias ES, Araujo EF, Guimaraes WV, Muchovej RMC (1996) Production and regeneration of protoplasts from the mycorrhizal fungus *Suillus granulatus*. W J Microbiol Biotechnol 12: 625-628

Dickinson DP, Isenberg I (1982) Preparation of spheroplasts from *Schizosaccharomyces pombe*. J Gen Microbiol 128: 651-654

Dooijewaard-Kloosterziel AMP, Sietma JH, Wooters JTM (1973) Formation and regeneration of *Geotrichum candidum* protoplasts. J Gen Microbiol 74:205-209

Eddy AA, Williamson DH (1957) A method for isolating protoplasts from yeast. Nature 179: 1252-1253

Eddy AA, Williamson DH (1959) Formation of aberrant cell-walls and of spores by the growing yeast protoplasts. Nature 183:1101-1104

Elbouami F (2000) Isolation and regeneration of protoplasts from mycelium of *Fusarium solani*. African Crop Sci J 9: 351-358

Färber P, Geisen R (2000) Karyotype of *Penicillium nalgiovense* and assignment of the penicillin biosynthetic genes to chomosome IV. Int J Food Microbiol 58: 59-63

Farkas V (1979) Biosynthesis of Cell-Wall of Fungi. Microbiol Ver 43: 117-144

Farkas V, Svoboda A (1980) Kinetics of â-glucan and chitin formation by cells and protoplasts of the yeast *Saccharomyces cerevisiae*. Curr Microbiol 4:99-104

Farman ML, Leong LA (1995) Genetic and physical mapping of telomeres in the rice blast fungus *Magnaporthe grisea*. Genetics 140: 479-492

Farquhar ML, Peterson RL (1990) Induction of protoplast formation in the ectomycorrhizal fungus *Paxillus involutus* by the root rot pathogen *Fusarium oxysporum*. New Phytol 116:107-113

Fawcett PA, Loder PB, Ducan MJ, Beesley TJ, Abraham EP (1973) Formation and properties of protoplasts from antibiotic producing strains of *Penicillium chrysogenum* and *Cephalosporium acremonium*. J Gen Microbiol 79: 293-309

Ferenczy L, Maraz A (1977) Transfer of mitochondria by protoplast fusion in *Saccharomyces cerevisiae*. Nature 268: 524-525

Fierro F, Gutiérrez S, Díez B, Martín JF (1993) Resolution of four large chromosomes in penicillin-producing filamentous fungi: the penicillin gene cluster is located on chromosome II (9.6 Mb) in *Penicillium notatum* and chromosome I (10.4 Mb) in *Penicillium chrysogenum*. Mol Gen Genet 241:573-578

Fincham JRS (1989) Transformation in fungi. Microbiol Rev 53:148-170

Finkelman MAJ, Zajic JE, Vardanis (1980) A New Method of Producing Protoplasts of *Aureobasidium pullulans*. Appl Environ Microbiol 39:923–925

Finkelstein DB (1992) Transformation. In: Finkelstein DB, Ball C (Eds) Biotechnology of Filamentous Fungi: Technology and Products. Butterworth-Heinemann, Boston pp 113-156

Foury F, Goffeau A (1973) Combination of 2-deoxyglucose and snail gut enzyme treatments for preparing spheroplasts of *Schizosaccharomyces pombe*. J Gen Microbiol 75: 227-229

Frank AB (1885) Ueber die auf Wurzelsymbiose beruhende Ernaehrung gewisser Baeume durch unterirdische Pilze. Ber Dtsch Bot Ges 3: 128-145

Fukuda H, Kirimura A (1991) Protoplast formation of a yeast *Hansenula jaldinii*, and release of hexokinase. Agric Biol Chem 55:1171-1173

Fukui K, Sagara Y, Yoshida N, Matsuoka T (1969) Analytical studies on the regeneration of protoplasts of the yeast *Saccharomyces cerevisiae*. Curr Microbiol 4: 99-104

Furlaneto MC, Pizzirani-Kleiner AA (1992) Intraspecific hybridisation of Trichoderma pseudokoningii by anastomosis and by protoplast fusion. FEMS Microbiol Lett 90: 191-196

Gems D, Aleksenko A, Belenky L, Robertson S, Ramsden M., Vinetsky Y, Clutterbuck AJ (1994) An 'instant gene bank' method for gene cloning by mutant complementation. Mol Gen Genet 242: 467-471

Gems D, Johnstone JL, Clutterbuck AJ (1991). An autonomously replicating plasmid transforms *Aspergillus nidulans* at high frequency. Gene 98: 61-67

Giaja J (1919) Emploi des ferments dans les etudes de physiologie cellulaire: Le globule de levure depouille de sa membrane. C R Soc Biol Fil Paris 82: 719-720

Gibson RK, Buckey CE, Peberdy JF (1976) Fungal Protoplasts: Isolation, Reversion, and Fusion. Protoplasma 89:381-387

Gokhale AV (1991) Fungal protoplast fusion: a tool for breeding industrial strains. J Sci Ind Res 95: 497-506

Goldman GH, Geremia R, Van Montagu M, Esterella A (1990) Transformation of lamentous fungi by high voltage electroporation. BioRad Laboratory Bulletin

Goosen T, Bos CJ, van den Broek H (1992) Transformation and gene manipulation in filamentous fungi: an overview. In: Arora DK, Elander RP, Mukerji KG (eds) Handbook of applied mycology, Fungal biotechnology, Marcel Dekker, Inc., New York, USA, pp 151-195

Gritz L, Davies J (1983) Plasmid encoded hygromycin B resistance:the sequence of hygromycin B phosphotransferase gene and its expression in *Escherichia coli* and *Saccharomyces cerevisiae*. Gene 25:179-188

Gu YH, Ko WH (2000) Occurrence of parasexual cycle in *Phytophthora parasitica* following protoplast fusion. Bot Bull Acad Sin 41: 225-230

Hamlinton JG, Calvet J (1964) Production of protoplasts in an osmotic mutant of *Neurospora crassa* without added enzyme. J Bacteriol 88:1084-1086

Hamlyn PF, Ball C (1979) Recombination studies with *Cephalosporium acremonium*. In: Subek OK, Laskin AI (eds) Third International Symposium on the Genetics of Industrial Micro-organisms, American Society for Microbiology, Washington DC, pp 185-191

Hamlyn PF, Bradshaw RE, Mellon FM, Santiago CM, Wilson JM Peberdy JF (1981) Efficient protoplast isolation from fungi using commercial enzymes. Enzyme Microbial Technol 3: 321-325

Harris GM (1982) Protoplasts from *Gibberella fujikaroi*. Phytopathology 72: 1403-1407

Hawksworth DL, Kirk PM, Sutton BC, Pegler DN (1995) Dictionary of the fungi. 8th ed. Cambridge: International Cambridge

Hebraud M, Fevre M (1988) Protoplast production and regeneration from mycorrhizal fungi and their use for isolation of mutants. Can J Microbiol 34:157-161

Hoh YK, Tan TK, Chua SL, Lim G (1992) Protoplast fusion of â-glucosidase producing *Aspergillus niger* strains. Appl Biochem Biotechnol 37: 81-88

Hondel Van den CAMJJ, Punt PJ (1991) Gene transfer systems and vector development for filamentous fungi. In: Peberdy JF, Caten CE, Ogden JE, Bennett JW (eds) Applied Molecular Genetics of Fungi. Cambridge University Press, pp 1-28

Huang D, Bahiri S, Staples RC (1989) A transformation procedure for *Botryotinia squamosa*. Curr Genet 15: 411-414

Hynes JM (1986) Transformation of filamentous fungi. Exp Mycol 10: 1-8

Isaac S, Gokhale AV (1982) Autolysis: A tool for protoplast production from *Aspergillus nidulans*. Trans Br Mycol Soc 78:389-394

Ito H, Fukuda Y, Murata K, Kimura A (1983) Transformation of intact yeast cells treated with alkali cations. J Bacteriol 153:163-168

Jain S, Durand H, Tiraby G (1992). Development of a transformation system for the thermophilic fungus *Talaromyces* sp. CL240 based on the use of phleomycin resistance as a dominant selectable marker. Mol Gen Genet 234: 489-493

Kahmann R, Basse C (1999) REMI (Restriction Enzyme Mediated Integration) and its impact on the isolation of pathogenicity genes in fungi attacking plants. Eur J Plant Pathol 105: 221-229

Kaldorf M, Koch B, Rexer K-H, Kost G, Varma A (2005) Patterns of Interaction between Populus Esch5 and Piriformospora indica: A Transition from Mutualism to Antagonism. Plant Biol 7: 210-218

Kaster KR, Burgett SG, Rao RN, Ingolia TD (1983) Analysis of a bacterial hygromycin B resistance gene by transcriptional and translational fusions and by DNA sequencing. Nucleic Acids Res 11: 6895-6911

Kaul W, Rossow U, Emeis CC (1993) Screening for microorganisms with cell-wall lytic activity to produce protoplast forming enzymes. Appl Microbiol Biotechnol 39: 574-576

Kayser T, Schulz G (1991) Electrophoretic karyotype of cellulolytic *Penicillium janthinellum* strains. Curr Genet 20: 289-291

Kevei F, Peberdy JF (1977) Interspecific hybridization between *Aspergillus nidulans* and *Aspergillus rugulosus* by fusion of somatic protoplasts. J Gen Microbiol 102:255-262

Kevei F, Peberdy JF (1979) Induced segregation in interspecific hybrids of *Aspergillus nidulans* and *Aspergillus rugulosus* obtained by protoplast fusion. Mol Gen Genet 170: 213-218

Khedkar R, Patil A, Rai, MK (2005) Isolation and regeneration of protoplasts from *Cantharellus cibarius* Fr. edible ectomycorrhizal mushroom. Int J Med Mush 7:1-213

Kirimura K, Nakajima I, Lee SP, Kawabe S, Usami S (1988) Citric acid production by the diploid strains of *Aspergillus niger* obtained by protoplast fusion. Appl Microbiol Biotechnol 27: 504-506

Kitamoto Y, Mori N, Yamamoto M, Ohiwa T, Ichikawa Y (1988) A simple method for protoplast formation and improvement of protoplast regeneration from various fungi using an enzyme from *Trichoderma harzianum*. Appl Microbiol Biotechnol 28: 445-450

Kovac L, Subik J (1970) Some aspects of the preparation of yeast protoplasts and isolation of mitochondria. Acta Fac Med Uni Brun 37: 91-94

Kreger DR, Kopecka M (1976) On the nature and formation of the fibrillar nets produced by protoplasts of *Saccharomyces cerevisiae* in liquid media: an electronmicroscopic, X-ray diffraction and chemical study. J Gen Microbiol 92: 207–220

Kropp BR, Fortin JA (1986) Formation and regeneration of protoplasts from the ectomycorrhizal basidiomycetes *Laccaria bicolor*. Can J Bot 64: 1224-1226

Larraya LM, Pérez G, Peñas MM, Baars JJP, Mikosch TSP, Pisabarro AG, Ramírez L (1999) Molecular karyotype of the white rot fungus *Pleurotus ostreatus*. Appl Environ Microbiol 65: 3413-3417

Layton AC, Kuhn DN (1988) Heterokaryon formation by protoplast fusion of drug- resistant mutants in *Phytophthora megasperma* f. sp. Glycinea Exp Mycol 12: 180-194

Lewis LA (1969) Genetic evidence for hybridization in an interspecific cross in the genus *Sordaria*. J Gen Microbiol 59: 359-367

Lopes JFF, Araujo EF de, Queiroz MV de (2004) Easy detection of green florescent protein transformants in *Penicillium griseoroseum*. Genet Mol Res 3: 449-455

Louis EJ, Naumova ES, Lee A, Naumov G, Haber JE (1994) The chromosome end in yeast: its mosaic nature and influence in recombinational dynamics. Genetics 136: 789-802

Lucas JA, Greer G, Oudemens PV, Coffey MD (1990) Fungicide sensitivity in somatic hybrids of *Phytopthora capsici* obtained by protoplast fusion. Physiol Mol Plant Pathol 36:175-187

Maier FJ, Schafer W (1999) Mutagenesis via insertional or restriction enzyme-mediated-integration (REMI) as a tool to tag pathogenicity related genes in plants pathogenic fungi. Biol Chem 380: 855-864

Malla R, Prasad R, Kumari R, Giang PH, Pokharel U, Oelueller R and Varma A (2005) Phosphorus solubilizing symbiotic fungus: *Piriformospora indica*. Endocytobiosis Cell Res 15: 579-600

Marmeisse R, Gay G, Debaud JC, Casselton LA (1992) Genetic transformation of the Basidiomycete fungus *Hebeloma cylindrosporum*. Curr Genet 22: 41-45

Martínez AI, Castillo L, Garcerá A, Elorza MV., Valentín E, Sentandreu R (2004) Role of Pir1 in the construction of the *Candida albicans* cell-wall. Microbiology 150: 3151-3161

Martinková L, Musilkova M, Ujcova E, Machek F, Seichert L (1990) Protoplast fusion in *Aspergillus niger* strains accumulating citric acid. Folia Microbiol Prague 35: 143-148

McQuillen K (1960) Bacterial Protoplasts.In: Gunsalus C, Stainer RY (eds) The bacteria. Academic Press, London, pp 249-349

Meinecke G (1960) Protoplasts from *Penicillium glaucum*. Nature 188: 426

Mills D, McCluskey K (1990) Electrophoretic karyotypes of fungi: the new cytology. Mol. Plant-Microbe Interact 3: 351-357

Mishra NC, Tatum EL (1973) Non-mendelian inheritance of DNA-induced inositol independence in *Neurospora*. Proc Natl Acad Sci 70: 3875-3879

Moore PM, Peberdy JF (1976) Release and regeneration of protoplasts from the conidia of *Aspergillus flavus*. Trans Br Mycol Soc 66: 421-425

Morton JB, Franke M, Bentivenga SP (1995) Developmental foundations for morphological diversity among endomycorrhizal fungi Glomales. In: Varma A, Hock B (eds) Mycorrhiza, Springer-Verlag, Germany, pp 669-684

Musilkova M, Fencl Z (1966) Formation of protoplasts in *Aspergillus niger*. Folia Microbiol 11: 472-474

Musilkova M, Fencl Z (1968) Some factors affecting the formation of protoplasts in *Aspergillus niger*. Folia Microbiol 13: 235-239

Necas O (1956) Regeneration of yeast cells from naked protoplasts. Nature 177: 898-899

Necas O (1971) Cell wall synthesis in yeast protoplasts. Bacteriol Rev 35:149-170

Necas O (1980) Advances in protoplast research. In: Ferenczy L, Farkas GL (eds) Akademiai Kiado, Budapest: Pergammon Press, Oxford, pp 151-161

Necas O, Svoboda A (1981) In: Arnold WN (ed) Yeast cell envelopes: Biochemistry, Biophysics and Ultrastructure. CRC Press, Boca Raton, pp 105-128

Necas O, Svoboda A (1985) Cell-wall regeneration and protoplast reversion. In: Peberdy JF, Ferenczy L (eds) Fungal Protoplasts, Dekker, New York, pp 115-133

Necas O, Svoboda A, (1974) Proceedings of the Fourth International Symposium on Yeasts, Vienna, pp D13

Nelson CE (1987) The water relations of vesicular-arbuscular mycorrhizal system. In: Saif GR (ed) Ecophysiology of VA mycorrhizal plants, CRC Press, Boca Raton, pp 71-91

Oelmüller R, Peškan-Berghöfer T, Shahollari B, Trebicka A, Sherameti Irena, Varma A (2005) MATH-domain proteins represent a novel protein family in *Arabidopsis thaliana* and at least one member is modified in roots in the course of a plant/microbe interaction. Physiol Plant 124:152-166

Ogawa K, Yoshida E N, Gesnara W, Omumasaba C A (2000) Hybridization and breeding of the benomyl resistant mutant, *Trichoderma harzianum* antagonized to phytopathogenic fungi by protoplast fusion. Biosc Biotechnol Biochem 64:833-836

Orbach MJ, Porro EB, Yanofsky C (1986) Cloning and characterization of the gene for â-tubulin from a benomylresistant mutant of *Neurospora crassa* and its use as a dominant selection marker. Mol and Cell Biol 6: 2452-2461

Peberdy (1985) Mycolytic enzymes. In: Peberdy JF, Ferenczy L (eds) Fungal Protoplasts, Dekker, New York, pp 31-44

Peberdy JF (1976) Microbial and plant protoplasts. In: Peberdy JF, Rose AH, Rogers HJ, Cocking EC (eds) Academic Press, New York, pp 39-50

Peberdy JF (1979a) Fungal protoplast: isolation, reversion and fusion. Ann Rev Microbial 33: 21-39

Peberdy JF (1979b) Fungal walls and hyphal growth. In: Burnett JH, Trinci APJ (eds) British Mycological society symposium series-2, held 6-7April,1978,Queen Elizabeth college London, ISBN,0521-2249-9,Cambridge University Press

Peberdy JF (1989) Fungi without coats-protoplasts as tools for mycological research. Mycol Res 93: 1-20

Peberdy JF (1995) Fungal protoplasts. In: Kueck (ed) The Mycota II. Genetics and Biotechnology, Springer-Verlag Berlin, pp 49-60

Peberdy JF, Gibson RK (1971) Regeneration of *Aspergillus nidulans* protoplasts. J Gen Microbiol 69: 325-330

Peng M, Lemke PA, Shaw JJ (1993) Improved conditions for protoplast formation and transformation of *Pleurotus ostreatus*. Appl Microbiol Biotechnol 40: 101-106

Peraza L, Ortiz MA, Peberdy JF, Aguilar G (2003) Growth and pectinase production by *Aspergillus* Mexican strain protoplast regenerated under acidic stress Appl Biochem Biotechnol 111:15-27

Pigac J, Hranueli D, Tamara S and Alacevic M (1982) Optimal cultural and physiological conditions for handling *Streptomyces rimosus* protoplasts. Appl Environ Microbiol 44: 1178-1186

Popov B, Reuter G, Meyer HW (1980) Cell-wall regeneration of Canadida specs. protoplasts.Z Alleg Mikrobiol 20:47-62

Price JS and Strock R (1975) Production, purification and characterization of an extracellular chitosanase from *Streptomyces*. J Bacteriol 124:1574-1585

Pukkila PJ (1992) Methods of genetic manipulation in Coprinus cinereus. In: Chang ST, Buswell JA, Miles PJ (eds) Culture collection and breeding of edible mushrooms. Gordon and Breach, Philadelphia, pp 249-264

Pukkila PJ, Skrzynia C (1993) Frequent changes in the number of reiterated ribosomal RNA genes throughout the life cycle of the basidiomycete *Coprinus cinereus*. Genetics 133: 203-211

Pukkila, PJ, Casselton LA (1991) Molecular genetics of the agaric Coprinus cinereus. In: Bennet JW, Lasure LL (eds) More gene manipulation in fungi. Academic Press Inc, San Diego, California, pp125-150

Rai M, Varma A (2002) Field performance of *Withania somnifera* Dunal after inoculation with three species of Glomus. J Basic Appl Mycol 1:74-80

Rai M, Varma A (2005) Arbuscular Mycorrhiza-like biotechnological potential of *Piriformospora indica*, which promotes the growth of *Adhatoda vasica Nees*. Electronic J Biotechnol 8: 107-112

Rai MK, Singh A, Arya D, Varma A (2001) Positive growth responses of *Withania somnifera* and *Spilanthes calva* were cultivated with *Piriformospora indica* in field. Mycorrhiza 11: 123-128

Redman RS, Rodriguez RJ (1992) Molecular transformation and genome analysis of *Colletotrichum* In: Bailey JA, Jeger M (eds) *Colletotrichum*: biology, pathology, and control. CAB, Oxford, pp 47-66

Richey MG, Marek ET, Schardl CL, Smith DA (1989) Transformation of lamentous fungi with plasmid DNA by electroporation. Phytopathology 79: 844-847

Rincones J, Meinhardt LW, Vidal BC, Pereira GA (2003) Electrophoretic karyotype analysis of *Crinipellis perniciosa*, the causal agent of witches' broom disease of *Theobroma cacao*. Mycol Res 107: 452-458

Robinson M, Sharon A (1999) Transformation of the bio-herbicide *Colletotrichum gloeosporioides* f. sp. Aeschynomene by electroporation of germinated conidia. Curr Genet 36: 98-104

Rodriguez Aguirre MJ, Garcia Acha I, Villanueva JR (1964) Formation of protoplasts from *Fusarium culmorum* by strepzyme. Antonie van Leeuwenhoek J Microbiol Serol 30: 33-44

Rolland S, Jobic C, Fevre M, Bruel C (2003) Agrobacterium-mediated transformation of *Botrytis cinerea*, simple purification of monokaryotic transformants and rapid conidia-based identification of the transfer-DNA host genomic DNA flanking sequences. Curr Genet 44: 164-171

Rowley BI, Bull AT (1977) Isolation of a yeast-lysing *Arthrobacter* species and the production of lytic enzyme complex in batch and continuous flow fermentors. Biotechnol Bioeng 19: 879-899

Roy A (1999) Immobilization of *Piriformospora indica*. M. Phil. thesis submitted to SLS, JNU, New Delhi

Rubinder K, Chadha BS, Singh S, Saini HS (2000) Amylase hyper-producing haploid recombinant strains of *Thermomyces lanuginosus* obtained by intraspecific protoplast fusion. Can J Microbiol 46: 669-673

Ruiz-Díez B (2002) Strategies for the transformation of filamentous fungi. J Appl Microbiol 92: 189-95

Sahay NS, Varma A (1999) *Piriformospora indica*: a new biological hardening tool for micropropagated plants, FEMS Microbiol Lett 181: 297-302

Sahay NS, Varma A (2000) Biological approach towards increasing the survival rates of micropropagated plants. Curr Sci 78: 126-129

Sanchez O, Aguirre J (1996) Efficient transformation of *Aspergillus nidulans* by electroporation of germinated conidia. Fungal Genet Newslett 43: 48-51

Sandhu DN, Wadhwa V, Bagga PS (1989) Use of lytic enzymes for protoplast production in *Trichoderma reesei* QM 9414. Enz Microbiol Technol 11:21-25

Sanford JC (1988) The biolistic process. Trends Biotechnol 6: 299-302

Santos M, Vallejo I, Rebordinos L, Gutiérrez S, Collado IG, Cantoral JM (1996) An autonomously replicating plasmid transforms *Botrytis cinerea* to phleomycin resistance. FEMS Microbiol Lett 137: 153-158

Sarachek A, Rhoads DD, Schwarzhoff RH (1981) Hybridization of *Candida albicans* through fusion of protoplasts. Arch Microbiol 129:1–8109

Sawicka-Zukowska R, Juszczakiewicz D, Misiewicz A, Krakowiak A, Jedrychowska B (2004) Intensification of lipase biosynthesis as a result of electrofusion of *Rhizopus cohnii* protoplasts. J Appl Genet 45:37-48

Schwencke J, Magana-Schwencke N, Laporte J (1977) Yeast protoplasts from stationary and starved cells: preparation, ultrastructure and vacuolar development. Ann Microbiol 128: 3-18

Selitrennikoff CP, Bloomfield EC (1984) Formation and regeneration of protoplasts of wild-type *Neurospora crassa*. Curr Microbiol 11: 113-118

Singh A (2001) Intergeneric hybridization between a yeast strain and a plant growth promoting endophytic fungus by isolation, fusion and regeneration of somatic protoplasts. Ph. D. thesis, Microbial Technology, School of Life Sciences, Jawaharlal Nehru University, New Delhi

Singh A, Sharma J, Rexer KH, Varma A (2000) Plant productivity determinants beyond minerals, water and light. *Piriformospora indica*: a revolutionary plant promoting fungus. Curr Sci 79:101-106

Sipiczki M, Ferenczy L (1977) Fusion of *Rhodosporidium* (Rhodotorula) protoplasts. FEMS. Microbiol Lett 2: 203-205

Smith SE, Gianinazzi-Pearson V (1988) Physiological interactions between symbionts in vesicular arbuscular mycorrhizal plants. Ann Rev Plant Physiol and Plant Mol Biol 39: 221-244

Smith SE, Read DJ (1997) Mycorrhizal symbiosis, 2nd edn, Academic Press, London

Solís S, Flores ME, Huitrón C (1996) Protoplasts from pectinolytic fungi: isolation, regeneration and pectinolytic enzyme production. Lett Appl Microbiol 23: 36-42

Solís S, Flores ME, Huitrón C (1997) Improvement of pectinase production by interspecific hybrids of *Aspergillus* strains. Lett Appl Microbiol 24: 77-81

Sonnenberg ASM, Groot PD, Schaap PJ, Baars JJ, Visser J, Griensven LJV (1996) Isolation of expressed sequence tags of *Agaricus bisporus* and their assignment to chromosomes. Appl Environ Microbiol 62: 4542-4547

Spencer JFT, Bizeau C, Reynolds N, Spencer DM (1985) The use of mitochondrial mutants in hybridization of industrial yeast strains. Curr Genet 9: 649-652

Stephen ER, Nasim A (1981) Production of protoplasts in different yeasts by mutanase. Can J Microbiol 27: 550-553

Stewart GG (1981a) The place of yeast in biotechnology. Ind J Biotechnol 21: 171-210

Stewart GG (1981b) The genetic manipulation of industrial yeast strains. Can J Microbiol 27: 973-990

Stinchcomb DT, Strhul K, Davies RW (1979) Isolation and characterization of yeast chromosomal replicator. Nature 282: 39-43

Suarez T, Eslava AP (1988) Transformation of Phycomyces with a bacterial gene for kanamycin resistance. Mol Cell Biol 212:120-123

Sun CB, Kong QL, Xu WS (2002) Efficient transformation of *Penicillium chrysogenum* mediated by *Agrobacterium tumefaciens* LBA4404 for cloning of *Vitreoscilla* hemoglobin gene. Electronic J Biotechnol 5: 1-8

Svoboda A (1978) Fusion of yeast protoplasts induced by polyethylene glycol. J Gen Microbiol 109:169-175

Svoboda A, Piedra D(1983) Reversion of yeast protoplasts in media containing polyethylene glycol. J Gen Microbiol 129: 3371-3377

Tahoun MK (1993) Gene manipulation by protoplast fusion and penicillin production by *Penicillium chrysogenum*. Appl Biochem Biotechnol 39: 445-453

Takada H, Yamamoto BT (1963) Regeneration Fragmentierter, Nackter Protoplasten In Hefezellen. Protoplasma 57:730-741

Tamaki H (1982) Genetic properties of abortive products resulting from the protoplast fusion in yeasts. Mol Gen Genet 187:177-179

Thomas KR, Davis B (1980) The effect of calcium on protoplast release from species of *Aspergillus*. Microbios 28: 69-80

Tisdall JM (1994) Possible role of soil micro-organisms in aggregation in soils. Plant and Soil 159:115-121

Trappe JM (1987) Phylogenetic and ecological aspects of mycotrophy in the Angiosperms from an evolutionary standpoint. In: Safir GR (ed) Ecophysiology of VA mycorrhizal plants. CRC Press, USA, pp 5-25

Tsujibaka Y, Tominga Y, Iwai M (1975) Purification and some properties of the lytic enzyme from *Bacillus* R-4 that acts on the *Rhizopus* cell-wall. Agric Biol Chem 39:145-152

Tully M, Gilbert HA (1985) Transformation of *Rhodosporidium toruloides*. Gene 36: 235-240

Typas MA (1983) Heterokaryon incompatibility and interspecific hybridization between *Verticillium albo-atrum* and *Verticillium dahliae* following protoplasts fusion and microinjection. J Gen Microbiol 129: 3043-3056

Valk van der P, Wessels JGH (1977) Mitotic synchrony in multinucleate *Schizophyllum* protoplasts. Protoplasma 78: 427-432

Varavallo MA, Queiroz de MV, Pereira JF, Araújo de EF (2004) Isolation and regeneration of *Penicillium brevicompactum* protoplasts. Acta Scientiarum 26: 475-479

Varma (1999) Functions and application of arbuscular mycorrhizal fungi in arid and semi-arid soils. In: Varma A, Hock B (eds) Mycorrhiza: Structure, function and molecular biology, 2nd edition, Springer-Verlag, Germany, pp 521-556

Varma A (1995) Arbuscular mycorrhiza fungi: The state of art. Critical Reviews in Biotechnology, CRC Press, USA 15:179-199

Varma A, Singh A, Sudha, Sahay N, Sharma J, Roy A, Kumari M, Rana D, Thakran S, Deka D, Bharti K, Franken P, Hurek T, Blechert O, Rexer K-H, Kost G, Hahn A, Hock B, Maier W, Walter M and Strack D, Kranner I (2001) *Piriformospora indica*: a cultivable mycorrhiza-like endosymbiotic fungus. In: Mycota IX, Springer Series, pp 125-153

Varma A, Singh A, Sudha, Sahay NS, Sharma J, Roy A, Kumari M, Rana D, Thakran S, Deka D, Bharti K, Hurek T, Blechert O, Rexer K-H, Kost G, Hahn A, Maier W, Walter M, Strack D, Kranner I (2001) *Piriformospora indica*: an axenically culturable mycorrhiza-like endosymbiotic fungus. In: Hock B (ed) The Mycota IX, Springer-Verlag, Berlin, Heidelberg pp 125-150

Varma A, Verma S, Sudha, Sahay N, Britta B, Franken P (1999b) *Piriformospora indica* – a cultivable plant growth promoting root endophyte with similarities to arbuscular mycorrhizal fungi. Appl and Environ Microbiol 65: 2741-2744

Verdoes JC, Punt PJ, van den Berg P, Debets F, Stouthamer A, Hondel van den CAMJJ, (1994) Characterization of an efficient gene cloning strategy for *Aspergillus niger* based on an autonomously replicating plasmid: cloning of the nicB gene of *A. niger*. Gene 146: 159-165

Verma S, Varma A, Rexer KH, Hassel A, Kost G, Sarabhoy A, Bisen P, Bütenhorn B Franken P (1998) *Piriformospora indica*, gen. et sp. nov., a new root colonizing fungus. Mycologia 90: 896-903

Vermeulen CA, Wessels JGH (1984) Ultrastructural differences between wall apices of growing and non-growing hyphae of *Schizophyllum commune*. Protoplasma 120: 123-131

Viaud M, Couteaudier Y, Riba G (1998) Molecular analysis of hypervirulent somatic hybrids of the entomopathogenic fungi *Beauveria bassiana* and *Beauveria sulfurescens*. Appl Environ Microbiol 64: 88-93

Vries OMH, Wessels JGH (1973a) Effectiveness of lytic preparation from *Trichoderma viride* resulting in spheroplasts from fungi, particularly basidiomycetes. J Gen Serol 39: 397-400

Vries OMH, Wessels JGH (1973b) release of protoplasts of *Schizophyllum commune* by combined action of purified b-1,3 glucanase and chitinase derived from *Trichoderma viride*. J Gen Microbiol 76: 319-330

Waller F, Achatz B, Baltruschat H, Fodor J, Becker K, Fischer M, Heier T, Hückelhoven R, Neumann C, von Wettstein D, Franken P, Kogel K-H (2005) The endophytic fungus *Piriformospora indica* reprograms barley to salt-stress tolerance, disease resistance, and higher yield. Procd Natl Acad Sci 102:13386-13391

Weaver JC (1995) Electroporation theory: concepts and mechanisms. In: Nickolo J (ed) Electroporation protocols for microorganisms. Humana Press, Totowa, pp 1-26

Weibull C (1953) The isolation of protoplasts from *Bacillus megaterium* by controlled action of lysozyme. J Bacteriol 66: 688-695

Wessels JGH (1994) Developmental Regulation of Fungal Cell-wall Formation. Annual Rev Phytopatho 32:413-437

Woestmeyer A, Woestmeyer J (1998) Fungal protoplasts: relics or modern objects of molecular research? Microbiol Res 153: 97-104

Yamamoto S, Kobayashi R, Nagasaki S (1974) Physicochemical, chemical and enzymatic properties of a crystalline yeast cell-wall lytic enzyme from a *Rhizopus* mould. Agric Biol Chem 38:1563-1573

Young C, Itoh Y, Johnson R, Garthwaite I, Miles CO, Munday-Finch SC, Scott B (1998) Paxilline-negative mutants of *Penicillium paxilli* generated by heterologous and homologous plasmid integration. Curr Genet 33: 368-377

Zhao K, Zhou D, Ping W, Ge J (2004) Study on the Preparation and Regeneration of Protoplast from Taxol-producing fungus *Nodulisporium sylviforme*. Nat Sci 2:52-59

Zhou DP, Ping WX (1990) Protoplast fusion of micro-organism, Hei Longjiang, Publishing House of the Science Technology

Zhou QW, Zhang YC, Zhou LZ (1984) Studies on the isolation and regeneration of *Acremonium chrysogenum* protoplasts. Acta Microbiologica Sinica 24: 345-351

Zolan ME (1995) Chromosome-length polymorphism in fungi. Microbiol Rev 59: 686-698

Zolan ME, Heyler NK, Stassen NY (1994) Inheritance of chromosome-length polymorphisms in Coprinus cinereus. Genetics 137: 87-94

Fungal Phytases in Ameliorating Nutritional Status of Foods and Combating Environmental Phosphorus Pollution

B SINGH, P KAUR and T SATYANARAYANA*

1. INTRODUCTION

In biological systems, hydrolysis of phytic acid to myo-inositol and inorganic phosphate by phytases (myo-inositol hexakis-phosphate phosphohydrolase) is an important reaction for energy metabolism, metabolic regulation and signal transduction pathways. Phytic acid (*myo*-inositol-hexakis-dihydrogenphosphate) is an organic form of phosphorus, which is abundantly present in plants comprising 1-5% (by weight) of edible legumes, cereals, oilseeds, pollens and nuts. It is largely unavailable to monogastrics such as poultry, pigs, fish and humans, due to the lack of adequate levels of phytases. The phytic acid present in the plant derived food acts as an anti-nutritional factor, since it causes mineral deficiency due to efficient chelation of metal ions such as Ca^{2+}, Mg^{2+}, $Zn^{2+}$and Fe^{2+}, forms complexes with proteins, thus affecting their digestion and also inhibits some digestive enzymes like α-amylase, trypsin, acid phosphatase and tyrosinase (Boling et al. 2000). Due to the lack of adequate levels of phytases in monogastric animals (poultry, pigs, fishes and humans), phytic acid is excreted in faeces, which is degraded by soil micro-organisms, releasing phosphorus in the soil. This phosphorus reaches aquatic bodies, leading to eutrophication. Phytic acid can be removed by some physical (autoclaving, cooking) and chemical (ion exchange, acid

Department of Microbiology, University of Delhi South Campus, Benito Juarez Road, New Delhi-110 021, India. E-mail: tsnarayana@vsnl.net

hydrolysis) methods, but these methods decrease the nutritional value of the food. Therefore, the reduction of phytic acid content in foods and feed by enzymatic hydrolysis using phytase is desirable as it improves the nutritional value of the food. This enzyme also has potential applications in other fields, and is of immense commercial value primarily in feed and food industries. The annual sale of commercial supplemental phytase is estimated as US$50 million, which is one third of the entire feed enzyme market and is still increasing (Sheppy 2001).

During the last fifteen years, phytases have attracted considerable attention from both scientists and entrepreneurs in the areas of nutrition, environmental protection, and biotechnology. Undoubtedly, increasing public concern regarding the environmental impact of high P-levels in animal excreta has driven the biotechnological development of phytase and its application in animal nutrition. Numerous experiments have shown the effectiveness of supplemental microbial phytases in improving utilization of phytate-P and the phytate-bound minerals by swine and poultry (Lei and Stahl 2001). Nutritionally, inorganic P supplementation in the diets for swine and poultry can be obviated by including adequate amounts of phytase, along with appropriate manipulation of other dietary factors (Han et al. 1997). As a result, the P excretion of these animals may be reduced by up to 50% (Lei et al. 1993a,b). Nevertheless the cost and thermo-tolerance constraints of the current commercial phytases have precluded widespread use of these enzymes in animal feeds. This article describes the role of fungal phytases in improving nutritional value of foods, and further in combating environmental phosphorus pollution.

2. PHOSPHORUS AND ITS ENVIRONMENTAL IMPACT

There are numerous indispensable biochemical roles of phosphorus (P) in living organisms as it forms the vital components of the genetic material i.e. DNA and RNA, and of the biospheric currency of metabolism i.e. ATP and ADP. Hence, no life is possible without phosphorus (Deevey 1970). The biogeochemical cycling of P is very slow and thus, P tends to be growth-limiting element in most soils and aquatic systems. Mineral rocks like apatites are the primary source of P in the environment, but P in these is usually present in poorly soluble, and hence, unutilizable forms. On weathering, P is released in solution and forms various orthophosphate forms (PO_4^{3-}, HPO_4^{2-} or $H_2PO_4^-$). If these are not immediately taken up by living organisms, they tend to react with various cations in soil and become fixed (Khasawneh et al. 1980). Erosion and run-off from soils causes transport of these insoluble P salts into water bodies, where P is released by microbial activities, leading to phosphorus pollution problems. Addition of fertilizers, plant residues, agricultural and animal wastes also contribute to the build up of excess P in soils and later in water bodies (Smil 2000).

The high P levels are a threat to the water quality. As in unfertilized soils, P is often the limiting nutrient in aquatic systems, and hence, its excess tends to promote the growth of algae and other aquatic microbes and plants. This in turn leads to higher oxygen requirement and growth continues till either oxygen or phosphorus becomes limiting. Limitation of dissolved oxygen tends to affect the aerobic organisms in the ecosystem and leads to the death of fish, thus leading to further increase in demand for oxygen required for decomposition until it eventually depletes (*anoxia*). Blooms of blue-green algae produce *neurotoxins* and *hepatotoxins*, thus causing further death in aquatic ecosystems as well as serious public health problems (Martin and Cooke 1994). This changes the entire system from aerobic to anaerobic, further leading to more unpleasant changes like surface scums, odours, and increased population of insects and pests. Thus phosphorus pollution leads to eutrophication, which is essentially the process of a lake's biological death due to depleted available oxygen.

One pound of P can result in the growth of 350-700 lbs. of green algae. These include blooms of cyanobacteria (*Anabaena*, *Aphanizomenon*, *Oscillatoria*), siliceous algae (*Asterionella*, *Melosira*), scum-forming algae (*Phaeocystic pichetii*) and potentially toxic algae like *Dinophysis* and *Gonyaulux* (Smil 2000). Thus enrichment of surface waters with phosphorus is clearly undesirable. The harmful effects of eutrophication on economy includes increased water treatment costs to remove odour, turbidity and colour; negative impact on navigational and recreational activities like fishing, boating and swimming, thus adversely affecting tourism and property values. Reversal of eutrophication is a very tedious process requiring phosphorus reduction of 70-90% to cause any significant change. As P is the key nutrient to manage water bodies as 'clean' or 'green', controlling the amount of phosphorus entering the aquatic systems is important to prevent excessive growth. In the US, the United States Environmental Protection Agency (USEPA) has recommended a limit of 0.05 ppm and 0.1 ppm of total P in lakes and flowing streams, respectively, as the critical values to control eutrophication (USEPA 1986).

3. PHYSIOLOGY OF PHYTATE AND ITS ROLE IN NUTRITION

Phytate can exist in a metal-free form or in metal–phytate complex, depending on the pH of the solution and the concentration of metal cations (Fig. 1A). At acidic pH, protonation of the phosphate groups of phytate generates the metal-free form. At neutral pH, in contrast, deprotonation of

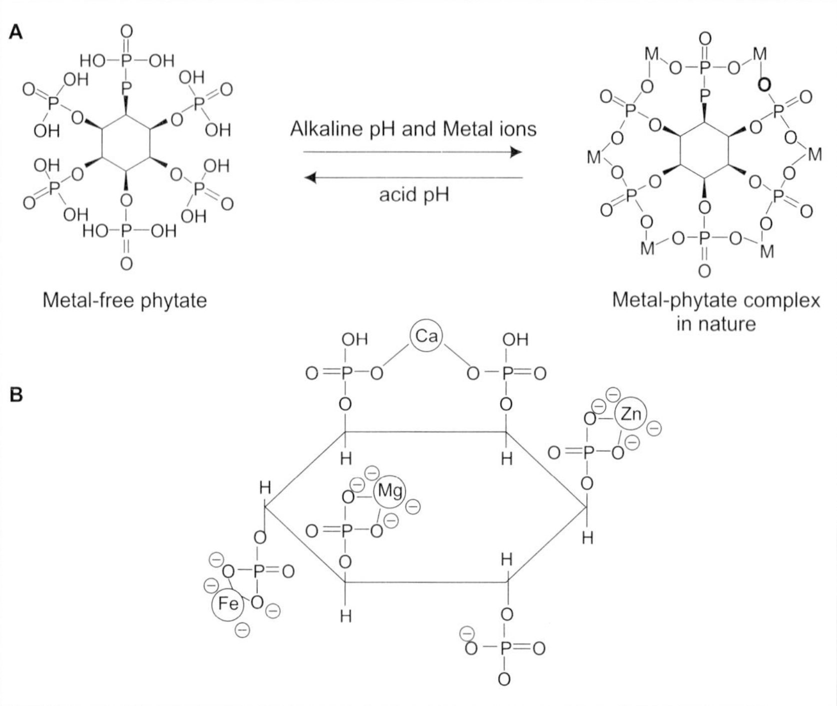

Fig. 1 Effect of divalent metal cations and pH on physiological nature of phytate

the phosphate groups of phytate enhances the affinity for divalent metal cations and, thus, phytate forms metal–phytate complexes with divalent metal cations, mostly Mg^{2+} and Ca^{2+} (Cheryan 1980; Maenz et al. 1999). The binding pattern of metals depends upon the ionic radii of the metal ions. The divalent metal cations with large ionic radii (Ca^{2+} and Sr^{2+}) bind two oxianions from the phosphate groups of phytate in a bidentate fashion (Martin and Evans 1986). However, divalent metal cations with small radii, such as Mg^{2+} (0.65 Å), Fe^{2+} (0.74 Å), and Zn^{2+} (0.71 Å), bind in a monodentate fashion within two oxygen atoms from the phosphate groups of phytate (Fig. 1B). Therefore, bidentate metal-complex formation prefers divalent cations with large ionic radii (Jonson and Tate 1969; Cheryan 1980). In addition to its role in phosphate storage, phytate acts as a strong chelator for divalent metal cations and exists as a stable metal–phytate complex with metal ions in plants (Asada et al. 1969; Reddy et al. 1982).

Due to the interaction of *phytic acid* with other compounds, it acts as an anti-nutritional factor in several ways as described below:

1. Six reactive groups in the molecules of IP_6 make it a strong chelating agent, which binds cations such as Ca^{2+}, Mg^{2+}, Fe^{2+}, Zn^{2+}. Under gastrointestinal pH conditions, insoluble metal phytate complexes are formed which make the metal unavailable for absorption in the intestinal tract of animals and humans (Maga 1982).
2. Phytates reduce digestibility of proteins, starch and lipids. Phytate complexes with proteins, and thus, making them insoluble. There is an evidence for the fact that phytate-protein complexes are less subject to proteolytic digestion than the same protein alone (Harland and Morris 1995).
3. The action of certain enzymes such as amylase, trypsin, acid phosphatase and tyrosinase has been shown to be inhibited by phytic acid and also by inositol pentaphosphate (Harland and Morris 1995).

3.1 Phytases

Phytases (myo-inositol hexaphosphate phosphohydrolase EC 3.1.3.8 & EC 3.1.3.26) hydrolyze phytic acid to myo-inositol and inorganic phosphates through a series of myo-inositol phosphate intermediates, and eliminate anti-nutritional characteristics of phytic acid. There are two phytases as classified by Nomenclature Committee of the International Union of Biochemistry and Molecular Biology (NC-IUBMB) in consultation with the IUPAC-IUBMB Joint Commission on Biochemical Nomenclature (JCBN):

3-phytase (EC 3.1.3.8), which first hydrolyses the ester bond at the 3 position of myo-inositol hexakisphosphate. It is typical of micro-organisms.

6-phytase (EC 3.1.3.26), which first hydrolyses the ester bond at the 6 position of myo-inositol hexakisphosphate. It is typical of plants. But recently it has been reported from some Basidiomycetous fungi (Lassen et al. 2001).

Besides this classification, recently phytases have also been classified as HAP (Histidine acid phosphatase), BPP (β-Propeller phytase) and PAP (purple acid phosphatase) depending upon their catalytic properties (Mullaney and Ullah 2003).

3.2 Histidine Acid Phosphatase Phytases (HAP)

HAPs (EC 3.1.3.8) are the most commonly studied phytases, which share a common active site motif, RHGXRXP, and a two-step mechanism that hydrolyzes phosphomonoesters (Ullah et al. 1991). The substratum specificity of all known HAPs for phytic acid varies from one to another as described and explained by Wyss et al. (1999). They proposed two classes of HAP phytases on the basis of the catalytic properties of several fungal phytases. One class has broad substratum specificity but a lower specific activity for phytic acid, and the second class has narrow substratum specificity but a high specific activity for phytate. *A. niger* NRRL 3135 phytase (phyA) is widely known for its high specific activity for phytic acid (Wodzinski and Ullah 1996). Another phytase (phyB) has been isolated from *A. niger* NRRL 3135 (Ullah and Cummins 1987), which showed distinct catalytic properties as compared to *A. niger* NRRL 3135 phyA. It was later identified as an *A. niger* acid phosphatase with an optimum pH 2.5 (Ullah and Phillippy 1994). Kostrewa et al. (1999) explained the high specific activity for phytate by revealing its substratum specificity site (SSS) that is specific for phytic acid. This model also offers a reason that other less charged substrates do not bind as effectively to the SSS of *A. niger* NRRL 3135 phyA. Kostrewa et al. (1999) identified the SSS of phyB, which was different from the SSS of phyA by having just two amino acids; in *A. niger* T213 phyB they are D75 and E272. This means the phyB SSS is more electrostatically neutral, and therefore, can accommodate a broader substrata spectrum (Kostrewa et al. 1999, Wyss et al. 1998) than *A. niger* phyA. At pH 2.5, the SSS of *A. niger* T213 phyB is uncharged and will accept negatively charged phytate as a substratum; however, at pH 5.0, it is negatively charged and would thus repel a negatively charged substratum (Kostrewa et al. 1999). Another difference between *A. niger* phyA and phyB is that the active form of phyA is a monomer, whereas the active form of phyB is a tetramer (Wyss et al. 1998). HAPs have been reported in filamentous fungi, bacteria, yeasts and plants (Mullaney et al. 2000).

3.3 β-Propeller Phytase

BPP (EC 3.1.3.8) is a recently discovered class of enzyme with a novel mechanism for hydrolyzing its substratum. They have a unique three-dimensional model, with their molecules display a basic form similar to a propeller with six blades, that is why the name BPP (Ha et al. 2000). They have been reported in *Bacillus subtilis* (phyC) [Kerovuo et al. 1998] and *Bacillus amyloliquefaciens* (TS-Phy) [Kim et al. 1998]. Unlike HAP, BPP requires Ca^{2+} for thermostability and catalytic activity (Oh et al. 2001). BPP has two phosphate binding sites viz. cleavage and affinity site (Shin et al. 2001). The hydrolysis of its substrate occurs at the 'cleavage site', while the 'affinity site' enhances the binding affinity for substrates like phytic acid. Recently, a class of enzymes, pyrophosphatase (PPase), has been identified which shares some structural features with β-propeller phytase (Hamelrych 2003). Both types of enzymes have similar catalytic mechanism. As in BPP, in PPase too, a water nucleophile that is coordinated to two metal ions, attacks the phosphorus atom of its substrate. Moreover, both enzymes contain a 'cleavage site' and an 'affinity site'. The nucleophilic attack by the water molecule occurs in the former and the binding of a second phosphate group in the latter (Hamelrych 2003).

3.4 Purple Acid Phosphatase: Soya bean (*Glycine max* L. Merr.) phytase (GmPhy)

Another phytase, GmPhy (EC 3.1.3.2), has recently been isolated from the cotyledons of germinating soya beans (Hegeman and Grabau 2001). GmPhy has the active site motif of a purple acid phosphatase (PAP). This class of metalloenzyme has been widely studied (Klabunde et al. 1994). Both its three-dimensional structure (Strater et al. 1995) and a proposed mechanism of catalysis are known (Klabunde et al. 1996). Searches of genomic databases have revealed PAP-like sequences in plants, mammals, fungi and bacteria (Schenk et al. 2000). The estimated size of purified GmPhy, 70–72 kDa, suggests a molecular mass similar to other plant PAPs (Hegeman and Grabau 2001). However, GmPhy is the only known PAP reported to have significant phytase activity. An *A. niger* NRRL 3135 PAP has previously been reported that displays only a minimum ability to utilize phytate as a substratum (Ullah and Cummins 1988). The lower catalytic activity of GmPhy than that of *A. niger* NRRL 3135 phyA may be necessary during germination in soybeans because the germination process requires a steady breakdown of phytate over a period of several days (Gibson and Ullah 1988). While a three dimensional model of GmPhy is not available, a model of another PAP, kidney bean purple acid phosphatase (KBPAP), is available. Both GmPhy and kidney bean PAP share the purple acid phosphatase active site motif and a common catalytic mechanism. Amino acid sequence comparison revealed 33% homology between the two enzymes. The structural differences in these three classes of enzymes are shown in Fig. 2.

3.5 Sources of Phytases

Phytases can be derived from a host of sources including plants, animals and micro-organisms (bacteria, yeasts and fungi), although microbial sources are more promising for the production of phytases on a commercial scale (Pandey et al. 2001; Vohra and Satyanarayana 2003; Vats and Banerjee 2004). Over 200 fungal isolates belonging to the genera *Aspergillus, Mucor, Penicillium* and *Rhizopus* have been shown to produce phytases extracellularly. Shieh and Ware (1968) screened 2000 cultures for

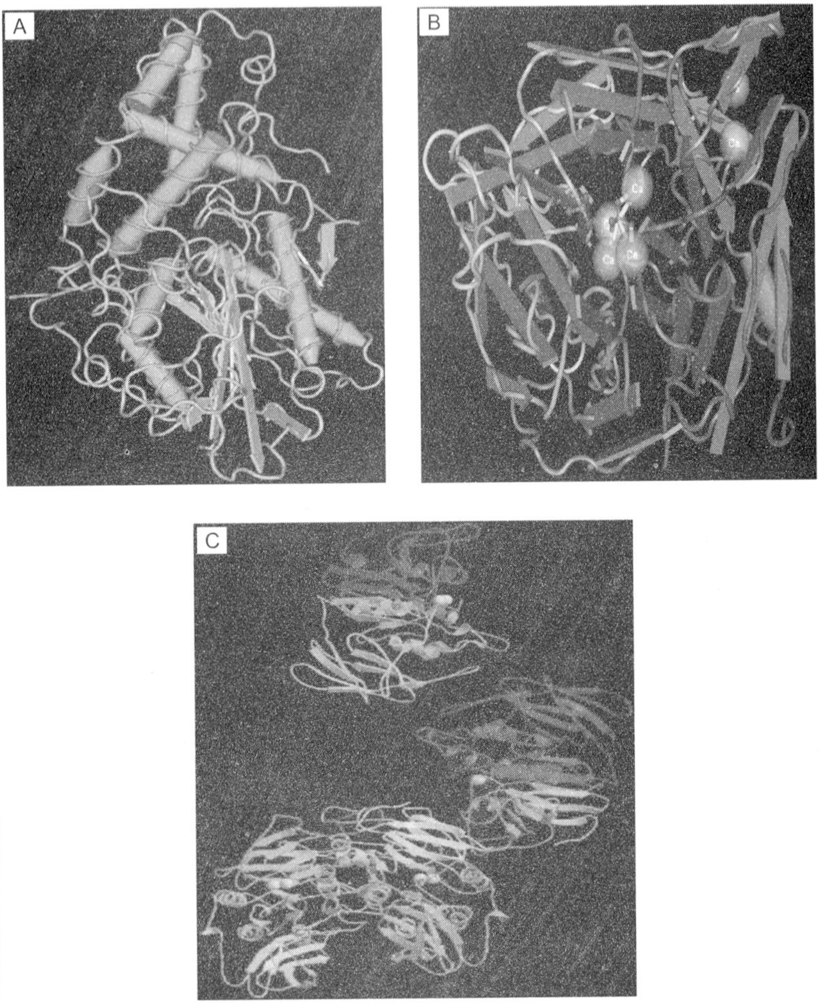

Fig. 2 Computer generated molecular models HAP (A), BPP,(B) and PAP(C) from National Center for Biotechnology Informatics web site [from Mullaney and Ullah, 2003]

phytase production from 68 soil samples, while Howson and Davis (1983) surveyed 84 fungal species for phytase production. Of all the organisms surveyed, *A. niger* NRRL 3135 was identified as the most potent phytase producer in corn starch (Shieh and Ware 1968) and semisynthetic (Howson and Davis 1983) media. It produced two different phytases, phyA and phyB with pH optima at 5.5 and 2.5 and the other optimally active at pH 2.0 and temperature optima at 55°C, respectively. Phytase from *Aspergillus fumigatus* was optimally active at pH 6.0-6.5, 37°C and 64% moisture (Pasamontes et al. 1997). Phytase activity has been found most frequently in fungi, such as *Aspergillus terreus* (Yamada et al. 1968), *A. ficuum* (Gibson 1987), and *A. niger* (Shieh and Ware 1968). Phytase has been reported from many yeasts like *Schwanniomyces castellii* (Lambrechts et al. 1992), *Arxula adeninivorans* (Sano et al. 1999), *Pichia anomala* (Vohra and Satyanarayana 2001), *Candida krusei* (Quan et al. 2001) and others. Phytase was detected in whole cells in fungi such as *Aspergillus clavatus* J239, *A. flavipes* Fla A-14, *A. flavus, A. nidulans* QM-329, *A. niger* NRRL 67, *A. niger* P330, *A. niger, A. oryzae* QM228, *A. phoenicus* QM 329, *A. repens* QM-44C, *A. terreus* Fla.C-93, *A. tamarii* J1008, *Mucor* spp., *Penicillium* spp. P-320 and *Rhizopus* spp. (Casida 1959).

Besides the above mentioned mesophilic fungi, thermophilic fungi also produce phytases. *Thermomyces lanuginosus* phytase exhibited optimum activity at 65°C and pH of 6.0 (Berka et al. 1998). Another thermophilic fungus *Sporotrichum thermophile* produced phytase optimally at 45°C and at pH 6.0 (Ghosh 1997). The fungi *Chaetomium thermophilum* (ATCC 58420), *Rhizomucor miehi* (ATCC 22064), *Thermomucor indicae-seudaticae* (ATCC 28404) and *Myceliophthora thermophila* (ATCC 48102) (Mitchell et al. 1997) are also known to produce phytases. *Rhizomucor pusillus* secreted phytase optimally at 50°C and pH 5.5 in SSF using wheat bran (Chadha et al. 2004). *Thermoascus aurantiacus* produced phytase in a semisynthetic medium comprising glucose, starch and wheat bran (Namapoothiri et al. 2004), while Pasamontes et al. (1997) cloned phytase gene from a thermophilic fungus *Talaromyces thermophilus.*

3.6 Production of Phytases

Both *solid-state fermentation* (SSF) and *submerged fermentation* (SmF) are being employed for phytase production (Pandey et al. 2001; Vohra and Satyanarayana 2003; Vats and Banerjee 2004). Commercially, however, phytases are produced using submerged fermentation (SmF). But recently scientists all over the world are focusing on solid-state fermentation (SSF) due to its advantages over SmF (Pandey et al. 1999; Pandey et al. 2001). The culture conditions, type of strain, nature of substratum and availability of nutrients should be taken into consideration for selecting a particular production technique, as they are the critical factors affecting the yield. The production of phytase from *Aspergillus ficuum* NRRL 3135 has been achieved by three different cultivation methods, viz. solid state (Bogar et al. 2003a,b), semi-solid (Han et al. 1987) and submerged (Howson and Davis 1983; Ullah and Gibson 1987) fermentations. It was reported that there was a complete reduction of phytic acid content in canola meal by

A. niger NRRL 3135 using SSF (Nair and Duvnjak 1990). Ebune et al. (1995) also studied phytase production by *A. ficuum* using canola meal and found that the age of inoculum had profound effect on enzyme synthesis. Krishna and Nokes (2001) studied the effect of culture conditions, particularly inoculum age, media composition and duration of SSF on phytase production by *A. niger*. Bogar et al. (2003) reported phytase production by *A. ficuum* NRRL 3135, *Mucor racemosus* NRRL 1994 and *Rhizopus oligosporus* NRRL 5905 on canola meal, cracked corn, soya bean meal and wheat bran in SSF. Optimization studies carried out using statistical designs like Plackett-Burman and response surface methodology (RSM) showed improvement in phytase production when wheat bran was supplemented with starch and ammonium sulphate. The fermentation conditions (pH 5.3, 30°C, 54.5% moisture content) of phytase production in SSF using canola oil cake with no additional nutrients by *R. oligosporus* were reported in literature (Sabu et al. 2002). Mayer et al. (1999) developed a pilot scale process (2000 L) for the low cost production of phytase, using recombinant *Hansula polymorpha* containing phytase genes of *A. fumigatus* (Pasamontes et al.1997) and *A. terreus* (Mitchell et al. 1997). Kim *et al.* (1999) studied phytase production by *Aspergillus* sp. 5990 in SmF at 37°C and pH 7.0, where five-fold higher activity in liquid culture was attained. Papagianni et al. (2000) investigated qualitative relationship between medium composition, morphology and phytase production by *A. niger*. *Mucor racemosus* NRRL 1994 secreted phytase on sesame oil cake but maximal production was achieved on coconut oil cake in solid-state fermentation (Bogar et al. 2003). A high phytase production in mixed substrata fermentation was recorded using coconut and sesame oil cake (Ramchandra et al. 2005). *Aspergillus niger* NCIM563 produced phytase maximally on cowpea meal followed by wheat bran (Mandviwala and Khire 2000), while *A. niger* PD synthesized phytase on cassava dregs in SSF (Hong et al. 2001). *Aspergillus ficuum* NRRL3135 and *Rhizomucor pusillus* produced phytase maximally on wheat bran (Bogar et al. 2003a; Chadha et al. 2004). It is evident from these observations that fungi have varied preferences for substrata for the production of phytase in SSF. Martin et al. (2003) had cloned and expressed phyA gene of *Aspergillus awamori* and *A. fumigatus* under the transcriptional control of glaA promoter of *A. awamori*. A Kex-2 protease cleavage site was inserted between native glucoamylase and heterologous protein for the efficient processing of chimeric proteins by endogenous Kex-2 protease. A high phytase expression (200 U/ml) was achieved in SmF.

Phytase production from some yeasts like *Pichia anomala* has also been extensively studied. A synthetic medium containing glucose (4%) and beef extract (1%), supplemented with Fe^{2+} (0.15 mM) supported high phytase titres when incubated at 20°C for 24 hrs. (Vohra and Satyanarayana 2001).

Further enhancement in the titres was achieved using the statistical approach, response surface methodology (RSM), whereby the interaction of 3 variables (glucose, beef extract and inoculum density) was studied. The final concentrations of glucose (2%) and beef extract (0.5%) were half of those initially used (Vohra and Satyanarayana 2002b). A medium consisting of cane molasses, a by-product of sugarcane industry, was also formulated that supported an improved phytase yield with reduced production cost as compared to that in the synthetic glucose-beef extract medium (Vohra and Satyanarayana 2004). A significant increase in cell-bound phytase content in cane molasses medium (176 U/g dry biomass) as compared to synthetic medium (100 U/g dry biomass), and an overall 86.6% enhancement in phytase yield was attained in the optimized cane molasses medium in fed-batch fermentation. This economical cane-molasses medium was further optimized using statistical approaches, Plackett-Burman and RSM, for attaining a higher biomass yield and cell-bound phytase by *P. anomala* (Kaur and Satyanarayana 2005). An overall 5- and 1.6-fold enhancement in phytase titres and biomass production were attained due to statistical optimization, respectively. Maximum phytase yield by the yeast, *C. krusei* WZ-001 was attained in 48 hrs. (late exponential phase) at 30°C and pH 7.0 in a medium comprising glucose (5%) and polypeptone (0.7%) as suitable carbon and nitrogen sources, respectively; however, phytase synthesis was repressed by the presence of phosphate in the medium (Quan et al. 2001).

High phosphate conditions are known to repress the synthesis of acid phosphatases and phytases, while limiting phosphate conditions result in their expression (Vohra and Satyanarayana 2003; Vats and Banerjee 2004). In a survey of phytase producing micro-organisms, *A. ficuum* was found to produce highest amount of phytase, when the inorganic phosphorus content was in the range of 0.0001–0.005%, the optimum being 0.4 mg/100 ml with 8% cornstarch (Shieh and Ware 1968). Han and Gallagher (1987) also confirmed that high phosphorus concentration inhibited phytase synthesis by *A. niger* NRRL 3135. Gibson (1987) further confirmed the effect of phosphorus level in the medium and compared the production from several sources, speculating the phosphoester linkage in some starch sources may be more resistant to cleavage than others, resulting in low but steady supply of phosphorus. Vats and Banerjee (2002) have also reported a sharp decline in phytase production by *A. niger* even at 0.05% phosphorus in the medium with absolute no production at 0.1% and above, indicating end product inhibition in phytase synthesis. Han et al. (1987) observed similar trend for phytase production by *A. ficuum* on semisolid substrate using soybean meal where 10 mg P/100 g substrate in the growth medium resulted in high phytase secretion (82.5 U/g substrate) as compared to a control without added phosphate (8.0 U/g substratum), while higher phosphate levels inhibited phytase production. Kim et al. (1999) showed that extracellular phytase production by *Aspergillus* sp. 5990 was maximum at lower phosphate concentration (50 mg/l), while at higher concentration (100 mg/l), enzyme production was greatly reduced.

Surfactants are known to increase cell-membrane permeability, thus affecting enzyme secretion. Al-asheh and Duvnjak (1994) studied the effect of surfactants such as Tween-80, Triton-X-100 and Na-oleate on the phytase production and reduction of phytic acid content in canola meal by *Aspergillus carbonarius* in SSF. The phytase production increased in the presence of sodium oleate (1%) and Tween-80, suggesting alteration of the cell-membrane permeability thus resulting in higher release of enzyme. Han and Gallagher (1987) tested the same surfactants for their affect on phytase production by *A. ficuum* in liquid medium and reported that besides dispersed growth of mycelium, there was also a resultant increase in phytase level of 1.3, 1.7 and 4.8 times, when 0.5% of Triton-X-100, Tween-80 and Na-oleate were added to the medium, respectively. Similarly, Mandviwala and Khire (2000) reported 30% increase in phytase activity of *A. niger* NCIM 563 when 0.5% Triton-X-100 was added to the production medium. Enhanced phytase production by a thermophilic mould *Thermoascus aurantiacus* was reported in a semi-synthetic medium using Tween 20 and Tween 80 (Namapoothiri et al. 2004). However, the effect was high in case of Tween 20, but Triton X 100 exerted a negative effect on enzyme production. The conditions that favour phytase production by various fungi are given in Table 2.

3.6 Biochemical Properties of Phytases

Phytases widely exist in a variety of micro-organisms and plants and in some animal tissues (Liu et al. 1998). Most phytases belong to either the acid phytases or the alkaline phytases, depending on their optimal pH for catalytic activity. HAPs from *A. niger* (Howson and Davis 1983) and *A. fumigatus* (Ullah et al. 2000) have an optimal pH range of 4.5–5.5. All phytases are monomeric proteins, except for phytase B from *A. niger*, which is a tetramer. The molecular masses of the enzymes are quite variable, within the range of 38–100 kDa. Glycosylation has no effect on the specific activity and thermostability of phytases. The higher molecular weights of fungi and yeast enzymes are due to glycosylation of the enzymes (Wyss et al. 1999b). Most phytases have an optimal temperature of 44–60°C. In contrast, phytases from *A. fumigatus* has an optimum temperature of about 70°C (Table 1). To use phytases as animal feed additives, thermostability of the enzyme is a highly desirable property during the animal feed-pelleting process (80–100°C). Phytases are high

Table 1 The biochemical properties of phytases from various fungi

Source	*MW (kDa)*	T_{opt}	pH_{opt}	K_m *(mM)*	*pI*	*Specificity*	*Reference*
Aspergillus carneus	-	40	5.6	-	-	-	Ghareib, 1990
A. fumigatus	75	58	5.0	-	-	-	Mullaney *et al.*, 2000
A. fumigatus	85–100	58	5.0	-	-	-	Ullah *et al.*, (2000)
A. niger	85	58	2.5, 5.0	0.04	4.5	P	Ullah and Gibson (1987)
A. niger	85–100	60	2.5	-	-	-	Ullah and Phillippy (1994)
A. niger SK-57	60	50	5.5, 2.5	0.0187	-	P	Nagashima *et al.*, 1999
A. niger	-	55	5.5	0.20	4.9	-	Berka *et al.*, 1998
A. niger	353	55	2.5	0.606	-	P	Vats and Banerjee 2005
A. terreus	214	70	4.5	-	-	-	Wyss *et al.*, (1999a)
A. oryzae	120–140	50	5.5	0.33	4.15	B	Shimizu (1993)
A. nidulans	77.8	55	5.5	-	-	-	Wyss *et al.*, (1999b)
Rhizopus oligosporus	-	55	4.5	0.15	-	-	Sutardi and Buckle, 1988
R. oligosporus	124	65	5.00	0.010	-	B	Casey and Walsh, 2004
R. niger ATCC9142	84	65	5.0	0.10	-	B	Casey and Walsh 2003
Peniophora lycii	72	50-55	4-4.5	-	3.61	-	Lassen *et al.*, 2001
Ceriporia sp.	59	55-60	5.5-6.0	-	7.36-8.01	-	Lassen *et al.*, 2001
Agrocybe pediades	59	50	5.0-6.0	-	4.15-4.86	-	Lassen *et al.*, 2001
Trametes pubescens	62	50	5.0-5.5	-	3.58	-	Lassen *et al.*, 2001
Thermomyces lanuginosus	60	65	7.0	0.11	4.7-5.2	B	Berka *et al.*, 1998
Thermoascus aurantiacus	-	55	-	-	-	-	Nampoothiri *et al.*, 2004
Rhizomucor pusillus	-	70	5.4	-	-	B	Chadha *et al.*, 2004
Myceliopthora thermophila	-	37	6.0	-	-	B	Mitchell *et al.*, 1997

Contd.

Table 1

Source	MW (kDa)	T_{opt}	pH_{opt}	K_m (mM)	pI	Specificity	Reference
Saccharomyces cerevisiae	-	45	4.6	-	-	-	Nayini (1984)
Schwanomyces castellii	490	77	4.4	0.038	-	B	Segueilha *et al.*, (1992)
Arxula adeninivorans	-	75	4.5	0.23	-	P	Sano *et al.*, 1999
Clavispora lusitaniae	-	70	4.0	-	-	-	Nakamura *et al.*, 2000
Pichia anomala	64	60	4.0	0.20	-	B	Vohra and Satyanarayana 2002
P. rhodanensis	-	70-75	4.0-4.5	0.25	-	-	Nakamura *et al.*, 2000
P. spartinae	-	75-80	4.5-5.0	0.33	-	-	Nakamura *et al.*, 2000

B= broad substrate and p= phytate-specific

Table 2 Conditions for the production of phytase by various fungi

	Production conditions					
Source	*pH_{opt}*	*T_{opt}*	*Fermentation*	*C-source*	*N-source*	*Reference*
Fungi						
A. fumigatus SRRC 322	5.0	37	SmF	Hylon starch	$NaNO_3$	Mullaney *et al.*, 2000
A. niger SK-57	5.0	30	SSF	wheat bran	–	Nagashima *et al.*, 1999
A. niger	5.5	30	SmF	glucose starch	–	Vats and Banerjee 2005
A. niger	5.0	30	SmF	corn starch, glucose	peptone	Papagianni *et al.*, 2001
A. ficuum	5.0	30	SSF	canola meal, glucose	–	Ebune *et al.*, 1995
A. ficuum	5.0	30	SmF	Corn starch, glucose	$NaNO_3$	Shieh and Ware, 1968
A. oryzae	6.4	37	SmF	glucose	$(NH_4)_2SO_4$	Shimizu (1993)
*A. oryzae*AK 9	—	30	SSF	rice flour	soyameal	Chanatasartrasamee *et al.*, 2005
Rhizopus oligosporus	5.5	27	SmF	corn starch, glucose	$NaNO_3$	Casey and Walsh, 2004
R. oligosporus	5.5	30	SSF	coconut oil cake	–	Sabu *et al.*, 2002
R. oryzae	5.5	30	SSF	Glucose	NH_4NO_3	Ramchandaran *et al.*, 2005
Mucor racemosus	5.5	30	SSF	starch	$NaNO_3$	Roopesh *et al.*, 2005
Peniophora lycii	5.5	26	SmF	maltodextrin, soya flour	peptone	Lassen *et al.*, 2001
Ceriporia sp.	"	"	"	"	"	"
Agrocybe pediades	"	"	"	"	"	"
Trametes pubescens	"	"	"	"	"	"
Thermoascus aurantiacus	5.5	45	SmF	starch, glucose, wheat bran	peptone	Nampoothiri *et al.*, 2004

Contd.

Table 2

	Production conditions					
Source	*pH_{opt}*	*T_{opt}*	*Fermentation*	*C-source*	*N-source*	*Reference*
Rhizomucor pusillus	8.0	50	SSF	wheat bran	asparagine, CSL	Chadha *et al.*, 2004
Myceliopthora thermophila	5.5	45	SmF	glucose	$NaNO_3$	Mitchell *et al.*, 1997
Pichia anomala	6.0	25	SmF	glucose	beef extract	Vohra and Satyanarayana 2001
Schwanomyces castellii	4.4	77	SmF	galactose	$(NH_4)_2SO_4$	Segueilha *et al.*, (1992)
Arxula adeninivorans	5.5	28	SmF	galactose	Yeast extract	Sano *et al.*, 1999
P. rhodanensis	4.5	70	SmF	glucose	-	Nakamura *et al.*, 2000
P. spartinae	4.5	75	SmF	glucose	-	Nakamura *et al.*, 2000
Candida krusei	4.6	40	SmF	glucose	Polypeptone	Quan *et al.*,, 2001

molecular-weight proteins ranging from 40-500 kDa. It can be a monomer as in *Pichia anomala* with 64 kDa (Vohra and Satyanarayana 2002a) and *Candida krusei* Wz-001 with 330 kDa (Quan et al. 2002) or a tetramer like from *Schwanniomyces castelli* with 490 kDa (Segueilha et al. 1992). The biochemical properties of phytases from various sources are summarised in Table 1.

4. AMELIORATION OF NUTRITIONAL STATUS OF FOODS

Phytases are useful in a large number of ways (Fig. 3) including in food and feed industries, preparation of myo-inositol phosphate intermediates, and combating phosphorus pollution (Vohra and Satyanarayana 2003, Kaur et al. 2003). The major food supplements in animal feeds are derived from plant sources such as cereals, legumes, etc. The presence of phytate in plant food stuffs (De Boland et al. 1975) is well known where they act as anti-nutritional factors and cause mineral deficiency. Canola meal contains 4-6% phytic acid, which reduces nutrition value of meal. This phytic acid has been shown to bind with multivalent cations and hence reduce their bioavailability. Following are the important roles of phytases in ameliorating the nutritional status of foods:

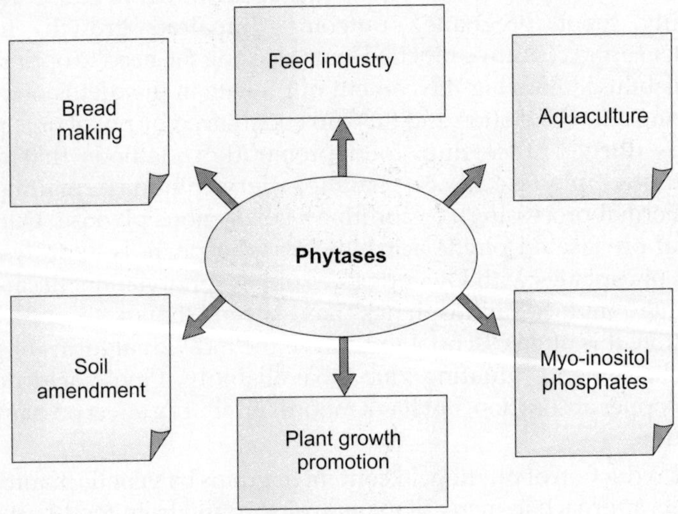

Fig. 3 Applications of Microbial Phytases

4.1 Effect of Phytase on Bioavailability of Minerals

Phytate makes complexes with various di- and trivalent cations as well as with proteins (Wise 1983). For example, calcium-bound phytate increases chelation with trace minerals, especially zinc, to form co-precipitates that make the zinc unavailable to animals. Phytase added to diets improves the bioavailability of copper and zinc in pigs (Adeola et al. 1995) and poultry (Yi et al. 1996). Microbial phytase also improves the apparent absorption of magnesium, zinc, copper and iron in pigs. Similar results have also been reported for fish. Phytase addition increases the concentration of minerals like magnesium, phosphorus, calcium, manganese and zinc in plasma, bone and the whole body (Vielma et al. 1998). Channel catfish fed phytase-supplemented diets had higher concentrations of ash, calcium, phosphorus and manganese in their bones than the control (Yan and Reigh 2002). Yan and Reigh (2002) further demonstrated that phytase supplementation at 500 units per kilogram of diet was sufficient to improve the retention of calcium, phosphorus and manganese by catfish fed with an all-plant protein diet. The microbial phytase supplementation significantly improved the digestibility of Ca, Mg, Mn, total-P, phytate-P, and gross energy (Cheng and Hardy 2002). Studies in animals and human subjects have shown that diets high in phytic acid can cause zinc deficiency, and that the phytate content is negatively correlated to zinc absorption. Sub-optimal zinc status has been shown to cause increased morbidity, poor pregnancy outcome, impaired growth, immune competence and cognitive function, emphasizing the need to optimize zinc bioavailability. Reducing the content of phytate in the diet is one way of improving zinc absorption and this can be achieved by novel precipitation methods during processing, food preparation methods that activate endogenous phytase (e.g. baking, fermentation, malting and hydrothermal processing), or addition of exogenous phytase. During the action of phytase on phytic acid, the hexaphosphate is hydrolysed into inositol phosphates with lower degrees of phosphorylation. Because only the penta- and hexaphosphates have been shown to inhibit zinc absorption, it is often essential to analyze the individual forms of phytate in the diet when evaluating zinc bioavailability. Phytic acid does not inhibit copper absorption, but has a modest inhibitory effect on manganese absorption.

The reduction of phytic acid content in grains by genetic manipulation is a novel approach to increase mineral absorption from food-based diets. Low phytic acid corn, rice, barley and soya bean genotypes have been generated and mineral absorption has been evaluated. Genetically modified low phytic acid plants could be a novel contribution to the reduction of micronutrient malnutrition and animal waste phosphorus.

But some more research needs to be done to understand the molecular biology and genetics of phytic acid accumulation during seed development and to know the negative and positive roles of dietary phytic acid in human health and the feasibility and effectiveness of the sustainable implementation of this approach at the community level (Mendoza 2002).

4.2 Effect of Phytase on Bioavailability of Phosphorus

The addition of phytase to high phytate containing diets improves the absorption and utilization of phosphorus (Hughes and Soares 1998). Dietary phytase also improves the nutritive value of canola protein concentrate and decreases phosphorus output in case of rainbow trout (Forster et al. 1999). Similar reports have been documented for different species like rainbow trout (Rodehutscord and Pfeiffer 1995), channel catfish (Li and Robinson 1997), African catfish (Van Weerd et al. 1999), and common carp (Schafer et al. 1995). Robinson et al. (2002) reported that 250 units of phytase per kilogram of diet could effectively replace dicalcium phosphate supplement in the diet of channel catfish without affecting growth, feed efficiency or bone phosphorus deposition. Microbial phytase is effective in enhancing the bioavailability of phosphorus considerably, thereby reducing the fecal phosphorus output.

4.3 Effect of Dietary Phytase on Protein Digestibility

Phytase treatment of soya-protein concentrate was found to improve protein digestibility and retention in Atlantic salmon (Storebakken et al. 1998). In addition, phytate binds trypsin in vitro and thus reduces protein digestibility (Singh and Krikorian 1982). Digestibility of dry matter (Papatryphon et al. 1999) and crude protein (Storebakken et al. 1998) were also improved by dietary phytase supplementation. The negative effect of phytate on protein utilization has been observed in fish. Phytase supplementation in plant-based practical diets has been reported to increase protein digestibility (Vielma et al. 1998). In poultry, phytase was reported to improve protein and amino acid utilization through breakdown of phytin-protein complexes (Kornegay 1995).

4.4 Effect of Phytase on Growth Performance of Monogastrics

Phytic acid is abundantly present in plant-derived foods, which are commonly used as animal feed ingredients. The presence of phytic acid (an anti-nutritional factor) makes all the minerals and protein unavailable to animals and forces external addition of inorganic phosphate into the diets. Therefore, the supplementation of phytases in the animal diets enables the farmers to use cheaper plant derived feed and enhances the bioavailability of all minerals and proteins for animals. Moulds commonly used in oriental food fermentations have been examined for their ability to produce phytase. Tempeh is a popular oriental fermented food made from soya beans inoculated with moulds (*Rhizopus oligosporus*) in the Koji process. The digestibility, vitamin content and flavour of soya bean were improved by the mould fermentation (Fardiaz and Markakis 1981). Soya beans are used in the animal diets as a good source of protein, but the presence of high phytate content deprives the animals from the protein content, since phytate binds to proteins and forms insoluble protein-phytate complex. Simell et al. (1989) used. Finase S phytase for the preparation of phytate-free soya-protein isolates. These protein isolates were more soluble at low pH (pH 3.0) than the control protein. The finase phytase can also be used in the production of phytate-free soya-milk. Anno et al. (1985) eliminated phytate from soya-milk before its consumption using wheat phytase from Sigma, while Khare et al. (1994) successfully hydrolyzed soya-milk phytate using immobilized wheat phytase. Extracellular phytase from *A. ficuum* NRRL3135 brought about dephytinization in legume products (Shieh et al. 1969). A 78% phytate loss occurred when *A. niger* phytase was mixed with soya bean meal and incubated for 15h (Han 1988). A crude preparation of intracellular acid phosphatase rich in phytase obtained from *A. niger* caused nearly complete dephytinization of protein isolates from soya bean in few hours (Zyta et al. 1989). Addition of *A. niger* phytase to the flour containing wheat bran increased iron absorption in humans (Sandberg et al. 1996). The use of phytase was suggested for producing low phytin bread. In commercial whole wheat bread, phytic acid is present at levels of 0.29 to 1.05% (w/w). By adding mould phytases during bread making, dough phytate could be almost completely eliminated. The desirable properties of phytase include Ca^{2+} independence, pH optimum of 4.5 to 5.0 and a high reaction rate at 30°C (Knorr et al. 1981). Caransa et al. (1988) reported that microbial phytase could accelerate the process of steeping required in the wet milling of corn, thereby improving the properties of corn steep liquor.

4.5 Role of Phytase in Aquaculture

The weight gain rates and specific growth rates of Indian major carp, *Labeo rohita* were significantly decreased when phytic acid was included in diet (Alvi 1994). Similar effects are evident on the growth performance and body composition of *Cirrhinus mrigala* fry (Usmani and Jafri 2002). When Chinook salmon, *Oncorhynchus tshawytscha*, was fed with semipurified diets containing various levels of calcium, phosphorus, zinc and sodium phosphate with a high dietary phytic acid, it exhibited depressed growth (Richardson et al. 1985). In contrast, the growth performance was increased when microbial phytase was supplemented in the diets. An increase in weight gain has been reported in channel catfish fed with phytase supplemented diets containing only plant protein or a combination of plant and animal protein sources (Jackson et al. 1996). Weight gain and feed consumption increased by 23.52 and 11.59%, respectively, compared to a control group. Similar performance of African catfish, *Clarias gariepinus* (Van Weerd et al. 1999) was also reported. The better performance of fish-fed phytase-supplemented diets implies that either the phosphorus requirement was met along with other nutrients or that phytase has other positive effect on performance. It has been reported that phytic acid inhibits some enzymes such as a-amylase (Sharma et al. 1978), trypsin, tyrosinase and pepsin (Graf 1986). This organic form of phosphorus is poorly utilized by man and other monogastric animals because either they lack phytase or have low level of phytase activity than required to catalyze the phytic acid hydrolysis. So hydrolysis of phytic acid prior to animal consumption would increase the availability of inorganic phosphorus and minerals in the animal diet. Phytic acid can be removed by several chemical and physical methods, such as autoclaving, cooking, and ion-exchange chromatography etc., but all these methods reduce the quality of food by destroying some nutrients. So the main solution of all these problems is the removal or degrading of phytic acid with the help of enzymes i.e. phytases. These enzymes not only degrade phytic acid but also make the availability of inorganic P and other minerals to the animals.

The effect of a commercial phytase (Natuphos®) from *A. niger* on growth, body minerals, phosphorus retention and phosphorus excretion was investigated by Schafer et al. (1995) in *Cyprinus carpio* (common carp). There was improved utilization of phytate-P and reduced phosphorus excretion. Body weight, body ash content and phosphorus content were enhanced after feed was supplemented with the enzyme. Phytase supplementation in extruded and expelled soya bean increased apparent digestibility coefficient (ADC) of magnesium, total phosphorus, phytate-phosphorus, manganese, zinc, crude protein (CP) and sulphur (Chang and Hardy 2002). A feeding trial was conducted for sixty days to study the effects of exogenous microbial phytase supplementation on the growth and nutrient digestibility of *Pangasius pangasius* fingerlings. Maximum weight gain, specific growth rate, protein efficiency ratio, apparent protein utilization, energy retention value and feed conversion efficiency were observed in diets supplemented with phytase. Apparent dry matter and protein digestibility in phytase-supplemented groups were significantly higher that the control diets (Debnath et al. 2005). Addition of phytase in the diet of rainbow trout fed with soya bean meal-based diets not only decreased phytic acid content of feces but also improved the apparent digestibility coefficient of phosphate, protein and Zn (Vielma et al. 2004). Rainbow trout was fed with microbial phytase supplemented into barley, canola meal, wheat and wheat middlings at 500 FTU per kg diet, to test the effectiveness of the phytase on digestibility of crude protein (CP), gross energy (GE) and minerals for rainbow trout. Results indicated that phytase supplementation significantly improved the digestibility of Ca, Mg, Mn, total-P, phytate-P, and GE (Cheng and Hardy 2002).

Phytase was added into the diets of Atlantic salmon to determine the separate and combined effects of phytic acid and phytase on feed intake, trypsin activity, digestibility and growth. The addition of phytic acid had no significant effect on feed intake or weight gain, it significantly reduced protein digestibility although there was no reduction in trypsin activity. Phytase inclusion neutralized the effect of phytic acid on protein digestibility. Phytase significantly enhanced growth whether included with or without phytic acid. Feed efficiency ratio was significantly improved for fish fed with the diet containing both phytase and phytic acid, but not separately (Sajjadi and Carter 2004). Effects of thermal and enzymatic treatments of soya bean meal on apparent absorption of total phosphorus, phytate phosphorus, nitrogen (protein), ash, calcium, magnesium, copper, iron, manganese, strontium and zinc were examined using rainbow trout, *Oncorhynchus mykiss* (Walbaum). Thermal treatments (microwaving, dry roasting, steam heating, cooking) had no measurable effect on the apparent absorption of phosphorus and other minerals. Phytase supplementation increased the apparent absorption of phosphorus, nitrogen (protein), ash, calcium, magnesium, copper, iron, strontium and zinc in low-ash diets containing soya bean meal, but had little effect in high-ash diets containing both soya bean and fish meal. Phytase supplementation also reduced the phosphorus content in the excreta (Sugiura et al. 2001). Effect of phytase, dietary protein, and citric acid was studied on intestinal digesta pH, bone ash and bone mineral contents in *Labeo rohita* juveniles. Addition of citric acid in the crude protein feed significantly decreased feed pH with concurrent decrease in intestinal digesta pH and increased the bone ash content. Dietary supplementation of microbial phytase significantly increased bone Na, Ca, K, P and Fe contents, whereas bone P and Mn content was significantly increased by addition of citric acid. Addition of phytase to plant-based diets increased the bioavailability of minerals, thereby increasing bone mineralization. This effect of phytase was enhanced by adding citric acid (Baruah et al. 2005).

4.6 Role of Phytase in Poultry

The supplementation of waste tea fungal biomass containing 179.38 g of crude protein, 120 g crude fibre, 4.82 g phosphorus, 6.56 g of calcium, phytase activity of 23 IU/mg protein and 8.92 MJ metabolizable energy per kilogram of biomass, at 150 g/kg poultry feed increased the feed consumption, body weight and performance efficiency factor. The histopathological examination of liver showed no abnormalities and the mortality rate (Murugesan et al. 2005). The inclusion of phytase to broilers diets with a low concentration of non-phytate phosphorus increased the coefficient of phosphorus retention and reduced the presence of this element in broiler excreta, thus, indicating a favourable environmental effect (Juanpere et al. 2004).

Brenes et al. (2003) investigated the effect of microbial phytase (Natuphos® 500) supplementation in chicks fed with different levels of available phosphorus (AP) and citric acid (CA) on performance, mineral retention (Ca, P, Mg, and Zn), bone and plasma minerals (Ca, P, Mg, and Zn), plasma total protein (TP), and serum *aspartate aminotransferase* (AST), *alanine aminotransferase* (ALT), *alkaline phosphatase* (ALP), and *lactate dehydrogenase* (LDH) activities. Phytase and citric acid supplementation increased Ca, P, and Zn retention in a linear fashion. Phytase supplementation increased tibia ash, tibia Ca, P and Zn contents, tibia weight and relative tibia and liver weights. Citric acid increased tibia ash and tibia Ca and P contents. By decreasing AP levels in the diet, plasma Ca and Zn concentrations as well as AST, ALP, and LDH activities increased. However, plasma P and TP content reduced. Phytase supplementation increased the plasma Ca, P, Mg, Zn and TP content, and serum AST, ALT, and LDH activities, but reduced serum ALP activity in linear fashion. Citric acid addition increased plasma Ca, Mg, and Zn content and reduced ALP activity. In conclusion, these results indicated that the addition of phytase to maize and soybean meal low-AP diets improved the performance and increased Ca, P, and Zn utilization in chicks. However, the inclusion of citric acid depressed the performance and caused an increase in mineral utilization. Growth response to phytase was negatively affected by citric acid. Maize and soya bean meal diets were supplemented with Phytase of *Aspergillus niger* and fed to chicks. The effects of enzyme on growth performance, apparent availability of P and Ca, tibia-and-toe ash and mineral contents of tibia were studied. Microbial phytase treatment of a low-P diet increased growth and relative retention of P and Ca, and improved bone mineralization in broiler chickens (Ahmad et al. 2000).

A basal poultry diet of corn-soya meal was supplemented with Zn and Mn in the presence or absence of microbial phytase. The addition of microbial phytases increased Zn and Mn availability in broilers (Mohanna and Nys, 1999). Phytate phosphorus in a mixture of ground maize, soya bean meal and wheat bran was decreased by 81%, when treated with native phytase from wheat bran and ground maize. This mixture was fed to chicks that resulted in increase in tibia bone ash weights as compared to control diet (Zhu et al. 1990).

The supplementation of feed of broiler chicks with cell-bound phytase of *Pichia anomala* resulted in improved growth (77.7% gain in control over 90.2% in biomass fed), better phosphorus retention in the body (29% in control over 73.6% in biomass fed) and reduced excretion of phosphorus in the faeces [Satyanarayana and Vohra 2004]. Thus the FCR (feed conversion ratio defined as the ratio of feed consumed per unit gain in body weight) of biomass fed chicks was lower than the control chicks, proving the economic viability of the *P. anomala* phytase (Vohra et al. 2005).

4.7 Role of Phytase in Piggery

The effects of *Aspergillus niger* phytase, organic acids, and their interaction was studied on animal performance, nutrient digestibility and urine composition. Microbial phytase positively affected the animal performance and their daily gain and feed conversion ratio were enhanced by the organic acids, and there was no synergistic effect. The apparent total tract digestibility of dry matter, ash, Ca and P were significantly enhanced synergistically by both. Microbial phytase affected Ca and P content in urine, but had no effect on pH, osmolarity and Mg content, where as the acids had no effect on urine parameters (Jongbloed et al. 2000).

The addition of microbial phytase and amino-acids to low-protein and low-phosphorus diets of barrows enhanced apparent digestibility of P, Ca and Zn (Walz and Pallauf 2002). Piglets were fed with maize and soya bean meal based diets supplemented with microbial phytase. Microbial phytase resulted in enhanced plasma alkaline phosphatase activity, plasma zinc and bone zinc concentrations. The supplementation of phytase also reduced the external supplementation of Zn in the diets (Revy et al. 2005).

The maize-tapioca-soya bean based diets of pigs were supplemented with phytase (500 FTU/kg). Though no lower inositol phosphates were obtained, substantial phytase activities were detected in the ileal digesta and faeces. The addition of feed phosphate increased the proportion of inorganic phosphorus, but reduced the phytase activity in the small intestine. Breakdown of IP_6 at the terminal ileum was 16.2% for the diets without phytase supplementation and this was due to microbial activity. Supplementation with phytase enhanced the breakdown of the pre-caecal IP_6 by 3-fold. However, the liberated *Pi* along the small intestine was not absorbed by the animal, but incorporated in microbial biomass as shown by lower organic matter disappearance and unaffected P disappearance, while increased phytase activity led to higher organic non-phytate P-fraction and higher amounts of bacterial residues or intestinal cell debris residues in the small intestine (Seynaeve et al. 2000). These results indicated that phosphorus absorption from feed-phosphate takes place to a large extent proximally to the ileo-caecal valve. The phosphorus that is liberated by the added microbial phytase from phytate in feedstuffs causes an increase in the microbial population in the small intestine of pigs but only becomes available for absorption in the caecum/colon region (Seynaeve et al. 2000).

A wheat-based diet for pigs was supplemented with *xylanase* (Porzyme® 9300), phytase (Phyzyme™ XP) and xylanase plus phytase. Xylanase plus phytase synergistically improved the coefficient of total tract apparent digestibility of P and Ca (Kim et al. 2005). As they are used as growth promoters or because large safety margins are applied, Cu and Zn are often oversupplied in pig diets. Consequently, manure is highly concentrated in these elements, which may concentrate in topsoil and cause toxicity to plants and micro-organisms. The reduction of Cu and Zn dietary supplies is one of the means to limit this environmental risk. The annual accumulation of Cu and Zn in top soils could be reduced by 35% if Cu and Zn concentrations were reduced from 100 to 20 ppm and from 250 to 100 ppm, respectively, in fattening pig diets. However, to safely reduce Cu and Zn supplies, the dietary factors and mechanisms that significantly affect Cu and Zn availability should be better understood and ranked. In addition, ways to improve the availability of Cu and Zn, by the use of organic supplements and/or phytase, should be considered and their actual effectiveness in controlling pollution assessed. Particularly, if microbial phytase seems promising in reducing the Zn supply in pig feeding, the actual decrease in dietary Zn remains to be assessed (Jondreville et al. 2003). High-density livestock facilities lead to a concentration of livestock wastes and subsequent leakage of pollutants into the environment, resulting in public concern about their effects. Nitrogen (N) and phosphorus (P) are the most harmful components of animal manure, but odour from the manure itself and the livestock facilities is also a problem. Improving the nutrient efficiency of the livestock helps to decrease excretion of these environmental contaminants. Pigs and chickens are mainly used in studies to improve nutrient efficiency to reduce excretion of environmental contaminants. Addition of feed supplements and modifying feeding programmes to improve nutrient efficiency can result in significant decreases in the N, P, odour, and dry matter (DM) weight of manure. Examples of these methods include the following: (1) The addition of synthetic amino-acids and reducing the protein contents resulted in N-reductions from 10 to 27% in broilers, 18 to 35% in chicks and layers, 19 to 62% in pigs, and a 9 to 43% reduction in odour from pigs. (2) Enzyme supplementation resulted in a 12 to 15% reduction in DM weight of broiler manure. (3) Phytase supplementation resulted in P-reductions of 25 to 35% in chickens and 25 to 60% in pigs. (4) The use of growth-promoting substances resulted in a 5 to 30% reduction in N and a 53 to 56% reduction in odour from pigs. (5) Formulating diets closer to requirements (diet modification) reduced N and P by 10 to 15% each in chickens and pigs, and odour by 28 to 79% in pigs. (6) Phase feeding reduced N and P excretion by chicken and pigs from 10 to 33% and 10 to 13% each, as well as odour in growing and finishing pigs by 49 to 79%. (7) Use of highly digestible raw materials in feed reduced N and P excretion by 5% in chickens and pigs. Certain feed manufacturing techniques (grinding feed-grains and proper particle size, feed uniformity in rations, or expanding and pelleting), when done properly, can significantly reduce N, P, and odour contents and DM weight of chicken and pig manure. Feed with proper grinding reduced 27% of N in finishing pigs and 22 to 23% reduction of N in piglets fed with pelleting, 60% reduction of NH_3 emission fed with finely ground Zeolites in pig, and a 26% reduction of DM weight in finishing pigs fed with proper grinding were reported, but further research is needed in this area. Coordinating actual feed analytical results with production technique modifications is needed to reduce environmental contamination by animal manure, but specialists may need to be consulted for the successful implementation of these efforts (Nahm et al. 2002). Late-finishing pigs with an average initial weight of 84 kg were used to evaluate the effects of supplemental microbial phytase to maize–soya-diets in which sources of supplemental phosphorus (P), zinc (Zn), copper (Cu), and manganese (Mn) were removed. The four dietary treatments employed were: (1) positive-control which included a standard trace-mineral premix and inorganic P-supplementation (1.6 g kg^{-1} available P, 4.6 g kg^{-1} Ca); (2) negative-control in which a trace-mineral premix without Zn, Cu, and Mn was fed, and no inorganic P was added (0.6 g kg^{-1} available P, 4.6 g kg^{-1} Ca); and the negative-control diet supplemented with either (3) 300; or (4) 500 U kg^{-1} microbial phytase. With the exception of available P, Zn, Mn and Cu, diets were formulated to meet or exceed National Research Council (NRC) nutrient recommendations for late-finishing pigs. Each supplementation regimen was fed to 102 pigs (6 pens of 17 pigs comprising triplicate replicates of both castrates and gilts) from 84 to 123 kg body weight. Removing inorganic P and selected trace minerals, or the addition of either 300 or 500 U kg^{-1} phytase to the negative-control diet did not affect ($P>0.10$) weight gain, feed intake, or feed efficiency. Moreover, carcass characteristics were not affected ($P>0.10$) by any of the supplementation strategies employed in this experiment. Metacarpal III and IV bone ash weight, however, was reduced ($P<0.05$) in pigs fed with the negative-control diet compared to the fully-supplemented positive-control diet and the diets containing the added phytase. These observations indicated that supplemental levels of inorganic P, Zn, Cu, and Mn can be reduced or eliminated without deleteriously affecting growth performance and carcass characteristics of late-finishing pigs (Peter et al. 2001). Two experiments were conducted to determine the effects of feeding microbial phytase, vitamin D3 and/or citric acid on growth performance and nutrient digestibility in pigs. In experiment 1, thirty crossbred pigs were fed one of five diets (23.4 kg) during a four-week trial. The basal diet (negative-control) was based on corn and soya bean meal and contained 6.9 g kg^{-1} calcium, 551 IU vitamin D but no inorganic phosphorus (3.2 g kg^{-1} total phosphorus). The experimental diets were supplemented with either vitamin D3 (2000 IU kg^{-1}), phytase (750 phytase units kg^{-1}) or both. A positive-control diet, containing monocalcium phosphate to supply a normal phosphorus level (5.1 g kg^{-1} P), was also used. Daily gain, feed intake and feed efficiency of pigs fed with a low phosphorus diet were improved by the addition of phytase ($p<0.05$). The addition of phytase increased serum phosphorus, but decreased alkaline phosphatase activity ($p<0.05$) by. Although pigs' performance was not improved by supplementing vitamin D3 (+2000 IU kg^{-1}), but serum phosphorus increased, while alkaline phosphatase activity decreased. Addition of vitamin D3 (+2000 IU kg^{-1}) to the diet containing phytase tended ($p>0.05$) to increase pig performance. In the second experiment, 12 castrates weaned at twenty eight days of age were used in a 6×6 incomplete latin square design experiment involving six diets. A corn-soya bean meal basal diet, containing no inorganic phosphorus, provided 3.8 g kg^{-1} total phosphorus. The experimental diets were similar to the basal diet but were supplemented with phytase (750 phytase units kg^{-1}) alone or in combination with either 15.0 g kg^{-1} citric acid or 2000 IU kg^{-1} of added vitamin D3. An additional diet provided all three additives in combination while a positive control diet, containing 10.6 g kg^{-1} dicalcium phosphate, was formulated to provide 5.6 g kg^{-1} total phosphorus. Each pig was fed a restricted quantity of feed, three times daily. The apparent digestibility of dry matter, phosphorus and calcium was significantly ($P<0.05$) improved by the addition of phytase. The addition of vitamin D and/or citric acid tended ($p>0.05$) to further increase the digestibility of these nutrients. Nitrogen digestibility was increased ($p<0.05$) by phytase in combination with vitamin D and/or citric acid but not when supplemented alone. Phosphorus excretion from pigs fed with the low phosphorus (3.8 g kg^{-1} P) diet plus phytase, alone or in combination with citric acid or vitamin D, was 27% less than pigs fed with the positive-control diet. Fecal nitrogen excretion was 8.3% lower for pigs fed phytase compared with the positive-control diet while further reductions were obtained when fed in combination with citric acid or vitamin D. These results indicated that the addition of phytase, to a corn-soya diet containing no inorganic phosphorus, liberated enough phosphorus from phytate to allow pig performance similar to that achieved with a diet containing supplemental inorganic phosphorus. There was no further increase in the effectiveness of phytase as a result of the addition of vitamin D3 and/or citric acid (Li et al. 1998).

Supplementation of phytase in the diet of broilers enhanced the coefficient of phosphorus retention and reduced the element in the excreta up to 45%, indicating a favourable environmental effect (Juanpere et al. 2004).

5. COMBATING ENVIRONMENTAL PHOSPHORUS POLLUTION

Phosphorus (P) is an essential ingredient in animal and plant production; however too much or too little P can be a problem both for animal production and the environment. Researchers all over the world are finding ways for poultry to better utilize P, thus increasing productive efficiency and protecting the environment. The U.S. poultry industry, which contributes more than $12 billion annually to the economy, includes some 75,000 growers nationwide who produce more than 6.5 billion broilers, 270 million layers, 285 million turkeys, and 20 million ducks. These operations generate 20 million tons of manure annually, which must be disposed of in an environmentally safe manner. Generally the waste is applied to the land as a fertilizer. This waste contains phosphorus, which is used by a wide range of plants; however, excess P can run off land and enter lakes and streams causing severe environmental, health, and economic problems. Ruminant animals sustain the microflora that enzymatically releases inorganic phosphorus from phytic acid. However, monogastric animals such as humans, chickens and pigs produce little or no phytase in the intestine. Hence, the phytic acid phosphorus is unavailable and the phytin-P is excreted (Mullaney et al. 2000). Phytic acid present in the manure of these animals is enzymatically cleaved by soil and water-borne micro-organisms. The phosphorus thus released is transported into the water bodies causing eutrophication. This results in oxygen depletion due to excessive algal growth. Pretreatment of animal feed with phytases would increase the availability of inorganic phosphorus, thereby improving the nutritional status of food and also help in combating phosphorus pollution (Bali and Satyanarayana 2001).

Coordinating actual feed analytical results with production technique, modifications are needed to reduce environmental contamination by animal manure, but specialists may need to be consulted for the successful implementation of these efforts (Nahm 2002).

Phytases are very well known to reduce pollution caused by excess of phosphorus accumulation in soil and water. Phytic acid (myo-inositol hexakisphosphate) is the major storage form of phosphorus in plant seeds. During germination, stored reserves are used as a source of nutrients by plant seedlings. Phytic acid is degraded by the activity of phytases to yield inositol and free phosphate. Due to the lack of phytases in the non-ruminant digestive tract, *monogastric animals* cannot utilize dietary phytic acid and it is excreted into manure. High phytic acid content in manure results in elevated phosphorus levels in soil and water and accompanying environmental concerns. The use of phytases to degrade seed phytic acid has the potential for reducing the negative environmental impact of livestock production.

The excretion of phosphorus can be reduced by 30% by replacing feed phosphate with phytase and by equally calculated digestible P-content. Application of phytase to all the pig and poultry feed in the Netherlands would result in 20 million kg less phosphate in the manure (Gist-brocades NV 1991).

The addition of phytase to the feed of piglets gives positive technical results in some experiments such as a significant increase of growth rate and feed intake and a significantly better feed conversion ratio in comparison with conventional feed. An explanation has not yet been found (Beers 1990). Phytase can also liberate zinc from phytate. Less of inorganic phosphate supplementation, such as monocalcium phosphate, dicalcium phosphate and monosodium phosphate, in feed is needed as excess of these components is polluting.

The assessment of the environmental impact of the aquaculture industry is getting more attention and rigorous restrictions are being set on this industry by governments and environmentalists. Farmers engaged in freshwater aquaculture and coastal marine operations are facing increasing pressure from various organizations to control farm-discharge into the surrounding ecosystems. This discharge, particularly with high phosphorus load, leads to eutrophication. The phosphorus in the feed ingredients occurs in a number of forms. It occurs in inorganic form as well as phosphate complexes of protein, lipid and carbohydrate. These forms are available to the fish. Phosphorus present in most grain and seed by-products is generally unavailable to fish and monogastric animals as mentioned earlier. Fish excrete phosphorus in soluble and particulate forms. The soluble forms, organic phosphorus and phosphates, affect water quality directly. The particulate forms accumulate in the sludge and phosphorus is released slowly to the water. Dissolved reactive phosphorus is usually regarded as the most important factor affecting water quality, because it is most available for phytoplankton growth. Microbial phytase supplementation in the diet of fish can overcome this problem. It makes the chelated phosphorus available to fish and hence there is less faecal excretion, thereby reducing environmental pollution. The environmental benefits of using this enzyme in fish-feed are:

- Reduced requirement of mineral supplements, thereby reducing chances of excess inorganic phosphorus getting into the aquatic system.
- Reduced organic phosphate (phytic acid) outputs.

Use of phytase in feeds reduces or sometimes eliminates the necessity of mineral supplementation, which also decreases the cost of feeds. Although phytase was first used for environmental reasons, it is now realized that there are a range of other nutritional and health benefits from using these enzymes.

CONCLUSION

Modern genetic and molecular technologies provide a number of tools that can be utilized for the development of staple foods with a higher iron and zinc content and improved bioavailability of the minerals and proteins. Adding phytase to the animal diets not only improves the bioavailability of proteins and minerals, but also plays an important role in combating environmental phosphorus pollution in the areas of intensive livestock population.

ACKNOWLEDGEMENTS

We gratefully acknowledge financial assistance from DBT and ICAR during the course of writing this review. Mr Bijender Singh and Ms Parvinder Kaur wish to thank CSIR for awarding fellowship.

REFERENCES

Adeola O, Lawrence BV, Sutton AL, Cline TR. (1995) Phytase-induced changes in mineral utilization in zinc-supplemented diets for pigs. J Anim Sci 73(11): 3384-3391

Ahmad T, Rasool S, Sarwar M, Haq A, Hasan Z (2000) Effect of microbial phytase produced from a fungus *Aspergillus niger* on bioavailability of phosphorus and calcium in broiler chickens. Anim Feed Sci Technol 83: 103-114

Al-asheh S, Duvnjak Z (1994) Effect of glucose concentration on the biomass and phytase production and reduction of phytic acid content in canola meal by *Aspergillus carbonarius* during solid-state fermentation process. Biotech Prog 10: 353–359

Alvi AS (1994) Adventitious toxins in plant origin feedstuffs: Quantification and tolerance levels in fish. Masters dissert Aligarh Muslim University, Aligarh, India

Anno T, Nakanishi K, Matsuno R, Kamikubo T (1985) Enzymatic elimination of phytate in soya bean milk. J Japan Soc Food Sci Technol 32: 174-180

Asada K, Tanaka K, Kasai Z (1969) Formation of phytic acid in cereal grains. Ann N Y Acad Sci 165(2): 801-814

Bali A, Satyanarayana T (2001) Microbial phytases in nutrition and combating phosphorus pollution. Everyman's Sci 4: 207-209

Baruah K, Pal AK, Sahu NP, Jain KK, Mukherjee SC, Debnath D (2005) Dietary protein level, microbial phytase, citric acid and their interactions on bone mineralization of *Labeo rohita* (Hamilton) juveniles. Aquacult Res 36 (8): 803-812

Beers S, T Koorn en (1990) Effect of microbial phytase in diets for piglets on their performance and phosphorus digestibility. Report IVVO no. 223

Berka RM, Rey MW, Brown KM, Byun T, Klotz AV (1998) Molecular characterization and expression of a phytase gene from the thermophilic fungus *Thermomyces lanuginosus*. Appl Environ Micro 64: 4423–4427

Bogar B, Szakacs G, Linden JC, Pandey A, Tengerdy RP (2003a) Optimization of phytase production by solid substrate fermentation. J Ind Microbiol Biotechnol 30, 183–189

Bogar B, Szakacs G, Pandey A, Abdulhameed S, Linden JC, Tengerdy RP (2003b) Production of phytase by *Mucor racemosus* in solid-state fermentation. Biotech Prog 19(2): 312-319

Boling SD, Douglas MW, Johnson ML, Wang X, Parsons CM, Koelkebeck KW, Zimmerman RA (2000) The effects of dietry available phosphorus levels and phytase performance of young and older laying hens. Poult sci 79: 224-30

Brenes A, Viveros A, Arija I, Centeno C, Pizarro M, Bravo C (2003) The effect of citric acid and microbial phytase on mineral utilization in broiler chicks. Anim Feed Sci Technol 110: 201-219

Caransa A, Simell M, Lehmussari M, Vaara M, Vaara T (1988) A novel enzyme application in corn wet milling. Starch 40: 409-411

Casey A, Walsh G (2003) Purification and characterization of extracellular phytase from *Aspergillus niger* ATCC 9142. Bioresour Technol 86: 183–188

Casey A, Walsh G (2004) Identification and characterization of a phytase of potential commercial interest. J Biotechnol 110(3): 313-22

Casida, L E Jr (1959) Phosphatase activity of some common soil fungi. Soil Sci 87: 305-310

Chadha BS, Gulati H, Minhas M, Saini HS, Singh N (2004) Phytase production by the thermophilic fungus *Rhizomucor pusillus*. World J Microbiol Biotechnol 20:105-109

Cheng ZJ, Hardy RW (2002) Effect of microbial phytase on apparent nutrient digestibility of barley, canola meal, wheat and wheat middlings, measured in vivo using rainbow trout (*Oncorhynchus mykiss*). Aquacult Nutr 8: 271-277

Cheryan M (1980) Phytic acid interactions in food systems. Crit Rev Food Sci Nutr 1980 13(4): 297-335

De Boland AR, Garner GB, O'Dell BL (1975) Identification and properties of 'phytate' in cereal grains and oilseed products. J Agri Food Chem 23: 1186-1189

Debnath D, Pal AK, Sahu NP, Jain KK, Yengkokpam S, Mukherjee SC (2005) Effect of dietary microbial phytase supplementation on growth and nutrient digestibility of *Pangasius pangasius* (Hamilton) fingerlings. Aquacult Res 36: 180-187

Deevey ES (1970) Mineral cycles. Sci American 223: 148-158

Ebune A, Asheh S Al, Duvnjak Z (1995) Effect of phosphate, surfactants and glucose on phytase production and hydrolysis of phytic acid in canola meal by *Aspergillus ficuum* during solid-state fermentation. Biores Technol 53: 7-12

Fardiaz D, Markakis P (1981) Degradation of phytic acid in oncom (fermented pea-nut press cake). J Food Sci 46: 523-525

Forster I, Higgs DA, Dosanjh BS, Rowshandeli M, Parr J (1999) Potential for dietary phytase to improve the nutritive value of canola protein concentrate and decrease phosphorus output in rainbow trout (*Oncorhynchus mykiss*) held in 11°C fresh water Aquacult 179: 109-125

Ghosh S (1997) Phytase of a thermophilic mould *Sporotrichum thermophile* Apinis. M.Sc. dissertation, Department of Microbiology, University of Delhi, Delhi

Gibson DM (1987) Production of extracellular phytase from *Aspergillus ficuum* on starch media. Biotech Lett 9: 305–310

Gibson DM, Ullah AHJ (1988) Purification and characterization of phytase from cotyledons of germinating soya bean seeds. Arch Biochem Biophys 260: 503–513

Gist-brocades NV (1991) Agro Business group; Natuphos de fosforvrije fosforbron

Graf E (1986) Phytic acid-chemistry and application. The Pillsbury Co Pilatus Press, Minneapolis, pp 42-44

Ha NC, Oh BC, Shin S, Kim HJ, Oh TK, Kim YO, Choi KY, Oh BH (2000) Crystal structures of a novel, thermostable phytase in partially and fully calcium-loaded states. Nat Struct Biol 7: 147–153

Hamelrych T (2003) Efficient identification of side-chain patterns using a multidimensional index tree. Proteins 51: 96–108

Han YM, Yang F, Zhou AG, Miller ER, Ku PK, Hogberg MG, Lei XG (1997) Supplemental phytases of microbial and cereal sources improve dietary phytate phosphorus utilization by pigs from weaning through finishing. J Anim Sci 75: 1017-1025

Han YW (1988) Removal of phytic acid from soya bean and cotton-seed meals. J Agric Food Chem 36: 1181-1183

Han YW, Gallagher DJ (1987) Phosphatase production by *Aspergillus ficuum*. J Ind Microbiol 1: 295–301

Han YW, Gallagher DJ, Wilfred DJ (1987) Phytase production by *Aspergillus ficuum* on semisolid substrate. J Ind Microbiol 2: 195–200

Harland BF, Morris ER (1995) Phytate: A good or a bad food component. Nutr Res 15(5): 733-754

Hegeman CE, Grabau EA (2001) A novel phytase with sequence similarity to purple acid phosphatases is expressed in cotyledons of germinating soya bean seedlings Plant Physiol 126: 1598–1608

Hong K, Ma Y, Li M (2001) Solid-state fermentation for phytase from cassava dregs. Appl Biochem Biotechnol 91-93: 777-785

Howson SJ, Davis RP (1983) Production of phytate hydrolyzing enzymes by some fungi. Enzyme Microb Technol 5: 377–382

Hughes KP, Soares Jr JH (1998) Efficacy of phytase on phosphate utilization in practical diets fed to striped bass, *Morone sexatilis*. Aqua Nutr 4: 133-140

Jackson LS, Li MH, Robinson EH (1996) Use of microbial phytase in channel catfish *Lactalurus punctatus* diets to improve utilization of phytate phosphorus. J World Aquacult Soc 27: 309-313

Johnson LF, Tate ME (1969) The structure of myo-inositol pentaphosphates. Ann N Y Acad Sci 165(2): 26-32

Jondreville A, Revy PS, Dourmad JY (2003) Dietary means to better control the environmental impact of copper and zinc by pigs from weaning to slaughter. Livestock Prod Sci 84: 147-156

Jongbloed AW, Mroz Z, van der Weij-Jongbloed R, Kemme PA (2000) The effects of microbial phytase, organic acids and their interaction in diets for growing pigs. Livestock Prod Sci 67: 113-122

Juanpere J, Pérez-Vendrell AM, Brufau J (2004) Effect of microbial phytase on broilers fed barley-based diets in the presence or not of endogenous phytase. Animal Feed Sci Technol 115: 265-279

Kaur P, Satyanarayana T (2005) Production of cell-bound phytase by *Pichia anomala* in an economical cane molasses medium: Optimization using statistical tools. Proc Biochem 40 (9): 3095-3102

Kaur P, Singh B, Vohra A, Satyanarayana T (2003) Fabulous phytases: Diverse functions in the living world and commercial prospects. The Botanica 53: 35-42

Kerovuo J, Lauraeus M, Nurminen P, Kalkkinen N, Apajalahti J (1998) Isolation, characterization, molecular gene cloning and sequencing of a novel phytase from *Bacillus subtilis*. Appl Environ Microbiol 64: 2079–2085

Khare SK, Jha K, Gupta MN (1994) Entrapment of wheat phytase in polyacrylamide gel and its application in soya-milk phytate hydrolysis. Biotechnol Appl Biochem 19: 193-198

Khasawneh FE, Sample EC, Kamprath EJ (1980) The role of phosphorus in agriculture. Am Soc Agron, Madison, WI

Kim DS, Godber JS, Kim HR (1999) Culture conditions for a new phytase producing fungus. Biotechnol Lett 21: 1077–1081

Kim JC, Simmins PH, Mullan BP, Pluske JR (2005) The effect of wheat phosphorus content and supplemental enzymes on digestibility and growth performance of weaner pigs. Anim Feed Sci Technol 118: 139-152

Kim YO, Kim HK, Bae KS, Yu JH, Oh TK (1998) Purification and properties of thermostable phytase from *Bacillus* sp. DS11. Enzyme Microb Technol 22: 2–7

Klabunde T, Stahl B, Suerbaum H, Hahner S, Karas M, Hillenkamp F, Krebs B, Witzel H (1994) The amino-acid sequence of the red kidney bean Fe(III)–Zn(II) purple acid phosphatase: determination of the amino-acid sequence by a combination of matrixassisted laser desorption/ionization mass spectrometry and automated Edman sequencing Eur J Biochem 226: 369-375

Klabunde T, Strater N, Frohlich R, Witzel H, Krebs B (1996) Mechanism of Fe (III)–Zn(II) purple acid phosphatase based on crystal structures. J Mol Biol 259: 737–748

Knorr D, Watkins T R, Carlson B L (1981) Enzymatic reduction of phytate in whole wheat breads. J Food Sci 46: 1866-1869

Kornegay ET (1995) In: Proc Second Symp Feed Enzymes (ESFE2) [eds. van Hartingsveldt W, Hessing M, van der Lugt JP and Somers WAC] TNO Nutrition and Food Research Institute, Zeist, Noordwijkerhout, Netherlands. pp 189-197

Kostrewa A, Grueninger-Leitch F, D'Arcy A, Broger C, Mitchell D, vanLoon APGM (1997) Crystal structure of phytase from *Aspergillus ficuum* at 2.5 Å resolution. Nat Struct Biol 4: 185–190

Krishna C, Nokes SE (2001) Predicting vegetative inoculum performance to maximize phytase production in solid-state fermentation using response surface methodology. J Ind Microbiol Biotechnol 26: 161–170

Lambrechts C, Boze H, Moulin G, Galzy P (1992) Utilization of phytate by some yeasts. Biotech Lett 14(1): 63-66

Lassen SF, Breinholt J, Ostergaard PR, Brugger R, Bischoff A, Wyss M et al. (2001) Expression, gene cloning and characterization of five novel phytases from four basidomycete fungi: *Peniophora lycii, Agrocybe pediades, Ceriporia* sp., and *Trametes pubescens*. Appl Environ Microbiol 67: 4701–4707

Lei XG, Ku PK, Miller ER, Yokoyama MT (1993b) Supplementing corn-soya bean meal diets with microbial phytase linearly improves phytate phosphorus utilization by weanling pigs. J Anim Sci 71(12): 3359-3367

Lei XG, Ku PK, Miller ER, Yokoyama MT, Ullrey DE (1993a) Supplementing corn-soya bean meal diets with microbial phytase maximizes phytate phosphorus utilization by weaning pigs. J Anim Sci 71(12): 3368-3375

Lei XG, Stahl CH (2001) Biotechnological development of effective phytases for mineral nutrition and environmental protection. Appl Microbiol Biotechnol 57(4): 474-81

Li D, Che X, Wang Y, Hong C, Thacker PA (1998) Effect of microbial phytase, vitamin D3, and citric acid on growth performance and phosphorus, nitrogen and calcium digestibility in growing swine. Anim Feed Sci Technol 73: 173-186

Li MH, Robinson EH (1997) Microbial phytase can replace inorganic phosphorus supplements in channel catfish *Lactalurus punctatus*. J World Aquacult Soc 28: 402-406

Liu BL, Jong CH, Tzeng YM (1999) Effect of immobilization on pH and thermal stability of *Aspergillus ficuum* phytase. Enzyme Microb Technol 25: 517–521

Maenz DD, Classen HL (1998) Phytase activity in the small intestinal brush-border membrane of the chicken. Poult Sci 77: 557–563

Maga JA (1982) Phytate: Its chemistry, occurrence, food interactions, nutritional significance, and methods of analysis. Crit Rev Food Sci Nutr 16(1):1-48

Mandviwala TN, Khire JM (2000) Production of high activity thermostable phytase from thermotolerant phytase from thermotolerant *Aspergillus niger* in solid-state fermentation. J Ind Microbiol Biotechnol 24: 237–243

Martin A, Cooke G D (1994) Health risks in eutrophic water supplies. Lake Line 14:24-26.

Martin CJ, Evans WJ (1986) Phytic acid-metal ion interactions. II. The effect of pH on Ca(II) binding. J Inorg Biochem 27(1): 17-30

Martin JA, Murphy RA, Power RF (2003) Cloning and expression of fungal phytases in genetically modified strains of *Aspergillus awamori*. J Ind Microbiol Biotechnol 30: 568–576

Mayer AF, Hellmuth K, Schlieker H, Lopez-Ulibarri R, Oertel S, Dahlems U (1999) An expression system matures: a highly efficient and cost-effective process for phytase production by recombinant strains of *Hansenula polymorpha*. Biotechnol Bioeng 63: 373–381

Mendoza C (2002) Effect of genetically modified low phytic acid plants on mineral absorption Int J Food Sci Technol 37: 759-767

Mitchell DB, Vogel K, Weimann BJ, Pasamontes L, van Loon AP (1997) The phytase subfamily of histidine acid phosphatase: isolation of genes for two novel phytases from fungi *Aspergillus terreus* and *Myceliophthora thermophila*. Microbiology 143 (Pt 1): 245-252

Mohanna A, Nys Y (1999) Changes in zinc and manganese availability in broiler chicks induced by vegetal and microbial phytases. Anim Feed Sci Technol 77: 241-253

Mullaney EJ, Daly CB, Ullah AH (2000) Advances in phytase research. Adv Appl Microbiol 47: 157–199

Mullaney EJ, Ullah AH (2003) The term phytase comprises several different classes of enzymes. Biochem Biophys Res Commun 312: 179–184

Murugesan GS, Sathishkumar M, Swaminathan K (2005) Supplementation of waste tea fungal biomass as a dietary ingredient for broiler chicks. Biores Technol (In Press)

Nagashima T, Tange T, Anazawa H (1999) Dephosphorylation of phytate by using the *Aspergillus niger* phytase with a high affinity for phytate. Appl Environ Microbiol 65: 4682–4684

Nahm K H (2002) Efficient Feed Nutrient Utilization to Reduce Pollutants in Poultry and Swine Manure. Crit Rev Env Sci Technol 32: 1-16

Nair VC, Duvnjak Z (1990) Reduction of phytic acid content in canola meal by *Aspergillus ficuum* in solid-state fermentation process. Appl Microbiol Biotechnol 34: 183–188

Nakamura Y, Fukuhara H, Sano L (2000) Secreted phytase activities of yeasts. Biosci Biotechnol Biochem 64: 841–844

Nampoothiri KM, Tomes G J, Roopesh K, Szakacs G, Nagy V, Soccol CR, Pandey A (2004) Thermostable phytase production by *Thermoascus aurantiacus* in submerged fermentation. Appl Biochem Biotechnol 118: 205-214

Oh BC, Chang BS, Park KH, Ha NC, Kim HK, Oh BH, Oh TK (2001) Calcium-dependent catalytic activity of a novel phytase from *Bacillus amyloliquefaciens* DS11. Biochem 40: 9669–9676

Pandey A, Szakacs G, Soccol CR, Rodriguez-Leon JA, Soccol VT (2001) Production, purification and properties of microbial phytases. Biores Technol 77(3): 203-214

Pandey P, Selvakumar P, Soccol CR, Nigam P (1999) Solid state fermentation for the production of industrial enzymes. Curr Sci 77: 149-162

Papagianni M, Nokes SE, Filer K (2000) Production of phytase by *Aspergillus niger* in submerged and solid state fermentation. Proc Biochem 35: 397–402

Papatryphon E, Howell RA, Soares Jr. JH (1999) Growth and mineral absorption by a striped bass *Morone sexatilis* fed a plant feedstuff based diet supplemented with phytase. J World Aquacult Soc 30: 161-173

Pasamontes L, Haiker M, Wyss M, Tessier M, van Loon APGM (1997) Gene cloning, purification and characterization of a heat stable phytase from the fungus *Aspergillus fumigatus* Appl Environ Microbiol 63: 1696–1700

Peter CM, Parr TM, Parr EN, Webel DM, Baker DH (2001) The effects of phytase on growth performance, carcass characteristics and bone mineralization of late-finishing pigs fed maize–soya bean meal diets containing no supplemental phosphorus, zinc, copper and manganese. Anim Feed Sci Technol 94: 199-205

Quan, CS, Difan S, Zhang L H, Wang Y J, Ohta Y (2002) Purification and properties of a phytase from *Candida krusei* WZ-001. J Biosci Bioeng 94 (5): 419-425

Quan, CS, Zhang LH, Wang YJ, Ohta Y (2001) Production of phytase in a low phosphate medium by a novel yeast *Candida krusei*. J Biosci Bioeng 92(2): 154-160

Ramachandran S, Roopesh K, Nampoothiri KM, Szakacs G, Pandey A (2005) Mixed substratum fermentation for the production of phytase by *Rhizopus* spp. using oilcakes as substrata. Proc Biochem 40 (5): 1749-1754

Reddy NR, Sathe SK, Salunkhe DK (1982) Phytases in legumes and cereals. Adv Food Res 82: 1–92

Revy PS, Jondreville C, Dourmad JY, Nys Y (2005) Assessment of dietary zinc requirement of weaned piglets fed diets with or without microbial phytase. J Animal Physiol Animal Nutr (In Press)

Richardson NL, Higgs DA, Beames RM, McBride JR (1985) Influence of dietary calcium, phosphorus, zinc and sodium phytate level on cataract incidence, growth and histopathology in juvenile chinook salmon *(Oncorhynchus tshawytscha)*. J Nutr 115: 553-567

Robinson EH, Li MH, Manning BB (2002) Influence of dietary calcium, phosphorus, zinc and sodium phytate level on cataract incidence, growth and histopathology in juvenile chinook salmon (*Oncorhynchus tshawytscha*).Comparison of Microbial Phytase and Dicalcium Phosphate for Growth and Bone Mineralization of Pond-Raised Channel Catfish, *Ictalurus punctatus*. J Appl Aquacult 12: 81-88

Rodehutscord M, Pfeffer E (1995) Effects of supplemental microbial phytase on phosphorus digestibility and utilization in rainbow trout (*Oncorhynchus mykiss*). Water Sci Technol 31: 143-147

Roopesh K, Ramachandran S, Nampoothiri KM, Szakacs G, Pandey A (2006) Comparison of phytase production on wheat bran and oilcakes in solid-state fermentation by *Mucor racemosus* Biores Technol 97(3): 506-511

Sabu A, Sarita S, Pandey A, Bogar B, Szakacs G, Soccol CR (2002) Solid-state fermentation for production of phytase by *Rhizopus oligosporus*. Appl Biochem Biotechnol 102–103: 251–260

Sajjad M, Carter CG (2004) Effect of phytic acid and phytase on feed intake, growth, digestibility and trypsin activity in Atlantic salmon (*Salmo salar*, L.). Aqua Nutr 10: 135-142

Sandberg AS, Hulthen LR, Turk M (1996) Dietary *Aspergillus niger* phytase increases iron absorption in humans. J Nutr 126: 476-480

Sano L, Fukuhara H, Nakamura Y (1999) Phytase of the yeast *Arxula adeninivorans*. Biotech Lett 21: 33–38

Satyanarayana T, Vohra A (2003) A synergistic feed composition to enhance phosphorous availability, assimilation and retention in non-ruminants. Indian Patent Appl no. 976/DEL/2003 Schafer A, Koppe WM, Meyer-Burgdorff KH, Gunther KD (1995) Effects of a microbial phytase on the utilization of native phosphorus by carp in a diet based on soya bean meal. Water Sci Technol 31: 149-155

Schenk A, Guddat LW, Ge Y, Carrington LE, Hume DA, Hamilton S, de Jersey J (2000) Identi?cation of mammalian-like purple acid phosphatase in a wide range of plants. Gene 250: 117–125

Segueilha L, Lambrechts C, Boze H, Moulin G, Galzy P (1992) Purification and properties of phytase from *Schwanniomyces castellii*. J Ferment Bioeng 74: 7–11

Seynaeve M, Janssens G, Hesta M, Van Nevel, De Wilde RO (2000) Effects of dietary Ca/P ratio, P level and microbial phytase supplementation on nutrient digestibilities in growing pigs: breakdown of phytic acid, partition of P and phytase activity along the intestinal tract. J Anim Physiol Animal Nutr 83: 193-204

Sharma C B, Goel M, Irshad M (1978) Myoinositol hexaphosphate as a potential inhibitor of á-amylases. Phytochem 17: 201-204

Sheppy C (2001) The current feed enzyme market and likely trends. In: Bedford MR, Parridge GG (eds.) Enzymes in Farm Animal Nutrition. CABI, Publishing, Oxon, U.K, pp 1-10

Shieh TR and Ware JH (1968) Survey of micro-organism for the production of extracellular phytase. Appl Microbiol 16(9): 1348-51.

Shieh TR, Wodzinski RJ, Ware JH (1969) Regulation of the formation of acid phosphatases by inorganic phosphate in *Aspergillus ficuum*. J Bacteriol 100: 1161-1165.

Shimizu M (1993) Purification and characterization of phytase and acid phosphatase produced by *Aspergillus* oryzae K1. Biosci Biotechnol Biochem 57: 1364–1365

Shin S, Ha NC, Oh BC, Oh TK, Oh BH (2001) Enzyme mechanism and catalytic property of β-propeller phytase. Structure 9: 851–858

Simell M, Turunen M, Pironen J, Vaara T (1989) Feed and food applications of phytase. Lecture at 3rd Meet. Industrial Applications of Enzymes, Barcelona, Spain

Smil V (2000) Phosphorus in the environment: Natural flows and human interferences. Ann Rev Energy Environ 25: 53-88

Storebakken T, Shearer KD, Roem AJ (1998) Availability of protein, phosphorus and other elements in fish meal, soya-protein concentrate and phytase-treated soya-protein-concentrate-based diets to Atlantic salmon, *Salmo salar*. Aquacult 161: 365-379

Strater N, Klabunde T, Tucker P, Witzel H, Krebs B (1995) Crystal structure of a purple acid phosphatase containing a dinuclear Fe(III)–Zn(II) active site. Science 268: 1489–1492

Sugiura SH, Gabaudan J, Dong FM, Hardy RW (2001) Dietary microbial phytase supplementation and the utilization of phosphorus, trace minerals and protein by rainbow trout [*Oncorhynchus mykiss* (Walbaum)] fed soya bean meal-based diets. Aquacult Res 32: 583-592

Sutardi S, Buckle KA (1988) Characterization of extra and intracellular phytase from *Rhizopus oligosporus* used in tempeh production. Int J Food Microbiol 6(1): 67-79

Ullah AHJ, Cummins BJ (1987) Purification, N-terminal amino acid sequence and characterisation of pH 2.5 optimum acid phosphatase (E.C.3.1.3.2) from *Aspergillus ficuum*. Prep Biochem 17: 397–422

Ullah AHJ, Cummins BJ (1988) *Aspergillus ficuum* extracellular pH 6.0 optimum acid phosphatase: puri?cation, N-terminal amino-acid sequence and biochemical characterization. Prep Biochem 18: 37–65

Ullah AHJ, Cummins BJ, Dischinger Jr HC (1991) Cyclohexanedione modification of arginine at the active site of *Aspergillus ficuum* phytase. Biochem Biophys Res Commun 178: 45–53

Ullah AHJ, Gibson DM (1987) Extracellular phytase (E.C.3.1.3.8) from *Aspergillus ficuum* NRRL 3135: purification and characterization. Prep Biochem 17: 63–91

Ullah AHJ, Phillippy BQ (1994) Substrate selectivity in *Aspergillus ficuum* phytase and acid phosphatases using myo-inositol phosphates. J Agric Food Chem 42: 423–425

US Environmental Protection Agency (USEPA) (1986) U.S. Environmental protection agency report 440/5-86-001, Quality control for water, Washington D.C.

Usmani N, Jafri AK (2002) Influence of dietry phytic acid on growth, conversion efficiency and carcass composition of mrigal *Cirrhinus mrigala* (Hamilton) fry. J World Aquacult Soc 33: 199-204

Van Weerd JH, Khalaf KHA, Aartsen FJ, Tijssen PAT (1999) Balance trials with African catfish *Clarias gariepinus* fed phytase-treated soybean meal-based diets. Aquacult Nutr 5: 135-142

Vats P, Banerjee UC (2002) Studies on the production of phytase by a newly isolated strain of *Aspergillus niger* van teigham obtained from rotten wood logs. Proc Biochem 38: 211–217

Vats P, Banerjee UC (2004) Production studies and catalytic properties of phytases (myo-inositolhexakisphosphate phosphohydrolases): an overview. Enzyme Microb Technol 35(1): 3-14

Vats P, Banerjee UC (2005) Biochemical characterisation of extracellular phytase (myo-inositol hexakisphosphate phosphohydrolase) from a hyper-producing strain of *Aspergillus niger* van Teighem. J Ind Microbiol Biotechnol 32 (4): 141 – 147

Vielma J, Lall SP, Koskela J, Schöner FJ, Mattila P (1998) Effects of dietary phytase and cholecalciferol on phosphorus bioavailability in rainbow trout (*Oncorhynchus mykiss*). Aquacult 163: 309-323

Vielma J, Ruohonen K, Gabaudan J, Vogel K (2004)Top-spraying soya bean meal-based diets with phytase improves protein and mineral digestibilities but not lysine utilization in rainbow trout, *Oncorhynchus mykiss* (Walbaum). Aquacult Res 35: 955-964

Vohra A, Rastogi SK, Satyanarayana T (2005) Amelioration in growth and phosphate assimilation of poultry birds using cell-bound phytase of *Pichia anomala*. World J Microbiol Biotechnol (In press)

Vohra A, Satyanarayana T (2001) Phytase production by the yeast *Pichia anomala*. Biotech Lett 23: 551 – 554

Vohra A, Satyanarayana T (2002a) Purification and characterization of a thermostable and acid-stable phytase from *Pichia anomala*. World J Microbiol Biotechnol 18: 687-691

Vohra A, Satyanarayana T (2002b) Statistical optimization of the medium components by response surface methodology to enhance phytase production by *Pichia anomala*. Proc Biochem 37: 999-1004

Vohra A, Satyanarayana T (2003) Phytases: Microbial Sources, Production, Purification, and Potential Biotechnological Applications. Crit Rev Biotechnol 23(1): 29-60

Vohra A, Satyanarayana T (2004) A cost-effective cane molasses medium for enhanced cell-bound phytase production by *Pichia anomala*. J Appl Microbiol 97: 471-476

Walz OP, Pallauf J (2002) Microbial phytase combined with amino-acid supplementation reduces P and N excretion of growing and finishing pigs without loss of performance. Int J Food Sci Technol 37: 835-848

Wise A (1983) Dietry factors determining the biological activities of phytase. Nutr Abstr Rev 53: 791-806

Wodzinski RJ, Ullah AHJ (1996) Phytase. Adv Appl Microbiol 42: 263–301

Wyss M, Brugger R, Kronenberger A, Remy R, Fimbel R, Oesterhelt O (1999b) Biochemical characterization of fungal phytases (myo-inositolhexakisphosphate-phosphohydrolases): catalytic properties. Appl Environ Microbiol 65: 367–373

Wyss M, Pasamontes L, Friedlein A, Remy R, Tessier M, Kronenberger A (1999a) Biophysical characterization of fungal phytases (myo-inositolhexakisphosphate-phosphohydrolases): molecular size, glycosylation pattern and engineering of proteolytic resistance. Appl Environ Microbiol 65: 359–366

Wyss M, Pasamontes L, Remy R, Kohler J, Kusznir E, Gadient M (1998) Comparison of the thermostability properties of three acid phosphatases from molds: *Aspergillus fumigatus* phytase, *A. niger* phytase and *A. niger* pH 2.5 acid phosphatase. Appl Environ Microbiol 64: 4446–4451

Yamada, K, Minoda Y, Kobayashi T, Hidaka Y, Motuo H, Kobayashi M (1968) Phytase from *Aspergillus terreus* : production, purification and some general properties of the enzyme. Agric Biol Chem 32: 1275-1282

Yan W, Reigh RC (2002) Effects of fungal phytase on utilization of dietary proteins and minerals and dephosphorylation of phytic acid in the alimentary tract of channel catfish, *Lactalurus punctatus* fed an all plant-protein diet. J World Aquacult Soc 33: 10-22

Yi Z, Kornegay ET, Denbow DM (1996) Effect of microbial phytase on nitrogen and amino acid digestibility and nitrogen retention of turkey poultry fed corn-soya bean meal diets. Poult Sci 75: 540-546

Yoon SJ, Choi YJ, Min K, Cho KK, Kim JW, Lee SC (1996) Isolation and identification of phytase producing bacterium, *Enterobacter* sp. 4 and enzymatic properties of phytase enzyme Enzyme Microb Technol 18: 449–454

Zhu XS, Seib PA, Allee GL, Liang YT (1990) Preparation of a low-phytate feed mixture and bioavailability of its phosphorus to chicks. Animal Feed Sci Technol 27: 341-351

Zyta K, Koreleski J, Kujawski M (1989) Dephosphorylation of phytate compounds by means of acid phosphatase from *Aspergillus niger*. J Sci Food Agric 49: 315-324

Microbial Intervention in Arsenic Rich Environment

JAISHREE PAUL[1] and KUMAR SURANJIT PRASAD[2]

1. INTRODUCTION

Arsenic catastrophes occurring today are quite alarming and have taken a huge dimension, most notably as the high arsenic levels present in drinking water in East Bengal and West Bengal, where over 40 million people are being exposed to more than 50 ppb of arsenic whereas, according to EPA, the limit is set to 10 ppb (Chowdhury et al. 1999). Besides the natural phenomena of weathering of rocks, volcanic activity various *anthropogenic activities* like use of arsenic in *pesticides*, herbicides, *wood preservatives* and dye stuffs are the major sources of arsenic contamination. In addition, arsenic can accumulate in groundwater and well-water from natural sources. Certain geological formations contain high levels of arsenic that can easily leach into groundwater and find their way into wells and other public water supplies. This has been a major problem in certain parts of the world including areas of Taiwan, South America, India, and Pakistan. Epidemiological studies of these populations have demonstrated a significant increase in the risk of lung, skin, liver, bladder, and other cancers associated with high levels of arsenic in drinking water, and most of the world's arsenic standards are based on risk assessment models of these data from high-exposure populations.

1. School of Life Sciences, Jawaharlal Nehru University, New Delhi 110067
Email: jpaul33@hotmail.com; Tel.No. 91-011-26704156 (O)

2. School of Environmental Sciences, Jawaharlal Nehru University, New Delhi 110067, India

In the present review we have concentrated on the broad diversity of microbes able either to reduce or to oxidize arsenic compounds and their mechanism of action. Emphasis has been given on the enzymes and the corresponding genes responsible for the transformations.

1.1 Arsenic Geocycle

Just as there are well-studied geocycles for carbon, nitrogen, oxygen, sulphur and other elements that are components of all living cells, there are also geocycles for toxic elements including arsenic. Living cells (especially microbes) carry out redox and covalent bond chemistry and are important players in the arsenic geocycle (Labrum et al. 2003; Quinn and McMullan 1995). Existence of different compounds of arsenic encountered in nature and their formation is represented in (Fig. 1).

Higher plants and animals bio-accumulate compounds to levels far above those of the environments in which they live. Arsenate (the main arsenic compound in seawater) is taken up by *marine organisms*, ranging from *phytoplankton*, algae, *crustaceans*, *mollusks* and fish (Knowles and Benson 1983), and converted to small organic compounds (such as

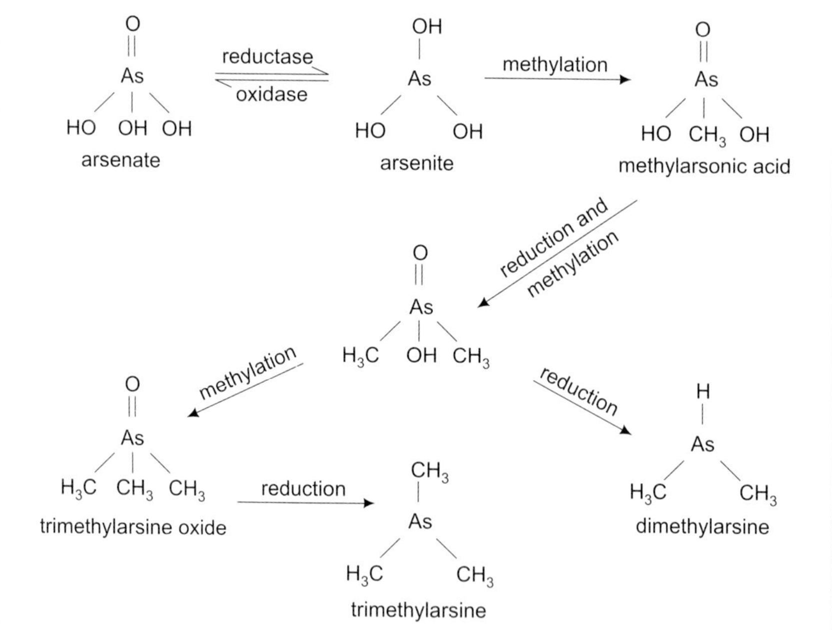

Fig. 1 Formation of different compounds of Arsenic in nature

methylarsonic acid or *dimethylarsinic acid* or is converted to organic storage forms that are then secreted into the environment (Challenger 1951). However, some arsenic is retained by phytoplankton and metabolized into complex organic compounds. The transformation of inorganic arsenic into lipid-soluble compounds might be an adaptive mechanism for marine phytoplankton to compensate for limited nitrate availability (Labrum et al 2003) More complex algal *organoarsenical compounds* include water-soluble arsenosugars (i.e. *dimethylarsenosugars*) and lipid-soluble compounds (arsenolipids). While phytoplankton and macroalgae are the primary producers of complex organoarsenic compounds in the sea, these organisms are themselves consumed and metabolized by marine animals. The major organoarsenic compound isolated from marine organisms is arsenobetain (Cervantes et al. 1994; Craig 1989; Stolz and Oremalnd 1999).

1.2 Arsenic Contamination and Toxicity Level

Arsenic is a classified *carcinogenic* (Bates et al. 1992; Pershang 1985) semi-metallic chemical element having valencies -3(arsine,) 0(elemental), +3 (arsenite) and +5(arsenate). Interestingly the differential toxicity of arsenic greatly depends upon its oxidation and reduction state i.e. reduced arsine is a deadly poisonous gas whereas comparing to As^{+5} (a moderately toxic ion), As^{+3} is approximately hundred times more toxic (Nidhubhghaill and Sadler 1991). While both, arsenite and arsenate are poisonus, the former is more toxic due to its affinity for thiols, and in particular lipoic acid of pyruvate dehydrogenase. The lesser toxicity of arsenate is due to its activity as a phosphate analogue (Hoke et al. 2004). Organisms respond to arsenicals either by lowering the intracellular concentration through transport mechanism or by chemical modification to a less toxic form (Conrads et al. 2002). Global Prevalence of arsenic ranges from West Bengal (India) Bangladesh, Southern China province, Mongolia, South Korea, Taiwan to name few. WHO announced the safe permissible limit to 0.01 mg/l from 0.05 mg/l in 1993, while Bangladesh and India still maintain an allowable limit of 50 ppb(Welch et al. 2000). The worst affected parts are southern West Bengal and southern and eastern part of Bangladesh where elevated concentration like 0.2mg/l in subsurface water has been frequently noticed and in a close estimate, over 40 million people are at risk of getting cancer (Ahsan et al. 2000; McArthur et al. 2004; Nickson et al. 1998; Milton et al.2001). This is why arsenic contamination in natural system as well as humanly impacted system and its toxicity for human being has become serious concern of current public health.

Arsenic Release and Contribution of Microbes

The ultimate source of arsenic on the earth's surface is igneous activity (Nriagu 1994). It becomes increasingly clear that severe arsenic pollution of ground water in most alluvial *aquifers* worldwide is driven by the microbially-mediated metabolism of organic matter, with $Fe(OH)_2$ acting as the source of oxygen: the oxyhydroxide is reduced during the process and its sorbed arsenic is released to ground water. Despite the widespread acceptance of this mechanism, much about it remains obscure (McArthur et al. 2004).

In addition to energy generation, a second important task for micro-organisms is to protect themselves from toxic substances. Arsenate, with its structural similarity to phosphate, enters microbial cells readily through phosphate uptake proteins. Its primary mode of toxicity is then to displace phosphate in the production of adenosine triphosphate (ATP), the primary energy currency of the cell. The resulting molecules hydrolyze spontaneously, causing the cell to deplete its energy stores rapidly (Winship 1984). Although this mechanism of toxicity is quite effective, many cells are able to induce highly phosphate-specific uptake proteins that improve the exclusion of arsenate (Willsky and Malamy 1980). Arsenite, in contrast, is uncharged at neutral pH and appears to gain access to the cytoplasm by less specific mechanisms, possibly including diffusion across the membrane. Once inside, it crosslinks sulfhydryl groups on enzymes, forming stable adducts that permanently disable the enzyme. This mechanism is even more destructive to the cell than that of arsenate. A *microcosm* based approach was used to understand the mechanism of arsenic release in sediments (Islam et al. 2004). Anaerobic metal-reducing bacteria was found to play a key role in the mobilization of toxic arsenic (As III) and it was proved that the release took place after Fe(III) reduction rather than occurring simultaneously.

1.3 Respiratory Arsenic Transformations

Aerobic and anaerobic respiratory processes form one central class of processes that strongly influence arsenic biogeochemistry, both directly and indirectly. Arsenite may function as an electron donor at the start of a membrane respiratory chain (Fig. 2A) whereas arsenate functions as a terminal electron acceptor for an anaerobic respiratory chain (Fig. 2B), as do other minerals, such as Fe and Mn with some microbes. Microbes possessing cytoplasmic arsenate reductase as an intracellular defense mechanism (Fig. 2C) is also widespread in nature. Within the past eight years, micro-organisms have been discovered in a great diversity of anoxic environments that are able to generate energy by coupling the oxidation of H_2 or organic carbon to the reduction of inorganic As(V), arsenate, forming

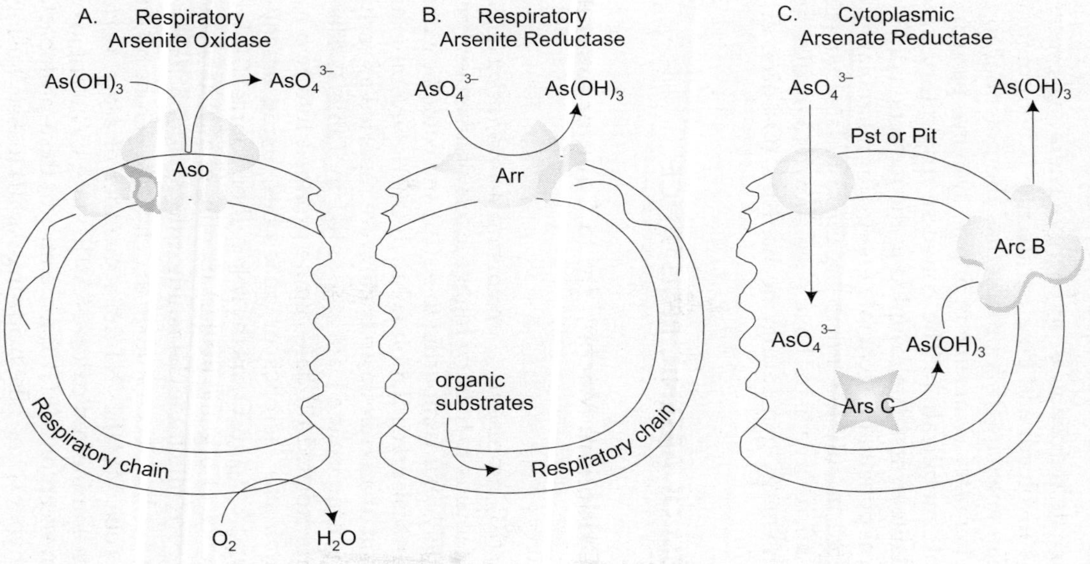

Fig. 2 Cellular locations and functions of bacterial respiratory arsenite oxidase, respiratory arsenate reductase, and cytoplasmic arsenate reductase (adopted from Silver and Phung 2005)

inorganic As(III), arsenite (Ahmann et al. 1994; Cummings et al. 1999). Arsenite behaves much differently than arsenate in natural environments; in particular, its sorption onto clay minerals and metal oxides appears to be less rapid and/or less stable, with the result that As (III) is generally much more mobile than As(V) in aqueous systems.

Because arsenate reduction is an energy-generating process for the micro-organisms involved, and because arsenite is both more toxic and more mobile than arsenate, this process has the potential to influence greatly the geochemistry of arsenic in anoxic systems, particularly with respect to arsenic mobilization. The converse respiratory process, the oxidation of arsenite to arsenate, coupled to the reduction of O_2 to water, has the theoretical potential to generate energy for microbial growth, but has been indicated in only few micro-organism todate. Nevertheless, a variety of other micro-organisms have been shown to oxidize arsenite to arsenate by non-energy-generating mechanisms (Osborne et al. 1976; Phillips et al. 1976).

2. MECHANISM OF ARSENIC RESISTANCE

2.1 Arsenite Oxidation: Mechanism to Counter Arsenite Toxicity

Oxidation of As(III) represents a promising *detoxification* process that allows micro-organisms to tolerate higher levels of arsenite. The product As(V) is moderately toxic comparing to As(III) and could be extracted out followed by chemical precipitation (Ehrlich 2001). Several examples of bacterial oxidation of arsenite to arsenate were reported as early as 1918. The organisms so far isolated are presented in Table 1. The arsenite oxidizing bacteria isolated till date can be grouped into two categories: (I) *chemolithoautotrophs* (aerobes or anaerobes, using arsenite as the electron donor and CO_2/HCO_3^- as the sole carbon source) (II) *heterotrophs* (growth in presence of organic matter) (Santini et al. 2000; Santini et al. 2004). There are currently three chemolithoautotrophic bacteria reprted so far, out of which two have been studied in detail : the aerobe NT-26 and the facultative anaerobe MLHE1. NT-26, a member of á-*protobacteria*, was isolated from a goldmine and oxidizes As(III) to As(V) using oxygen as a terminal electron acceptor. MLHE1, a member of the ã-protobacteria, was isolated from a hyper saline lake oxidising As(III) to As(V) using NO_3^- as the terminal electron acceptor (Vanden and Santini 2004; Oremland et al 2002). Several heterotrophic arsenite oxidizing bacteria have been isolated that include *Alcaligenes faecalis*, ULPAs1, *Agrobacterium albertimagni* and three *Thermus* species (Table 1). In 1992, a *periplasmic soluble enzyme* capable

Table 1

Micro-organism	*Place of Isolation*	*Ambient As conc.*	*Experimental [As](mM)*	*Km(μM)*	*Vmax*	*References*
Bacillus Arsenooxidans	Cattle dipping fluid	NR*	20-100	NR	NR	HH Green (1918)
Pseudomonas arsenooxidans	Cattle dipping fluid	NR	20-100	450	31 μM/mg dry wt/hr	JW Legge and AW turner (1954)
Achromobacter arsenooxydans	Soil	NR	2.5-40	NR	NR	Quastal and Scholefield (1953)
Alcaligenes faecalis	Raw sewage	NR	10-20	450	0.05 μmol/mg protein/min	Philips and Talyor (1976)
Alcaligenes strain	soil	NR	0.24-2.4	1540	-	Osborn and Ehrlich (1976)
Pseudomonas arsenitooxidans	Mine water	NR	13.3-26.7	NR	NR	Ilyaletdinov and Abdrashitova (1981)
Sea water consortia	Coastal sea water	<70 nM	0.0013	70-144	3.6-9.2 μM/hr	Scudlark and Jhonson (1982)
As1-As6	Mine water	173 μM	0.67-6.7	NR	NR	Wakao et al. (1988)
Sulfolobus acidocaldarius	From deposit	NR	1	NR	NR	Sehlin and Lindstorm (1992)
Alcaligenes faecalis	From deposit	NR	0.20	NR	0.023 μM/mg protein/min	Anderson et al. (1992)
ULPAs1	Contaminated water	0.47 mmol /Kg drywt	1.33	NR	NR	Weeger et al. (1999)

Contd.

Table 1

Micro-organism	*Place of Isolation*	*Ambient As conc.*	*Experimental [As](mM)*	*Km(μM)*	*Vmax*	*References*
NT-25 and NT-26	Gold mine arsenopyrite	NR	5-10	NR	NR	Santini et al. (2000)
Thiomonas (strain b6)	Mine water	NR	NR	NR	NR	Battaglia-Brunet et al. (2002)
Agrobacterium albertimagni AOL 15	Macropyte surface	2.7 μM	0.002-5.0	3.4±2.2	0.043± 0.017 μM/mg protein/min	Salmassi et al. (2002)
Bacillus selenitireducens strain MLS10	Mono Lake, CA,USA		10	34 μM	2.5 μmol/min/mg	Afkar et al. (2003)
Hydrogenophaga *strainNT-14*	Australian gold mine		0.1-2.5	35 μM	6.1 μmol /min/mg	Hoven et al. (2004)
Thermus sp. HR 13	Hot spring, North California	1-10 mg/l	NR	NR	Nr	Gihiring and Banfield (2001)

*NR- Not reported

of oxidizing arsenite As (III) was purified from â protobacterium, *Alcaligenes faecalis* (Anderson et al 1992). Expression of this so-called arsenite oxidase was induced by presence of As(III) in the growth medium and purified enzyme exhibits arsenite oxidation activity measured biochemically in the presence of azurin or cytochrome *c* as electron acceptor (Anderson et al. 2001; Ellis et al. 2001).

2.2 Arsenite Oxidase

The enzyme catalyzes the two electron oxidation of arsenite to arsenate as the first step in detoxification pathway that is important in cycling if arsenic in the environment, as well as providing an alternate respiratory chain in certain organism (Hoke et al. 2004; Labrum et al. 2003). *In vitro* studies indicated that arsenite oxidase transfers the electron obtained from oxidation of arsenite towards the soluble periplasmic electron carriers cytochrome *c* or *amicyanin*. The recently reported three-dimensional (3D) structure of this enzyme showed that arsenite oxidase is a *heterodimeric enzyme* containing a small and a large subunit (Fig.3A) The small subunit belongs to the structural class of the Rieske protein found in Rieske/cyt*b* complexes in *dioxygenase* (Ellis et al. 2001). The large catalytic subunit harbours the molybdopterin cofactor and the [3Fe-4S] cluster and is structurally related to the family of *molybdopterin enzyme* (Anderson et al. 1992) [Fig 3]. The Mo-pterin cofactor is released on denaturation, like that from other molybdenum proteins (McEwan et al. 2002). The structure of arsenite oxidase shows two subunits, a larger 88-kDa polypeptide containing the Mo-pterin and a HiPIP 3Fe-4S center and a smaller 14-kDa subunit with the Rieske 2Fe-2S center (Fig. 3A) (Ellis et al. 2001). Arsenite oxidase is thus unique in that the reduction or oxidation of active site occurs without accumulation of Mo(V) is consistent with failure to observe a Mo(V) EPR signal for the enzyme under a variety of conditions and is an indicative of an obligate two-electron centre. That is why arsenite oxidase is an unusual example of a highly cooperative two-electron Molybdenum centre (Conrads et al. 2002). The amino-acid sequence deduced from the DNA sequence of small subunit aoxA and large subunit aoxB correspond to two proteins of 174 and 826 amino acid (aa) respectively. The 134 aa of the C-terminal end of the putative AoxA protein displayed 65% identity with the small sub-unit of the enzyme of *A. faecalis* (Muller et al. 2003). The consensus sequence Cys-X-His-X_{15}-Cys-X_2-His, which coordinate the Riske type[2Fe-2S] cluster in the small sub-unit of *A.faecalis*, was detected at equivalent position in AoxA. However, the predicted Aox protein of stain ULPA-1 was larger than the small Rieske sub-unit of *A.faecalis* (174 Vs 134 aa). An additional sequence characteristic of Tat (twin-arginine translocator) secretion signal petide was detected at N-terminus of

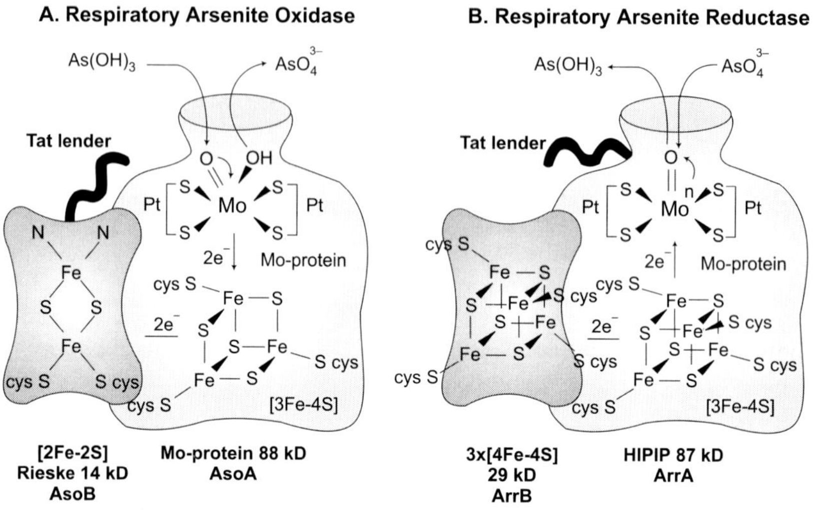

Fig. 3 Models for heterodimer arsenite oxidase (A) and arsenate reductase (B) Funnel-shaped active sites are shown at the top. Also shown are embedded Mo-pterin and [Fe-S] cofactors, proposed two-electron(2e$^-$) transfer pathways and amino-acids (Cys or His) linking the [Fe-S] cofactors to the polypeptides. HPIP, high-potential iron protein. The structure and proposed reaction cycle of arsenite oxidase. Reaction steps are (1) binding of arsenite to the enzyme, (2) two-electron transfer to Mo, oxidizing AS(III) to AS(V) and reducing MO(VI) to MO(IV), (3) release of arsenate, (4) two-electron transfer from 3Fe-4S center in large subunit to 2Fe-2S Rieske centre of small subunit, and (6) electron transfer from the 2Fe-2S centre of arsenite oxidase to the respiratory chains to oxygen. (adopted from Silver and Phung 2005)

FIG. 3. Genes for the arsenite oxidase region in *A. faecalis* (NCBI accession number AY297781; http://www.uic.edu/depts/mcmi/faculty/silver.html), a Sargasso Sea *meta*-genome environmental isolate (NCBI AACY01082423) (59), *C. arsenoxidans* (NCBI AF509588) (37), and chemolithoautotrophic strain NT-26 (NCBI AY345225) (51) and upstream and downstream genes. Presumed gene product lengths (in amino-acids [aa]) and functions are indicated, as are per cent amino-acid identities between homologous products and those of *A. faecalis*.

AoxA (Fig)(Muller et al 2003). The protein sequence deduced from aoxB (826 aa) showed 72% identity with the large sub-unit (825 aa) of the alcaligenes faecalis enzyme. No signal sequence was detected for this sub-unit. The [3Fe-4S] cluster binding motif Cys-X_2-Cys-X_3 –cys-X_{70}-Ser of *A. faecalis* and the majority of aminoacid interacting with the molybdenum centre are conserved in AoxB of strain ULPAs1 (Muller et al. 2003). In another α-protobacteria NT-26 Aro subunit share ≤ 52% identity with the respective subunits of arsenite oxidases. Tat-translocated proteins in the periplasm are exported already folded in final tertiary form with bound cofactors (unlike the Sec system which exports unfolded polypeptides that then fold outside the cell membrane) (Berks et al 2000; Yahr and Wickner 2001). The hypothesis from the preliminary gene sequence is then that a Tat signal sequence of the small subunit suffices for Tat export of the heterodimer, consisting of small and large AsoA and AsoB sub-units, with inserted Mo-pterin and Fe-S clusters that were synthesized, assembled and inserted in the cytoplasm. This follows from the primary sequence of the unprocessed protein translated from the asoAB genes plus extensive studies on other members of the DMSO reductase family (McEwan et al. 2002). Phylogenies for the two constituent sub-units (i.e molybdopterin–containing and the Rieske sub-unit) of the heterodimeric enzyme and their respective homologous in DMSO reductase, formate dehydrogenase, nitrate reductase, and the Rieske/cytb were calculated from multiple sequence alignments. The obtained phylogenetic trees indicates an early origin of arsenite oxidase before the divergence of archaea and bacteria (Labrum et al. 2003).

2.3 Gene Cluster

The *Alcaligenes* arsenic-related genes called *'arsenic gene island'* are presented in Fig. 4. Though the details are incomplete, but the overall conclusion is that arsenite oxidase is encoded in a gene island of over twenty functionally related genes, a major change in the understanding of cellular arsenite resistance, from a smaller operon to a larger 'island' with multiple related phenotypes. A cluster of four contiguous genes including those encoding arsenite oxidase was identified (GenBank accession number AF509588) (Muller et al. 2003) from *Cenibacterium arsenoxidans*, a newly named member of the β-Proteobacteria isolated from industrial wastewater (Weeger et al.1999). The four identified genes were named aoxABCD (for arsenite oxidase); a fifth, a partial gene upstream of aoxA was also found (Fig. 3). Unfortunately, the current names for the *A. fecalis* genes and the homologous genes from *C. arsenoxidans* are different, although the asoA gene product is 73% identical at the amino-acid level to the aoxB gene product; similarly, the asoB and aoxA gene products are 62% identical. Yet another set of genes named as aroA and aroB, isolated from chemolithoautotrophic a-Proteobacterium strain NT-26, were homologous to those of AsoA and asoB from *A. fecalis* (Santini et al. 2004). The chemolithoautotrophic strain NT-26 is thought to derive useful energy for growth from arsenite oxidation, although it is debatable whether obligatory heterotrophic arsenite-oxidizing strains derive useful energy in

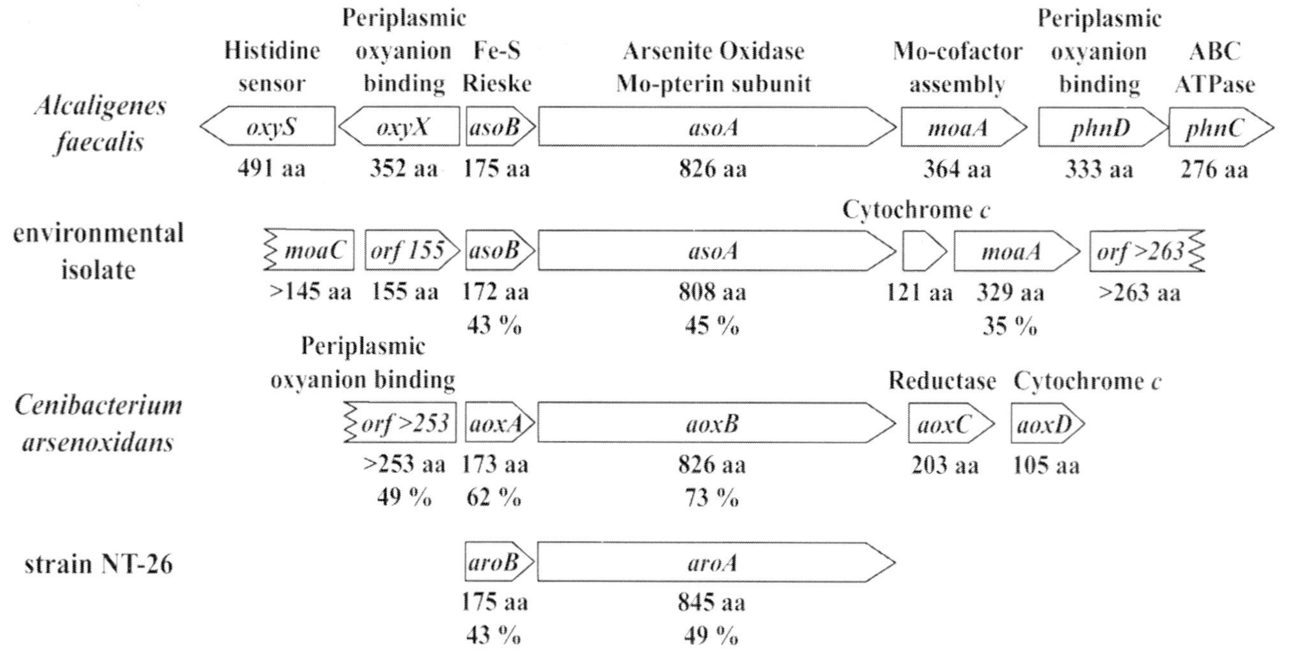

Fig. 4 Genes for the arsenite oxidase region in A. faecalis (NCBI accession number AY297781; http://www.uic.edu/depts/mcmi/faculty/silver.html), a Sargasso Sea *meta*-genome environmental isolate (NCBI AACY01082423), *C. arsenoxidans* (NCBI AF509588) and chemolithoautotrophic strain NT-26 (NCBI AY345225) and upstream and downstream genes. Presumed gene product lengths (in amino acids [aa]) and functions are indicated, as are per cent amino-acid identities between homologous products and those of *A. faecalis*. (adopted from Silver and Phung 2005)

this way. Researchers are clearly at an early stage of understanding arsenite-oxidizing microbes. Downstream from asoBA and aoxAB, the *A. fecalis*, *C. arsenoxidans* are unrelated both at the DNA level as well as at the protein level (Fig. 4). In addition to bacterial sequences, reasonable candidate for arsenite oxidase have been identified in the genomes of two hyperthermophilic Archaea, *Aeropyrum pernix* (Genbank accession number NC_000854) and *Sulfolobus tokodaii* (Accession no. NC_003106).

3. ARSENATE REDUCTASE: A CELLULAR MECHANISM FOR DETOXIFICATION

Arsenate-respiring bacteria affect the specification and mobilization of arsenic as they have been shown to release asrenite from sediment and ferrihydrite as well as grow on arsenate containing mineral (Newman et al. 1997, 1998).

3.1 Cytoplasmic Arsenate Reductase

Arsenic resistance in bacteria is conferred by mechanisms involving proteins encoded by the *ars* operons (Carlin et al. 1995), depicted in Fig. 5 a and b. The two most common types of these operons contain either five (*ars*RDABC) or three genes (*ars*RBC). The *ars*RDABC operons are found in the plasmids of Gram-negative bacteria, such as *E. Coli* R773, and *ars*RBC is generally in the plasmids of Gram-positive bacteria such as *Staphylococcus aureus* pI258, or in the bacterial chromosome (Diorio et al. 1995). The *ars*DR genes encode transacting proteins that are responsible for operon regulation (Wu and Rosen 1993). *ars*R controls the basal levels of expression in response to arsenite, and *ars*D controls the upper and basal levels of expression. Arsenate and phosphate are chemically similar, which allows the arsenic ion to utilize phosphate transport systems to enter the cell.

Operons, which encode arsenic resistance, have been found in multicopy plasmids from both gram-positive and gram-negative bacteria. The resistance mechanism is encoded from a single operon which typically consists of an arsenite ion-inducible repressor that regulates expression of an arsenate reductase and inner membrane-associated arsenite export system. Using a *lac*Z transcriptional gene fusion library, authors (Diorio et al. 1995) have identified an *Escherichia coli* operon whose expression is induced by cellular exposure to sodium arsenite at concentrations as low as 5 micrograms/litre. This *chromosomal operon* was cloned, sequenced, and found to consist of three cistrons which were named *ars*R, *ars*B, and *ars*C because of their strong homology to plasmid-borne *ars* operons. These

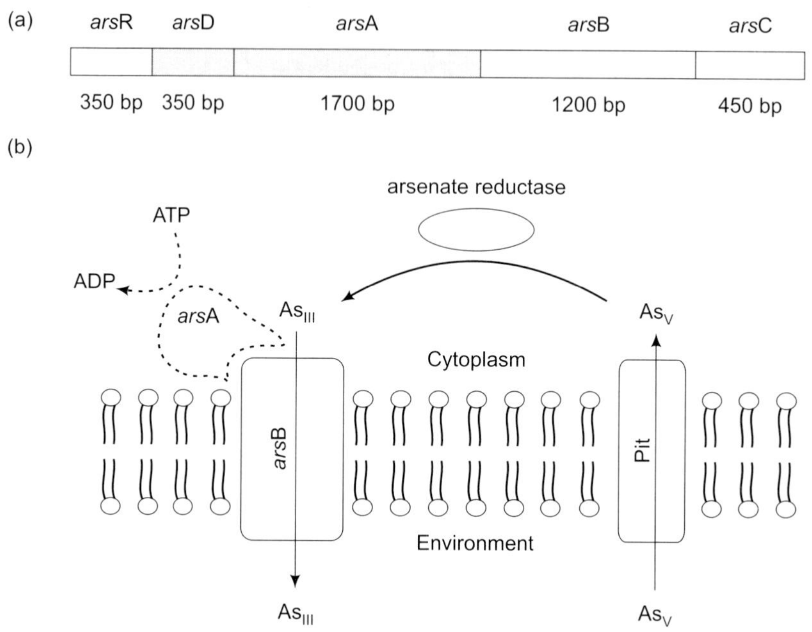

Fig. 5 Conceptual illustration of the genes of the ars operon (a) and the actions of the proteins involved in arsenic resistance (b). Arsenate can be taken up by bacterial cells via none specific phosphate transport, such as the Pit system (b). Arsenate reductase (arsC) converts arsenate to arsenite, which is extruded from the cell via the arsB protein. arsA codes for an ATPase which enhances arsenite extrusion in some organisms.

results suggested that the chromosomal ars operon may be the evolutionary precursor of the plasmid-borne operon, as a multicopy plasmid location would allow the operon to be amplified and its products to confer increased resistance to this toxic metalloid.

In some plasmid-determined systems of Gram-negative bacteria, the efflux pump consists of a two-component ATPase complex. The *ars*A gene product is a soluble ATPase subunit, which physically associates with an integral membrane protein, the product of the *ars*B gene (Dey et al.1994; Tisa and Rosen (1990). Prior to efflux, arsenate is enzymatically reduced to arsenite (the substrate of *arsB* and the activator of *ars*A ATPase activity) by the small cytoplasmic arsenate reductase, the product of the *ars*C gene (Martin et al. 2001). In most chromosomal arsenic resistance systems of

Gram-negative bacteria and the plasmids and chromosomes of Gram-positive bacteria, contiguous *ars*B and *ars*C genes are found, but there is no *ars*A gene (Rosen 1999).

The same determinants are found also on bacterial chromosomes, including those of *E. coli, Pseudomonas aeruginosa, Bacillus subtilis* and *Mycobacterium tuberculosis* (Tisa and Rosen 1990; Zegers et al. 2001; Oden et al. 1994). As more and more bacterial genomes are sequenced, it has become clear that arsenic resistance operons are ubiquitous. The chromosomal systems are functional and provide arsenic tolerance; inactivating these *ars* operons leads to 'hypersensitivity' to arsenic compounds. Bacterial *ars* systems confer arsenic resistance primarily by encoding a specific efflux pump that extrudes As(III) from the cytoplasm (Rosen 1999), thus lowering the intracellular concentration of arsenic.

The resistance mechanism controlled by the *ars* operon comprises a specific efflux pump that removes As(III) from the cytoplasm. The specific efflux pump in most plasmids of Gram-negative bacteria is a two-component ATPase complex coded by the *ars*A and *ars*B genes (Rosen et al. 1999; Wu et al. 1993; Gatti et al. 2000). *ars*B is the potential-driven membrane arsenite efflux protein that is associated with the *ars*A gene product, a soluble ATPase subunit, to form a complex responsible for the removal of arsenite throughout the membrane. In the Gram-negative bacterial chromosome as well as in the plasmids and chromosomes of Gram-positive bacteria, the arsenic operons do not possess the *ars*A gene and the operons have only the *ars*RBC genes (Dey and Rosen 1995). In these cases, the *ars*B protein is solely responsible for arsenite removal from the cell.

Prior to efflux, arsenate is reduced to arsenite by an arsenate reductase, the gene product of *ars*C (Gladysheva et al. 1994; Oden et al. 1994). Bacterial arsenate reductases can be grouped into two families according to their structure and consequent catalytic mechanisms, but both share a need to be associated with proteins that promote thiol oxidation/reduction, such as glutaredoxin (Grx) or thioredoxin (Trx), in order to catalyze disulphide bond reduction (Mukhopadhyay et al. 2002). The best-studied group is the *E. coli* resistance plasmid R773 family (Fig. 6A). This arsenate reductase is dependent on Grx and reduced glutathione (GSH) to convert arsenate to arsenite. Cys12 is the amino-acid residue that is thought to be the catalyst site, and some crystallographic evidence indicates the formation of two intermediates, (Cys12) S-As(V) and (Cys12) S-As(III) (Martin et al. 2001). A third intermediate in the catalytic cycle, (Cys12) S-As(V)-S (GSH), has also been proposed.

The first step in the catalytic cycle involves the formation of a thioarsenate binary adduct (Cys12) S-As(V). This compound reacts with GSH to form the (Cys12) S-As(V)-S (GSH) intermediate. In the next step of

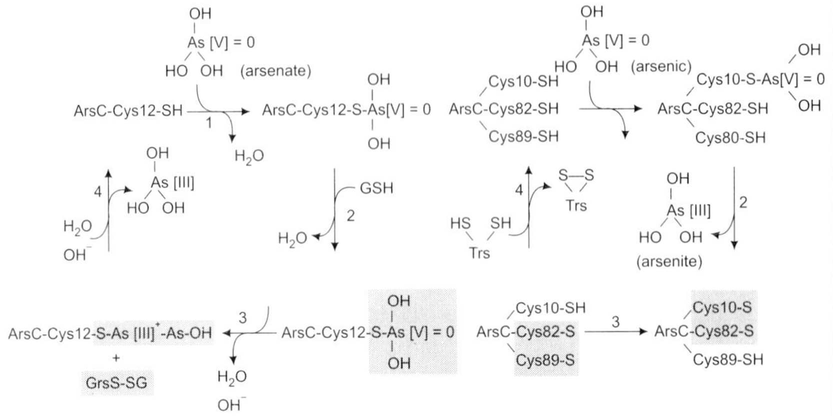

Fig. 6 The proposed reaction mechanism pathways of ArsC arsenate reductases from (A) plasmid R7739 from *E. coli* and (B) plasmid pl258 from (*Staphylococcus aureus*). The figure is highlighted to emphasize the differences in proposed intermediates.

catalysis, arsenate is reduced to arsenite, and Grx is the electron donor, forming a novel covalent As(III) intermediate, (Cys12) S-As^+-OH^-, which is hydrolyzed, releasing As(III). The crystal structure of R773 arsenate reductase indicates that the amino-acid residues Arg60, Arg94 and Arg107 are close to the catalytic Cys12 (Martin et al. 2001). The concentration of positive charge stabilizes the bound substratum residue and lowers the pKa.

In the *Staphylococcus* Trx family (Fig. 6B) the *S. aureus* plasmid p1258 arsenate reductase has the PTPase I-fold that is typical of low-molecular weight tyrosine phosphatases (Zegers et al. 2001). In this *ars*C enzyme, in addition to Cys10 (the equivalent cysteine residue of R778's Cys12), there are two other cysteine residues involved in catalysis, Cys82 and cys89. The active site Cys10 attacks arsenate nucleophylically with protonated oxygen from Asp105. Cys10 provides electrons for the reduction of arsenate to arsenite and forms a disulfide bond with cys82. Cys89 then attacks cys82, reforming the Cys10 thiolate in a step that utilizes Trx. *Bacillus subtilis* arsenate reductase also belongs to this family, and it has a similar catalytic mechanism (Bennett et al. 2001).

Chromobacterium violaceum possesses a chromosomal arsenic resistance operon of the *ars*RBC type (ORFs CV2438, CV2439 and CV2440) that comprises a regulatory protein *ars*R, a membrane-bound protein responsible for arsenite efflux *ars*B, and an arsenic reductase, *ars*C (Vasconcelos et al. 2003). The amino-acid sequence of the *ars*R protein from

C. violaceum was compared with four sequences of other *ars*R proteins found in the NCBI database, following alignment with the Clustal W programme (Fig. 7).

The *ars*R sequence of *C. violaceum* did not contain the conserved cysteine residues (ELCVDCL), which are considered to be the metal binding domain present in typical *ars*R proteins, such as chromosomal *E. coli ars*R (Shi et al. 1998, 1999). The absence of this domain places this protein in the atypical group of *ars*R proteins, which is represented by the *ars*R protein from *Acidithiobacillus ferrooxidans* (Butcher et al. 2000). The *C. violaceum ars*R protein is most similar to a hypothetical protein from *Ralstonia metallidurans* (58% homology, E-value of 8E-28). The putative regulator *ars*R found in the NCBI that is most similar to *C. violaceum* is from *Ralstonia solanacearum* (54% homology, E-value of 9E-24). Although the binding motif is absent in these atypical proteins, other conserved residues appear in this group of regulator proteins, such as two cysteine residues close to the C-terminal of the protein and the conserved Gly-X-L-(A/G) motif located immediately downstream of the region corresponding to the metal-binding motif of typical *ars*R proteins. As they do not possess the metal binding motif, the way in which regulation is performed by these proteins is not yet well established. However, in *A. ferrooxidans*, the *ars*R protein is able to regulate the expression of the operon by responding to either As(III) or As(V) (Butcher et al. 2000).

Families of Arsenic Transporters:

Bacterial arsenic resistance (*ars*) operons encode an arsenite-efflux system that can be a secondary carrier protein (*ars*B) or an anion – translocating ATPase (ArsAB). Yeast extrude arsenite using Acr3p, a plasma membrane carrier protein, or sequester it in vacuoles as the glutatione conjugate using Ycf1p, an ABC transporter. Both the mechanisms are illustrated in Fig.8. The transport of arsenate into bacterial cells as oxy-anions comparable to those of phosphate is carried out by phosphate transport membrane systems, for example the Pit and Pst systems of *Escherichia coli*. $As(OH)_3$ is transported into cells at neutral pH by aqua-glyceroporins (glycerol transport proteins) in bacteria, yeast and mammals (Rosen 1999; Rosen et al 1999), since $As(OH)_3$ resembles the inorganic equivalent of a polyol. GlpF, which was originally identified as the glycerol facilitator in *E. coli*, is a member of the aqua-glyceroporin family. Disruption of the *glpF* gene confers resistance to antimonite, consistent with the GlpF channel allowing translocation of $Sb(OH)_3$ (Cai et al. 1998). It seems likely that $As(OH)_3$ is a GlpF substrate also, but arsenite also may enter *E. coli* by another system. The structure of the *E. coli* GlpF protein has been solved at 6.9 Å resolution (Dey et al. 1994) and shows a tetrameric assembly of sub-units, comparable to aquaporins, but with a larger central channel in each sub-unit. The

```
                 ....|....|  ....|....|  ....|....|  ....|....|  ....|....|  ....|....|
                     5           15          25          35          45          55
C. violaceum     ---- E  A   T AAA D     TR -A R      GPEG A G    IGER AAN    AT  FH  E
A. ferrooxidans   EP DPA I   AR EA A P    R EIPR     E EPTG  G    DIAEH G PH  NGI FH  N
R. solanacearum  ---- EETDA  IR  AA AH    R R FR      AGPAG TPG   AIAE  D PG  AT  FH  E
E. coli ch.      ----  F  P  I  F I ADE  TR GI       E G--E C C   D CTA D     P I RH A

                 ....|....|  ....|....|  ....|....|  ....|....|  ....|....|  ....|....|
                     65          75          85          95          105         115
C. violaceum     HAG I  R    EGRFI   AN   E  NA  GF   TENCCRG-E   T C T-------  -PANN PPCD
A. ferrooxidans  HAG  T R    EGR  R RAA   P  RA  A    TENCCHGTR   D C A------    GETR P
R. solanacearum  NAA  T ER   DGRH I RAA  FDH NG  GF   TENCC G-E   A C--------  -PEF AAGC
E. coli ch.      RE G   DR    G  H R     -PHIP  AA   IIE A RCE   E   I RN      AR NC  D

                 ....

C. violaceum     GTD-
A. ferrooxidans  EGNQ
R. solanacearum  --C-
E. coli ch.      NTCS
```

Fig. 7 Sequence alignment of a selection of arsR proteins isolated from the chromosomes of different organisms, including *Chromobacterium violaceum*, *Acidithiobacillus ferrooxidans*, *Ralstonia solanacearum* and *Escherichia coli*. Sequences were obtained from the NCBI data bank. Boxed residues are conserved and are possibly directly involved in regulation. The alignment was performed using the CLUSTAL W-based optimal alignment tool. (adopted from Carepo et al. 2004)

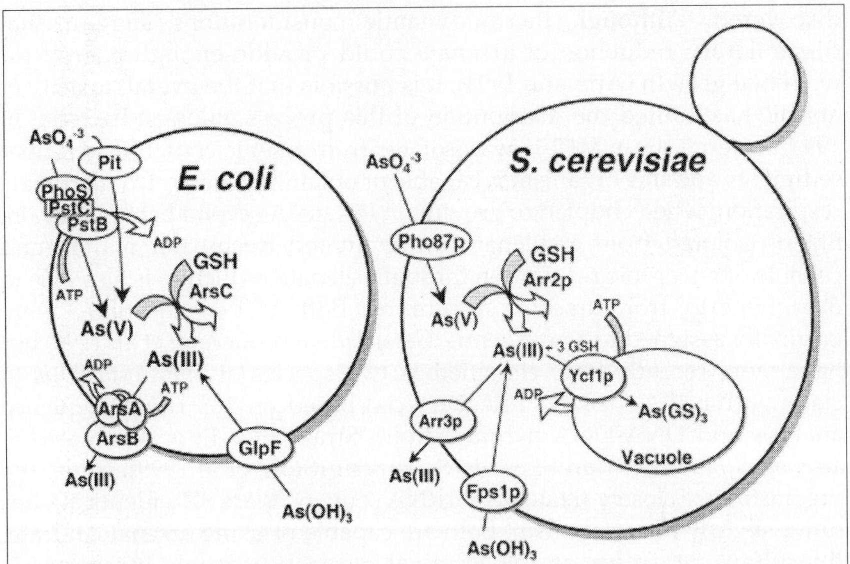

Fig. 8 Arsenical detoxification: Arsenite and arsenate transport in *E. coli* and *S. cerevisiae.* Arsenate As(V) is taken up by phosphate transporters, and As(III) is taken up by aquaglceroproteins (GlpF in *E. coli* and Fps1p in yeast). In both *E. coli* and *S. cerevisiae,* arsenate is reduced to arsenite by the bacteria ArsC or yeast Acr2p enzymes, the cytoplasmic arsenate reductases. ArsB and Arr3p, the potential-driven membrane arsenite efflux proteins (in bacteria coupled with ArsA to form an ATPase). Pit and Pho87p, the potential-coupled phosphate (and arsenate) uptake transporters. PstB, PstC, PhoS, the three-component Pst ATP-coupled phosphate (and arsenate) uptake system. In both organisms, glutathione and glutaredoxin serve as the source of reducing potential. Ycf1p, the As(III)-3 GSH adduct carrier that transports the adduct complex into the yeast cell vacuole compartment, functioning as an ATPase. GSH, glutathione. (adopted from Rosen 1999)

problem for a glyceroporin membrane protein is how to allow glycerol (and arsenite) movement across the membrane while excluding the smaller water molecules. Deletion of the gene for yeast aqua-glyceroporin Fps1p similarly confers resistance to Sb(III) and to As(III) (Wysocki et al. 1997).

3.2 Arsenic Breathing Bacteria: Dissimilatory Reduction of Arsenate

While a number of bacteria are capable of reducing arsenate as a form of detoxification, it was only recently that organisms capable of using arsenate as the terminal electron acceptor in anaerobic respiration were discovered. Although thermodynamic considerations suggest that dissimilatory reduction of arsenate could provide enough energy for microbial growth (Ahmann 1994), it is possible that the overall toxicity of arsenic has limited the distribution of this process amongst bacteria. In 1994, bacterial strain MIT-13 was isolated from arsenic-contaminated river sediments and this organism is capable of obtaining energy from arsenate respiration, when coupled to growth on lactate. A second bacterial strain, SES-3, isolated from a selenate contaminated freshwater marsh (and capable of anaerobic respiration through selenate reduction is also able to obtain energy from arsenate respiration. Both MIT-13 and SES-3 were originally assigned to a new genus, *Geospirillum* (Lonergan et al. 1996) but have more recently been classified as two species of *Sulfurospirillum* (a clade within the epsilon Proteobacteria) based on 16S rRNA sequence analysis and DNA-DNA hybridizations. Strain MIT-13 is designated *S. arsenophilum* and strain SES-3 is *S. barnesii* (Stolz et al.1999). Thus, the organisms are closely related (16SrRNA sequences are 97% identical), but differ slightly in metabolism. Both are capable of using arsenate, nitrate, thiosulfate, or sulfur as the terminal electron acceptor in anaerobic respiration, and can also grow microaerobically with low levels of oxygen or fermentatively on fumarate. *S. barnesii* is also capable of respiratory iron or selenate reduction (23,26), while *S. arsenophilum* can reduce sulphate. In terms of arsenate reduction, *S. arsenophilum* shows optimal growth at around 10 mM AsV (Ahmann 1994), whereas *S. barnesii* shows optimum growth at 5 mM AsV. Growth at higher arsenate concentrations may be inhibited by accumulating levels of arsenite. A third dissimilatory arsenate reducing bacterium was isolated from lake sediments that had low levels of arsenic contamination (Newman et al. 1997). This organism (originally referred to as strain OREX-4) is capable of respiring lactate when using either arsenate or sulphate as the terminal electron acceptor, with arsenate being the acceptor of choice. Unlike the other two isolates, this organism was phylogenetically affiliated with the low G+C Gram-positive bacteria, and has been designated *Desulfotomaculum auripigmentum*. The specific epithet *auripigmentum* refers to its ability to form the yellow colored arsenic trisulphide (As2S3) through the joint reduction of arsenate and sulphate (Newman et al. 1997a). The arsenic trisulphide precipitates both intra- and extra-cellularly, being found near the cell-membrane and on the surface of the cell-wall. Apart from growing on sodium arsenate in laboratory cultures, *D. auripigmentum* was capable of respiring arsenate released from the mineral scorodite, suggesting that naturally occurring rocks might serve as a source of AsV for dissimilatory arsenate reducers (Newman et al. 1997a). Two other dissimilatory AsV reducing bacteria that are phylogenetically affiliated with the low G+C Gram-positive bacteria were isolated from an alkaline, arsenic-rich, saline lake, and have been designated *Bacillus arsenicoselenatis* and *Bacillus selenitireducens* (Blum et al. 1998). Both isolates are alkaliphiles that are also capable of growth through the respiratory reduction of selenium compounds.

An organism that represents a novel phylogenetic group of bacteria was isolated from a reed bed exposed to goldmine wastewater (Macy et al. 1996). This bacterium is strictly anaerobic, using arsenate, nitrate, or nitrite as the terminal electron acceptor in respiration. 16S rRNA sequence analysis for this organism suggests that it is the first representative of a deeply branching lineage of Domain Bacteria, and the organism has been named *Chrysiogenes arsenatis*. Unlike the other arsenate reducers, *C. arsenatis* can use acetate, which combined with its unique phylogeny, suggests a novel mechanism of arsenate reduction. The respiratory arsenate reductase from this organism has been characterized and is inducible by arsenate, does not recognise alternative electron acceptors (i.e. it is arsenate specific), and is located in the periplasm (Kraft and Macy 1998). This is in contrast to the respiratory arsenate reductase of *S. barnesii*, which is thought to span the cell-membrane with its active site facing the cytoplasm (Newman et al. 1998). Among the archaea, a strictly anaerobic hyperthermophile was isolated from a hot spring in Italy, and this organism (*Pyrobaculum arsenaticum*) is capable of respiratory growth using arsenate, sulphur, or selenate (Huber et al. 2000). The isolate can also grow chemoautotrophically using carbon dioxide, hydrogen as an electron donor, and arsenate or sulphur as the electron acceptor. 16S rRNA gene sequence analysis showed that this organism belongs to the Thermoproteales order of archaea, and when tested, another species of this order (*Pyrobaculum aerophilum*) was also able to grow anaerobically in the presence of arsenate or selenate. Other recently discovered arsenate respiring organisms include a species (strain GBFH) of *Desulfitobacterium* (belonging to the low G+C Gram positive bacteria) isolated from arsenic-contaminated lake sediments (Niggemyer et al, 2001), and a new strain of *Thermus* (strain HR13; *Deinococcus/Thermus* phylum of Bacteria) isolated from the drainage channel of an arsenic-rich hot spring (Gihring 2001).

The most detailed report of the purification and characterization of the respiratory arsenate reductase enzyme (Fig. 2B) (Kraft and Macy 1998) showed that this enzyme-like arsenite oxidase, is a heterodimer periplasmic or membrane associated protein consisting of a larger molybdopterin sub-unit (*Arr*A) which contains an iron-sulphur center, perhaps a high potential [4Fe-4S] cluster, and a smaller [Fe-S] centre protein (*Arr*B) that is not homologous to the Rieske polypeptide of arsenite oxidase. The respiratory arsenate reductase of gram-positive *Bacillus* differs from that of gram-negative bacteria in that it is anchored to the membrane of the Gram-positive cell (Afkar et al. 2003), which lacks a periplasmic compartment. Genetic determinants of a respiratory arsenate reductase system has been analysed lately from a γ-Proteobacterium, Shewanella strain ANA-3 (Saltikov et al. 2003). Interestingly, the DNA sequence consists of two divergently transcribed operons (Fig. 9) followed by a predicted transcriptional termination signal and two unrelated genes. Upstream of *arrA* and *arrB*, encoding the two subunits of respiratory reductase, is a standard *arsDABC* operon for arsenate and arsenite resistance. The transcriptional regulatory gene, *arsR*, is absent in the sequence and is predicted to be present elsewhere in the chromosome which is unusual as *arsR* generally occurs at the beginning of the operon.

4. FUTURE BIOTECHNOLOGICAL POTENTIALS

Inorganic arsenic primarily exists as oxidized arsenate or reduced arsenite. A number of micro-organisms have been identified that show arsenic redox activity and are capable of transforming arsenic between these two states. Microbial metabolism as illustrated in the above review, undoubtedly aggravates environmental arsenic problems, perhaps by releasing arsenic into drinking water in shallow wells (as in East Bengal, West Bengal, the American Midwest and the Canadian Maritime Provinces). However, understanding the mechanisms may help to minimize the impact. We have also got a glimpse of the arsenic detoxification mechanisms that exist in living organisms. The common themes are a) uptake of As(V) in the form of arsenate by phosphate transporters, b) uptake of As(III) in the form of arsenite by *aquaglyceroporins*, c) reduction of As (V) to As (III) by arsenate reductases, and d) extrusion or sequestration of As(III).

While the mechanisms underlying these processes are well understood in many cases, and their geochemical influences are potentially great, the ability to quantify and, more importantly, to predict the rates and extents of these processes in natural environments, remains a tremendous challenge for the future. Further work is needed for designing strategies for practical bioremediation of drinking water contaminated with arsenic. We propose the areas need to be explored further:

- Designing microbial batch reactors to remove arsenic by oxidation of As(III) to As(V) (Lievremont et al. 2003).
- Use of bacterial arsenate reductase genes in transgenic plants for potential phytoremediation by intracellular sequestration after reduction from As(V) to As(III) (Dhanker et al. 2002).
- Devising a sensing system for arsenite, based on bacterial bioluminescence in which a single plasmid that incorporates the regulatory gene of the extrusion system, *arsR* and the genes of

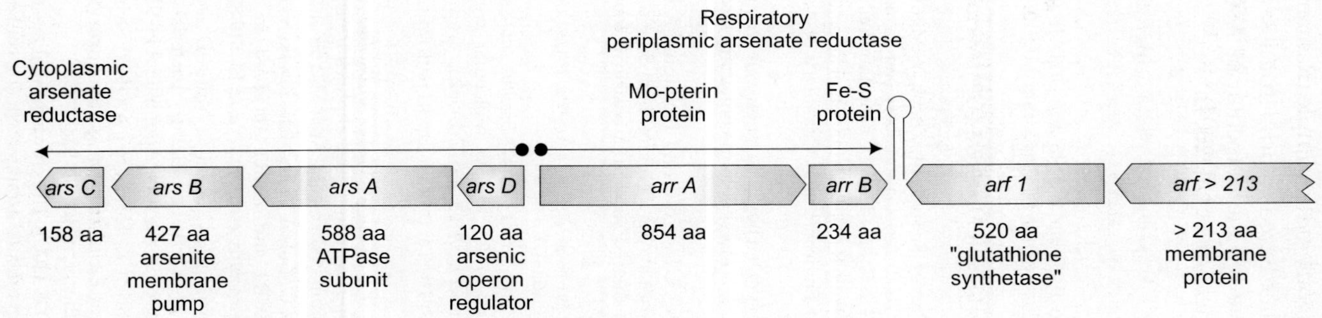

Fig. 9 Genes for respiratory (*arrAB*) and cytoplasmic (*arsC*) arsenate reductases of *Shewanella* strain ANA-3 (from GenBank accession number (AY271310). Upstream and downstream regions are divergently oriented from the *arrA* and *arrB* genes for respiratory arsenate reductase is a four-gene canonical *ars* operon with the *arsC* gene for cytoplasmic arsenate reductase. aa, amino-acid.

bacterial luciferase in a manner that is dependent on the concentration of arsenite in the sample (Ramanathan et al. 1997).

- An efficient microplate based colorimetric assay for fast screening of bacteria, sensitive for the detection of As(III) oxidisers and As(V) reducers (Simeonova et al. 2004).

REFERENCES

Afkar E, Lisak J, Saltikov C, Basu P, Oremland RS and Stolz JF (2003) The respiratory arsenate reductase from *Bacillus selenitireducens* strain MLS10. FEMS Microbiol Letts 226: 107-112

Ahmann D, Roberts A, Krumholz LR and Morel FM (1994) Microbe grows by reducing arsenic. Nature 371: 750

Ahsan H, Perrin M, Rahman A, Parvez F, Stute M, Zheng Y, Milton AH, Brandt-Rauf P, VanGreen A and Graziano J (2000) Associations between drinking water and urinary arsenic levels and skin lesions in Bangladesh. J Occup Environ Med 42: 1195-1201

Anderson GL, Ellis PJ, Kuhn P and Hille R (2001) Oxidation of arsenite by *Alcaligenes faecalis*. In: Frankenberger WT Jr (ed) Environmental Chemistry of Arsenic. Marcel Dekker, New York, pp 343-362

Anderson GL, Williams J, Hille R (1992) The purification and characterization of arsenite oxidase from *Alcaligenes faecalis*, a molybdenum-containing hydroxylase. J Biol Chem 267: 23674-23682

Aslund F, Ehn B, Miranda-Vizuete A, Pueyo C and Holmgren A (1994) Two additional glutaredoxins exist in *Escherichia coli* : glutaredoxin-3 is a hydrogen donor for ribonucleotide reductase in a thioredoxin/glutaredoxin-1 double mutant. Proc Natl Acad Sci USA 91: 9813-9817

Bates MN, Smith AH and Hopenhayn-Rich C (1992) Arsenic ingestion and internal cancers: a review. Am J Epidemiol 135: 462-476

Bennett MS, Guan Z, Laurberg M and Su XD (2001) *Bacillus subtilis* arsenate reductase is structurally and functionally similar to low molecular weight protein tyrosine phosphatases. Proc Natl Acad Sci USA 98: 13577-13582

Berks BC, Sargent F, Palmer T (2000) The Tat protein export pathway. Mol Microbiol 35: 260-274

Blum JS, Bindi AB, Buzzeli J, Stolz JF, Oremland RS (1998) *Bacillus arsenicoselenatis* sp nov, and *Bacillus selenitireducenes* sp nov: two haloalkaliphiles from mono lake, California that respire oxyanion of selenium and arsenic. Arch Microbiol 17: 19-30

Bobrowicz P, Wysocki R, Owsianik G, Goleau A and Ulaszewski S (1997) Isolation of three contiguous genes ACR1, ACR2 and ACR3, involved in resistance to arsenic compounds in the yeast *Saccharomyces cerevisiae*. Yeast 13: 819-828

Brunet Battaglia F, Dictor MC, Garrido F, Crouzet C, Morin D, Dekeyser K, Clarens M, Baranger P (2002) An arsenic(III)-oxidizing bacterial population:selection characterization and performance in reactors. Appl microbiol 93: 1-12

Bushweller JH, AR slund F, Wuthrich K, Holmgren A (1992) Structural and functional characterization of the mutant *Escherichia coli* glutaredoxin (C14_S) and its mixed disulphide with glutathione. Biochemistry 31: 9288-9293

Butcher BG, Deane SM, Rawlings DE (2000) The chromosomal arsenic resistance genes of *Thiobacillus ferrooxidans* have an unusual arrangement and confer increased arsenic and antimony resistance to *Escherichia coli*. Appl Environ Microbiol 66: 1826-1833

Cai J, Salmon K, DuBow MS (1998) A chromosomal *ars* operon homologue of *Pseudomonas aeruginosa* confers increased resistance to arsenic and antimony in *Escherichia coli*. Microbiology 144: 2705-2713

Carepo MSP, Juliana S, Nina de Azevedo, Porto JIR, Bentes-Sousa AR, Batista JS, Silva ALC, Schneider MPC (2004) Identification of *Chromobacterium violaceum* genes with potential biotechnological application in environmental detoxification. Genet Mol Res 3: 181-195

Carlin A, Shi W, Dey S, Rosen BP (1995) The ars operon of *Escherichia coli* confers arsenical and antimonial resistance. J Bacteriol 177: 981-986

Cervantes C, Ji G, Ramrez JL, Silver S (1994) Resistance to arsenic compounds in micro-organisms. FEMS Microbiol Rev 15: 355-367

Challenger F (1951) Biological methylation. Adv Enzymol 12: 429- 491

Chowdhury TR, Basu GK, Mandal Bk, Samanta G, Chowdhury UK, Chanda CR, Lodh D, Roy SL, Saha KC, Roy S, Kabir S, Quamruzzaman Q and Chakraborti D (1999) Arsenic Poisoning in the Ganges delta. Nature 401: 545-547

Conrads T, Hemann C, George GM, Pickering IJ, Prince RC, Hille R (2002) The active site of arsenite oxidase from *Alcaligenes faecalis*. J Am chem Soc 124 :11276-11277

Craig PJ (1989) Biological and environmental methylation of metals. In: Hartley FR (ed) The Chemistry of the Metal-Carbon Bond, John Wiley and Sons, London, Vol 5, pp 437-463

Cummings DE, Caccavo Jr F, Fendorf S, Rosenzweig RF (1999) Arsenic mobilization by dissimilatory Fe(III)- Reducing bacterium *Shewanella alga* BrY. Environ Sc Technol 33: 723-729

Denu JM, Dixon JE (1998) Protein tyrosine phosphatases: mechanisms of catalysis and regulation. Curr Opin Chem Biol 2: 633-641

Dey S, Dou D, Tisa LS, Rosen BP (1994) Interaction of the catalytic and the membrane sub-units of an oxy-anion-translocating ATPase. Arch Biochem Biophys 311: 418-424

Dey S, Rosen BP (1995) Dual mode of energy coupling by oxyanion-translocation *arsB* protein. J Bacteriol 177: 385-389

Dhankher OP, Li Y, Rosen BP, Shi J, Salt D, Senecoff JF, Sashti NA, Meagher RB (2002) Engineering tolerance and hyperaccumulation of arsenic in plants by combining arsenate reductase and gamma-glutamylcysteine synthetase expression. Nat Biotechnol 20: 1140-1145

Diorio C, Cai J, Marmor J, Shinder R, DuBow MS (1995) An *Escherichia coli* chromosomal *ars* operon homolog is functional in arsenic detoxification and is conserved in gram-negative bacteria. J Bacteriol 177: 2050- 2056

Ehrlich HL (2001) Bacterial oxidation of As(III) compounds In: Frankenberger WT, Jr (eds) Environmental Chemistry of Arsenic Marcel Dekker, New York pp 313-328

Ellis PJ, Conrads T, Hille R, Kuhn P (2001) Crystal structure of the 100 kDa arsenate oxidase from *Alcaligenes faecalis* in two crystal forms at 1.64 AR and 2.03 AR. Structure 9: 125-132

Galperin MY, Walker DR, Koonin EV (1998) Analogous enzymes: independent inventions in enzyme evolution. Genome Res 8: 779-790

Gatti D, Mitra B, Rosen BP (2000) *Escherichia coli* soft metal ion-translocating ATPase. J Biol Chem 275: 34009-340012

Ghosh M, Shen J, Rosen BP (1999) Pathways of As(III) detoxification in *Saccharomyces cerevisiae*. Proc Natl Acad Sci USA 96: 5001-5006

Gihring TM, Banfield JF (2001) Arsenite oxidation and arsenate respiration by a new *Thermus* isolate. FEMS Microbiol Lett 204 : 335-340

Gihring TM, Druschel GK, Mccleskey RB, Hamer RJ, Banfield JF (2001) Rapid arsenite oxidation by *Thermus aquaticus* and *Thermus thermophilus*:field and laboratory investigation. Env Sci Technol 35: 3857-3862

Gladysheva TB, Oden KL, Rosen BP (1994) Properties of the arsenate reductase of plasmid R773. Biochemistry 33: 7288-7293

Green HH (1918) Description of a bacterium that oxidizes arsenite to arsenate and one which reduces arsenate to arsenite, isolated from cattle dipping tank. South African J Sci 14: 456-467

Hofmann K, Bucher P, Kajava AV (1998) A model of Cdc25 phosphatase catalytic domain and Cdk-interaction surface based on the presence of a rhodanese homology domain. J Mol Biol 282:195-208

Hoke KR, Cobb N, Armstrong FA, Hille R (2004) Elecrochemical studies of Arsenite oxidase: An Unusual example of a Highly cooperative Two-Electron Molybdenum Centre. Biochemistry 43: 1667-1674

Hoven N, Vanden R, Santini JM (2004) Arsenite oxidation by the heterotrophs

Huber R, Sacher M, Vollman A. Huber H, Rose D (2000) Respiration of arsenate and selenate by hyperthermophylic archaea. Syst. Appl. Microbiol. 23: 305-314

Hydrogenophaga sp.str.NT-14: the arsenite oxidase and its physiological electron acceptor. Biochemica et Biophysica Acta 1656: 148-155

Ilyaletdinov AN, Abdrashitova SA (1981) Autotrophic oxidation of arsenic by a culture of *Pseudomonas arsenitoxidans*. Mikrobiologiya 50:197-204

Islam FS, Gault AG, Boothman C, Polya DA, Charnock JM, Chatterjee D, Lloyd JR (2004) Role of metal-reducing bacteria in arsenic release from Bengal delta sediment. Nature 430: 68- 71

Jacobs DM, Messens J, Wechselberger RW, Brosens Willem R, Wyns L, Martins JC (2001) 1H, 13C and 15N backbone resonance assignment of arsenate reductase from *Staphylococcus aureus* in its reduced state. J Biomol NMR 20: 95-96

Ji G, Silver S (1992) Reduction of arsenate to arsenite by the *arsC* protein of the arsenic resistance operon of *Staphylococcus aureus* plasmid pI258. Proc Natl Acad Sci USA 89: 9474-9478

Ji G, Garber EA, Armes LG, Chen CM, Fuchs JA, Silver S (1994) Arsenate reductase of *Staphylococcus aureus* plasmid pI258. Biochemistry 33: 7294-7299

Ji G, Silver S (1992) Regulation and expression of the arsenic resistance operon from *Staphylococcus aureus* plasmid pI258. J Bacteriol 174: 3684-3694

Kennelly PJ (2002) Protein kinases and protein phosphatases in prokaryotes: a genomic perspective. FEMS Microbiol Lett 206: 1-8

Knowles FC, Benson AA (1983) The biochemistry of arsenic. Trends Biochem Sci 8: 178-180

Kraft T, Macy JM (1998) Purification and characterization of the respiratory arsenate reductase of *Chrysiogenes arsenatis*. Eur J Biochem 255: 647-653

Labrum E, Brugna M, Baymann F, Muller D, Lievermont D, Lett MC, Nitschke (B) (2003) Arsenite oxidase, an Ancient Bioenergetic Enzyme. Mol Biol Evol 20: 686-693

Legge JW, Turner AW (1954) Bacterial oxidation of arsenite. III. Cell-free arsenite dehydrogenase. Aust J Biol Sci 7: 496-503

Lievremont D, N'Negue MA, Behra P, Lett MC (2003) Biological oxidation of arsenite: batch reactor experiments in presence of kutnahorite and chabazite. Chemosphere 51: 419-428

Liu J, Gladysheva TB, Lee L, Rosen BP (1995) Identification of an essential cysteinyl residue in the *arsC* arsenate reductase of plasmid R773. Biochemistry 34: 13472-13476

Lonergan DJ, Jenter H, Coates JD, Schmidt T, Lovley DR (1996) Phylogenetic analysis of dissimilatory Fe(III)-reducing bacteia. J Bacteriol 178: 2402-2408

Macy JM, Nunan K, Hagen KD, Dixon DR, Harbour PJ, Cahill M, Sly LI (1996) *Chrysiogenes arsenatis* gen.nov, sp. Nov., a new arsenate respiring bacterium isolated from gold mine waste water. Int J Syst Bacteriol 46: 1153-1157

Martin P, DeMel S, Shi J, Rosen BP, Edwards BFP (2001) Insights into the structure, solvation, and mechanism of *arsC* arsenate reductase, a novel arsenic detoxification enzyme. Structure 9: 1071-1081

McArthur JM, Banerjee DM, Hudson-Edwards KA, Mishra R, Purohit R, Ravenscroft P, Cronin A, Howarth RJ, Chatterjee A, Talukder T, Lowry D, Houghton S, Chadha DK (2004) Natural organic matter in sedimentary basins and its relation to arsenic in anoxic ground water: the example of West Bengal and its world-wide implication. Applied Geochemistry 19: 1255-1293

McEwan A, Ridge JP, McDevitt CA, Hugenholtz P (2002) The DMSO reductase family of microbial molybdenum enzymes: molecular properties and role in the dissimilatory reduction of toxic elements. Geomicrobiol 19: 3-21

Messens J, Hayburn G, Desmyter A, Laus G, Wyns L (1999) The essential catalytic redox couple in arsenate reductase from *Staphylococcus aureus*. Biochemistry 38: 16857-16865

Messens J, Martins JC, Brosens E, Van Belle K, Jacobs DM, Willem R, Wyns L (2002) Kinetics and active site dynamics of *Staphylococcus aureus* arsenate reductase. J Biol Inorg Chem 7: 146-156

Messens J, Martins JC, Van Belle K, Brosen E, Desmyter A, De Gieter M, Wieruszeski JM, Willem R, Wyns L, Zegers I (2002) All intermediates of the arsenate reductase mechanism including an intramolecular dynamic disulphide bond cascade. Proc Natl Acad Sci USA 99: 8506-8511

Milton AH, Hasan Z, Rahman A, Rahman M (2001) Chronic arsenic poisoning and respiratory effects in Bangladesh. J Occup Health 43: 136-140

Mukhopadhyay R, Rosen BP (1998) *Saccharomyces cerevisiae* ACR2 gene encodes an arsenate reductase. FEMS Microbiol Lett 168: 127-136

Mukhopadhyay R, Rosen BP, Phung LT, Silver S (2002) Microbial arsenic: from geocycle to gene and enzyme. FEMS Microbiol Rev 26 :311-325

Mukhopadhyay R, Shi J, Rosen BP (2000) Purification and characterization of ACR2p, the *Saccharomyces cerevisiae* arsenate reductase. J Biol Chem 275: 21149-21157

Muller D, Lievermont D, Simeonova DD, Hubert JC, Lett MC (2003) Arsenite oxidase aox gene from a metal resistant â-protobacterium. J Bacteriol 185: 135-141

Newman DK, Ahmann D, Morel FMM (1998) A brief review of microbial arsenate respiration. Geomicrobiology 15: 255- 268.

Newman DK, Beveridge TJ, Morel FMM (1997a) Precipitation of arsenic trisulphde by *Desulfotomaculum auripigmentum*. Appl Environ Microbiol 63: 2022–2028

Newman DK, Kennedy EK, Coates JD, Ahmann D, Ellis DJ, Lovley DR, Morel FM (1997b) Dissimilatory arsenate and sulphate reduction in *Desulfotomaculum auripigmentum sp. nov.* Arch Microbiol 168: 380-388

Nickson R, McArthur J, Burgess W, Ahmed KM, Ravenscroft P, Rahman M (1998) Arsenic poisoning of Bangladesh groundwater. Nature 395: 338

Nidhubhghaill OM, Sadler PJ (1991) The structure and reactivity of arsenic compounds: biological activity and drug design. Struct Bond 78: 129-190

Niggemyer A, Spring S, Stackebrandt E, Rosenzweig RF (2001) Isolation and charecterisation of a novel As(V)- reducing bacterium: implications for arsenic mobilization and the genus desulfobacterium. Appl Environ Microbiol 67: 5568-5580

Nriagu JO (2001) Arsenic poisoning through the ages. In: Frankenberger WT (ed)Environmental Chemistry of Arsenic. Marcel Dekker, New York pp 1-26

Oden KL, Gladysheva TB, Rosen BP (1994) Arsenate reduction mediated by the plasmid-encoded ArsC protein is coupled to glutathione. Mol Microbiol 12: 301-306

Oremland RS, Hoeft SE, Santini JM, Bano N,Hollibaugh RA, Hollibaugh JT (2002) Anaerobic oxidation of arsenite in Monolake water and by a facultative arsenite oxidizing chemoautotroph, strain MLHE -1 Appl Environ Microbiol 68 :4795-4802

Oremland RS, Stolz JF (2003) The ecology of arsenic. Science 300939: 944

Osborne FH, Ehrlich FH (1976) Oxidation of arsenite by a soil isolate of Alcaligenes. J Appl Bacteriol 41: 295

Pershang G (1985) Lung cancer mortality among men living near arsenic-emitting smelters. Am J Epidemiol 122: 684-694

Phillips SE, Talylor ML (1976) Oxidation of arsenite to arsenate by Alcaligenes faecalis. Appl Environ Microbiol 32: 392-399

Quastal JH, Scholefield PG (1953) Arsenite oxidation in soil. Soil Sci 75: 279-285

Quinn JP, McMullan G (1995) Carbon-arsenic bond cleavage by a newly isolated Gram-negative bacterium, strain ASV2. Microbiology 141: 721-727

Ramanathan S, Shi W, Rosen BP, Daunert S (1997) Sensing antimonite and arsenite at the subatomole level with genetically engineered bioluminescent bacteria. Anal. Chem. 69: 3380-3384

Rosen BP (1999) Families of arsenic transporters. Trends Microbiol 7: 207-212

Rosen BP, Bhattacharjee H, Zhou TQ, Walmsely AR (1999) Mechanism of the ArsA ATPase. Biochim Biophys Acta 1461: 207-215

Salmassi TM, Venkateswaren K, Satomi MK, Nealson, Newman DK, Hering JG (2002) Oxidation of Arsenite by *Agrobacterium albertimagni* AOL 15 sp nov., isolatd from Hot Creek California. Geomicrobiol J 19: 53-66

Saltikov CW, Cifuentes A, Venkateswaran K, Newman DK (2003) The *ars* detoxification system is advantageous but not required for As(V) respiration by the genetically tractable *Shewanella* species strain ANA-3. Appl Environ Microbiol 69: 2800-2809

Santini JM, Sly LI, Schnagl RD, Macy JM (2000) A new chemolithoautotrophic Arsenite-oxidising bacterium isolated from gold mine: phylogenetic,physiological and prelimnary biochemical studies. Appl Env microbiol 66: 92-97

Santini JM, Hoven N, Vanden R (2004) Molybdenum containing arsenite oxidase of chemolithoautotrophic arsenite oxidizer NT-26. J Bacteriol 186: 1614-1619

Sato T, Kobayashi Y (1998) The *ars* operon in the skin element of *Bacillus subtilis* confers resistance to arsenate and arsenite. J Bacteriol 180: 1655-1661

Scudlark JR, Johnson DL (1982) Biological oxidation of arsenite in sea water.Estuarine. Coastal and Shelf Science 14: 693-706

Sehlin HM, Lindstrom EB (1992) Oxidation and reduction of arsenic by *Sulpholobus acidocaldarius* strain BC. FEMS Microbiol Lett 93: 87-92

Shi J, Vlamis-Gardikas A, AR Slund F, Holmgren A, Rosen BP (1999) Reactivity of glutaredoxins 1, 2, and 3 from *Escherichia coli* shows that glutaredoxin 2 is the primary hydrogen donor to *arsC*-catalyzed arsenate reduction. J Biol Chem 274: 36039-36042

Shi L, Potts M, Kennelly PJ (1998) The serine, threonine and/or tyrosine-specific protein kinases and protein phosphatases of prokaryotic organisms: a family portrait. FEMS Microbiol Rev 22: 229-253

Silver S, Budd K, Leahy KM, Shaw WV, Hammond D, Novick RP, Willsky GR, Malamy MH, Rosenberg H (1981) Inducible plasmid-determined resistance to arsenate, arsenite and antimony (III) in *Escherichia coli* and *Staphylococcus aureus*. J Bacteriol 146: 983-996

Simeonova DD, Lievremont D, Lagarde F, Muller DAE, Groudeva VI and Lett MC (2004) Microplate screening assay for the detection of arsenite-oxidizing and arsenate reducing-bacteria. FEMS Microbiol Lett 237: 249-253

Stolz JF, Oremland RS (1999) Bacterial respiration of arsenic and selenium. FEMS Microbiol Rev 23: 615-627

Suzuki K, Wakao N, Kimura T, Sakka K, Ohmiya K (1998) Expression and regulation of the arsenic resistance operon of *Acidiphilium multivorum* AIU 301 plasmid pKW301 in *Escherichia coli.* Appl Environ Microbiol 64: 411-418

Tisa LS, Rosen BP (1990) Molecular characterization of an anion pump: the *arsB* protein is the membrane anchor for the *arsA* protein. J Biol Chem 265: 190-194

Turner AW (1954) Bacterial oxidation of arsenite, a description of bacteria isolated from arsenical cattle dipping fluid. Austral J Biol Sci 7: 452-467

Vasconcelos ATR et al. (2003) The complete genome sequence of *Chromobacterium violaceum* reveals remarkable and exploitable bacterial adaptability. Proc Natl Acad Sci USA 100: 11660-11665

Wakao N, Hiroyansu K YK, Hiroshi S, Yonekichi S, Shhiota H (1988) Microbial oxidation of arsenite and occurance of arsenite oxidizing bacteria in acid mine water from a sulphur pyrite mine. Geomicrobiolol J 6: 11-24

Weeger W, Lievermont D, Perret M, Lagarde F, Hubbert JC, Leroy M, MC Lett (1999) Oxidation of arsenite to arsenate by a bacterium isolated from an aquatic environment. Biometal 12 :141-149

Welch AH, Westjohn DB, Helsel DR, Wanty RB (2000) Arsenic in ground water of the United States: occurrence and geochemistry. Groundwater 38:589-604

Willsky GR, Malamy MH (1980) Effect of arsenate on inorganic phosphate transport in *Escherichia coli.* J Bacteriol 144: 366-374

Winship KA (1984) Toxicity of inorganic arsenic salts. Adv Drug React Ac Pois Rev 3: 129-60

Wu J, Rosen BP (1993) The *arsD* gene encodes a second trans-acting regulatory protein of the plasmid-encoded arsenical resistance operon. Mol Microbiol 8: 615-623

Wysocki R, Bobrowicz P, Ulaszewski S (1997) The Saccharomyces cerevisiae ACR3 gene encodes a putative membrane protein involved in arsenite transport. J Biol Chem 272: 30061-30066

Yahr TL, Wickner WT (2001) Functional reconstitution of bacterial Tat translocation *in vitro*. EMBO J 20: 2472-2479

Zegers I, Martins JC, Willem R, Wyns L and Messens J (2001) Arsenate reductase from S. aureus pI258 is a phosphatase drafted for redox duty. Nature Struct Biol 8 : 843-847

Applications of Alkalistable and Thermostable Microbial Xylanolytic Enzymes in Pulp and Paper Industry

T SATYANARAYANA* and S ADHIKARI

1. INTRODUCTION

The pulp and paper industry is emerging as one of the largest areas for enzyme application in the world. The world market for enzymes applicable in the pulp and paper industry is about 10 million Euros and growing by an estimated 25% annually. Increased pulp yield, improved fibre properties, enhanced paper recycling, reduced processing and environmental problems are all consequences of the application of enzymes in the pulp and paper industry. Traditional bleaching methods in the pulp and paper industry rely on chlorine and its derivatives, and thus, place heavy burden on the environment. The bleaching sequence involves chlorination and alkali extraction followed by hypochlorite treatment. The effluent generated from the bleaching section contains oxygenated halogens and other associated compounds. The process based on chlorine or peroxide bleaching increases the adsorbable organic halides (AOX) discharge, biochemical/chemical oxygen demand (BOD/COD) and also adds colour and toxicity to the effluent generated. Thus, alternative strategies based on the use of biological agents may prove to be the most suitable processes. Xylanases are the key enzymes applied for the enzyme aided bleaching as it removes xylan, the most abundant natural

Department of Microbiology, University of Delhi South Campus, Benito Juarez Road, New Delhi-110 021, India. Tel.: 091-11-24102008; Fax.: 091-11-26885270
E-mail: tsnarayana@vsnl.net, tsnarayana@gmail.com

polysaccharide after cellulose. It simultaneously enhances the removal of lignin in the subsequent bleaching process. Thus it helps in the significant reduction in the use of chlorine compounds utilized in the bleaching process. Since chlorine compounds are toxic, mutagenic, persistent, bio-accumulating and potentially carcinogenic, reduction in the level of chlorine consumption through the enzyme-based process is a significant step towards alleviating environmental degeneration and degradation. Current bleaching processes are relatively inefficient due to chemical bonds that exist between hemicellulose and lignin. The application of xylanases may facilitate the removal of residual lignin by removing the residual and re-precipitated xylan (Iversen and Wännström 1986). The incorporation of xylanases into pulp and paper mill bleaching sequence may be more effective and will prove to be an ecofriendly process.

Xylanase application in the pulp and paper industry commenced in 1986, when Viikari et al. (1986) first demonstrated its utility in pulp and paper industry. Enzymatic applications are generally considered to be environmentally benign. The limitations of the use of enzymes in pulping and paper making processes are related to the size and properties of the enzymes. The conditions used in many stages in pulping and paper manufacture have led to the development of enzyme preparations having pH and temperature ranges suitable for this target process. The successful introduction of xylanase into pulp and paper process apparently requires the following characteristics:

(i) Low molecular weight ensures the enzyme access to the pulp matrix,
(ii) Thermal stability ensures activity at or beyond 70°C,
(iii) Activity at alkaline pH ensures the action on kraft pulps,
(iv) Specificity for xylan and cellulase-free nature avoids cellulose viscosity losses,
(v) Affinity for acidic side chains to maximise Hex A (hexenuronic acid) removal, and
(vi) Alkaline iso-electric point to bind enzyme more readily to the pulp fibres.

Microbial xylanases devoid of cellulase, optimally active and stable at alkaline pH and elevated temperatures have tremendous potential for application because of the nature of cellulose extraction in the kraft process (Bansod et al. 1993). The use of thermostable alkaline xylanases for enzyme-assisted pulp bleaching could greatly reduce the need for pH and temperature readjustment that offers enormous technical and economic advantages (Bastawde 1992; Bansod et al.1993). This review deals with the alkalistable and thermostable microbial xylanolytic enzymes and their applications in prebleaching of paper pulps.

2. STRUCTURE OF XYLAN

Wood is the main source of fibre for pulp and paper production. It is composed of cellulose, hemicellulose, lignin and extractives in different proportions. Cellulose is the major component of the pulp, and *hemicellulose* includes *xylan, mannan, galactan,* and *arabinan* as the main components. Removal of xylan and consequently of lignin, from the pulp greatly improves the quality of paper.

Xylans are hetero-polymers comprising mainly D-xylose as its monomeric units linked by β-1,4-glycosidic bonds, and traces of L-arabinose. The main chain of xylan is composed of β-xylopyranose residues (Whistler and Richards 1970) (Fig. 1). The total dry weight of xylan in softwood and hardwood is approximately 15-30% and 7-12%, respectively Wong et al.1988; Puls 1997). The xylan from hardwood is O-acetyl-4-O-methylglucuronoxylan consisting of at least 70 β-xylopyranose residues (average degree of polymerization (DP) between 150 and 200), linked by β-1,4-glycosidic bonds and is highly acetylated. *Acetylation* is more frequent at C-3 than at the C-2 position. The presence of these acetyl groups is responsible for the partial solubility of xylan in water. These acetyl groups are readily removed when xylan is subjected to alkali extraction (Sunna and Antranikian 1997). Xylan from softwoods is composed of arabino-4-O-methylglucuroxylans. They have higher 4-O-methylglucuronic acid residues attached to the C-2 position. Soft wood xylans are not acetylated, and instead of an acetyl group, they have α-1,3-glycosidic bonds at the C-3 position of xylose (Puls and Schuseil 1993). The softwood xylans are shorter than hardwood xylans, with a DP between 70 and 130 and are less branched (Sunna and Antranikian 1997).

The location and structure of hemicellulose in the fibres affect the delignification of pulps as well as the technical properties of the fibre products. The removal of residual lignin in kraft pulps appears to be both physically and chemically restricted by hemicelluloses in the fibre matrix. Lignin-carbohydrate linkages have been suggested to restrict the chemical removal of residual lignin from pulp fibre (Viikari et al. 1993). During pulping process, natural softwood and hardwood xylan solubilizes and relocates, and interlinks the hemicelluloses and lignin physically and chemically. In the natural woods and grasses, hemicelluloses appear to be the cementing material between cellulose and lignin. Hence, hemicellulases such as *xylanases, mannanases* and others serve to degrade this cementing layer, rendering the cellulose free of lignin (Coughlan and Hazlewood 1993).

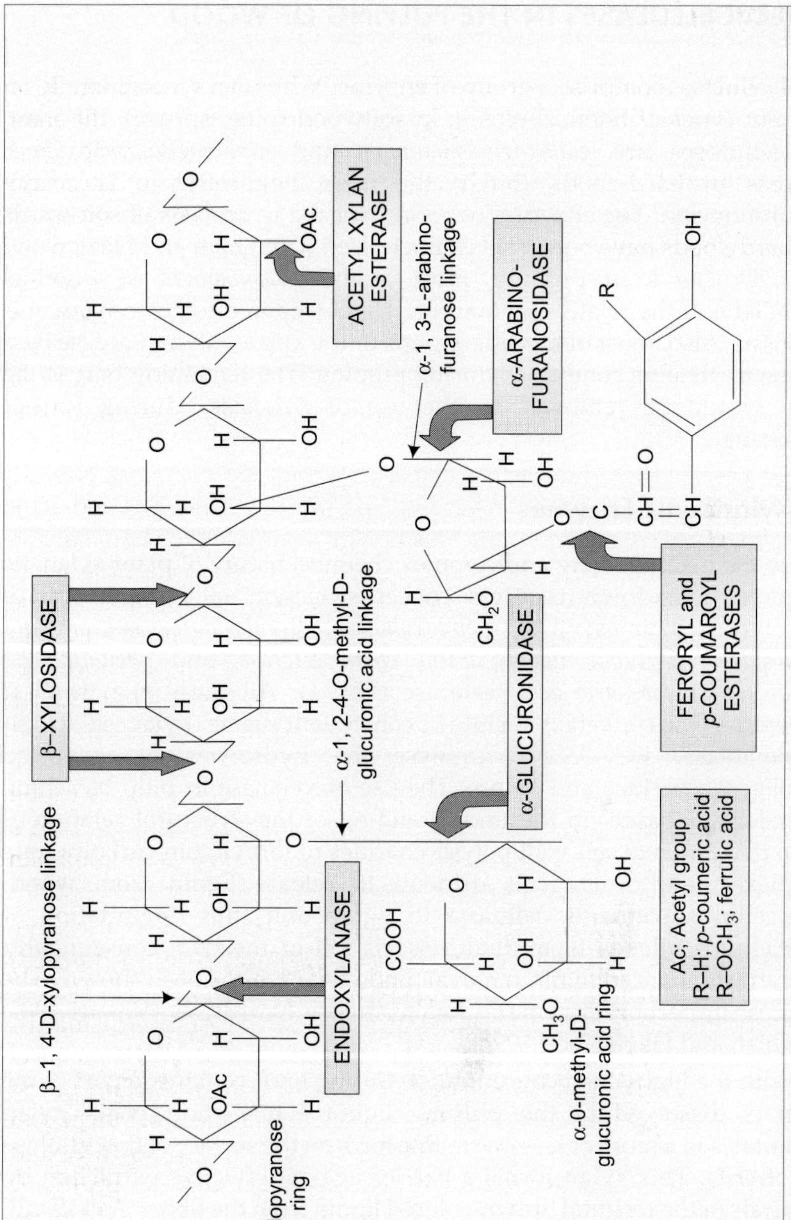

Fig. 1 A hypothetical plant xylan structure showing different substituent groups with sites of attack by microbial xylanolytic enzymes.

3. HEMICELLULASES IN THE PULPING OF WOOD

Hemicellulases comprise a group of enzymes which act synergistically on different types of hemicelluloses. In softwood (pine, spruce), the main hemicelluloses are *galactoglucomannans* and *arabinoglucuronoxylans*, whereas in hardwoods (birch) the main hemicellulose is acetyl-glucuronoxylan. The enzymes necessary for the hydrolysis of softwoods and hardwoods have been well characterized (Coughlan and Hazlewood 1993). During kraft pulping, most of the *glucomannan* of wood is degraded and the relative amount of xylan compared to glucomannan is increased. Also, most of the side groups of the xylan polymer are cleaved off due to alkaline conditions during pulping. The remaining part of the xylan would be removed by the use of xylanases during further processing.

3.1 Xylanolytic Enzymes

Due to the heterogeneity and complex chemical nature of plant xylan, its complete breakdown requires concerted action of a repertoire of hydrolytic enzymes: β-1, 4-*endoxylanase*, β-*xylosidase*, α-*L-arabino-furanosidase*, α-*glucuronidase*, *acetyl xylan esterase*, and *phenolic acid* (*ferulic and p-coumaric acid*) esterase (Fig. 1). All these enzymes act cooperatively to convert xylan into its constituent sugars. Xylanases (β-1,4-endoxylanase, EC 3.2.1.8) catalyse the hydrolysis of xylan to xylooligosaccharides and xylose. The use of xylanase in pulp bleaching technology is based on the understanding of the structural relation of lignin that binds to cell-wall polysaccharides to form lignin-carbohydrate complexes, and thus, it is difficult to release lignin from wood. Hemicellulose cements cellulose to lignin and thus degradation of hemicelluloses leads to mutual dissociation of the two, consequently facilitating enhanced lignin removal. Endoxylanase has been shown to be the most important enzyme in hemicellulose hydrolysis (Viikari 1987; Coughlan and Hazlewood 1993).

With the high-alkali concentration during kraft cooking, a part of the xylan is dissolved in the pulping liquor while short chain xylan precipitates in a more or less crystalline form on the surface of the cellulose microfibrils. This xylan forms a barrier against effective extraction by chemicals of the residual brown-colored lignin from the fibres. As a result, large quantities of chlorine or chlorine-containing compounds are required to be used for effective reduction in the kappa number, and to increase pulp brightness. In most of the investigations, crude enzyme mixtures have been employed in the solubilization of hemicellulose that has re-precipitated on the pulp fibres. The culture filtrates, however, contained predominantly xylanases as the main component (Paice et al. 1988), and attacked hemicellulose and altered the interface between the cellulose and lignin (Fig. 2). Increased de-lignifications during enzymatic pretreatment of pulp could be due to the hydrolysis of re-precipitated xylan in the inner layer. Side group cleaving enzymes have been shown to further enhance the *delignification* processes if xylan is attached to lignin molecules through side groups (Kantelinen et al. 1988).

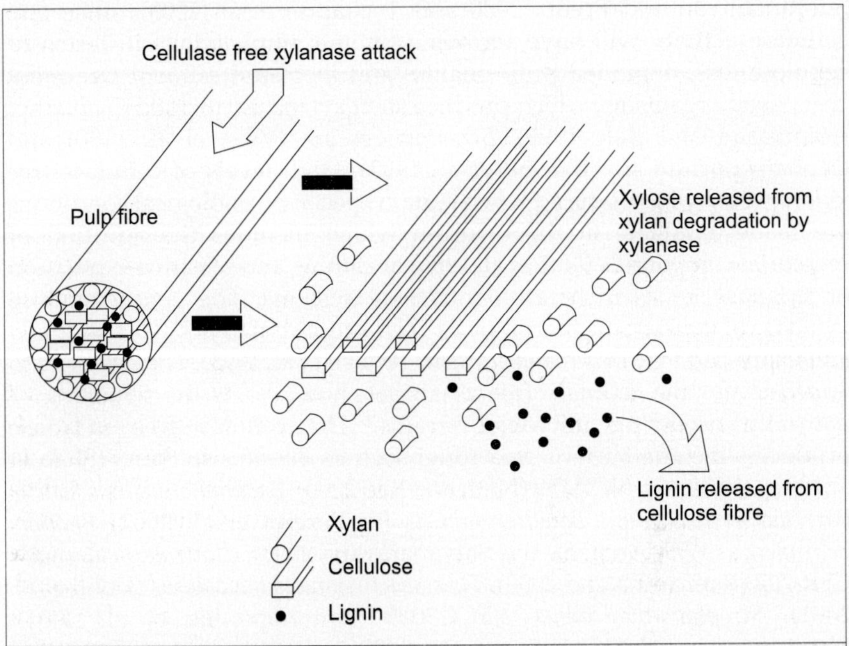

Fig. 2 Lignin associated hemicellulose fraction removal from pulp by the action of cellulase free-xylanase (Techapun et al. 2003)

4. CHARACTERISTICS OF MICROBIAL XYLANASES FOR PULPING

Xylanases have been produced by the vast variety of prokaryotes and eukaryotes including bacteria, fungi, protozoa, insects, *crustaceans* and germinating seeds (Dekker and Richards 1976). The demand for microbial xylanases used in pulp and paper processing has increased tremendously, making a sensible economic choice in bleaching. In keeping with the requirements of the pulping operations, the search for cellulase-free, alkalistable and thermostable xylanases from diverse microbial strains has gained momentum for the last few years (Srinivasan and Rele 1995).

4.1 Cellulase-Free Xylanases

An important prerequisite for the utilization of the xylanase in the pulp processing with a target to produce superior quality dissolving pulp is to be free of contamination from the cellulase activity (Eriksson et al. 1990; Srinivasan and Rele 1995; Archana and Satyanarayana 1999; Subramaniyan and Prema 2000 and Techapun et al. 2003), since any cellulase activity will have serious economic implications in terms of cellulose loss, degraded pulp quality, and increased effluent treatment cost. Some organisms, which produce such xylanases, include *Chainia* sp. (Srinivasan and Rele 1995), *Streptomyces* sp. (Vyas et al. 1990) and Cephalosporium sp. (Bansod et al. 1993). High levels of cellulase-free xylanases may be produced when certain special physiological conditions are made available in the medium which includes the addition of mercurial compounds (Noe et al. 1986) or cloning and selective expression of xylanase genes in heterologous host systems. The gene encoding xylanase of the extreme thermophile *Thermotoga* strain FjSS3B1 was cloned and expressed in *Kluyveromyuces lactis* (Walsh et al. 1998). The best way to approach for the cellulase-free xylanases, however, is the screening of naturally occurring microbial strains. The cellulase-free xylanase producers include bacteria and fungi such as *Bacilllus* sp Sam3 (Shah et al.1999), *Bacillus* sp NCIM59 (Nath and Rao 2000), *Bacillus amyloliquefaciens* (Breccia et al. 1998). *Bacillus subtilis* (Sa-Pereira et al. 2002) *Bacillus licheniformis A99* (Archana and Satyanarayana 2003), *Clostridium absonum* CFR-702 (Rani and Nand 2000), *Thermoactinomyces thalophilus* (Kohli et al. 2001), *Streptomytces albus* ATCC3005 (Antonopoulos et al. 2001), *Streptomyces* sp Ab106 (Techapun *et al.* 2001; Techapun et al. 2002) and *Streptomyces lividans* (Morosoli et al. 1986; Kluefel et al. 1990) and *Aspergillus oryzae* NRRL 1808 (Christov et al. 1999). A list of such organisms and the characteristics of their enzymes is presented in Table 1.

4.2 Alkalistable Xylanases

Alkaline xylanases have gained importance due to their applications in the development of eco-friendly technologies used in pulp and paper industries. The enzymes would be in a better position to hydrolyze xylan, which is soluble under alkaline conditions. First report on xylanase from alkaliphilic *Bacillus* sp.C.59-2 was published in 1973 (Horikoshi and Atsukawa 1973). Alkalistable xylanases have been produced by many alkaliphiles (Honda et al. 1985; Okazaki et al. 1984; Nakamura et al. 1993).

Table 1 Cellulase-free xylanase producers and their xylanase properties

Source	*Optimum conditions*				References
	(Growth)		*(Enzyme Activity)*		
	pH	*Temp (°C)*	*pH*	*Temp (°C)*	
Aspergillus fumigatus AR1	9	30	6-6.5	60	Anthony et al. 2003
Aspergillus oryzae NRRLI1808	5.5	28	5-6	60	Angelo et al. 1997
Bacillus sp Sam 3	7	28	8	60	Shah et al. 1999
Bacillus sp NCIM 59	10	50	7	60	Kulkarni et al.1996; Nath and Rao 2000
B. licheniformis A 99	7.0	60	7.0	50	Archana and Satyanarayana, 2003
B. subtilis	6	50	5-8	50-65	Sa-Pereira et al. 2002
Geobcillus thermoleovorans	7.5	70	8.5	80	Sharma 2000
Clostridium absonum CFR-702	8.5	75	8.5	75	Rani and Nand 2000
Emericella nidulans NK 62		45	4-8	50-70	Kango et. al. 2003
Penicillium canescens CP10	6	35	5.5	55	Curotto et al. 1998
Penicillium janthinellum	5.5	30	5.5	45	Curotto et al. 1994; Palma et al.1996
Streptomyces sp. Ab106	7.5	55	7	60	Techapun et al. 2001, 2002
Streptomyces albus ATCC3005	7.6	30	6.5	60	Antonopoulos et al. 2001
Streptomyces lividans	7	34	6	60	Morosoli et al. 1986; Kluefel et al. 1990
Thermomyces lanuginosus	7	45	–	75	Damaso et al. 2002
Thermoactinomyces thalophilus	8.5	50	8.5	65	Kohli et al. 2001

Four strains (W1, W2, W3, W4) of alkaliphilic and thermophilic bacteria, which produced alkaline xylanases, were isolated from soils (Okazaki et al. 1984). Archana and Satyanarayana (1998) reported a thermoalkalistable endoxylanase from *Bacillus licheniformis* A99. Morales et al. (1995) reported a bacterial xylanase from *Bacillus polymyxa*, while Nakamura et al. (1993) recorded the production of an alkaline xylanase by an alkaliphilic *Bacillus* sp. Alkaline xylanase has also been produced by *Aeromonas* sp, that exhibited activity in a broad pH range (Ohkoshi et al. 1985). Xylanase from strictly anaerobic and non-sporulating bacterium, *Dictyoglomus* sp. R146B1 was reported by Mathrani and Ahring (1992) that exhibited a high activity in alkaline conditions. A list of xylanase producing alkaliphilic microbes is presented in Table 2.

Table 2 Properties of xylanase produced by alkaliphilic and/or thermophilic microbes

Source	*Optimum conditions*				*References*
	(Growth)		*(Enzyme Activity)*		
	pH	*Temp (°C)*	*pH*	*Temp (°C)*	
Bacillus circulans AB16	8	55	6	80	Dhillon et al. 2000; Dhillon and Khanna 2000
Bacillus firmus	10.5	37	7	37	Tseng et al. 2002
Bacillus pumilus	10	45	8-9	55-60	Duarte et al. 1999, 2000; Santos et al. 2002
B. stearothermophilus	9.0	60	6.0-7.0	60-70	Rajaram and Varma 1990
B. stearothermophilus T-6	7.0-7.3	60	9.0	65	Khasin et al. 1993
Geobacillus thermoleovorans	7.5	70	8.5	80	Sharma 2000
Bacillus sp	8	37	10	60	Zheng and Zhang 2000
Bacillus sp.	9	37	9	50	Yang et al. 1988
Bacillus C-59-2	8.0	37	5.5-9.0	60	Horikoshi and Atsukawa 1973
Bacillus C-125	10.5	-	6.0-10	70	Honda et al. 1985a
Bacillus sp. K-1	10.5		5.5	60	Ratanakhanokchi et al. 1999
Bacillus 41 M-1	10.3	37	9.0	50	Nakamura et al. 1993a
Bacillus sp NCIM 2128	9	28	8	60	Balkrishnan et al. 1992
Bacillus sp NCIM 59	10	50	7	60	Kulkarni and Rao. 1996; Nath and Rao 2000
Bacillus sp. NG-27	9.0-10.0	27	7.0-8.4	70	Gupta et al. 1992
Bacillus sp. Sam-3		28	8.0	60	Shah et al. 1999
Bacillus sp. SPS-0	8.2	60	6	70	Bataillon et al. 2000
Bacillus TAR-1	10.5	50	9.0	70	Nakamura et al. 1993b
Bacillus sp.		45-50			Okazaki et al. 1984
W1			6.0	65	
W2			6.0	65	

Contd.

Table 2

Source	Optimum conditions (Growth)		(Enzyme Activity)		References
	pH	Temp (°C)	pH	Temp (°C)	
W3			7.0-9.5	70	
W4			6.0-7.0	70	
Clostridium absomum CFR-702	8.5	75	8.5	75	Rani and Nand, 2000
Dictyoglomus thermophilum B1	7.0	68	7.0	80	Mathrani and Ahring 1992
Dictyoglomus sp. B1	8.0	70	8	73	Adamsen et al. 1995
Fusarium oxysporum	8.0	30	6	55-60	Christakopoulos et al. 1996
Staphylococcus sp. SG-13	8.0	37	7.5	50	Gupta et al. 2000, 2001
Thermoactinomyces thalophilus sub gr.*C*	8.5-9	50	8.5-9	65	Kohli et al. 2001
Thermomonospora *fusca* YX	8.0	50	6.0-8.0	70	Irwin et al. 1994
Thermomonospora sp.	9	50	7	70	George et al. 2001
Thermotoga chromogena MT 814	8.0	50	5.0-8.0	75	McCarthy et al. 1985
T.fusca BD 21	8.0	50	6.0-8.0	65	Bachmann and Mc Carthy 1991
Thermus thermophilus		75	6	100	Lyon et al 2000

4.3 Thermostable Xylanase

Since the pulp processing is carried out at high temperature, the enzyme should be stable at that temperature. Xylanase treatment of the pulp at elevated temperatures opens up cell-wall structure, thereby facilitating lignin removal in the subsequent bleaching stages. Mostly thermophilic microbes have been found to be suitable sources, since xylanases secreted by them are frequently quite thermostable (Brodel et al. 1990). The xylanases of various thermophilic *Bacillus* spp. could be useful in pulp and paper industry (Horikoshi and Atsukawa 1973; Okazaki et al. 1984; Rajaram and Verma 1990; Nakamura et al. 1993; Ratto et al. 1994). Thermotolerant xylanases have been reported from many thermophilic organisms (*Bacillus stearothermophilus* (Khasin et al. 1993); *Clostridium sterocorarium* (Berenger et al. 1985); *Caldocellum saccharolyticum* (Luthi et al. 1990) and *Streptomyces* sp. QG-11-3 (Beg et al. 2000). *Dictyoglomus* sp. produced xylanase optimally active at 90°C (Mathrani and Ahring 1992).

The xylanase of thermophilic *Thermotoga* sp. was extremely stable at 105°C, which is the most thermostable xylanase (Bragger et al. 1989). High values of temperature and pH optima have been reported for *Bacillus* xylanases (Dey et al. 1992; Ratto et al. 1994; Nakamura et al. 1993; Gupta et al. 1992). Xylanases with a half-life of a few to 90 minutes at 80°C have been reported in *Bacillus thermophilus* (Gruninger and Fiechter 1986), *B. licheniformis* (Archana and Satyanarayana 1997), *Geobacillus thermoleovorans* (Sharma 2000) and thermophilic actinomycetes *Thermomonospora fusca, T. curvata* and *T. chromogena* (McCarthy et al. 1985). *Thermomyces lanuginosus,* formerly known as *Humicola lanuginosa,* has been reported by a number of laboratories to produce a highly thermostable xylanase based on the $t_{1/2}$ of the enzyme (Lischnig et al. 1993; Gomes et al. 1993; Singh et al. 2000; Singh et al. 2003; Kamra and Satyanarayana 2004). The xylanase of *T. languginosus* strain SSBP was reported to be the most stable ($t_{1/2}$=337 min at 70°C), whereas the DSM 5826 strain ($t_{1/2}$=201 min at 70°C), and other strains showed lesser degrees of stability ($t_{1/2}$=126 min or less at 70°C). Most microbial xylanases are stable at 50-70°C, and this is within the range of prevailing temperatures in pulp mills. The combination of alkali and thermal stability is, however, more difficult to come by. A list of thermophilic micro-organisms producing thermostable xylanases is given in Table 2.

5. PRODUCTION OF XYLANASES

Development of suitable medium and culture conditions is obligatory in order to obtain maximum yield of an enzyme (Narang and Satyanarayana 2000). Xylanase production has been studied in both, submerged as well as solid-state fermentations by bacteria and fungi. List of some micro-organisms producing thermostable and alkalistable xylanases is presented in Table 3.

5.1 Submerged Fermentation (SmF)

Submerged fermentation involves the growth and fermentation by micro-organisms in presence of sufficient water so as to dissolve the whole medium components in it and is well characterized with homogenous conditions maintained throughout the processing. The physical parameters such as pH, temperature and dissolved oxygen can be effectively controlled and scaling up of the process is feasible due to defined conditions. The choice of carbon and nitrogen sources varies from organism to organism. Xylanase production by microbes may be growth-associated or growth-independent. Dey et al. (1992) reported non-growth

Table 3 Xylanase production by some micro-organisms in submerged and solid-state fermentations

Organisms	*Mode of fermentation*	*Xylanase production*	*References*
Aspergillus niger	Submerged	74.5 U/ml	Gawande and Kamat 1999
A. niger A3	Solid-state	5147 U/g	Cai et al. 1997
A. niger KK2	Solid-state	14,790 U/g	Park et al. 2002
Aspergillus terreus	Submerged	68.9 U/ml	Gawande and Kamat 1999
Bacillus circulans	Submerged	11.5 U/ml	Ratto et al. 1992
B. licheniformis A99	Submerged	0.78 U/ml	Archana 1995
B. licheniformis A99	Solid-state	19.13U/ml	Archana and Satyanarayana 1997
B. licheniformis 77-2	Submerged	46.47 U/ml	Damiano et al. 2003
B. stearothermophilus	Submerged	2.33 U/ml	Khasin et al. 1993
Bacillus sp AR-009	Solid-state	720 U/g	Gessesse and Mamo 1999
Bacillus SSP-34	Submerged	379 U/ml	Subramaniyam et al. 2000
Bacillus sp	Submerged	11.5 U/ml	Paul and Verma 1993
Humicola lanuginosa	Solid-state	7832 U/g	Kamra and Satyanarayana 2004
Melanocarpus albomyces IIS 68	Solid-state	7760 U/g	Narang et al. 2001
Streptomyces. roseiscleroticus NRRL-B-11019	Submerged	16.2 U/ml	Grabski and Jeffries 1991
Streptomyces sp.QG-11-3	Solid-state	2360 U/g	Beg et al. 2002
Streptomyces sp. 106	Submerged	13.0 U/ml	Techapun et al. 2002
Streptomyces sp.	Submerged	3.5 U/ml	Techapun et al. 2001
Thermoactinomyces thalophilus P2	Submerged	42.0 U/ml	Kohli et al. 2001
Trichoderma reesei	Submerged	2172 U/ml	Purkarthofer et al. 1993
T. reesei	Solid-state	20220 U/g	Purkarthofer et al. 1993

associated xylanase production by *Bacillus* sp., while Esteban et al. (1982) and Nakamura et al. (1993a) observed xylanase production coupled with bacterial exponential phase of growth. There are very few reports on the production of xylanases that are cellulase-free, thermostability and alkalistability properties. Sharma (2002) has studied thermoalkalistable xylanase in *Geobacillus thermoleovorans* AP7 (syn. *Bacillus thermoleovorans*) by using submerged fermentation. Techapun et al. (2002) reported thermostable, alkali-tolerant and cellulase-free xylanase from *Streptomyces* sp. 106 in submerged fermentation. Most of the bacterial xylanases are produced by this process, and the production is optimized by controlling various physical and nutritional parameters.

5.1.1 Physical Parameters

The most important physical parameters suitable for the growth and production of industrially important xylanases are temperature, pH, agitation, and dissolved oxygen.

5.1.1.1 Temperature

Xylanases have been reported from both mesophiles and thermopiles. More reports pertain to thermophilic bacteria because thermostable enzymes are needed in paper bleaching processes. Intensive investigations have been carried over with xylanaolytic enzymes from mesophilic bacteria and fungi (Wong et al. 1988; Coughlan and Hazelwood 1993). Most of the xylanases from fungi and bacteria show their growth and optimum activity between 40-70°C, but the other thermophiles or the extremophiles like *Dictyoglomus*, *Geobacillus* and *Thermotoga* sp. show their optima beyond this temperature.

5.1.1.2 pH

pH has a profound effect on the production as well as stability and activity of the extracellular xylanases. In general fungal xylanases are less stable under alkaline conditions. Different organisms have a different optimal pH for the production of enzyme and its activity. Alkaliphiles are reported to frequently produce xylanases with pH optima near neutral range (Horikoshi and Atsukawa 1973; Okazaki et al. 1984; Tsujibo et al 1990).

5.1.1.3 Agitation and Aeration

Mechanical agitation and aeration are crucial factors for the production of xylanases, since these aid in uniform distribution of the nutrients and supply oxygen for the growth of the organisms. Agitation rate of 250 rpm supported higher xylanase production by *Bacillus* sp. (Okazaki et al. 1984). Xylanase production as well as growth rate were favoured at 150 rpm and 1 vvm aeration in *Thermomyces lanuginosus* (Purkarthofer et al. 1993). Agitation at 200 rpm was optimum for xylanase production in *Bacillus* Sam-3 strain (Shah et al. 1999) and *B. licheniformis* (Archana and Satyanarayana 1998). Techapun et al. (2003) recorded 1 vvm of aeration and agitation of 150 rpm for the production of thermostable and cellulase-free xylanase by *Streptomyces* sp. Ab 106.

5.1.2 Nutritional Parameters

5.1.2.1 Carbon Sources

Different sources of carbon as well as their concentrations are important factors not only for the optimal production of enzymes but also their localization (extracellular or cell bound). Xylan has been widely reported to support xylanase production (Esteban et al. 1982; Okazaki et al. 1984 Nakanishi et al. 1992). Among lignocellulosic substrates, wheat bran was reported to be a good carbon source for xylanase production (Wong et al. 1988; Dey et al. 1992; He et al. 1993). Rice straw was found to be the best carbon source for xylanase production in *Bacillus* AB 16 (Dhillon et al. 2000).

5.1.2.2 Nitrogen Sources

The source of nitrogen in the culture medium is another important parameter influencing the growth and production of metabolites. Organic forms of nitrogen such as yeast extract, tryptone, peptone, soya bean meal and corn steep solids have been extensively used for the production of xylanases. Yeast extract in combination with peptone enhanced xylanase production in *Bacillus* sp. SSP-34 significantly (Subramaniyan and Prema, 2000). Similarly, tryptone supported maximum xylanase secretion in *Bacillus* sp. B16 (Dhillon et al. 2000). Soya bean meal increased the production by 25% in *Bacillus* Sam-3 (Shah et al. 1999). Corn steep solids supported good production levels of xylanase in *T. reesei* (Lappalainen et al. 2000).

5.1.2.3 Trace Elements and Vitamins

Trace elements and vitamins have been reported to be important for the production of enzymes, especially by thermo-anaerobes (Antranikian et al. 1987) and some Bacilli (Ara et al. 1996). Besides carbon and nitrogen sources, hyper-thermophiles usually require the addition of different trace elements and vitamins to the medium. *Thermotoga* sp. FjSS3-B.1 required casamino acid in the culture medium. A requirement for amino-acids was reported for the production of xylanase by *Streptomyces* sp QG-11-3 (Beg et al. 2000). Vitamin solution and trace elements were required for xylanase production in *Bacillus* sp. AB16 (Dhillon et al. 2000). However, Dey et al. (1992) reported xylanase production in wheat bran and yeast extract medium that provided required trace elements and vitamins.

5.2 Solid-State Fermentation (SSF)

In contrast to submerged fermentation, the solid-state fermentation involves the growth and fermentation by micro-organisms, especially fungi on moist, water insoluble and solid substr in the absence or near absence of free water. It offers distinct advantages as it requires no fermentation controls, and lesser water volumes lead to greater product titrae and is considered as the self-control process. The SSF is useful in the area of solid waste management, biomass energy conservation and production of various primary and secondary metabolites. In SSF, the solid substratum in the form of particles serves as source of carbon, nitrogen, salts and growth factors and also provide mechanical support and anchorage to microbial cells.

There are several factors (physical, chemical and biochemical) which one needs to consider for any SSF (Pandey et al. 2001). The major factors that affect microbial growth and activity in SSF include selection of suitable micro-organism and substr, pretreatment of the, particle size (inter particle space and surface area) of the substr, water content and water activity (a_w) of the substr, relative humidity, type and size of inoculum and temperature of the fermenting matter/removal of metabolic heat, period of cultivation, maintenance of uniformity in the environment of SSF, and the gaseous atmosphere (oxygen consumption rate and carbon dioxide evolution rate).

Alam et al. (1994) reported production of a thermostable and cellulase-free xylanase by *T. lanuginosa* in SSF stable at 70°C. A thermostable xylanase preparation from *Humicola* sp. exhibited temperature optima at 75°C (Da-Silva et al. 1994). A xylanase from *Thermomonospora* sp. was stable at 80°C (Srivastava, 1993). Bacteria, in general, are considered to be less amenable to SSF (Lonsane and Ramesh, 1990). Few bacteria belonging to genera *Bacillus, Streptomyces, Clostridium* and *Cellulomonas* have been used for the production of thermostable hemicellulases (Uchino and Nakane, 1981; Kumar and Singh, 1992; Kanko et al. 1994; Shao et al.1995; Babu and Satyanarayana, 1996). Dunlop (1995) described a bacterium, isolated from wood compost, producing xylanase that was active at 80°C.

Agro-industrial residues are generally considered the best substratum for the SSF processes (Pandey et al. 2001). A number of such substratum have been employed for the cultivation of micro-organisms to produce enzymes. Some of the substr that have been used included sugar cane bagasse, wheat bran, rice bran, maize bran, gram bran, wheat straw, rice straw, rice husk, corn cobs and others. Wheat bran was the best among the various substr used in SSF for the production of xylanases. This could be attributed to its different and more suitable physiochemical structure than other lignocellulosics (Krik et al.1983; Jaleel et al. 1992). Some *Bacillus* have been shown to grow and produce enzymes in SSF (Archana and Satyanarayana 1997; Lonsane and Ramesh 1990). Xylanase production by SSF led to 22-folds increase in enzyme levels in *B. licheniformis* (Archana and Satyanarayana 1997). High-level xylanase production was achieved by an alkaliphilic *Bacillus* sp. by using wheat bran as substratum (Gessesse and Mamo 1999). Narang et al. (2001) and Karma and Satyanarayana (2004) reported a high enzyme titres using wheat straw and wheat bran as the substr by thermophilic fungi, *Melanocarpus albomyces* IIS68 and *Humicola lanuginose*, respectively. Production of a thermostable xylanase in SSF using wheat bran and eucalyptus kraft pulp as primary substratum was reported in *Streptomyces* sp. QH-11-3 (Beg et al. 2000a). Extremely thermophilic bacteria were not able to grow in solid-state fermentation due to requirement of higher levels of available water than is possible in SSF, and also due to high evaporation rate at elevated temperatures.

6. MOLECULAR APPROACHES FOR XYLANASE PRODUCTION

Isolation of xylanase producing organisms from natural resources and their improvement by molecular approaches for hyper-production of enzymes is needed. Cloning and expression of xylanase gene through recombinant DNA technology, random and site directed mutagenesis is the most commonly used method for strain improvement as part of the gene technology.

The isolation and cloning of the xylanase genes is an essential step in the engineering of most efficient organisms (Kulkarni et al. 1999). Cloning and sequencing of the genes encoding xylanases from different microbes, bacteria, fungi and actinomycetes has been attempted by various groups and most of them have succeeded in that. Nakai et al. (1994) reported a detailed account of nucleotide sequence and mutational analysis of the gene encoding the novel alkaline xylanases from an alkaliphilic *Bacillus* sp. 41M-A. Production of xylanase in *Bacillus subtilis* was enhanced successfully using a plasmid vector carrying the *B. pumilus* gene. The transformant produced approximately three times more extracellular xylanase than the donor strain (Panbangred et al.1985). Sung et al. (1993) successfully over-expressed xylanase encoding genes from *Bacillus subtilis* and *B. circulans* in *E.coli* by constructing synthetic gene with multiple unique restriction sites and achieved 10-100-fold increase in enzyme activity. Georis et al. (1999) have cloned a xylanase gene from *Streptomyces* sp. 538 in *Streptomyces lividans* TK24 and *Streptomyces parvulus* and achieved enzyme production 40-fold higher than the donor using plasmid pDML1000 and pDML1001, respectively.

Cloning and expression of a xylanase gene from the extreme thermophile *Dictyoglomus thermophile* Rt 46B.1 in *E. coli* has been reported (Gibbs et al.1995). The recombinant enzyme was optimally active at 85°C. Walsh et al. (1998) cloned the thermophilic xylanase from extreme thermophile *Thermotoga* in the yeast *Kluyveromyces lactis*. The xylanase cloned from *Thermotoga maritima* exhibited optimum activity at 90°C and at pH 5.5, and was stable upto 100°C (Chen et al.1997). The recombinant xylanase from *Thermotoga neapolitana* was found to be stable for 4 hrs at 90°C with a half-life of 2 hrs at 100°C. It was optimally active at 102°C and pH 5.5 (Veoikodvorskaya et al. 1997). Similarly, xylanase gene of *Bacillus polymyxa* had also been cloned and expressed in *E. coli* (Sadhu et al. 1984; Yang et al. 1998). Luthi et al. (1992) have cloned and over expressed a thermostable xylanase from *Caldocellum saccharolyticum* in *E.coli*. Ito et al. (2003) cloned and expressed *Xyn*5 gene encoding xylanase 5 (Xyn5) of *Paenibacillus* sp. strain W-61 in *Escherichia coli* and studied its sub-cellular location. Gallardo et al. (2004) have cloned *xyn A* gene encoding a xylanase from *Bacillus* sp strain BP-7 and expressed in *E. coli*. The recombinant xylanase showed a high activity on xylans from hard wood and cereals, and exhibited maximum activity at pH 6 and 60°C.

Commercially manufactured xylanases are typically produced by mesophilic filamentous fungi, such as *Trichoderma reesei* and *Aspergillus niger*, which are excellent protein secretors by nature. However, the xylanases produced by them may not be adequately thermostable for processes where high temperature (up to 80°C) is required, and hence, thermostable enzymes would have competitive advantage. Fungal expression systems provide a promising industrially relevant alternative to bacteria for heterologous enzyme production. Bergquist et al. (2000) developed a recombinant yeast *Kluyveromyces lactis* and filamentous fungus *Trichoderma reesei* for extracellular production of thermostable enzyme by inserting *Dictyoglomus thermophilum Xyn* A gene.

Hyper-producing mutants of industrially important organisms can be constructed by using mutagenic agents including UV irradiation and chemicals such as ethyl methane sulphate (EMS), nitrosoguanidine (NTG) and others. The secretion process involves signal peptide, signal recognization particle (SRP), translocation system in membrane and other features. Mutation in any of these steps may affect accumulation and secretion of the enzyme (Maruo and Tojo 1985; Wandersman 1992; Simonen and Palva 1993). The mutant *Thermomyces lanuginosus* QSI, developed by using UV/NTG, was reported to produce 2.5 folds high xylanase production than the parental strain (Chanda et al. 1999).

The enzyme active site residues could be determined by selective chemical modifications. The highly conserved amino-acid residues located at specific positions in xylanases play an important role for their properties. Site directed mutation could be used to improve the properties of the enzyme by replacing the key residue in the active site of the enzyme. The xylanase A gene from *Streptomyces lividans* was modified by site directed mutagenesis that improved the catalytic activity and thermostability of the enzyme (Moreau et al. 1994). The amino-acids at positions 155, 156 and 173 were replaced either by amino-acids having the polarity but a different side chain or by amino-acids having the same side chain with a different polarity. The thermostability of mesophilic xylanases especially from *T. reesei* and *Bacillus circulans* has been increased considerably by the designed mutations (Wakarchuk et al. 1994; Turunen et al. 2001). Several strategies to improve particular character of the organism can be achieved by introducing disulphide bridges at protein N-terminus, a helix and single amino-acid mutations in N-terminal region of xylanase (Turunen et al. 2004). pH – dependent properties of the xylanase is another important part and is influenced by several factors. The activity at low pH can be increased by modifying the environment of the acid/base catalyst *(Glu*-177 in *T. reesi* XYNII and *Glu*-172 in *B. circulans* xylanase*)*. Similarly, the pH optima can be shifted towards alkaline pH by increasing the pK_a value of the acid/base glutamate. Furthermore, the introduction of arginines into the *Ser/Thr* surface (Turunen et al. 2002) and modification of protein N-terminus (Sung et al. 1998) have improved the activity of *T. reesei* XYNII xylanase at alkaline pH. Other factors may also influence the pH dependence of the xylanases that needs further research (Turunen et al. 2004).

7. ROLE OF XYLANASES IN BLEACHING

Bleaching is the treatment of cellulosic fibre with chemicals to increase brightness. Brightness may be achieved by either lignin removal (delignification) or lignin decolonization from the pulp. Bleaching of fibres for decolonization has been practiced since early time. Sunlight was one of the earliest bleaching agents. Japanese paper makers are known to bleach fibres by soaking them in water from high mountain streams that contained ozone (the first use of oxygen for bleaching). In 1774, Karl Wilhelm Scheele discovered chlorine and its bleaching action on vegetable fibres. Several years later in 1799, Charles Tenanant invented 'bleaching powder' (calcium hypochlorite), thereby converting chlorine to an easily transportable form. Improvements in the manufacture of chlorine dioxide bleaching technology were developed in 1940s. By 1940, these developments led to the adoption of five-stage bleaching sequence that is still used extensively in the industry: (1) Chlorine; (2) alkali extraction;(3) chlorine dioxide; (4) alkali extraction and (5) chlorine dioxide. These sequences allowed the manufacture of bright fibre with minor losses in fibre strength.

In bleaching, the primary goal is to remove the low amount of residual lignin present in the pulp after cooking without decreasing the molecular weight of cellulose. Lignin in unbleached pulps represents typically only one per cent of the dry weight. During pulping, however, lignin is chemically modified and condensed, resulting in poorly degradable structures. Traditionally, the bleaching of chemical pulps has been carried out with elemental chlorine and chlorine dioxide and the typical sequence would consist of the cited above five stages.

Modern bleaching is usually carried out in a step-wise sequence utilizing different chemicals and conditions in each stage, with washing carried out between stages. The commonly used chemical treatments and the 'short hand' designations are listed as follows:

Chlorination (C)	-	Reaction with elemental chlorine in acidic medium
Alkaline Extraction (E)	-	Dissolution of reaction products with NaOH.
Hypochlorite (H)	-	Reaction with hypochlorite in an alkaline solution
Chlorine Dioxide (D)	-	Reaction with ClO_2 in acidic medium
Peroxide (P)	-	Reaction with peroxides in alkaline medium
Oxygen (O)	-	Reaction with elemental oxygen at high pressure in alkaline medium.
Ozone (Z)	-	Reaction with ozone (O_3)
Enzyme [Xylanase] (X)	-	Enzymatic hydrolysis of xylan
(D_C) or (C_D)	-	Admixtures of chlorine and chlorine dioxide

Bleaching sequence generally contains two phases within each sequence: 1) a delignification segment, whose function is to remove the lignin; and 2) a brightening segment, whose principle function is to increase the brightness of the pulp. Examples of delignification stages include oxidation by chlorine (C) followed by extraction of the dissolved lignin with sodium hydroxide (E). Brightening segments use sodium hypochlorite (H) and/or chlorine dioxide (D). Oxygen can be used for delignification and for reinforcing extraction of the dissolved lignin in the alkali stage.

To achieve 'full bleach' brightness, the bleaching is usually carried out in five or six stages, employing CEDED, CEHDED or OCEDED sequences. Lower brightness levels can be achieved with fewer stages as CEH sequence; intermediate levels can be achieved with CED, CEHH, CEHD or CEHP. Several of the more commonly used bleach sequences in U.S. and Canadian mills are: CEDED; CEDH; CEHDED; CEH and CED. Although these are the most prominent bleaching sequences currently in use, an increasing number of mills are now using oxygen in combination with alkali for extraction (E_O), and chlorine dioxide (C_D, D_C) in chlorination stages.

Chlorinated organic compounds are mainly formed in bleaching with elemental chlorine. The public concern together with tightened environmental regulations has driven the pulp and paper industry to search for and to utilize alternative bleaching processes. The major aim has been to replace chlorine gas with other chemicals. Reduction in bleach plant effluents can be achieved by reducing the lignin content of pulp prior to bleaching by modified cooking procedures or oxygen delignification (O), or replacing elemental chlorine with other chemicals such as chlorine dioxide, ozone (Z), oxygen (O), peroxide (P) and/or peroxyacids in bleaching (McDonough, 1995). The alternative bleaching sequences, the oxygen-based totally chlorine-free (TCF) and the chlorine dioxide-based elemental chlorine-free (ECF) sequences, are increasingly used in industrial pulp bleaching.

The effect of enzymes on pulp bleach ability has been studied by different methods. In the first phase, enzymes are usually characterized with isolated substrates, which are used in the determination of their activities. These substrates, however, vary extensively with respect to their origin and composition. Furthermore, a comparison of enzyme activities is complicated by the utilization of different analysis methods (Baily 1985). Hence in pulp applications, the action of enzymes must be compared on the actual substrates, the pulp. In these tests, the liberation of sugars into the pulp solution has usually been measured either by reducing sugar analysis or by high performance liquid chromatography (HPLC). In addition, increase in the liberation of lignin-derived compounds after enzymatic treatment (Yang and Eriksson 1992) or alkaline extraction (Hertling et al. 1994) has also been used for evaluation of different enzymes. The most reliable method for comparison of the effects of different enzymes is, however, to bleach the enzyme-treated pulps and to measure the brightness and final lignin content (Kappa number).

The action of enzymes is influenced by the electrochemical interactions between the fibres and enzymes (Buchert et al. 1993). The carboxyl groups within the fibre cell-wall are mainly responsible for the swelling of fibres and these have been reported to affect the action of xylanases. The more negative the surface charge, the less the pulp was hydrolyzed (Buchert et al. 1993). However, the swelling or surface charge may not be the primary factors affecting the hydrolysis. The type of the counter-ions and the degree of the substitution of the carboxyl groups in pulp were found to have a profound effect on the action of xylanases in the pulp matrix.

The effect of xylanases in bleaching is based on the modification of pulp hemicelluloses and enhancing the removal of lignin in chemical bleaching. Xylanases are being employed as enzymatic pre-treatment in kraft pulp bleaching process at mill scale in order to improve delignification by the degradation of hemicelluloses (Senior and Hamilton 1992). It has been proposed that the action of xylanases is due to the partial hydrolysis of reprecipitated xylan formed during delignification rendering the pulp more permeable, thus facilitating the removal of residual lignin (Kantelinen et al. 1993) or removal of xylan from the lignin-carbohydrate complex to facilitate further bleaching (Yang and Eriksson 1992). In addition, it has been suggested that the hemicellulase treatment removes chromophoric groups from the pulp (Wong et al. 1996). Reducing sugars, chromophore release, and kappa number have been widely monitored to check pulp solubilization following xylanase treatment (Jefferies 1981; Ratto et al. 1994; Shah et al. 1999).

Xylanases can be used at different stages of the pulping process, but specially in the prebleaching of kraft pulp. The process of kraft pulping consists of cooking the wood chips at 170°C with sodium sulphide and NaOH, which leads to solubilization of most of the lignin. The residual 3-5% lignin in hard wood as well as softwood pulp imparts an undesirable brown color to the pulp. Bleaching with Cl_2 or ClO_2 in conventional pulping process removes the brown colored alkali extract of chlorinated derivatives of lignin comprising of dioxin and related compounds. These are toxic, carcinogenic, and recalcitrant and pose serious hazards as environmental pollutants. Xylanase pretreatment of kraft pulp has been consistently shown to reduce the brown color of the pulp with concomitant reduction in the amounts of Cl_2 compounds.

Xylanase pretreatment has led to reduction in effluent AOX and dioxin concentration due to reduced chlorine requirement to achieve a given brightness (Murata et al. 1992; Iimori et al. 1994; Viikari et al. 1994; Iimori et al. 1996). It decreases the AOX in proportion to the decrease in chlorine compound usage, i.e., a 15% decrease in ClO_2 will decrease the bleach plant AOX discharge by 15%. The level of AOX in effluents was found to be significantly lower in xylanase pretreated pulps when compared with conventionally bleached control pulps (Viikari et al. 1986; Fujita et al. 1993; Iimori et al.1996) (Table 4). In another study, use of xylanase reduced the amount of chlorophenols and other forms of organically bound chlorine in the spent bleach liquor. It has also been reported that the total organic chlorine (TOCl) content in extraction-stage effluent was reduced by 30% when the pulp was first treated with xylanase and then subjected to CEH bleaching (Fujita et al. 1993; Bajpai et al. 1994). The acute toxicity problem could be tackled successfully by purifying waste bleach water or better still by avoiding the hazardous chlorine

Table 4 Effect of xylanase treatment on the effluent quality (Viikari et al. 1986)

Particulars	*Control*	*Treated*
Pretreatment	No	Yes
pH	–	4.8
Xylanase charge (unit/kg pulp)	–	5000
Time (h)	–	3
Temperature (°C)	–	37
Kappa number	32	31.3
Viscosity (mPa/s)	25.1	30.7
($C_{70}D_{30}$) Stage		
Cl_2 (kg/mt pulp)	19.2	15.0
ClO_2 (kg/mt pulp)	17.0	13.3
Active Cl_2 (kg/mt pulp)	64.0	49.9
(Eo) Stage		
NaOH (kg/mt pulp)	35.2	27.0
O_2 (kg/mt pulp)	5.0	5.0
Eo kappa number	4.8	4.4
Effluent properties		
Colour (kg/mt pulp)	155	118
AOX (kg/mt pulp)	2.20	1.68
BOD (kg/mt pulp)	15	11
COD (kg/mt pulp)	74	62

compounds in newer and modified pulp bleaching techniques. The elemental chlorine can be replaced by the less toxic chlorine dioxide, that decreases effluent colour and drastically reduces total organic chlorine (TOCl), adsorbable organic halogen (AOX), amount of dioxin and also chlorinated phenolics. Hydrogen peroxide and ozone are not suitable bleaching agents since they are very expensive at such a large scale (Perttula et al. 1993). Other biochemical methods like employing ligninolytic enzymes (lignin peroxidases, manganese peroxidases and laccases) have been found to be effective, but their practical utility has turned out to be limited primarily due to lack of understanding of enzyme degradation systems (Viikari et al. 1993).

Due to the increasing public concern about the environmental effects caused by chemical bleaching, papermaking process is moving towards total elimination of chlorine requirement as its ultimate goal. Increasing stringent regulations are causing bleach plant operators to modify the currently existing bleaching schemes. In elementally chlorine free (ECF) bleaching sequences, especially where the utilization of chlorine gas has been abandoned, the use of enzymes increases the productivity of the bleaching plant when the production capacity of chlorine dioxide is the limiting factor. The addition of enzymes in totally chlorine free (TCF) bleaching sequences increases the final brightness value and also leads to saving in the TCF bleaching chemicals, and this is important both in terms of cost and the strength properties of the pulp. Several alternative bleaching methods based on different bleaching chemicals have been developed. These chemicals are oxygen, ozone and peroxide. Frequently, enzymes are added to oxygen and delignified pulps to increase the brightness. Present day TCF technologies are usually based on bleaching of oxygen-delignified pulps with enzymes and hydrogen peroxide. Enzyme aided technology has been frequently used in many paper mills. Finnish forest companies have been pioneers in implementing the enzymatic pretreatment in pulp treatment with mill scale trials conducted way back in 1988. Optimization of microbial xylanase production, development of hyperxylanolytic strains, isolation of cellulase-free xylanase producing microbes, isolating thermoalkalistable xylanases or modifying the pre-existing ones by means of enzyme engineering and enzyme stabilization techniques may enhance their feasibility and usefulness towards the objective of turning paper technology, non-polluting and eco-friendly. The benefits of employing xylanase in different bleaching sequences are summarized in the Table 5.

Table 5 Benefits of xylanase pretreatment in different bleaching sequences

Type of bleaching sequence	*Benefits*
Traditional	Reduced Cl_2 consumption
	Reduced AOX
ECF	Reduced ClO_2 consumption
	Reduced AOX
	Increased productivity, when ClO_2 limiting
TCF	Increased brightness
	Reduced chemical consumption
	Retention of strength properties

8. COMMERCIALIZATION OF XYLANASES

Commercial enzymatic prebleaching has been successfully demonstrated at industrial scale in which 88% ISO brightness was achieved with the record of 82% ISO brightness without enzyme treatment.

In the last decade, the actual potential application of xylanases in the production of pulp and paper has steadily grown. Mills, generally in

Europe and America, are using xylanases on a daily basis for bleaching of kraft pulp to conserve energy. Many multinational companies are marketing enzymes. Most of the multinational companies have their commercial xylanases under different trade names and sources. Pulpzyme (*Bacillus* sp. VI-4) from Novo Nordisc. Denmark; Irgazyme 40 (*Trichoderma longibranchiatum*) from Genencor international USA; Cartazyme HS and HT (*Thermomonospor fusca*) from Sandoz UK; Ecopulp X, X-0014 and XM (*Trichoderma reesei*) from Primalco Biotech; Strernzyme HC40 (*Aspergillus niger*) from Solvay Enzymes GmbH & Co, KG, Germany; Xylanase GS35 (*Trichoderma reesei*) from Iogen Corp, Canada and Allzym PT (*Aspergillus niger*) from Alteh Inc. USA are some examples. In India, so far not a single indigenous xylanase is commercialized for paper pulp processing. BIOCON Industries, Bangalore have, however, developed and commercialized xylanase usefully in food industries.

9. CONCLUSION

Paper pulp bleaching involving microbial xylanases is a promising and environment friendly alternative to the conventional chemical bleaching. The requirement of such a replacement is becoming mandatory due to the pollution and long-term hazards caused by the organochlorines. Xylanase pretreatment of pulps prior to bleach plant reduces bleach chemical requirements and permits higher brightness. The reduction in chemical charges can translate into significant cost saving when high levels of chlorine dioxide and hydrogen peroxide are being used. A reduction in the use of chlorine chemicals clearly reduces the formation and release of chlorinated organic compounds in the effluents and the pulps themselves, which ultimately reduces the environmental pollution. The ability of xylanases to activate pulp and increase the effectiveness of the bleaching chemicals may allow new bleaching technologies to become more effective and sustains the traditional chemical industry with clear environmental benefits, and it is economically attractive. Xylanases used for this purpose must be free from cellulase activity, alkalistable and thermostable. Innovative approaches for the screening of novel xylanolytic microbial strains from the extreme environments must be undertaken with full vigour to explore, isolate and conserve in germplasm banks. Genetic engineering approaches can be used for obtaining xylanases with novel properties that can eventually be exploited commercially. Microbial xylanases thus offer an opportunity as well as challenge to microbiologists, biotechnologists and industrialists in the quest for global competitiveness for the utilization of sustainable technology.

REFERENCES

Adamsen AK, Lindhagen J, Ahring BK (1995) Optimization of extracellular xylanase production by *Dictyoglomus* sp. B1 in continuous culture. Appl Microbiol Biotechnol 44:327 -32

Alam M, Gomes I, Mohiuddin G, Hoq M M (1994) Production and characterization of thermostable xylanase by *Thermomyces lanuginosus* and *Thermoascus aurantiacus* grown on lignocellulose. Enz Microb Technol 16: 298-302

Angelo R, Aguirre C, Curotto E, Esposito E, Fontana JD, Baron M, Millagres AMF, Duran N (1997) Stability and chemical modification of xylanase from *Aspergillus* sp. (2M1 strain). Biotechnol Appl Biochem 25:19-27

Anthony T, Chandra Raj K, Rajendra A, Gunasekaran P (2003) High molecular weight cellulase-free xylanase from alkali-tolerant *Aspergillus fumigatus* AR1. Enz Microb Technol 32:647-654

Antonopoulos VT, Hernandez M, Arias ME, Mavrakos E, Ball AS (2001) The use of extracellular enzyme from *Streptomyces albus*ATCC3005 for the bleaching of eucalyptus kraft pulp. Appl Microbiol Biotechnol 54:92 -97

Antranikian G, Zablowski P, Gottschalk G (1987) Conditions for the overproduction and excretion of thermostable á-amylase and pullulanase from *Clostridium themohydrosulfuricum* DSM 567. Appl Microbiol Biotechnol 27: 75-81

Ara K, Igarashi K, Hagihara H, Sawada K, Kobayashi T, Ito S (1996) Separation of functional domains for the á-1-4 and á-1,6 hydrolytic activities of a *Bacillus* amylopullulanase by limited proteolysis with papain. Biosc Biotechnol Biochem 60(4): 634-639

Archana A (1995) Xylanolytic enzymes of a moderate thermophile *Bacillus licheniformis* A99. Ph.D. Thesis, University of Delhi

Archana A, Satyanarayana T (1997) Xylanase production by thermophilic *Bacillus licheniformis* A99 in solid-state fermentation. Enz Microb Technol 21(1):12-17

Archana A, Satyanarayana T (1998) Cellulase-free xylanase production by thermophilic *Bacillus licheniformis* A 99. Indian J Microbiol 38:135-139

Archana A, Satyanarayana T (1999) Bacterial thermostable cellulase-free xylanases in environment friendly paper pulp bleaching technology. In:Tiwari J.P.,Lakhanpal, T.N., Singh Jagjit, Gupta Rani, Chamola BP (eds) Advances in Microbial Technology. APH Publishing Corporation pp 131-139

Archana A, Satyanarayana T (2003) Purification and characterization of a cellulase-free of a moderate thermophile *Bacillus licheniformis* A99. World J Microbiol Biotechnol 19: 53-57

Babu KR, Satyanarayana T (1996) Production of bacterial enzymes by solid-state fermentation. J Sci Indust Res 55:564-567

Bachmann S L, McCarthy A J (1991) Purification and cooperative activity of enzymes constituting the xylan-degrading system of *Thermomonospora fusca*. Appl Env Microbiol 57:2121-2130

Baily P (1985) Microbial xylanolytic systems. Trends Biotechnol 3: 286

Bajpai P, Bhardwaj NK, Bajpai PK, Jauhari MB (1994) The impact of xylanases on bleaching of eucalyptus kraft pulp. J Biotechnol 38:106

Bajpai P, Bhardwaj NK, Maheshwari S, Bajpai PK (1993) Use of xylanase in bleaching of eukalpyptus kraft pulp. Appita J 46: 274-276

Balakrishnan H, Dutty-Choudhury M, Srinivasan MC, Rele MV (1992) Cellulase-free xylanse production from an alkalophilic *Bacillus* species. World J Microbiol Biotechnol 8:627 -31

Bansod SM, Chaudhary MD, Srinivasan MC, Rele M V (1993) Xylanase active at high pH from alkalotolerant *Cephalosporium* species. Biotechnol Lett 15: 965-970

Bastawde KB (1992) Xylan structure, microbial xylanases, and their mode of action. World J Microbiol Biotechnol 8:353-368

Bastawde KB, Tabatabia LB, Meagher MM, Srinivasan MC, Vartak HG, Rele MV, Reilly PJ (1991) Catalytic properties and partial amino acid sequence of an actinomycete endoxylanase from *Chainia* sp. American Chemical Society Symposium Series 460: 417-425

Bataillon M, Cardinali APN, Castillon N, Duchiron F (2000) Purification and characterization of a moderately thermostable xylanase from *Bacillus* sp. strain SPS-0. Enz Microb Technol 26:187-192

Beg QK, Bhushan B, Kapoor M, Hoondal, GS (2000a) Production and characterization of thermostable xylanase and pectinase from a *Streptomyces* sp. QG-11-3. J Ind Microbiol Biotechnol 24:396-402

Beg QK, Kapoor M, Bhushan B, Hondal GS (2000b) Enhanced production of a thermostable xylanase from *Streptomyces* sp. QG-11-3 and its application in biobleaching of eucalyptus kraft pulp. Enz Microb Technol 27(7): 557-466

Berenger JF, Frixon C, Bigliardi J, Creuzet N (1985) Production, purification and properties of thermostable xylanase of *Clostridium steroonarium*. Can J Micorbiol 31: 635-643

Bergquist PL, Te'o VSJ, Gibbs MD, Cziferszky ACE, de Faria FD,Azevedo MO, Nevalainen KMH (2002) Expression of thermophilic xylanases in fungal hosts.In: Biotechnology in the pulp and paper Industry. Elsevier Science BV pp 239-246

Bocchini DA, Alves-Prado HF, Baida LC, Roberts IC, Gomes E, Da-Silva R(2002) Optimization of xylanase production by *Bacillus circulans* D 1 in submerged fermentation using RSM. Process Biochem 38: 727-731

Bragger J M, Daniel RM, Coolbear T, Morgan H W (1989) Very stable enzymes from extremely thermophilic archaebacteria and eubacteria. Appl. Microbiol. Biotechnol 31: 556-561

Breccia JD, Sineriz F, Baigori MD, Castro GR, Hatti-kaul R (1998) Purification and characterization of a thermostable xylanase from *Bacillus amyloliquefaciens*. Enz Microb Technol 22(1): 42-49

Brodel B, Samain E, Debeire P (1990) Regulation and optimization of xylanase production from *Clostridium thermolacticum*. Biotechnol Lett 12: 65-70

Buchert J, Tenkanen M, Viikari L, Pitkanen M (1993) Role of surface charge and swelling on the action of xylanases on birch kraft pulp. TAPPI J 76: 131-135

Cai J, Wu K, Zhang J, He X, Pang R (1997) Production of xylanase by *Aspergillus niger* A3 using solid-state fermentation. Ind. Microbiol 27(2): 1-4

Chanda B S, Singh S, Arvind S, Saini H S (1996) Mutagenesis for hyperproduction of extracellular analysis by *Thermomyces lanuginosus*. Acta. Microbiol Polon 45: 31-37

Chen C, Adolphson R, Dean JFD, Eriksson KL, Adams MWW, Westpheling J (1997) Release of lignin from Kraft pulp by a hyperthermophilic xylanase from *Thermotoga maritima*. Enz Microb Technol 20: 39-45

Christakopoulos P, Nerinckx W, Kekos D, Macris B, Claeyssens M (1996) Purification and characterization of two low molecular mass alkaline xylanases from *Fusarium oxysporum* F3. J Biotechnol 51: 181-189

Christov LP, Szakacs G, Balakrishnan H (1999) Production partial characterization and use of fungal cellulase-free xylanases in pulp bleaching. Process Biochem 64: 511-7

Coughlan MP, Hazlewood GP (1993) β-1,4-D-xylan-degrading enzyme systems: biochemistry, molecular biology and application. Biotechnol Appl Biochem 17: 259-289

Curotto A, Nasal A, Aguirre A, Campos V, Duran N (1998) Enzymatic pretreatment of Kraft pulps from *Pinus radiata* D Don with xylanolytic complex of *Penicillium canescens* (CP10 fungi). Appl Biochem Biotechnol 73:29-42

Curotto E, Concha M, Campos V, Milagres AM, Duran N (1994) Production of extracellular xylanases by *Penicillium janthinellum*, effect of elected growth conditions. Appl Biochem Biotechnol 48(2):107-116

Damaso M C T, Andrade CMMC, Pereira Jr,Nei (2002) Production and properties of the cellulase-free xylanase from *Thermomyces lanuginosus* IOC-4145. Braz. J. Microbiol 33(4): 333-338

Damiano VB, Bocchini DA, Gomes E, Da Silva R (2003) Application of crude xylanase from *Bacillus licheniformis* 77-2 to the bleaching of eucalyptus Kraft pulp. World J Microbiol Biotechnol 19:139-144

Da-Silva R, Yim DK, Park YKJ(1994) Application of thermostable xylanase from *Humicola* sp. for pulp improvement. J Fermen Bioeng 77: 109-111

Dekker RFH, Richard GN (1976) Hemicellulases: Their occurance, purification, properties, mode of action. Adv Carbohyd Chem Biochem 32: 436-442

Dey D, Hinge J, Shendye A, Rao M (1992) Purification and properties of extracellular endoxylanases from alkaliphilic thermophilic *Bacillus* sp. Can J Microbiol 38(5): 436-442

Dhillon A, Gupta JK, Jauhari BM, Khanna S (2000a) A cellulase-poor, thermostable, alkalitolerant xylanase produced by *Bacillus circulans* AB16 grown on rice straw and its application in biobleaching of eucalyptus pulp. Bioresources Technol 73: 273-/7

Dhillon A, Gupta JK, Khanna S (2000b) Enhanced production, purification and characterisation of a novel cellulase-poor thermostable, alkalitolerant xylanase from *Bacillus circulans* AB16. Process Biochem 35: 849-856

Dhillon A, Khanna S (2000) Production of a thermostable alkalitolerant xylanase from *Bacillus circulans* AB16 grown on wheat straw. J Microbiol Biotechnol 16(4): 325-/7

Duarte MCT, Pellegrino ACA, Portugal EP, Ponezi AN, Franco TT (2000) Characterization of alkaline xylanases from *Bacillus pumilus* Bioresource Technol 31: 90-/4

Duarte MCT, Portugal EP, Ponezi AN, Bim MA, Tagliari CV, Franco TT (1999) Production and purification of alkaline xylanases. Bioresource Technol 68: 49-53

Dunlop RW, Wang B, Ball D (1995) PN-WO 9527779

Eriksson KEL, Blanchette RA, Ander P (1990) Microbial and enzymatic degradation of wood and wood components. Springer Verlag. Berlin, Heidelberg, New York

Esteban R, Villanueva JR, Villa TG (1982) β-D-Xylanases of *Bacillus circulans* WL-12. Can. J. Microbiol 28:733-739

Fujita K, Kondo R, Sakai K (1993) Biobleaching of softwood kraft pulp with white rot fungus IZU154. TAPPI J 76(1): 81-84

Gallardo Oscar, Diaz Pilar, Pastor Javier F I (2004) Cloning and characterization of xylanase A from the strain *Bacillus* sp. BP-7: Comparison with alkaline pI-low molecular weight xylanases of family 11.Current Microbiol 48: 276-279

Gawande P V, Kamat M Y (1999) Production of Aspergillus xylanases by lignocellulosic waste fermentation and its application. J Appl Microbiol 87: 551-519

George SP, Ahmad A, Rao MB (2001) A novel thermostable xylanase from *Thermomonospora* sp: influence of additives on thermostability. Bioresource Technol 78: 221-224

Georis J, Giannotta F, Lamotte-Brasseur J, Devreeese B, Beeumen JV, Granier B, Frere, J (1999) Sequence, overproduction and purification of the family 11 endo-b1,4-xylanase encoded by the *xylI* gene of *Streptomyces* sp. S38. Gene 237,123

Gessess A, Gashe BA (1997) Production of alkaline xylanase by an alkaliphilic *Bacillus* sp. isolated from an alkaline lake. J Appl Microbiol 83:402-406

Gessesse A, Mamo G. (1999) High-level xylanase production by an alkalophilic *Bacillus* sp. by using solid-state fermentation. Enz Microb Technol 25:68 -72

Gibbs MD, Reeves R A, Bergquist PK (1995) Cloning, sequencing and expression of a xylanase gene from the extreme thermophilic *Dictyoglomus thermophilum* Rt 46B.1 and activity of the enzyme on fibre-bound substrate. Appl Env Microbiol 61: 4403-4408

Gomes J, Gomes I, Terler K, Gubala N, Ditzelmuller G, Steiner W (2000) Optimization of culture medium and conditions for L-arabinofuranosidase production by the extreme thermophilic eubacterium *Rhodothermus marinus*. Enz Microb Technol 27: 414-22.

Gomes J, Purkarthofer H, Hayn M, Kapplmuller J, Sinner M, Steiner W (1993) Production of a high-level cellulase-free xylanase by the thermophilic fungus *Thermomyces lanuginosus* in laboratory and plot scales using lignocellulosic materials. Appl Microbiol Biotechnol 39: 700-707

Grabski AC, Jeffries TW (1991) Production, purification and characterization of α-(1$\rightarrow$4) endoxylanase of *Streptomyces roseiscleroticus*. Appl Environ Microbiol 57: 987-992

Gruninger H, Fiechter A (1986) A novel highly thermostable D-xylanase. Enz Microb Technol 8: 309-314

Gupta N, Vohra R M, Hoondal G S(1992) A thermostable extracellular xylanase from alkaliphilic *Bacillus* sp NG-27. Biotechnol Lett 14: 1045-1046

Gupta S, Bhushan B, Hoondal GS (2000) Isolation, purification and characterization of xylanase from *Staphylococcus* sp. SG-13 and its application in biobleaching of kraft pulp. J Appl Microbiol 88(2): 325-334

Gupta S, Kuhad RC, Bhushan B, Hoondal GS (2001) Improved xylanase production from a haloalkalophilic *Staphylococcus* sp.SG-13 using inexpensive agricultural residues. World J Microbiol Biotechnol 17(1): 5-8

He L, Bicherstaff GF, Pateerson A, Buswell A (1993) Purification and partial characterization of two xylanases that differ in hydrolysis of soluble and insoluble xylan fractions. Enz Microb Technol 15: 13-18

Hertling B, Korhonen M, Buchert J, Sundquist J, Viikari L (1994) The leachability of lignin from kraft pulps after xylanase treatment. Holzforschung 48: 441-446

Honda H, Kudo T, Horikoshi K (1985a) Purification and partial characterization of alkaline xylanase from *Escherichia coli* carrying pCX311. Agric Biol Chem 49: 3165-3169

Honda H, Kudo T, Horikoshi K (1985b) Molecular cloning and expression of the xylanase gene of alkaliphilic *Bacillus* sp. strain C125 in *Escherichia coli*. J Bacteriol 161(2): 784-785

Horikoshi K, Atsukawa Y (1973) Xylanase produced by alkaliphilic *Bacillus* No.C. 59-2. Agric Biol Chem 37, 2097

Iimori T, Kaneko R, Yoshikawa H, Machida M, Yoshioka H, Murakami K(1994) Screening of pulp bleaching fungi and bleaching activity of newly isolated fungus SKB-1152. Mokuzai Gakkaishi 40(7):733-737

Iimori T, Yoshikawa H, Kaneko R, Miyawaki S, Machida M, Murakami K (1996) Effects of treatment conditions on treatment times for biobleaching by SKB-1152. Mokuzai Gakkaishi 42:313-317

Irwin D, Jung ED, Wilson DB (1994) Characterization and sequence of *Thermomonospora fusca* xylanase. Appl Env Microbiol 60: 763-770

Ito Yasuko, Tomita Toshio, Roy Narayan, Nakano Akito, Sugawara-Tomita Noriko, Watanabe Seiji, Okai Naoko, Abe Naoki and Kamio Yoshiyuki(2003) Cloning, expression and cell-surface localization of *Paenibacillus* sp. strain W-61 xylanase 5, a multidomain xylanase. Appl Env Microbiol 69(12): 6960-6978

Iversen T, Wannstrom S (1986) Lignin-carbohydrate bonds in a residual lignin isolated from pine kraft pulp. Holzforschung 40: 19-22

Jaleel SA, Srikanta S, Karanth NG (1992) Production of fungal amyloglucosidase by solid-state fermentation: Influence of some parameters. J Microbiol Biotechnol 7: 1-8

Jeffries TW, Choi S, Kirk TK (1981) Nutritional regulation of lignin degradation by *Phanerochaete chrysosporium*. Appl Env Microbiol 41: 290-296

Kamra P, Satayanarayana T (2004) Xylanase k production by *Humicola lanuginosa* in solid-state fermentation. Appl. Biochem. Biotechnol. 119:145-157

Kango N, Agrawal SC, Jain PC (2003) Production of xylose by *Emericella nidulans* NK-62 on low-value lignocellulosic substrates. World J Microbiol Biotechnol 19(7): 691-694

Kantelinen A, Hortling B, Sundquist J, Linko M, Viikari L(1993) Proposed mechanism of the enzymatic bleaching of kraft pulp with xylanase. Holzforschung 47:318-324

Kantelinen A, Ranua M, Ratto M (1988) International pulp bleaching conference proceeding. TAPPI Press Atlanata P-1

Khasin A, Alchanati I, Shlham Y (1993) Purification and characterization of a thermostable xylanase Kirk from *Bacillus stearothermophilus* T-6. Appl. Env Microbiol 59(6): 1725-1730

Kluefel D, Vats-Mehta S, Aumont F, Shareck F, Morosoli R (1990) Purification and characterization of a new xylanase (xylanase B) produced by *Streptomyces lividans* 66. J Biochem 267:45-50

Kohli N, Singh P, Chaudhary D (2001) Thermostable, alkaliphilic and cellulase free xylanase production by *Thermoactinomyces thalophiles* sub group C. Enz Microb Technol 28: 606-610

Krik TK, Jeffries TW, Leathem GF (1983) Biotechnology, application land implications for the pulp and paper industry. TAAPI, 66:45-51

Kulkarni N, Rao M (1996) Application of xylanase from alkaliphilic thermophilic *Bacillus* sp. NCIM59 in biobleaching of bagasse pulp. J Biotechnol 51:167-173

Kulkarni N, Shendye A, Rao M (1999) Molecular and biotechnological aspects of xylanases. FEMS Microbiol Rev 23:411-456

Kumar N, Singh K (1992) Chemical and microbial changes during solid-state fermentation of wheat straw with *Corpinus fimetarius*. Biological Wastes 33: 231-242

Lappalainen A., Siika-Aho, Kalkkinen M, Fagerstrom R, Tenkanen M (2000) Endoxylanase II from *Trichoderma reesei* has several isoforms with different isoelectric points. Biotechnol Appl Biochem 31: 61-68

Lischinig T, Purkarthofer H, Steiner W (1993) Thermostability of endo-b-xylanase from the thermophilic fungus *Thermomyces lanuginosus*. Biotechnol Lett 15:411-414

Lonsane BK, Ramesh MV (1990) Production of bacterial thermostable á-amylase by SSF, a potential tool for achieving economy in enzyme production and starch hydrolysis. Adv Appl Microbiol 35: 1-56

Luthi E, Bhana J M, Bergquist PL (1990) Xylanase from the extremely thermophilic bacterium *Caldocellion saccharolyticum* over expression of the gene in *E.coli* and characterization of the gene product. Appl Env Microbiol 56: 2677-2683

Luthi E, Reif K, Jasmat NB, Bergquist PL (1992) In vitro mutagenesis of a xylanase from the extreme thermophile *Caldocellum saccharolyticum*: Over expression of the gene in *Escherichia coli* and characterization of the gene product. Appl Env Microbiol 56:2677-2683

Lyon PF, Beffa T, Blance M, Auling G, Arangno M (2000) Isolation and characterization of highly thermophilic xylanolytic *Thermus thermophilus* strains from hot composts. Can J Microbiol 46(11): 1029-35

Maruo B, Tojo T (1985) Stepwise enhancement of productivity of thermostable amylase in *Bacillus licheniformis* by a series of mutations. J Gen Appl Microbiol 31:323-328

Mathrani I M, Ahring BK (1992) Thermophilic and alkaliphilic xylanase from several *Dictyoglomus* isolates. Appl Microbiol Biotechnol 38: 23-27

McCarthy AJ, Peace E, Broda P (1985) Studies on the extracellular xylanase activity of some thermophilic Actinomycetes. Appl Microbiol Biotechnol 21: 138-244

McDonough T J (1995) Recent advances in bleached chemical pulp manufacturing technology part 1: Extended delignification, oxygen delignification, enzyme application, and ECF and TCF bleaching. TAPPI J 78:55

Morales P, Madrarro A, Flors A, Sendra JM, Gonzalez JAP (1995) Purification and characterization of a xylanase and *arabinofuranosidase* from *Bacillus polymyxa*. Enz Microb Technol 17:424-429

Moreau A, Shareck F, Kluepfel D, Morosoli R (1994) Increase in catalytic activity and thermostability of the xylanase A of *Streptomyces lividans* 1326 by site specific mutagenesis. Enz Microb Technol 16: 420-424

Morosoli RM, Bertrand J, Mondou F, Shareck F, Klueppel D (1986) Purification and properties of a xylanase from *Streptomyces lividans*. J Biochem 239:587-592

Murata S, Kondo R, Sakai K, Kashino Y, Nishida T, Takahara Y (1992) Chlorine-free bleaching process of kraft pulp using treatment with the fungus IZU-154 TAPPI J 75(132): 91-94

Nakai R, Wakahayoshi K, Asano T, Aono R, Horikoshi K, Nakamura (1994) In: Nucleic acid symposium series No. 31:235-236. Oxford Press

Nakamura S, Wakabayashi K, Nakai R, Aono R, Horikoshi K (1993a) Production of alkaline xylanase by a newly isolated alkaliphilic *Bacillus* strain 41 M-1. World J. Micorbiol Biotechnol 9: 221-224

Nakamura S, Wakabayashi K, Nakai R, Aono R, Horikoshi K (1993b) Purification and some properties of an alkaline xylanase from alkaliphilic *Bacillus* sp. strain 41 M-1. Appl Env Microbiol 59(7): 2311-2316

Nakanishi K, Marui M, Yasui T (1992) Comparison of xylan and methyl Beta-xyloside induced xylanases from *Streptomyces* sp. J Ferm Bioeng. 74(6): 392-394

Narang S, Sashi V, Bisaria VS (2001) Optimization of xylanase production by *Melanocarpus albomyces* IIS 68 in solid-state fermentation using Response Surface Methology. J Biosc Biotech 91:425-427

Narang S, Satyanarayana. T (2001) Thermostable α-amylase production by an extreme thermophile *Bacillus thermoleovorans*. Lett Appl Microbiol 32:31-35

Nath D, Rao M (2000) pH dependent conformational and structural changes of xylanase from an alkalophilic thermophilic *Bacillus* sp. (NCIM59). Enz Microb Technol 28:397-403

Noe P, Chevalier J, Mora F, Comtat J (1986) Action of xylanases on chemical pulp fibres. Part II, enzymatic beating. J Wood Sci Technol 6: 167-184

Ohakoshi A, Kudo T, Mase T, Horikoshi K (1985) Purification of three types of xylanases from an alkaliphilic *Aeromonas* sp. Agric Biol Chem 49: 3037-3038

Okazaki W, Akiba T, Horikoshi K, Akahoshi E (1984) Production and properties of two types of xylanases from alkaliphilic thermophilic *Bacillus* sp. Appl. Microbiol Biotechnol 19: 335-340

Paice MG, Bernier R Jr, Jurasek L (1988) Viscosity enhancing bleaching of hard wood kraft kpulp with xylanase from a cloned gene. Biotechnol Bioeng 32: 235-239

Palma MB, Milagres AMF, Prata AMR, Manchilha IM (1996) Influence of aeration and agitation rate on the xylanase activity from *Penicillium janthinellum*. Process Biochem 31:141-145

Panbangred W, Fukusaki E, Epifanio EC, Shinmyo A, Okada H (1985) Expression of a xylanase gene of Bacillus pumilus in *Escherichia coli* and *Bacillus subtilis,* Appl. Microbiol Biotechnol 22:259

Pandey A, Soccol CR, Rodriguez-Leon JA, Nigam P (2001) Solid-state fermentation in biotechnology: fundamentals and applications. Asiatech publishers, Inc. New Delhi

Park YS, Kang SW, Lee JS, Hong S I, Kim SW (2002) Xylanase production in SSF by *Aspergillus niger* mutatant using statistical designs. Appl Microbiol Biotechnol 58:761-766

Paul J, Verma AK (1993) Characterization of cellulose and hemicellulose degrading *Bacillus* sp. from termite infested soil. Curr Sci 64(4):262-266

Perttula M, Ratto M, Kondradsdothir M, Kristjansson JK, Viikari L (1993) Xylanases of thermophilic bacteria from Icelandic hot springs. Appl Microbiol Biotechnol 38: 592-595

Puls J (1997) Chemistry & biochemistry of hemicelluloses: relationship between hemicellulose structure and enzyme required for hydrolysis. Macromol Symp. 120,183

Puls J, Schuseil J (1993) Chemistry of hemicelluloses: relationship between hemicellulose structure and enzyme required for hydrolysis. In: Coughlan MP, Hazlewood GP(eds) Hemicellulose and hemicellulases. Portland Press, London, pp 1-28

Purkarthofer H, Sinner M, Steiner W (1993) Cellulase-free xylanase from *Thermomyces lanuginosus:* Optimization of production in submerged and solid-state culture. Enz Microb Technol 15:677-682

Rajaram S, Varma A (1990) Production and characterization of xylanase from *Bacillus thermoalkalophilus* grown on agricultural wastes. Appl. Microbiol Biotechnol 34: 141-144

Rani DS, Nand K (2000) Production of thermostable cellulase-free xylanase by *Clostridium absonum* CFR-702. Process Biochem 36:355-62

Ratanakhanokchai K, Kyu K L, Tanticharoen M (1999) Purification and properties of a xylan-binding endoxylanase from alkaliphilic *Bacillus* sp. strain K-1. Appl Env Microbiol 65:694-697

Ratto M, Mafthrani IM, Ahring B, Viikari L (1994) Application of thermostable xylanase of *Dictyoglomus* sp. in enzymatic treatment of kraft pulps. Appl Microbiol 41: 130-133

Sadhu JS, Kennedy JF (1984) Molecular cloning of *Bacillus polymyxa*(1→4)-β-D-xylanase gene in *Escherichia coli*. Enz Microb Technol 6:271-274

Santos ESD, Guirardello R, Franco TT (2002) Preparative chromatography of xylanase using expanded bed adsorption. J Chromatogr 944:217-24

Sa-Pereira P, Mesquita A, Duarte JC, Barros MRA, Costa-Ferreira M (2002) Rapid production of thermostable cellulase-freexylanase by a strain of *Bacillus subtilis* and its properties. Enz Microb Technol 30:924-33

Senior DJ, Hamilton J (1992) Use of xylanases to decrease the formation of AOX in kraft pulp bleaching. J Pulp Pap Sci 18(15): 165-168

Shah AK, Sidid SS, Ahmad A, Rele MV(1999) Treatment of baggasse pulp with cellulase-free xylanase from an alkaliphilic *Bacillus* sp. Sam-3. Bioresource Technol 68:133-140

Shao W, Deblois S, Wiegel J (1995) A high molecular weight, cell-associated xylanase isolated from exponentially growing *Thermoanaerobacterium* sp. strain JW/SL-YS 485. Appl Env Microbiol 61: 937-940

Sharma A (2000) Thermo-alkali stable cellulase-free xylanase of an extreme thermophilic *Bacillus thermoleovorans* AP7. Ph.D. Thesis. University of Delhi, South Campus New Delhi, India

Simonen M, Palva I (1993) Protein secretion in *Bacillus* species. Microbiol Rev 57: 109-137

Singh S, Pillay B, Prior BA (2000) Thermal stability of b-xylanases produced by different *Thermomyces lanuginosus* strains. Enzyme Microb Technol. 26, 502-508

Singh SM, Andreas M, Prior BA (2003) *Thermomyces lanuginosus*: Properties of strains and their hemicellulases. FEMS Microbiol Rev 27: 3-16

Srinivasan MC, Rele MV (1995) Cellulose-free xylanase from micro-organisms and their application to pulp and paper biotechnology: an overview. Indian J Microbiol 35:93-101

Srivastava KC (1993) Properties of thermostable hemicellulolytic enzymes from *Thermomonospora* strain 29 grown in solid-state fermentation on coffee processing solid waste. Biotechnol Adv 11(3): 441-65

Subramaniyan S, Prema P (2000) Cellulase-free xylanases from *Bacillus* and other micro-organisms. FEMS Microbiol Letts 183:1-7

Subramaniyan S, Prema P, Ramakrishan SV(1998) Isolation and screening for alkaline thermostable xylanases. J Basic Microbiol 37(6): 431-437

Sung WL, Luk CK, Zahab DM, Wakarchuyk W (1993) Over expression of the *Bacillus subtilis* and *circulans* xylanases in *Escherichia coli*. Prot. Expression Purif 4, 200

Sung WL, Yaguchi M, Ishikawa K (1998) U.S. Patent Number 5,866,408

Sunna A, Antranikian G (1997) Xylanolytic enzymes from fungi and bacteria. Crit Rev Biotechnol 17:39-67

Techapun C, Chareonrat T, Watanabe M, Poosaran N, Sasaki K (2002) Thermostable and alkaline-tolerant cellulase-free xylanases produced from thermotolerant *Streptomyces* sp. Ab106. J Biosci Bioeng 93(4): 431-433

Techapun C, Poosaran N, Watanabe M, Sasaki K (2003) Thermostable and alkaline-tolerent microbial cellulose-free xylanase produced from agricultutal wastes and the properties required for use in pulp bleaching processes: a review. Process Biochem 38:1327-1340

Techapun C, Sinsuwongwat S, Poosaran N, Watanabe M, Sasaki K(2001) Production of a cellulase-free xylanase from agricultural waste materials by a thermotolerant *Streptomyces* sp. Biotechnol Lett 23:1685-1689

Tseng M, Yap M, Ratanakanokchai K, Kyu KL, Chen S (2002) Purification and characterization of two cellulase-free xylanase from an alkalophilic *Bacillus firmus*. Enz Microb Technol 30 : 590-595

Tsujibo H, Sakamoto T, Nishino N, Hasegawa T (1990) Purification and properties of three types of xylanases produced by an alkaliphilic Actinomycete. J Appl Bacteriol 69: 398-405

Turunen O, Ethuatio K, Fenel F, Vehmaanpera J, Rouvinen Wu X, Leisola M (2001) A combination of weakly stabilizing mutation with a disulphide bridge in the α helix region of *Trichoderma reesei* endo-1,4-β-xylanase II increases the thermostability through synergism. J Biotechnol 88: 37-46

Turunen O, Vuorio M, Fenel F and Leisola M (2002) Engineering multiple arginines into Ser/Thr surface of *Trichoderma reesei* endo-1,4-β-xylanase increases the temperature optimum and shifts the pH optimum towards alkaline pH. Protein Eng 15: 141-145

Turunen Ossi, Janis Janne, Fenel fred and Leisola Matti (2004). Engineering the thermotolerance and pH optimum of family 11 xylanase by site-directed mutagenesis. In: Methods in Enzymology, Elsevier Inc. 388: 156-166

Uchino F, Nakane T(1981) A thermostable xylanase from a thermophilic *Bacillus* sp. Agric Biol Chem 45: 1121-1227

Veoikodvorskaya TV, Volkov IY, Vasilevko VT, Zverlov VV, Piruzian ES (1997) Purification and some properties of *Thermotoga neapolitana* thermostable xylanase B expressed in *E. coli* cells. Biochemistry (Moscow) 62: 66-70

Viikari L, Kantelinen A, Sundquist J, Linko M (1994) Xylanases in bleaching: from an idea to the industry. FEMS Microbiol Rev 13: 335-50

Viikari L, Ranua M, Kantelinen A, Linko M, Sundquist J (1987) Application of enzymes in bleaching. In: Proceedings of 4th International Symposium on Wood and Pulping Chemistry Vol.1 pp 69-90

Viikari L, Ranua M, Kantelinen A, Sunduist J, Linko M (1986) Bleaching with enzymes. In: Proc. 3rd Int. Conf. Biotechnology in the Pulp and Paper Industry, STFI, Stockholm, Sweden. 67-69

Viikari L, Tenkanen M, Buchart J, Ratto M, Bailey Siika-aho M, Linko M(1993) Hemicellulases for industrial application. In: Bioconversion of forest and agricultural plant residues. Suddler JN(eds) CAB, International Wallingford 131-182

Vyas P, Chauthaiwale V, Phadatare S, Deshpande V, Srinivasan MC (1990) Studies on the alkaliphilic *Streptomyces* with extracellular xylanolytic activity. Biotechnol Lett 12:225-228

Wakarchuk WW, Sung WL, Campbell RL, Cunningham A, Watson DC, Yaguchi M (1994) Thermostabilization of the *Bacillus circulans* xylanase by the introduction of disulphide bonds. Protein Eng 7:1379-1386

Walsh D, Gibbs MD, Bergquist PL (1988) Expression and secretion of a xylanase from the extreme thermophile, *Thermotoga* strain FjSS3B.1. in *Kluyveromyces lactis*. Extremophiles 2:9-14

Wandersman C (1992) Secretion across the bacterial outer membrane. Trends in Genetics 8:317-322

Whistler RL, Richards EL (1970) Hemicelluloses. In: Pigman W, Horton D (eds) The carbohydrates. Academic Press, New York, pp 447-469

Wong KKY, Clarke P, Nelson SL(1996) Possible roles of xylan derived chromophores in xylanase prebleaching of soft wood kraft pulp. ACS Sym. Ser. 618,352

Wong KKY, Tan LUL, Saddler JN(1988) Multiplicity of b-1,4-xylanase in micro-organisms: functions and applications. Microbiol Rev 52:305-317

Yang CA, Robert Mackenzie, C Roger, Bilous Doris, Seligy Verner L, Narag Saran A (1988) Molecular cloning and expression of a xylanase gene from *Bacillus polymyxa* in *Escherichia coli*. Appl Env Microbiol 54(4): 1023-1029

Yang JL, Lou G, Eriksson KE (1992) The impact of xylanase on bleaching of kraft pulps. TAPPI J 75(12): 95-101

Zheng L, Du Y, Zhang J (2000) Biobleaching effect of xylanase preparation from an alkalophilic *Bacillus* sp. on ramie fibres. Biotechnol Lett 22(17):1363-1367

Bioleaching and Microbial Mineral Degradation

G EBENA and E KOTHE

1. INTRODUCTION

When we go to work each morning by car or bus, enter a modern building or take a pen, we are probably not aware that we are depending on metals which has been mined and extracted from ore. This dependency has lasted for several thousand years as development of human society accelerated from the bronze age, when man first learned to use metals.

The process of transferring metals from solid minerals into solution has till recently been regarded as a geochemical reaction, so far covered by the fields of geology or chemistry. A recent literature survey of acid mine drainage and related issues showed that only about 10% of the more than 4000 articles found contained keywords related to microbiology or biology. A strikingly low number, since now it is widely accepted that these reactions are catalyzed by bacteria.

The importance of bacteria in acid mine drainage (AMD) production has been known for some time; Hallberg and Rickard (1973) cite work from the 1950s in their popular review. For example, micro-organisms can increase the rate of iron oxidation by up to three orders of magnitude as compared to chemical oxidation alone (Strömberg and Banwart 1994). This clearly shows that micro-organisms must not be neglected when looking for biotechnological applications in studying the negative environmental effects of mine waste. This is especially true for the reduced waste originating from sulphide mines.

The insight of the potential in bacterially mediated dissolution of minerals has led to the industrial application of *'bioleaching'*. The process is

Jena University, Jena, Germany

especially suitable for sulphidic ore because production of sulphate generates sulfuric acid which enhances the mobility of the reduced metals. This process is seen naturally in weathering of sulphidic rock exposed to air.

The term bioleaching' will be used throughout this text when referring to microbially aided metal recovery. Although sometimes referred to as biomining, since it is not necessarily the metal to be recovered that is leached; bioleaching is the most widespread and widely known term. The same is true for bio-oxidation. One example, where as leaching/oxidation does not directly target the metal to be recovered, is the recovery of gold from arsenopyrite, where arsenic, iron and sulphur are leached to enhance the subsequent extraction of gold with cyanide.

Whether microbial impact on mineral degradation is a possibility or a problem, is largely a matter on the side of the metal recovery process: a possibility, when making metals available for man to use; a potential problem, when the minerals in waste rock piles or remnants from the recovery process are degraded and release environmentally harmful substances like heavy metals and highly acidic seepage of water.

2. MICROBIAL MINERAL DEGRADATION

There are many processes that fit to the description of mineral degradation. In this context, however, we will disregard all kinds of physical break-down and erosion and focus on dissolution, that is the transformation from solid mineral to (metal) ions in solution.

The dissolution of a solid mineral is governed by a number of environmental parameters. Although there is a never-ending debate among scientists which factor is the most important in a certain situation, there are some that could be considered of major importance: pH, redox-conditions (including oxygen availability), water availability and quality as well as the composition of the mineral itself. Most of these factors are interconnected with each other and, more importantly, with the microbial ecosystem.

When considering the habitats of micro-organisms found in the mineral environment, the focus is often set on a single, isolated species and its metabolic capacities in pure culture. Although, often necessary for methodological reasons to learn as much as possible about the single players, this is only the first step in understanding the microbial ecosystems and its functions. The use of pure cultures to unravel metabolic pathways may even prove unfruitful due to complicating factors like syntrophy and co-metabolism (Atlas and Bartha 1993).

2.1 Mining Practices

The way that most people perceive a mine is more or less a hole in the ground. The hole in the ground is probably the only accurate part when describing modern underground mining. Today an underground mine could stretch as far as a kilometre deep into the ground. The ore, that is the mineral having a metal content high enough to be economically viable to extract, is removed with heavy machinery and explosives. The crushed ore is then transported to the surface. There are examples of the first sorting being carried out underground to minimize the transport costs.

The other method for ore extraction is open pit mining. It does not involve shafts and tunnels, but rather the removal of very large amounts of covering non-ore material. The pits created can be several hundred meters deep and kilometers across. Open pit operations are usually used when the ore has a lower metal content and the economic viability of the mine is dependent on the large scale, naturally also dependent on the shape and size of the ore body.

The processes described here are high throughput methods, which, by lack of time, limit microbial activities. Therefore, the bioleaching part in these operations is rather connected to the waste rock and tailings produced, and AMD is seen as an environmental hazard.

Every mining process gives rise to two kinds of waste: waste rock, originating from the uncovering of the ore, and tailings, the residues from the enrichment process (Fig. 1). Waste rock is the rock that previously surrounded the ore and is removed before extraction of the ore itself. Waste rock can make significant contributions to the environmental effects of the mining industry.

Tailings are the residues of the modern enrichment processes, in which the ore is ground and mixed with water. To the sludge thereby formed, flotation chemicals are added (*e.g.* pine oil, xanthates), which allow the metal containing sulphide mineral to float in a foam which can be removed (Walterson 1984) and further treated for purification of the metals. The residues, the tailings, are then pumped to an appropriate location.

2.2 The Ores/the Minerals

Metals mined include iron, copper, zinc, aluminum, lead, nickel, cadmium and precious metals such as silver and gold. This list is by no means complete. However, as will be discussed in the coming sections, iron ore or sulphide ore are used to harvest the majority of the metals. In particular, the sulphide ore is of interest in the sense of bioleaching and acid mine drainage production. In addition, coal recovery produces waste with properties similar to that of sulphide ore due to the sometimes high content of sulphide minerals, mostly pyrite, within the coal.

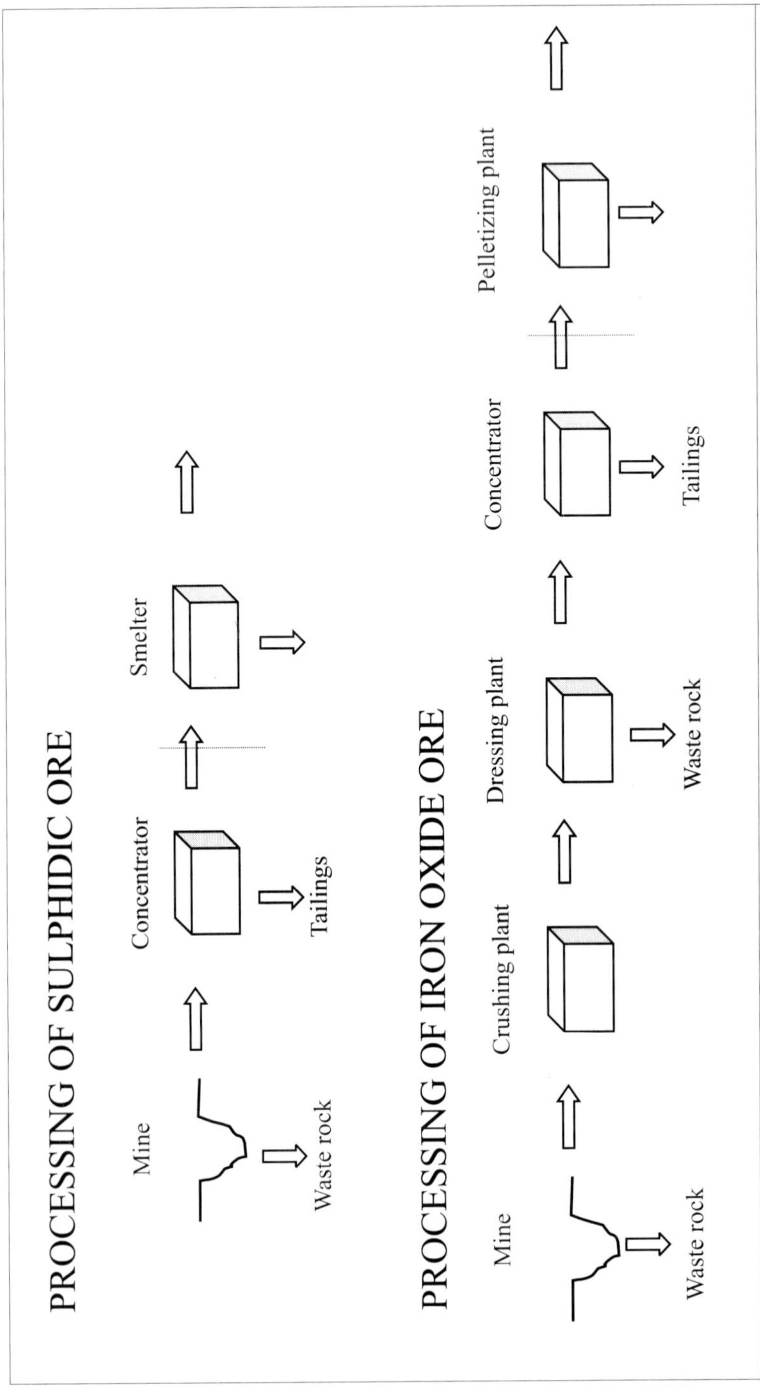

Fig. 1 A schematic flow chart for the two different mining processes carried out. Waste produced in processes shown to the left of the dashed lines is considered mine waste. From Naturvårdsverket (1998)

Although a tremendous amount of waste is produced from iron mines, both as waste rock and tailings, the impact on the environment is of only minor importance, because of the mineral constitution of the waste. The main ore (magnetite, Fe_3O_4, and hematite, Fe_2O_3), and therefore also the waste, is largely inert, due to its already oxidized chemical composition.

While at the same time the oxic form is also one of the reasons why bioleaching has not come to play a role in iron extraction, the main reason would be that the iron content in iron ore is already very high. The mined ore contains as much as 65-70% iron, making it suitable for direct smelting, as compared with, for example, copper that would be present at approximately 1% in mined ores.

There is a large variety of sulphidic minerals mined (for examples see Table 1). The low metal content is increasing the demand for more efficient extraction procedures, and the reduced state of both, the metal and sulphur component, makes these minerals ideal for bioleaching. An oxidation of the sulphur component generates acid, and under acidic conditions a metal containing solution is recovered which can be further processed for metal extraction. Besides copper bioleaching, which is the largest bioleaching process used, also uranium, zinc, nickel, molybdenum, cobalt, chromium, vanadium, gold and silver can be obtained using bioleaching.

Table 1 Some examples of sulphide minerals. All of these can be degraded by Acidithiobacillus ferro-oxidans (Ritcey 1989)

Mineral	*Composition*	*Mineral*	*Composition*
Arsenopyrite	- Fe_2AsS_2	*Marmatite*	- (ZnFe)S
Bornite	- Cu_5FeS_4	*Millerite*	- NiS
Bravoite	- $(Ni,Fe)S_2$	*Molybdenite*	- MoS_2
Chalcocite	- Cu_2S	*Orpiment*	- As_2S_3
Chalcopyrite	- $CuFeS_2$	*Pyrrhotite*	- Fe_7S_8
Cobalite	- CoAsS	*Sphlaerite*	- ZnS
Covellite	- CuS	*Stannite*	- Cu_2FeSnS_4
Enargite	- $Cu_3(As, Sb)S_4$	*Tetrahedrite*	- $Cu_8Sb_2S_7$
Marcasite	- FeS_2	*Violarite*	- $(Ni, Fe)_3S_4$

3. MICROBIAL PROCESSES

Bioleaching has a history of at least several hundred years, although the earliest miners using microbially mediated processes probably not were aware of the microbial contribution. It is difficult to find a figure describing the amount of bioleaching going on around the world, but as an example for the past twelve years there has been in excess of 30 million tonnes of copper ore treated each year, summing up to 15-20% of the production of copper in the US.

Apart from the previously mentioned gold-extraction, bioleaching is largely a matter of transferring the metals from the (low) grade ore into solution. This is achieved through oxidation of the metal sulphides, giving dissolved metal ions (e.g. Cu^{2+}) and sulphuric acid. The metal containing solution is then further treated, *e.g.* electrochemically to precipitate the desired metal.

3.1 The Organisms

There are a large number of different bacteria involved in bioleaching and acid mine drainage as well. A thorough description of the bacteria involved is far beyond the scope of this chapter. However, there are a number of excellent reviews on the matter (Rawlings 2002). Apart from the somewhat more in-depth presentation of the genera *Acidithiobacillus* and *Leptospirillum*, is the introduction to these bacteria limited to an overview of the functional groups of sulphur oxidizing and iron oxidizing bacteria.

The oxidation of sulphide minerals (using Pyrite, FeS_2, as an example) is commonly described by the following reactions (Holmström 2000):

(1) $2FeS_2 + 2H_2O + 7O_2 \rightarrow 2Fe^{2+} + 4H^+ + 4SO_4^{2-}$

(2) $2Fe^{2+} + \frac{1}{2} O_2 + 2\,H^+ \rightarrow 2\,Fe^{3+} + H_2O$

(3) $Fe^{3+} + 3H_2O \rightarrow Fe(OH)_3 + 3H^+$

While the entire process is exergonic, the second reaction is slow under acidic conditions and thought to be the rate-determining step in the formation of acid leachate from sulphide minerals (Singer and Stumm 1970). Iron oxidising bacteria may enhance the reaction rate of equation to several orders of magnitude. Most sulphide minerals could release metals in reactions analogous to (1). It is worth noting that the oxidation of iron (2), and to a smaller extent other metals, and the subsequent precipitation of iron (3) is greatly enhancing acid production. The low pH is beneficial for the process of microbial mineral degradation by increasing the solubility of metals and also through the direct effect on iron metabolism.

In the oxidation of pyrite (FeS_2), tetra- and pentathionates (S_4O_6 and S_5O_6) have been found as side-products. This indicates that there is more to microbial metabolism than merely the ability to oxidize both iron and sulphur in the 'classical manner'. Schippers et al. (1996) have proposed that cyclic degradation of pyrite may occur, based on an indirect attack mechanism (Fig. 2).

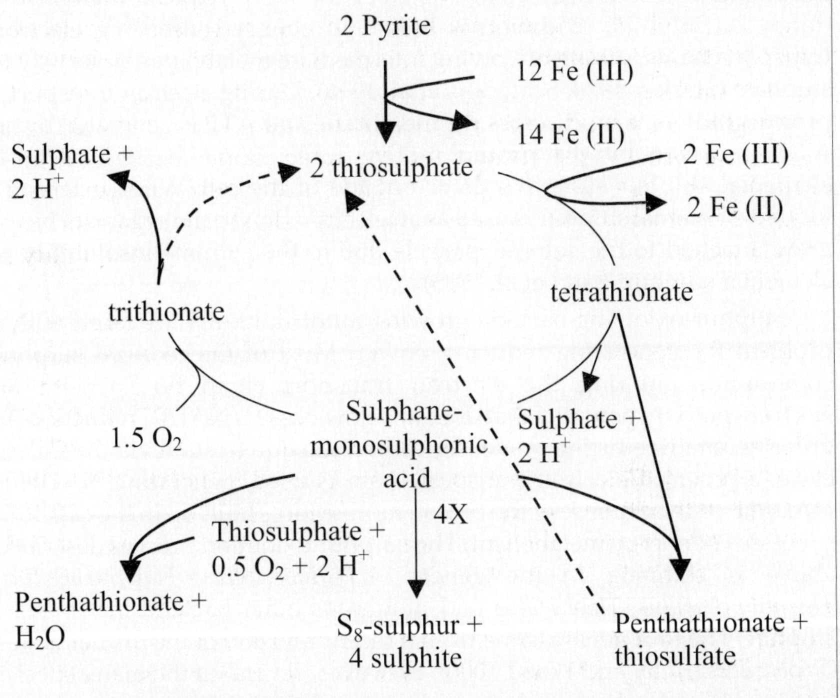

Fig. 2 Cyclical oxidative pyrite degradation by bacterial processes and/or chemical leaching. Note the role of Fe^{3+} in the oxidation of pyrite. Dashed lines indicate that thiosulphate may re-enter the cycle (Schippers et al. 1996).

In the process described above, the ferric ion (Fe^{3+}) acts as a powerful tool that is used in the primary attack on pyrite, thus enabling energy to be harvested from the sulphur oxidation. Bacterially formed $FeSO_4$ (1) can react to form $Fe_2(SO_4)_3$ (ferrisulphate).

(4) $2FeSO_4 + ½O_2 + H_2SO_4 \rightarrow Fe_2(SO_4)_3 + H_2O$

The $Fe_2(SO_4)_3$ chemically oxidizes many metal sulphides, thus releasing soluble sulphates (*e.g.* 5,6):

(5) $Cu_2S + 2Fe_2(SO_4)_3 \rightarrow CuSO_4 + 5FeSO_4 + 2S$

(6) $CuFeS + 2Fe_2(SO_4)_3 \rightarrow 2CuSO_4 + 4FeSO_4 + S$

Also applicable in uranium leaching (7):

(7) $UO_2 + Fe_2(SO_4)_3 + 2H_2SO_4 \rightarrow UO_2(SO_4)_3 + 2FeSO_4 + 4H^+$

3.1.1 Sulphur-oxidizing bacteria

A wide variety of sulphur compounds can be used as electron donors. Among the most common are (hydrogen) sulphide, elemental sulphur and thiosulphate. The energy yield is greater the more reduced the electron donor is. Sulphide oxidation is linked to energy-conserving electron transport chains, usually involving intermediate metabolites on its way to sulphate (Starkey 1934; Schippers et al. 1996). During electron transport a proton gradient is built across the membrane and ATP is generated by an ATPase driven by the proton motive force. Some bacteria deposit elemental sulphur either inside or outside of the cell. When externally located elemental sulphur is used as an electron donor, the organism has to grow attached to the sulphur particle due to the extreme insolubility of elemental sulphur (Sand et al. 1995).

Sulphur-oxidizing bacteria growing autotrophically are faced with a problem for generating reducing power. Most of the reduced sulphur compounds entering the electron transport chain do so with an electronegativity potential that does no allow NAD^+/$NADP^+$ reduction. In order to obtain reducing power for carbon dioxide fixation via the Calvin cycle, a reversed electron transport chain is used, generating $NADH^+$/ $NADPH^+$ at the expense of the proton motive force built up in the catabolic processes of energy metabolism. The sulphur oxidation process described above is common to the genera *Acidithiobacillus, Halothiobacillus, Thermithiobacillus, Thiobacillus* and numerous other bacteria that oxidize sulphur. The four genera come from a recent revision of the former genus *Thiobacillus* (Kelly and Wood 2000). However, several of the many species involved have further metabolic features, such as denitrification and iron-oxidizing capabilities.

The sulphur-oxidizing bacteria cover a wide range of genera, including archea and eubacteria, predominantly within the subdivision of proteobacteria. Since sulphuric acid is produced, most genera tolerate acidic pH, often with growth optimum at ph 3 to 4. *A. ferro-oxidans* for example growths at pH 1.8 and survives at pH 1.

3.1.2 Iron-oxidizing bacteria

Bacteria that can oxidize iron can be divided into two groups: acidophilic and neutrophilic. There are doubts that the neutrophilic iron-oxidizing bacteria (i.e. those that prevail at or around neutral pH) actually derive their energy from oxidation of iron (Nealson 1983). Ferrous ion (Fe^{2+}) is unstable in near-neutral environments and is, thus, only found at interfaces between anoxic and oxic substrata. Only in *Gallionella ferruginea* has true lithotrophy at near-neutral pH been observed so far (Brock et al. 1994). It is able to fix CO_2 through the Calvin cycle with energy derived from iron oxidation at neutral pH, but only at an interface where anoxic water with Fe^{2+} contents meet molecular oxygen. Several other bacteria can be found in neutral, iron-rich environments. However, these strains might not really live on oxidation of iron, but merely take advantage of this source of iron.

At pH below 4, Fe^{2+} is stable even in the presence of oxygen. At the same time, low pH increases the free energy of the iron/metal oxidation reaction, allowing bacterial growth (Lizama and Suzuki 1988). Thus, chemolithotrophic iron-oxidizers usually are acidophilic. There are several types of bacteria that are capable of growth on iron oxidation in acidic conditions. Most iron-oxidizing bacteria are autotrophs (Kelly 1988). A dual feature of some iron-oxidizing bacteria is their ability to oxidize not only iron, but also sulphur compounds. Two of the most well known iron-oxidizing bacteria have this ability: the Archean *Sulfolobus* sp. and the eubacterium *Acidithiobacillus ferro-oxidans*.

The iron metabolism is straightforward. A steep proton-gradient is formed between the acidic surroundings of the cell and the near-neutral pH of the cytoplasm. The proton translocating ATPase of the organism couples the natural proton-motive force over the membrane to the synthesis of ATP. The oxidation of iron is a proton-consuming reaction (Fig. 3). The oxidation of iron is, thus, only an indirectly energy producing reaction, as its major function is to maintain the proton gradient between the environment and the cytoplasm. The Fe^{3+} formed readily precipitates as iron hydroxide complexes outside the cell.

The metabolic process described above is aerobic, but there is evidence that anaerobic metabolism also occurs in *A. ferrooxidans* (Das and Mishra

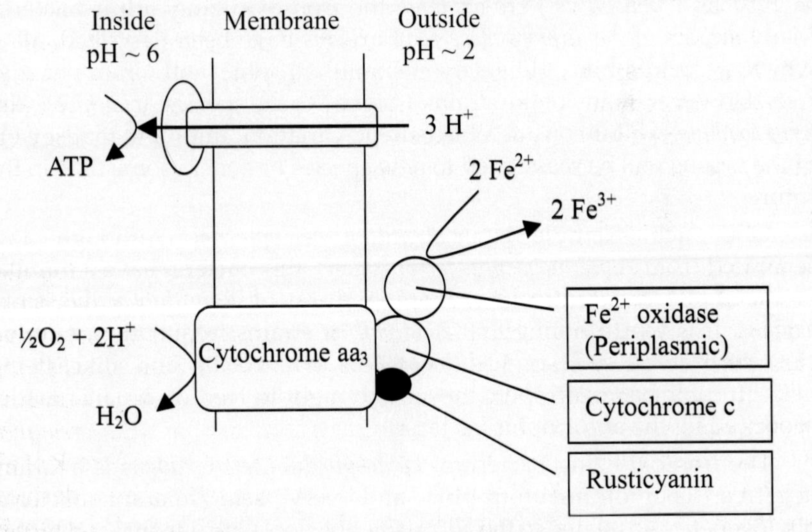

Fig. 3 Iron metabolism in a typical acidophilic iron-oxidizing bacteria.

1996; Donati et al. 1997). In this, the ferric ion, Fe^{3+}, acts as the electron acceptor, and the reduced sulphur compounds in the metal sulphide as electron donors, thus coupling iron reduction to sulphide oxidation (Das and Mishra 1996). There are also indications that the rate of weathering under these conditions is as high as in oxygenated environments (Donati et al. 1997).

A habitat for an organism may be defined simply as an environment in which it can live and form a population, either permanently or temporarily. The main natural habitats of *A. ferro-oxidans* are probably gleysols, for example sulphur-containing soils and gleyic podsols, where anaerobic conditions allow reduced sulphur and iron to occur. Bogs, where the roots of plants provide oxygen, would be another natural habitat, and roots are found to be covered with iron hydroxides (Küsel et al. 2003). Still another natural habitat for *A. ferrooxidans* would be areas with high natural concentrations of pyrite or other metal sulphides. Sulphidic mine waste is a human artifact, even if such waste may have existed for thousands of years, but it is nevertheless a habitat for *A. ferro-oxidans*. It is important to bear in mind that the habitat is in no way unrelated to the organisms it hosts; on the contrary, the organisms are probably the most important factors shaping their habitat (McNaughton et al. 1988; Naiman 1988). The low pH-conditions formed by *A. ferro-oxidans* would be an example of such an interaction.

Temple and Colmer (1951) first described *Acidithiobacillus ferro-oxidans* in 1951 as *Thiobacillus ferro-oxidans*, the iron-oxidizing sulfur bacteria. Many strains of *Acidithiobacillus ferro-oxidans* have been described, all of which are acidophilic, obligately chemolithotrophic, and Gram-negative rods. However, many of the strains assigned to the species *Acidithiobacillus ferro-oxidans* exhibit considerable genetic variation, implying that several of the strains will be reassigned to new species or genera some time in the future.

One such example is *Acidiphilum acidophilum*. Although now separated from *Acidithiobacillus ferro-oxidans,* this bacteria have a number of metabolic capabilities overlapping those of *Acidithiobacillus ferro-oxidans*. It is worth noting that *Acidiphilum* strains frequently are found close to bacteria such as *Acidithiobacillus ferro-oxidans* and alike. Being heterotrophic or mixotrophic they are thought to feed on organic matter produced by the autotrophic bacteria.

The iron-oxidizing bacterium *Leptospirillum ferro-oxidans* is a Gram-negative, chemolithoautotrophic and very acid tolerant bacteria, phylogenetically related to the *Nitrospira* division. One unusual and highly relevant characteristic of *L. ferro-oxidans* is its dependency on Fe^{2+} which is the sole electron donor. This naturally makes the organism an obligately anaerobic micro-organism. The iron metabolism of *L. ferro-oxidans* is not fully understood, it does, however, differ from that in *A. ferro-oxidans* in that it is not inhibited by high levels of Fe^{3+}. The Fe^{3+} produced is thought to chemically oxidize pyrite (Lengeler et al. 1999)

(8) $FeS_2 + 14Fe^{3+} + 8H_2O$ ® $15Fe^{2+} + 2SO_4^{2-} + 16H^+$

Several studies are indicating that *L. ferrooxidans* is one of the most common bacteria in bioleaching plants (Dew et al. 1997 and Lawson 1997).

3.2 Leaching Practices

The goal of all leaching techniques is to create an optimal environment for leaching bacteria, thus maximizing the yield of metals. Optimizing the environment would include ensuring oxygen and water supply, an appropriate pH and access to the mineral surface. Although some experiments with the goal of controlling the microbial community have been done, it has been proven more fruitful to focus on the conditions controlling the process and thus indirectly controlling the microbial populations (Rawlings 2002). That is possible because in these environments bacteria with leaching capability are omnipresent. The naturally present strains are likely to outcompete any introduced strain since they are adapted to the conditions at the site, as there is a continuous selection for the most efficient strains.

Heap-leaching is the simplest and least elaborate type of bioleaching. The material to be leached, either ore or dump material (low grade ore waste), is placed on an impermeable surface with a suitable topography. The purpose is that it should be possible to collect the leachate after passing through the material. This could, for example, be achieved at steep hillsides on an underlying impermeable bedrock. This operation is often chosen when former dumps, where the material was tipped over the edge, are taken up for leaching. Another example would be by shaping a small valley and add a layer of clay, having a bowl-like structure where the leaching solution can be readily collected (Fig. 4)

The material to be leached is subjected to cycles of irrigation – 'ripening' – washing – conditioning/rest – irrigation… The length of the cycles varies with regard to quality of the ore, amount and climate. Each step could be as long as a year. The desired metals are extracted from the leachate by means of electrochemical methods. Irrigation is normally done with recycled water from the previous cycle; this means that it is generally high in sulphate and iron and with a very low pH. The iron and sulphate is enriched with each cycle. The irrigation water could be amended with inorganic nutrients such as $(NH_4)_2SO_4$ and KH_2PO_4 in order to provide optimized conditions for the micro-organisms, especially when the ore has a comparatively high metal content.

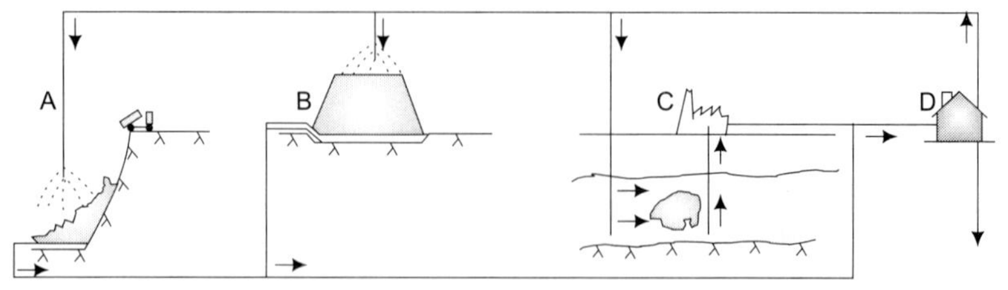

Fig. 4 Processig of ore in three different bioleaching schemes: A) Dump leaching of former waste or very low grade ore. B) Heap leaching with more controlled conditions and smaller batches. The height of the pile could be 10-50 meters. C) In-situ leaching. A well is drilled into the permeable rock through which the acid water is injected, the metal rich water is extracted through another well after passing through the ore body. D) The plant where the desired metal is removed from the leachate using electrochemical methods. The acid, iron-rich water is recycled for further irrigation/ injection

In situ leaching could be regarded as a special case of heap or dump leaching as the only large difference being the heap. The term *in situ* leaching is used when an acidic solution is pumped into the ore body without the ore being removed. The metal laden water is then collected through some kind of drainage system. The process is often used for mines no longer in use, hence the drainage system is already available through the old tunnels and shafts. The great advantage of not having to remove the ore to extract the desired metals has to be weighed against the draw-backs of a rather uncontrolled process with the possible loss of leachate through cracks and crevices infiltrating ground water and thus the risk of contaminating nearby aquifers with (heavy) metals.

Stirred tank leaching is another very elaborate and technical process used. The rate of mineral oxidation is increased through the use of a series of aerated and stirred bioreactors. Due to the cost of construction and maintenance this type of set-up is limited to high-value ores and concentrates. The tanks are typically arranged in a series with concentrate and fertilizer added to the first tank. A continuous flow from tank to tank until the bio-oxidation has provided sufficient level metal concentrations. Oxidation of minerals is an exothermic reaction, thus excess heat has to be removed which is expensive. Large volume of air blown into each tank provides oxygen, and large agitators ensure a homogenous suspension of the solid material.

In addition, leaching of industrial waste such as ashes and leaching of coal for removal of sulphides is used.

4. MITIGATION OF ACID MINE DRAINAGE

Due to the low metal content of the sulphidic ores, a large amount of waste is produced. In areas where sulphide minerals are mined, both the waste rock and the tailings may be readily degraded leading to AMD production. The waste rock contains low amounts of the mined metal sulphides and frequently also pyrite (FeS_2). This will, through microbially mediated weathering, frequently result in an acidic, metal containing drainage water with adverse environmental effects. If acidic waters containing high amounts of dissolved iron are contributories to near-neutral surface waters, the change of pH will lead to precipitation of iron.

Mining industry in the USA may serve as an example: US mines produce about 2.7 million metric tons of acid a year and Acid Mine Drainage pollutes over 26,000 kilometers of streams. (http://www.eco-web.com 2004) However, the problem is similar in all areas where metal mines are operated. Even a small country like Sweden has large amounts of mine waste accumulated over the years, today reaching close to 1,000 million tonnes of sulphidic mine waste (waste rock and tailings) (extrapolated from MiMi 1998; Naturvårdsverket 1998). Contrary to the common belief that the poor enrichment methods of the past generated the majority of this waste, the low-grade ores currently mined are responsible for by far the largest portion.

Mine waste can be treated in several ways to minimize the production of acid mine drainage. Some of these methods are directly based on manipulation of the microflora, since the microbial community has been shown to be the single largest causative factor affecting AMD (Strömberg and Banwart 1994; Ledin and Pedersen 1996). Other methods are more indirect and affect the biogeochemical cycle as a whole, but their effects on the microbial community still have to be taken into account. For society, a demand for long-term, low-maintenance solutions is rising which also has to be kept in mind.

Until recently, the main focus for AMD amelioration was to limit oxygen and water access to the material by application of covers. There, the microflora has only indirectly been the target for the means applied. More recent experiments and even full-scale operations include methods directly aimed at the microflora such as applications of bactericides and bioattenuation.

One of the first things to come to mind in mitigating the effects from AMD is to cover the waste. The basic idea of a cover is to limit the access of oxygen to the mine waste. This, in turn, will limit both the biological and chemical oxidation of the sulphides, which will substantially reduce the production of AMD. This could be achieved by a soil or water cover which could be called 'dilution in time' (Naturvårdsverket 1998), meaning that the yearly contribution of AMD may be reduced to sustainable levels.

There are several types of covers. Soil covers using till, clay or some other impermeable materials have been successfully employed at various mine waste locations (Ritcey 1989). The main intention is to create a water-saturated zone, which is more or less impermeable to oxygen; another aim is to decrease the amount of infiltrating water in order to decrease the amount of AMD generated. Subsurface deposition, or flooding of impoundments, that is employing a water cover, is a more cost-effective abatement technique than soil covers. Water is a very effective oxygen barrier, and thus allows reducing conditions to form, depending on the formation of anoxic sediments due to microbial respiration. As with soil covers, there are several examples of water being successfully used as an oxygen and erosion barrier, for instance at the Stekenjokk mine in northern Sweden (Holmström 2000). As in natural lakes, an organic sediment layer may form on top of the mine waste and act as a seal for metals by providing favourable conditions for sulphate-reducing bacteria. Most metals can then precipitate as metal sulphides.

There are two approaches to adding chemicals in order to ameliorate the formation of AMD. The first and most obvious is to add a bactericide, since the formation of AMD is largely biological. One such chemical is sodium dodecyl sulphate (SDS). Schippers et al. (1998) studied its effect on the microflora, and found profound reductions in both bacterial numbers and activity following an addition of 480 g SDS/ton tailings. Furthermore, field experiments have shown that application of bactericides can reduce AMD production by more than 50% (Olson et al. 2003). Advantages with bactericides include their rapid effects and low price. The major disadvantages are associated with doubts about their long-term performance (Schippers et al. 1996) and possible negative effects on the surroundings.

A second approach that can be adopted in attempts to ameliorate the effects of AMD with chemicals is to raise the pH. Dolomite, concrete and even CaO are examples of substances that are used. The basic idea is that a high pH will render the habitat unsuitable for the micro-organisms and inhibit the deleterious chemical reactions. They may also have additional, beneficial chemical effects, e.g. precipitation of metals that are dissolved under acidic conditions, and the possibility of hard-pan formation, whereby the precipitate forms an impermeable seal (Schippers et al. 1996).

Bioattenuation

Bioattenuation could in many respects be regarded as the opposite of bioleaching, hence the precipitation of free metals from a solution. As stated earlier iron can precipitate as Fe^{3+}-hydroxides at the low pH generally found in mineral leachates. Other metals, like Zn and Pb, are more prone to stay in solution under aerobic conditions; the stable precipitates are rather formed under reduced conditions and then as metal sulphides. Again largely a biological matter.

The most well-known and intensively studied genera of sulphate-reducing bacteria that can be used to form metal sulphides are *Desulfovibrio* and *Desulfotomaculum*. Sulphate is a powerful electron acceptor in anoxic environments and can be readily reduced by organic matter as follows:

(9) $2[CH_2O] + SO_4^{2-}$? $H_2S + 2HCO^{3-}$

Where $[CH_2O]$ represents organic matter, molecular hydrogen can act as an electron donor in a reaction analogous with (9). However, the sulphate-reducing bacteria are heterotrophs which lack the ability to fix CO_2, hence they need organic carbon for biomass production (Atlas and Bartha 1993). Among the most common electron donors are low molecular weight carbon compounds, such as pyruvate, lactate and acetate (Widdel 1988). The hydrogen sulphide in the reaction can react further with dissolved metal ions to form the highly insoluble metal sulphides (10):

(10) $M^{2+} + S^{2-}$? MS (where M is any bivalent metal)

The metal sulphide formed is generally precipitated due to the low solubility of most metal sulphides. The formation of metal sulphides thus immobilizes metals that can be precipitated as metal sulphides.

Sulphate reduction is inhibited by the presence of oxygen, nitrate or ferric ions. It has been suggested that sulphate-reducing bacteria might be out-competed by iron-reducing bacteria in mine waste environments (Ledin and Pedersen 1996). If so, this would imply that sulphate reduction the single described mechanisms that has a mitigating effect on the problems arising from sulphidic mine waste would be of minor importance in pyrite-containing tailings impoundments.

The sulphate-reducing bacteria are often limited by organic carbon availability, and addition of organic carbon to marine sediments can greatly enhance sulphate reduction (Atlas and Bartha 1993). This could be of importance in mine waste environments which usually are carbon-limited. Another problematic feature is that sulfate-reducing capacity is sensitive to low temperatures (Abdollahi and Nedwell 1979), which might favour other processes in cold climate including large mining districts in Europe and North America.

The possibility that lies within microbial sulfate reduction has been used for bioattenuation of AMD. The first example encompasses reactive barriers, where AMD is led through a covered filter containing organic matter and sulphate reducing bacteria (Blowes 2000). The other example would be wetlands, either natural or constructed. The idea is to use the sulphate reducing capability of the microbial community found in the reduced, anaerobic and organic-rich sediment. Wetlands also have the effect of slowing down water flow allowing sedimentation of metal pollutants transported as particulate matter.

REFERENCES

Abdollahi H, Nedwell DB (1979) Seasonal temperatures as a factor influencing bacterial sulphate reduction in a salt-marsh sediment. Microb Ecol 5:73-79

Atlas RM, Bartha R (1993) Microbial ecology - fundamentals and applications. The Benjamin/Cummings Publishing company Inc., Redwood city, CA, USA

Blowes DW, Ptacek CJ, Benner SG, McRae Che WT, Bennet TA, Puls RW (2000) Treatment of inorganic contaminants using permeable reactive barriers. J Contam Hydrol 45:123-137

Brock TD, Madigan MT, Martinko JM, Parker J (1994) Biology of micro-organisms. Prentice-Hall Inc., Englewood cliffs, NJ, USA

Das A, Mishra AK (1996) Role of *Thiobacillus ferrooxidans* and sulphur(sulphide)-dependent ferric-ion-reducing activity in the oxidation of sulphide minerals. Appl Microbiol Biotechnol 45: 377-382

Dew DW, Lawson EN, Broadhurst JL (1997) The BIOX(R) process for bio-oxidation of gold-bearing ores or concentrates In: Rawlings DE, ed. Biomining: theory, Microbes and Industrial processes. Springer-Verlag, Germany

Donati E, Pogliani C, Boiardi JL (1997). Anaerobic leaching of covellite by *Thiobacillus ferrooxidans*. Appl Microbiol Biotechnol 47: 636-639

Hallberg RO, Rickard DT (1973) De 'små' gruvarbetarna i Falun. In: B. Afzelius. Svensk naturvetenskap 1973 Allmänna förlaget, Stockholm, Sweden. (In Swedish)

Holmström H (2000) Geochemical processes in sulphidic mine tailings. Department of environmental engineering. Doctoral thesis, Luleå University of Technology, Luleå, Sweden

Kelly DP (1988) Evolution of the understanding of the microbiology and biochemistry of the mineral leaching habitat. In: Norris PR, Kelly DP(eds) Biohydrometallurgy: Science and Technology Letters Kew, Surrey 3-14

Kelly DP, Wood AP (2000) Reclassification of some species of *Thiobacillus* to the newly designated genera *Acidithiobacillus* gen. nov., *Halothiobacillus* gen. nov. and *Thermithiobacillus* gen. nov. Int J Syst Evol Microbiol 50: 511-516

Küsel K, Chabbi A, Trinkwalter T (2003) Microbial Processes Associated with Roots of Bulbous Rush Coated with Iron Plaques. Microb Ecol 46: 302-311

Lawson EN (1997) The composition of mixed populations of leaching bacteria active in Nickel and Gold recovery from sulphide ores. In: Aust. mineral found., International biohydrometallurgy symposium IBS97, pp QP4.1-4.10. Glenside, South Aust

Ledin M, Pedersen K (1996) The environmental impact of mine wastes – roles of micro-organisms and their significance in treatment of mine wastes. Earth Sci Rev 41:67-109

Lengeler JW, Drews G, Schlegel HG (1999) Biology of the prokaryotes, Georg Thieme Verlag, Stuttgart, Germany

Lizama HM, Suzuki I (1988) 'Bacterial leaching of a sulphide ore by *Thiobacillus ferrooxidans* and *Thiobacillus thiooxidans*: I. Shake flask studies.' Biotechnol Bioeng 32:110-116

McNaughton SJ, Ruess RW, Seagle SW (1988). Large mammals and process dynamics in African ecosystems. Bioscience 38:794-800

MiMi (1998) Programme plan for the period 1999-2000. Luleå University of Technology: 50. Sweden

Naiman RJ (1988) Animal influences on ecosystem dynamics. Bioscience 38(11): 750-752

Naturvårdsverket (1998) Gruvavfall - Miljöeffekter och behov av åtgärder. Stockholm, Naturvårdsverket: 67. (*In Swedish)*

Nealson KH (1983) The microbial iron cycle. In: Krumbein WE (ed) Microbial Geochemistry Blackwell scientific publications, Oxford

Olson GJ, Clark TR, Mudder TL, Logsdon M (2003) A novel approach for control and prevention of acid rock drainage. 6th ICARD, July 14-17 2003, July 14-17 2003, Cairns, Australia

Rawlings DE (2002) Heavy Metal Mining Using Microbes. Annu Rev Microbiol 56: 65-91

Ritcey GM (1989) Tailings Management-problems and solutions in the mining industry. Elsevier, Amsterdam-Oxford-New York-Tokyo, pp

Sand W, Gerke T, Hallmann R, Schippers A (1995) Sulphur chemistry, biofilm, and the (in)direct attack mechanism - a critical evaluation of bacterial leaching. Appl Microbiol Biotechnol 43:961- 966

Schippers A, Jozsa P-G, Sand W (1996) Sulphur Chemistry in Bacterial Leaching of Pyrite. Appl Environ Microbiol 62(9): 3424-3431

Schippers A, Jozsa P-G, Sand W (1998) Evaluation of the efficiency of measures for sulphidic mine waste mitigation. Appl Environ Microbiol 49:698-701

Singer PC, Stumm W (1970) Acidic mine drainage: The rate-determining step. Science 167: 1121-1123

Starkey RL (1934) Isolation of some bacteria which oxidize thiosulphate. Journal series paper of New Jersey Agricultural Experiment Station, New Jersey Agricultural Experiment Station, pp

Strömberg B, Banwart S (1994) Kinetic modelling of geochemical processes at the Aitik mining waste rock site in northern Sweden. Appl geochem 9: 583-595

Temple KL, Colmer AR (1951) The autotrophic oxidation of iron by a new bacterium, *Thiobacillus ferrooxidans*. J Bacteriol 62: 605-611

Walterson E (1984) Effekter av anrikningsreagenser - fördelning och spridning av xantater och xantatderivat vid anrikningsverk, IVL, Stockholm: 50 (*In Swedish)*

Widdel F (1988) Microbiology and ecology of sulphate and sulphur-reducing bacteria. In: Zehnder AJB (ed) Biology of anaerobic micro-organisms. John Wiley & Sons, New York

Environmental Benefits of Xylanase-Assisted Prebleaching of Kraft Pulps

R BISWAS, V SAHAI, S MISHRA and VS BISARIA

1. INTRODUCTION

The environment is contaminated by halogen compounds in the form of pesticides, pulp and paper mills' effluent, vinyl chloride from PVC mills, etc. Halogen compounds are responsible for most cases of ground water contamination. One ton of pulp carries a load of one kg of organic halides which flows out as effluent, expressed in terms of Adsorbable Organic Halides (AOX) (Salkinoja-Salonen et al.1995). Biomethylation of organic halides in soil, catalyzed by many soil bacteria and fungi, further increases health risk. The effluent from pulp and paper industry consists of approximately 700 organic and inorganic compounds (Eeroakova and E Golis 1994). The variety of toxic effects, the aquatic life is exposed to due to effluent of pulp and paper mills flowing into it, can be classified as carcinogenic, mutagenic and clastogenic. The toxic effect has also been recorded at the major planktonic and benthic trophic levels, reducing the diversity and abundance of *phyto-zooplankton* and *zoobenthos*. The fishes and their reproductive physiology have been affected by the endocrinic effect of organohalogens (Karrasch et al. 2005).

Presently, the Indian paper industry is having a mix of large and small paper mills, of capacities ranging from 5 to 600 tons per day, with a minimum turnover of 1800 tons per year. There are more than 600 pulp and paper mills producing nearly 6.2 million tons of paper per year and

Department of Biochemical Engineering and Biotechnology, Indian Institute of Technology Delhi, New Delhi, India. E-mail: vsbisaria@hotmail.com

turnover of more than $35 million. The total AOX present in the bleach plant effluent is in the order of 120,000 tons/annum which continues to wreak havoc on the surrounding ecosystems (Jain et al. 2005).

2. PULPING OF WOOD

Wood is made of cellulose fibres that are bound together by lignin. Cellulose can be 40-45%, hemicellulose 20-30% and lignin 15-25% of dry weight of wood (Sjöström 1993). The two main hemicelluloses in wood are xylans and glucomannans. The basic structure of xylan is a main chain of β-1, 4-linked *D-xylopyranosyl residues*. Typically, these linear chains carry short side chains in varying extent. The chemical composition of the substituent side groups and the frequency of their occurrence depend on the origin of xylan and the method of their isolation. Xylan of hard-wood is *acetyl-4-O-methyl glucuronoxylan* with a degree of polymerization of about 200. Approximately 10% β-*D-xylopyranose* backbone units are substituted at C-2 with a 1, 2-linked 4-O-methyl-α-D-glucuronic acid residue, while 70% are acetylated at C-2 or C-3 or both. Hard-woods contain a small amount of glucomannan and the ratio of glucose to mannose in it varies between 1:1 and 1:2 depending on the wood species. Soft-woods contain 10-15% xylan as *arabino-4-O-glucuronoxylan* with degree of polymerization of >120. It is not acetylated and contains β-D-xylopyranose, 4-O-methyl-α-D-glucuronic acid and L-arabinose in a ratio of 100:20:13. The 4-O-methyl-glucuronosyl residues are attached to C-2 and L-arabinofuranosyl residues to C-3 of xylopyranose backbone units. The backbone of soft-wood glucomannan is made of β-1,4-linked D-glucopyranose and D-mannopyranose units and is partially substituted by α-galactose and acetyl units. The ratio of glucose to mannose is 1:3 to 1:4 in these two fractions of soft-wood glucomannan (Saraswat 1997).

The xylan of grasses is also arabino-4-O-methyl glucuronnoxylan with a degree of polymerization of 70. It contains less 1, 2-linked 4-O-methyl-á-D-glucuronic acid than hard-wood xylan but have a large content of á-arabinofuranosyl side chains. These are linked to C-2 or C-3 or to both positions in the β-D-xylopyranose main chain residues. In addition, such xylans contain 2-5% by weight of α-acetyl groups linked to C-2 or C-3 of the xylopyranose units. Moreover, 6% of the arabinosyl side chains are themselves substituted at position C-5 with feruloyl groups, while 3% are substituted with p-coumaroyl residues. The relative proportions of the various components of grass arabinoxylans vary from species to species, and from tissue to tissue within a single species. In natural lignocellulosic materials some or all of the ferulosyl substituents may be engaged in covalent cross-linking of xylan molecules with lignin or with other xylan molecules (Saraswat 1997).

Pulping of wood is done to separate wood fibres to make them suitable for bleaching in paper making (Suurnäkki et al. 1997). The delignification of woody material can be done by sulphate (kraft) or sulphite processes (Rydholm 1965). In most part of the world, kraft process remains the preferred method of pulping of wood (Kirk and Jeffries 1996). In this process, wood chips are cooked with sodium hydroxide and sodium sulphide (Sjöström 1977). The acetyl groups and part of glucuronic acid side chains get removed from the xylan (Hamilton et al. 1958; Croon and Enström 1961). Soft-wood is more resistant to the kraft process than hard-wood due to the arabinose substituents present in it (Simonson 1971). During cooking process, part of the xylan is dissolved in the pulping liquor due to high alkali concentration. However, along the process, as alkali concentration decreases, degraded and short chain xylans precipitate on the surface of cellulose fibrils (Yllner et al. 1957). Therefore, in cooking process about 90% of the lignin is solubilized and removed. The remaining 10% lignin is removed by bleaching with elemental chlorine and chlorine dioxide. Elemental chlorine reacts with lignin and other organic matter present in the pulp and forms chlorinated compounds like chlorinated lignosulfonic acids, chlorinated resin acids, chlorinated phenols, chlorinated hydrocarbons, dioxins and furans. Therefore, the effluent from pulp and paper mills has a high AOX, BOD and COD (Ali and Sreekrishnan 2001). The AOX content of effluent depends on the amount of lignin in the pulp fibre before bleaching and the amount of chlorine applied to the pulp.

3. XYLANASES IN THE PREBLEACHING OF KRAFT PULPS

Two plausible explanations given for action of xylanase on pulp are: (i) the disruption of xylan chains by xylanases cleaves the lignin-carbohydrate bonds and improves the accessibility of bleaching chemicals to the pulps and facilitates easier removal of solubilized lignin in bleaching (Paice et al. 1992; Buchert et al. 1992) and (ii) the xylan dissolved in kraft process gets reabsorbed or reprecipitated on and within the pulp fibres at the end of the pulping process and thereby it shields the residual lignin from bleaching chemicals. Xylanases act on this redeposited xylan and help in making lignin accessible to bleach chemicals (Kantelinen et al. 1993). Still, experiments show that removal of redeposited xylan by *dimethylsulphoxide* (DMSO) did not improve bleachability of the pulp but treatment with xylanases did, indicating that DMSO-insoluble xylan is attached with lignin (Pederson et al. 1992).

Xylanase is added to kraft pulp in the treatment tower after the pH and temperature of the pulp have been brought down to optimum range of its action. The total chlorine dioxide required across a five-stage bleach plant to reach the desired brightness as a function of the kappa number decreases significantly as a result of xylanase prebleaching (Tolan and Guenette 1997). Adsorbable organic halides (AOX) and total organochlorine (TOX) in the effluent also decrease. Enzyme treatment decreases the AOX in proportion to the decrease in chlorine compound usage. The effluent colour also decreases as the colour of the effluent is due to the quantity of chlorine used. In one of the surveys, mills using enzyme treatment reported no change in the pulp strength and an increase in tear strength due to xylan reprecipitation (Tolan et al. 1995).

The effectiveness of enzyme on the pulp depends on the pH of pulp, temperature of pulp, dispersion of enzyme in the pulp and time of interaction of enzyme and pulp. The optimum pH of enzyme depends on the source of xylanase and pulp has to be acidified to make it conducive for the action of enzyme. But acidification of pulp has to be done carefully so that 10% pulp consistency is maintained. After chemical pulping, the temperature of the pulp is in range of 50-90°C depending on the extent of heat removal. Therefore, in pulp and paper industry thermostable xylanase is preferred. The adequate dispersion of enzyme and acid into the pulp is crucial for action of the enzyme and the residence time required for enzyme treatment is about 1-2 hr. (Tolan and Vega Canovas 1992). It has been found that treatment of chemical pulps with xylanase leads to savings in the consumption of bleaching chemicals, decreased environmental loadings and increased final brightness of pulp (Viikari et al. 1986; Viikari et al. 1987; Kantelinen et al. 1988).

4. PRODUCTION OF XYLANASE

Several micro-organisms produce xylanase in nature but the enzyme that can work optimally under harsh alkaline condition of pulp and paper industry is the most desired. Several bacteria and fungi produce enzymes that show optimum activity in alkaline pH and high temperature and are also free from cellulase (Table 1). The large scale production of xylanase can take place in submerged fermentation as well as in solid-state fermentation depending on the process conditions required for high productivity by the organism as shown in Table 2.

4.1 Xylanase Production by Submerged Fermentation

In submerged fermentation, the biomass remains evenly dispersed in liquid medium with equal excess to the dissolved nutrients and oxygen. Efficient heat and mass transfer also takes place. The scale-up from shake flask to fermentor is generally convenient in submerged cultivation than in

Table 1 A few important Xylanase producing microbes having optimum activity in alkaline pH and high temperature.

	Organism	Substrate	Optimum activity		Xylanase Activity	References
			pH	*Temp (°C)*		
1.	*Aspergillus terreus*	Wheat straw	7.0	50	16.16 IU/g	(Ghanem et al. 2000)
2.	Bacillus amyloliquefaciens	Xylan	7.0	80	10.00 IU/ml	(Breccia et al. 1998)
3.	Bacillus pumilus	xylan	9.0	60	328.00 IU/ml	(Duarte et al. 1999)
4.	*Bacillus* sp.	Oat spelt xylan	10.0	60	9.00 IU/ml	(Zheng et al. 2000)
5.	*Bacillus* sp. NCIM59	Wheat bran	7.0	60	500.00 IU/ml	(Kulkarni and Rao 1996)
6.	*Bacillus* sp. NCIM2128	Wheat bran	8.0	60	52.00 IU/ml	(Balakrishnan et al. 1992)
7.	*Bacillus* sp. NCIM2128	Wheat bran	8.0	60	120.00 IU/ml	(Balakrishnan et al. 1997)
8.	*Bacillus* sp. Sam 3	Wheat bran	8.0	60	131.00 IU/ml	(Shah et al. 1999)
9.	*Bacillus strearothermophilus*	Wheat bran	7.0	60	184.00 IU/ml	(Nammori et al. 1990)
10.	*Cellulomonas flavigena* PN-120	Sugar cane bagasse	9.0	55	-	(Martinez-Trujilo et al. 2003)
11.	*Cephalosporium* sp. RYM-202	Wheat bran	8.0	50	-	(Kang et al. 1996)
12.	*Clostridium absonum* CFR-702	Birch wood xylan	8.5	75	420.00 IU/ml	(Rani and Nand 2000)
13.	*Dictyoglomus* sp. B1	Birch wood xylan	8.0	73	2.30 IU/ml	(Adamsen et al. 1995)
14.	*Pleurotus ostreatus*	Wheat bran	7.0	50	24.98 U/ml	(Qinnghe et al. 2004)
15.	*Staphylococcus* sp.	Oat spelt xylan	7.5	50	0.80 IU/ml	(Gupta et al. 2000)
16.	*Thermomonospora* sp.	Corn cob	9.0	50	125.00 IU/ml	(George et al. 2001)
17.	*Thermomyces lanuginosus* DSM 10635	Oat husk extract	7.0	75	-	(Xiong et al. 2004)

Table 2 Production of Xylanase in Fermentor by Micro-organisms

S.No.	*Organism*	*Carbon source*	*Fermentation conditions*				*Xylanase activity*		*References*
			Temp. (°C)	*pH*	*Type*	*Scale (l)*	*(IU/ml or IU/g)*	*Time (h)*	
1.	*Aspergillus niger*	Corn cobs	28	3.5	SmF	20.0	290.00	80	(Qi-peng et al. 2005)
2.	*Aspergillus sulphureus*	Wheat bran	32	6.5	SSF	75.0	7.50	72	(Wenqing et al. 2003)
3.	*Bacillus coagulans* BL69	Fibrous soy residue	37	-	SSF	0.5	1.47	72	(Heck et al. 2005)
4.	*Bacillus circulans* BL53	Fibrous soy residue	37	-	SSF	12.0	8.25	96	(Heck et al. 2005)
5.	*Bacillus* sp.	Oat spelt xylan	40	8.0	SmF	1.5	65.00	24	(Chivero et al. 2001)
6.	*Bacillus subtilis*	Oat spelt xylan	50	6.0	SmF	2.0	1.73	18	(Sá-Pereira et al. 2002)
7.	*Fusaruim oxysporum* F3	Corn stover	30	7.0	SSF	10.0	1840.00	144	(Panagiotou et al. 2003)
8.	*Melanocarpus albomyces* IIS 68	Wheat Straw	45	7.0	SmF	150.0	160.00	120	(Bisaria et al. 2002)
9.	*Neocallimastix frontalis*	Cellulose	39	6.8	SmF	1.2	3.68	144	(Srinivasan et al.2001)
10.	*Penicillium brasilianum* IBT *20888*	Oat spelt xylan	30	5.0	SmF	5.0	-	111	(Jørgensen et al. 2003)
11.	*Rhizopus oryzae*	Corn cob	35	5.0	SmF	2.0	260.00	120	(Bakir et al. 2001)
12.	*Rhodothermus marinus*	Birchwood xylan	61	7.5	SmF	5.0	7.50	72	(Gomes et al. 2000)
13.	*Schizophyllum commune*	Avicel	50	5.0	SmF	9.5	4839.00	200	(Haltrich et al. 1993)
14.	*Streptomyces* sp. Ab106	Sugarcane bagasse	50	7.0	SmF	5.0	32.00	144	(Techapun et al.2003)
15.	*Thermoascus aurantiacus*	Sugarcane bagasse	45	-	SSF	0.2	1597.00	240	(Milagres et al. 2004)
16.	*Thermoascus aurantiacus*	Solka Floc	47	4.5	SmF	5.0	208.00	264	(Gomes et al. 2000)
17.	*Thermomyces lanuginosus* SSBP	Xylose	50	6.5	SmF	30.0	405.00	48	(Reddy et al. 2002)
18.	*Trichoderma reesei* Rut C-30	Lactose	28	6.0	SmF	2.0	94.70	120	(Xiong et al. 2004)

SmF: Submerged Fermentation (enzyme activity in IU/ml) SSF: Solid-State Fermentation (enzyme activity in IU/g solid substrate)

solid-state cultivation. In *Bacillus circulans* D1, optimization of xylanase production parameters like pH, temperature, substrate concentration, cultivation time and aeration improved enzyme productivity (Bocchini et al. 2002). Different xylanases were produced by *Trichoderma reesei* Rut C-30 between pH 3.5 to 7.5 in submerged cultivation. The xylanase activity of 94.7 IU/ml was obtained at pH 6.0 (Xiong et al. 2004). The scale-up of xylanase production from 15l to 30l required increased aeration and yielded more biomass and better productivity in *Thermomyces lanuginosus* SSBP. At an aeration rate of 0.75 vvm, maximum xylanase activity of 405 IU/ml in 48 hr. was obtained (Reddy et al. 2002). A novel halophillic eubacterium, strain SX15, resulted in 20-fold increase in xylanase activity to 174 IU/ml in 168 h when optimized by response surface methodology in shake flask (Wejse et al. 2003). The xylanase activity of 210 IU/ml was observed at the end of cultivation in bioreactor, which was higher than in shake flask when carbon source was replaced by soluble oat husk extract in *Thermomyces lanuginosus* DSM 10635 (Xiong et al. 2004). Optimization of production media of *Schizophyllum commune* increased xylanase production by 330%. The strain when cultivated in optimized media in 9.5l fermentor, a maximum xylanase activity of 4,839 IU/ml was obtained at 200 hr. having optimum pH of 5.0 and temperature 50°C (Haltrich et al. 1993).

4.2 Xylanase Production by Solid-State Fermentation

In Solid-State Fermentation (SSF), the solid waste residues from agriculture, forest, various mills etc. are used as support substratum on whose surface the dispersed biomass grows under controlled temperature, moisture and aeration. SSF offers several advantages over liquid cultivation, especially for the fungal cultures, as there is higher productivity per unit volume, reduced energy requirements, lower capital investment, low waste water output, higher concentrations of metabolites obtained and low downstream processing cost (Narang et al. 2001). Production of xylanase by *Fusarium oxysporum* under solid-state culture on corn stover was enhanced by optimization of the type of nitrogen source, initial moisture level, growth temperature and initial pH (Panagiotou et al. 2003). The fungi, *Thermomyces lanuginosus* and *Thermoascus aurantiacus*, both produced xylanase that was active at higher temperature by developing on inexpensive industrial waste of wheat bran (Alam et al. 1994). Comparison of optimization of xylanase production in submerged and solid-state culture by *Thermomyces lanuginosus* indicated that solid-state cultivation had 3.5-fold better yield (Purkarthofer et al. 1993). The SSF faces a major problem related to design and operation of large-scale bioreactors (Ashley et al. 1999). Various bioreactor types have been used in

SSF processes, including packed beds, rotating drums, gas-solid fluidized beds and other stirred bioreactors (Mitchell et al. 2000) but still they are not being able to overcome the mass and heat transfer limitations completely. A novel intermittent agitation rotating drum type bioreactor for SSF of thermophillic micro-organism was studied for xylanase production by *Thermoascus aurantiacus*. Important fermentation variable like initial moisture content of the medium, growth temperature and airflow rate were effectively controlled at the set values through this design and obtained xylanase activity of 4,490 U/g of dry wheat straw (Kalogeris et al. 2003).

5. *MELANOCARPUS ALBOMYCES*: A POTENTIAL SOURCE FOR LARGE-SCALE XYLANASE PRODUCTION

The fungus, *M. albomyces* IIS 68 (Maheshwari and Kamalam 1985), on which we have been working, is a filamentous, multinucleate, thermophilic, heterothallic and non-sporulating fungus. It has been found to be a good source of thermostable xylanase which also has xylosidase and xylan-debranching enzymes. The debranching enzymes produced include acetyl esterase, α-L-arabino-furanosidase and α-D-glucuronidase. Amongst various carbon sources tested, the inexpensive lignocellulosic residue, wheat straw, was found to be the best carbon source for production of extracellular xylanase which consisted of seven iso-enzymes. The iso-enzyme, Ic, was constitutive whereas the other six exhibited more specific inducibility, the magnitude of which depended on the nature of the inducer (Saraswat and Bisaria 1997). Using optimized culture conditions it has been possible to get 160 IU/ml of xylanase activity in 150l fermenter under submerged cultivation (Bisaria et al. 2002), (Fig. 1).

The purified xylanase isoenzymes of *M. albomyces* have been characterized in terms of various physico-chemical and kinetic parameters. The molecular weights of the iso-enzymes, as determined by SDS-PAGE, were in the range of 18,600 to 38,500 and pIs of isoenzymes Ia, Ib, Ic, IIa and IIb were in the range of 3.7 to 6.4. The pH and temperature optima were determined to lie in the range of 5.5 to 8.5 and 55 to 77°C, respectively. Two iso-enzymes, IIa and IIc, showed the maximum activity in alkaline range. Three iso-enzymes Ia, Ib, and Ic, showed maximum activity at 70°C. Out of the seven xylanase isoenzymes, Ia was found to be the most stable xylanase with half lives of 164.28, 16.67 and 6.56 min at 60, 70 and 80°C, respectively. The range of K_m for xylanase isoenzymes was 0.4 to 6.9 mg/ml for wheat straw whereas V_{max} varied from 16.39 to 198 μmol/(min.mg). The turnover number (k_{cat}) was computed to lie in the

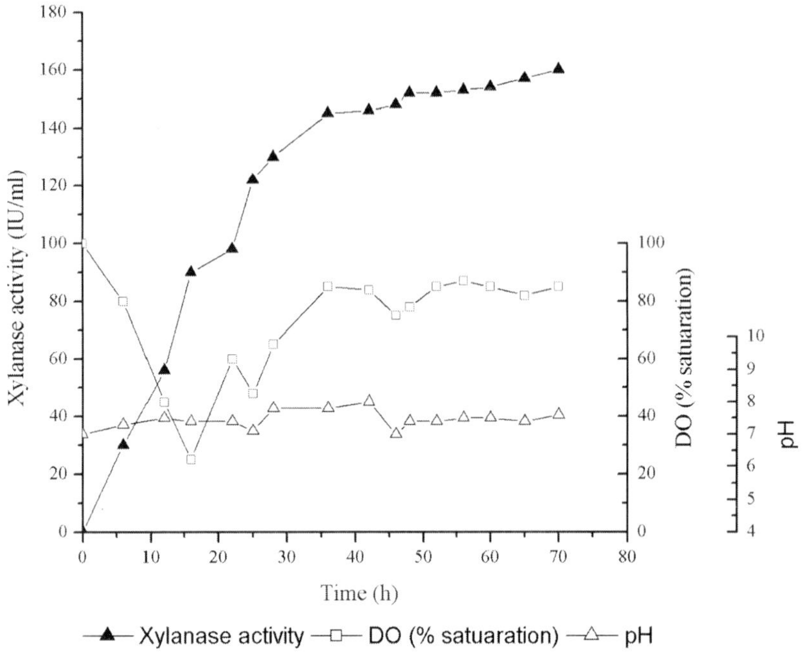

Fig. 1 Production of xylanase by *Melanocarpus albomyces* in 150 l fermentor.

range of 10.52 to 83.82 s^{-1} and k_{cat}/K_m in the range of 1.52 to 133.62 ml/mg.s. Five out of seven xylanase isoenzymes were found to be specific only for xylans. Xylanases Ic and IIa showed some activity on Solka Floc and p-nitrophenyl-β-D-xylopyranoside, respectively. The effect of seven purified xylanase isoenzymes, separately and in combination, was studied on three xylans, namely birchwood, larchwood and oat spelt xylan and the extent of their hydrolysis was compared with that of the crude extract of *M. albomyces*. All the seven xylanase isoenzymes acted synergistically and the presence of β-xylosidase and xylan-debranching enzymes in crude extract further increased xylan hydrolysis. The nature and extent of xylan hydrolysis products were also determined by individual and combined action of purified xylanases, as well as by the crude extract. The major product of xylan hydrolysis was xylose for Ib and IIa. Although xylose was the major reaction product, small amounts of xylobiose and xylooligosaccharides were also generated. Four xylanase iso-enzymes, namely Ia, Ib, Ic and IIa exhibited arabinose-releasing property (Bisaria et al. 2002; Saraswat and Bisaria 2000) (Table 3).

Table 3 Major products of xylan hydrolysis by individual and combined action of xylanases.

Enzyme	Relative concentration of sugars produced (% of total) by hydrolysis of xylan							
	Birchwood xylan				*Larchwood xylan*			
	X_1	X_2	X_r	A	X_1	X_2	X_r	A
I. Purified xylanase iso-enzymes	ND	ND	76.17	ND	ND	ND	54.98	1.52
Ia	67.96	11.75	20.30	ND	42.99	10.75	19.17	26.10
Ib	9.73	2.93	83.03	ND	7.86	1.40	82.21	2.64
Ic	23.41	3.71	51.25	ND	46.30	10.80	34.73	7.79
IIa	ND	9.29	57.55	ND	ND	10.45	73.93	ND
IIb	19.40	4.74	75.86	ND	14.31	2.96	74.04	ND
IIc	ND	11.49	67.07	ND	3.21	10.08	66.76	ND
IId	95.57	0.52	3.82	ND	87.83	0.85	4.07	7.25
II. Crude Extract								

X_1: Xylose; X_2: Xylobiose; X_r: *Xylooligosaccharides* (r >2); A: *Arabinose*; ND: Not detected

The solid state fermentation for production of xylanase by *M. albomyces* was optimized by applying fractional design such as the Box-Behnken design (Box and Behnken 1960), followed by response surface methodology to investigate and optimize six variables (inoculum age, initial moisture, Tween 80 level, urea level, yeast extract level and the harvest time). The optimum levels of the variables were determined to be 600-850 im particle size, 43 hr. inoculum age, 1.37% Tween 80, 86% initial moisture content, 5.1% urea, 0.74% yeast extract and a harvest time of 96 hr. Under these optimized conditions, xylanase activity of 7760 U/g initial dry substratum was obtained which was in very good agreement with the value predicted by the quadratic model (7890 U/g initial dry substratum) (Narang et al. 2001).

6. ASSESSMENT OF XYLANASE PRODUCED BY M. ALBOMYCES FOR PREBLEACHING OF KRAFT PULPS

The effectiveness of the xylanase enzyme produced by *M. albomyces* as prebleaching agent was assessed on eucalyptus + bamboo-based pulp, procured from M/S Star Paper Mills Ltd., Saharanpur. Different parameters such as Kappa number, pulp filtrate characteristics, viscosity, savings in bleach chemicals, strength and optical properties, and environment impact were obtained at Central Pulp and Paper Research Institute, Saharanpur through a collaborative project.

6.1 Kappa Number

There was reduction in Kappa number of unbleached kraft wood pulp after enzyme treatment which decreased by 1.5 points i.e. from 18.0 to 16.5 with gain in pulp brightness of 1.0 point i.e. from 24 to 25% ISO.

6.2 Characteristic of Pulp Filtrates

The extractability of the dissolved lignin and the chromophores in pulp filtrates after xylanase treatment and from the control pulp were studied and the solubilised lignin and chromophores were measured by UV at 280 nm and in visible range at 465 nm respectively. The filtrate after enzyme treatment was found to be more coloured as compared to the control pulp sample. Determination of lignin at 280 nm showed extraction of higher amount of lignin i.e. 1.03 kg/ton as against 0.39 kg/ton in control pulp. The chromophores released were also high i.e. 2.72 kg/ton after xylanase treatment as against 0.93 kg/ton in control pulp indicating the effectiveness of the xylanase enzyme for wood kraft pulp. The reduction in Kappa number of the enzyme treated sample from 18.0 to 16.0 could be attributed to the release of lignin and chromophores.

6.3 Viscosity of Pulp

There was no reduction in viscosity of the unbleached pulp after enzyme treatment when the pulp was pretreated with optimized dose of enzyme (10 IU/g). A little increase on CED viscosity was observed which was from 690 (control pulp) to 740 (enzyme treated pulp). As expected, this little increase in viscosity could be due to the fact that the xylan has a molar mass that is generally lower than that of cellulose. So its removal leaves behind cellulose that has a higher viscosity. Therefore, the conventional view that higher pulp strength is observed with higher pulp viscosity might not hold for xylanase-treated pulp.

6.4 Bleaching of Xylanase-treated Kraft Pulp

6.4.1 Saving in Bleaching Chemicals

From the results shown in Table 4a, it is clear that by xylanase treatment of wood kraft pulp, there was reduction in chlorine requirement from 4.1% (41 kg/t) to 3.5% (35 kg/t) due to xylanase treatment. The alkali usage during extraction stage was also reduced to some extent as reflected by consumption of alkali (60.1% against 68.4 for control pulp).

6.4.2 Strength and Optical Properties of Enzyme-treated Bleached Pulp

Strength and optical properties of the untreated and treated pulp, shown in Table 4b, were found to be almost at par in terms of tensile index and burst index which were 64 and 62 Nm/g and 4.4 and 4.2 kPa m^2/g respectively. A little drop in tear index could be noticed after enzyme treatment which dropped from 6.04 to 5.8 mN m^2/g. Such a drop can be arrested by reducing the treatment time and/or enzyme dose. Final brightness of the pulp was improved by 3 points i.e. from 80 to 83% ISO (Table 4a).

Table 4(a) Bleaching of xylanase-pretreated pulp using conventional CEH sequence

Particulars	*Control pulp*	*Enzyme-treated pulp*
Chlorination Stage:		
% Chlorine Applied	4.1	3.5
% Chlorine Consumed	98.0	91.0
Saving in Chlorine (%)	–	15.0
Alkali Extraction:		
% NaOH Applied	1.5	1.5
% NaOH Consumed	68.4	60.1
Final pH	11.0	11.2
Kappa Number	4.6	3.3
Hypo Stage:		
% Applied	2.0	2.0
% Consumed	98.0	93.0
Final Brightness of Pulp (% ISO)	80.0	83.0

Table 4(b) Strength and optical properties of bleached pulp

Particulars	*Control pulp*	*Enzyme-treated pulp*
Strength Properties:		
Revolution (PFI)	3000.00	3000.00
Freeness (CSF)	295.00	270.00
Apparent Density (g/cm^3)	0.78	0.81
Burst Index ($kPa.m^2/g$)	4.40	4.20
Tensile Index ($mN.m^2/g$)	64.00	62.00
Tear Index ($mN.m^2/g$)	6.04	5.80
Optical Properties:		
Brightness (% ISO)	80.00	83.00
Opacity (%)	82.10	79.00

6.4.3 Environmental Impact of Enzyme Treatment

Characterization of the bleach effluents after enzyme treatment showed an improved environment status in terms of AOX, color and COD. The AOX level in bleach effluents was reduced by more than 20% i.e. from 2.12 kg/t to 1.8 kg/t in enzyme-treated bleach effluent (Table 4c). There was also an improvement in terms of COD after enzyme treatment.

Table 4(c) Characteristics of bleach effluent (CE Stage) arising out of xylanase-treated bleached pulp

Particulars	*Control pulp*	*Enzyme-treated pulp*
Strength Properties:		
COD (kg/t)	32.00	27.0
AOX (kg/t)	2.12	1.8
AOX Reduction (%)	–	20.0

Comparative studies were carried out with commercially available xylanase (Bleachzyme F) from M/S Biocon India Limited, Bangalore. This enzyme formulation had similar pH optimum as the enzyme of *M. albomyces*. The results indicate that enzymes from the test organism had very similar effectivity as the commercial enzyme. Savings in chlorine were of the order of 15% for *M. albomyces* enzyme and 16% for the commercial enzyme. Slight improvement in final brightness of the pulp was observed with the fungal enzyme (increase of 3 percentage points) compared to the commercial enzyme (increase of 2.5 percentage points). The strength properties were also found to be similar for both, the *M. albomyces* as well as the commercial enzyme (Bisaria et al. 2002).

7. INDUSTRIAL APPLICATIONS OF XYLANASE-ASSISTED PREBLEACHING OF PULP

Xylanase treatment of pulps improved the strength properties of the fibres in some cases and also improved viscosity of the pulp along with savings in bleach chemicals (Bajpai and Bajpai 1997). The Enso Gutzeit Mill in Imatra, Finland conducted the first mill trial of xylanase enzyme and reported a bleach chemical reduction by 25-30% and AOX level reduction by over 50%. More notable was that the level of chlorinated dioxins formed was reduced below the detection threshold. Cellulase present with xylanase did reduce the pulp quality. Now xylanases are produced using microbes that are either naturally free of cellulase-producing ability or have been mutated or genetically engineered to eliminate the cellulases. Another mill, Metsa-Sellu Mill in Aanekoksi, Finland obtained a 12%

savings in total active chlorine by applying 35 tons of enzyme, Albazyme 10, on 35,000 tons of pulp in a month long trial (Grant 1991). In Bukoza Pulp Mill in Vranov, Czech and Slovak Federal Republic, consumption of chlorine was reduced by 30% and hypochlorite by 38% on 220 ton/day of kraft pulp (Siiiner and Preselmayr 1992). In Tasman Pulp and Paper Company Ltd., New Zealand, total chlorine dioxide was reduced by 20% with improvements in AOX level and pulp qualities like brightness in mill turnover of 500 ton/day of bleached pulp (Werthemann 1993). Many major players in the market are adapting to the enzyme treated pulp and conducting further research to develop chlorine-free bleaching which involves the use of enzymes, oxygen, peroxide and ozone. A significant number of pulp and paper industries in Europe, North America and Japan are doing enzymatic bleaching full time with improvement in brightness and tear strength of pulps and reduction in AOX level of mill effluent.

8. CONCLUSION

The pulp and paper industry effluent contaminates water resources with hazardous organic halides and their various derivatives, imposing great threat to the ecosystem. Application of xylanase during prebleaching of kraft pulp has evolved as a successful technology in curbing the amount of bleach chemicals required for paper-making. Xylanases that act optimally under the harsh alkaline and 50-90°C pulp temperature conditions without changing the pulp consistency are required by the paper mills. *Melanocarpus albomyces*, a thermophillic fungus, produces a thermostable xylanase along with various debranching enzymes, having optimum in the pH range of 5.5 to 8.5 and optimum temperature at 70°C. The enzyme can efficiently reduce the adsorbable organic halides (AOX), COD and BOD of pulp mill effluents and has the potential of being successfully produced at industrial scale.

The microbial enzyme treatment of pulp has come a long way from laboratory to successful adopting of the technology by the pulp and paper industry. Xylanases are sold as concentrated liquids and the amount required per metric ton of pulp is very low and cost of enzymes has decreased due to advances in production strains and technologies. The economy of the process makes it very attractive by not only saving money by consuming lesser bleach chemicals but also by improving the pulp quality and brightness along with environmental benefits. Biotechnological application of microbial xylanases thus have been shown to make a significant contribution towards healthier environment by reducing the environmental loadings of paper mill effluents. The technology, however, needs to be applied to more mills to realize its full potential.

REFERENCES

Adamsen AK, Lindagen J, Ahring BK (1995) Optimization of extracellular xylanase production by *Dictyoglomus* sp. B1 in continuous culture. Appl Microbiol Biotechnol 44: 327-332

Alam M, Gomes I, Mohiuddin G, Hoq MH (1994) Production and characterization of thermostable xylanases by *Thermomyces lanuginosus* and *Thermoascus aurantiacus* grown on lignocelluloses. Enzyme Microb Technol 16: 298-302

Ali M, Sreekrishnan TR (2001) Aquatic toxicity from pulp and paper mill effluents: review. Adv Environ Res 5: 175-196

Ashley VM, Mitchell DA, Howes T (1999) Evaluating strategies for overcoming overheating problems during solid-state fermentation in packed bed bioreactors. Biochem Eng J 3: 141-150

Bajpai P, Bajpai PK (1997) Realities and trends in enzymatic prebleaching of kraft pulp. Adv Biochem Eng 56: 1-31

Bakir U, Yavascaoglu S, Guvenc F, Ersayin A (2001) An endo-β-1, 4-xylanase from *Rhizopus oryzae*: production, partial purification and biochemical characterization. Enzyme Microb Technol 29: 328-334

Balakrishnan H, Dutty-Choudhury M, Srinivasan MC, Rele MV (1992) Cellulase-free xylanase production from an alkalophilic *Bacillus* species. World J Microb Biotechnol 8: 627-631

Balakrishnan H, Srinivasan MC, Rele MV (1997) Extracellular protease activities in relation to xylanase secretion in an alkalophilic *Bacillus* sp. Biotechnol Lett 19(7): 599-601

Bisaria VS, Mishra S, Sahai V (2002) Enzymatic prebleaching of kraft pulps for paper manufacture. In: Proc. of Int. Conference on Tropical Bioresources and Green Chemistry Strategy, Osaka Int. Symp., Osaka, Japan, pp 332-337

Bocchini DA, Alves-Prado HF, Baida LC, Roberto IC, Gomes E, Da Silva R (2002) Optimization of xylanase production by *Bacillus circulans* D1 in submerged fermentation using response surface methodology. Process Biochem 38: 727-731

Box GEP, Behnken DW (1960) Some new three-level designs for the study of quantitative variables. Technometrics 2: 455-475

Breccia JD, Sifieriz F, Baigori MD, Castro GR, Hatti-Kaul R (1998) Purifica-tion and characterization of a thermostable xylanase from *Bacillus amyloliquefaciens*. Enzyme Microb.Technol 22: 42-49

Buchert J, Kantelinen A, Rätto M, Siika-aho M, Ranua M, Viikari L (1992) Xylanases and mannanases in the treatment of pulp. In: 5th International Conference on Biotechnology in Pulp and Paper Industry, Kyoto, Japan, pp 139-144

Èeròáková M, Golis E (1994) Testing of the cytotoxic effects of sulphate pulp mill waste waters. Folia Microbiol 29: 1-9

Chivero ET, Mutukumira AN, Zvauyu R (2001) Partial purification and characterisation of a xylanase enzyme produced by a micro-organism isolated from selected indigenous fruits of Zimbabwe. Food Chem 72(2): 179-185

Croon I, Enström B (1961) The 4-*O*-Methyl-D-glucuronic Acid groups of birch xylan during Sulphate pulping. Tappi 44: 870-898

Duarte MCT, Portugal EP, Ponezi AN, Bim MA, Tagliari CV, Franco TT (1999) Production and purification of alkaline xylanases. Bioresource Technol 68: 49-53

George SP, Ahmad A, Rao MB (2001) A novel thermostable xylanase from *Thermomonospora* sp.: influence of additives on thermostability. Bioresource Technol 78: 221-224

Ghanem NB, Yusef HH, Mahrouse HK (2000) Production of *Aspergillus terreus* xylanase in solid-state cultures: application of the Plackett-Burman experimental design to evaluate nutritional requirements. Bioresource Technol. 73: 113-121

Gomes I, Gomes J, Gomes DJ, Steiner W (2000) Simultaneous production of high activities of thermostable endoglucanase and β-glucosidase by the wild thermophilic fungus *Thermoascus aurantiacus*. Appl Microbiol Biotechnol 53: 461-468

Gomes J, Gomes I, Terler K, Gubala N, Ditzelmüller G, Steiner W (2000) Optimization of culture medium and conditions for α-L-Arabinosidase production by the extreme thermophilic eubacterium *Rhodothermus marinus*. Enzyme Microb Technol 27: 414-422

Grant R (1991) First mill scale trials get underway. Pulp Paper Int 33(6): 61-73

Gupta S, Bhusan B, Hoondal GS (2000) Isolation, purification and characterization of xylanase from *Staphylococcus* sp. SG-13 and its application in biobleaching of kraft pulp. J Appl Microb 88: 325-334

Haltrich D, Preiss M, Steiner W (1993) Optimization of a culture medium for increased xylanase production by a wild strain of *Schizophyllum commune*. Enzyme Microb Technol 15: 854-858

Hamilton JK, Partlow EV, Thompson NS (1958) The behaviour of wood hemicellulose during pulping: I. Examination of the xylose-containing hemicellulose associated with hard-wood and soft-wood pulps. Tappi 41: 803-811

Heck JX, Flôres SH, Hertz PF, Ayub MAZ (2005) Optimization of cellulase-free xylanase activity produced by *Bacillus coagulans* BL 69. Process Biochem 40: 107-112

Heck JX, Hertz PF, Ayub MAZ (2005) Extraction optimization of xylanases obtained by solid-state cultivation of *Bacillus circulans* BL53. Process Biochem. 40: 2891-2895

Jain RK, Singh K, Kulkarni AG (2005) The Indian paper industry: towards sustainability. Pulp Paper Int 47: 3-6

Jørgensen H, Eriksson T, Borjesson J, Tjerneld F, Olsson L (2003) Purification and characterization of five cellulases and one xylanase from *Penicillium brasilianum* IBT 20888. Enzyme Microb Technol 32: 851-861

Kalogeris E, Iniotaki F, Topakas E, Christakopoulos P, Kekos D, Macris BJ (2003) Performance of an intermittent agitation rotating drum type bioreactor for solid-state fermentation of wheat straw. Bioresource Technol 86: 207-213

Kang MK, Maeng PJ, Rhee YH (1996) Purification and Characterization of Two Xylanases from Alkalophilic *Cephalosporium sp.* Strain RYM-202. Appl Environ Microbiol 62: 3480-3482

Kantelinen A, Hortling B, Sundquist J, Linko M, Viikari L (1993) Proposed mechanisms of the enzymatic bleaching of kraft pulp with mannanases. Holzforschung 47: 318-324

Kantelinen A, Rättö M, Sundquist J, Ranua M, Viikari L, Linko M (1988) Hemicellulases and their potential role in bleaching. In: Proc. of Tappi Int. Pulp Bleaching Conference, Orlando, pp 1

Karrasch B, Parra O, Cid H, Mehrens M, Pacheco P, Urrutia R, Valdovinos C, Zaror C (2005) Effects of pulp and paper mill effluents on the microplankton and microbial self-purification capabilities of the Biobio river Chile. Sci of the Total Environ. Available online 31 May 2005

Kirk TK, Jeffries TW (1996) Roles for microbial enzymes in pulp and paper processing. In: Enzymes for Pulp and Paper Processing, ACS Symposium series, pp 2- 10

Kulkarni N, Rao M (1996) Application of xylanase from alkalophilic thermophilic *Bacillus* sp. NCIM59 in biobleaching of bagasse pulp. J Biotechnol 51: 167-173

Maheshwari R, Kamalam PT (1985) Isolation and culture of a thermophilic fungus, *Melanocarpus albomyces*, and factors influencing the production and activity of xylanases. J Gen Microbiol 131: 3017-3027

Martinez-Trujilo A, Pérez-Avalos O, Ponce-Noyola T (2003) Enzymatic properties of a purified xylanase from mutant PN-120 of *Cellulomonas flavigena.* Enzyme Microb Technol 32: 401- 406

Milagres AMF, Santos E, Piovan T, Roberto IC (2004) Production of xylanases by *Thermomyces aurantiacus* from sugarcane bagasse in an aerated growth fermentor. Process Biochem 39: 1387-1391

Mitchell DA, Krieger N, Stuart DM, Pandey A (2000) New developments in solid-state fermentation. II. Rational approaches to the design operation and scale-up of bioreactors. Process Biochem 35: 1211-1225

Nammori T, Watanabe T, Shinke R, Kohno A, Kawamura Y (1990) Purification and properties of thermostable xylanase and β-xylosidase produced by a newly isolated *Bacillus stearothermophilus* strain. J Bacteriol 172: 6669-6672

Narang S, Sahai V, Bisaria VS (2001) Optimization of xylanase production by Melanocarpus albomyces IIS 68 in solid-state fermentation using response surface methodology. J Biosci Bioeng 91: 425-427

Paice MG, Gurnagul N, Page DH, Jurasil L (1992) Mechanisms of hemicellulose-directed prebleaching of kraft pulp. Enz Microb Technol 14: 272-276

Panagiotou G, Kekos D, Macris BJ, Christakopoulos P (2003) Production of cellulytic and xylanolytic enzymes by *Fusarium oxysporum* grown on corn stover in solid-state fermentation. Industrial Crops Products 18: 37-45

Pedersen LS, Kihlgren P, Nielsen AM, Munk N, Holm HC, Choma PP (1992) Enzymatic bleach boosting of kraft pulp: laboratory and mill scale experiences. In: Proc. of Tappi Pulping Conference, Boston, M.A., U.S.A, Tappi Press, Atlanta, Vol.1, pp 31

Purkarthofer H, Sinner M, Steiner W (1993) Cellulase-free xylanase from *Thermomyces lanuginosus*: optimization of production in submerged and solid-state culture. Enzyme Microb Technol 15: 677-682

Qinnghe C, Xiaoyo Y, Tiangui N, Cheng J, Qiugang M (2004) The screening of culture condition and properties of xylanase by white-rot fungus *Pleurotus ostreatus*. Process Biochem 39: 1561-1566

Qi-peng Y, Jian-dong W, Huai Z, Zhong-ming Q (2005) Effect of temperature shift on production of xylanase by *Aspergillus niger*. Process Biochem 40: 3255-3257

Rani DS, Nand K (2000) Production of thermostable cellulase-free xylanase by *Clostridium absonum* CFR-702. Process Biochem 36: 355-362

Reddy V, Reddy P, Pillay B, Singh S (2002) Effect of aeration on the production of hemicellulases by *Thermomyces lanuginosus* SSBP in a 30l bioreactor. Process Biochem 37: 1221-1228

Rydholm S (1965) Pulping Processes, Krieger Publishing Company, Malabar, Florida

Salkinoja-Salonen M, Uotila J, Jokela J, Laine M, Saski E (1995) Organic halogens in the environment: studies of environmental biodegradability and human exposure. Environ.Health Perspect. 103: 63-69

Sá-Pereira P, Mesquita A, Duarte JC, Barros MRA, Costa-Ferreira M (2002) Rapid production of thermostable cellulase-free xylanase by a strain of *Bacillus subtilis* and its properties. Enzyme Microb Technol 30: 924-933

Saraswat V (1997) Xylanases of Melanocarpus albomyces IIS 68 – biosynthesis, purification and characterization. PhD Thesis, Indian Institute of Technology Delhi, New Delhi, India, p12

Saraswat V, Bisaria VS (1997) Biosynthesis of xylanolytic and xylan-debranching enzymes in *Melanocarpus albomyces* IIS 68. J Ferment Bioeng 83: 352-357

Saraswat V, Bisaria VS (2000) Purification, characterization and substrate specificities of xylanase isoenzymes from *Melanocarpus albomyces* IIS 68 Biosci Biotechnol Biochem 64: 1173-1180

Shah AK, Sidid SS, Ahmad A, Rele MV(1999) Treatment of bagasse pulp with cellulase-free xylanase from an alkalophilic *Bacillus* sp. Sam-3. Bioresource Technol 68: 133-140

Siiner M, Preselmayr W (1992) Chlorine is out, bring in the enzymes. Pulp Paper Int 34: 87-102

Simonson R (1971) Hemicellulose in the Sulphate pulping process. Svensk Papperstidning 74: 691-700

Sjöström E (1977) The behaviour of wood polysaccharides during alkaline pulping process. Tappi 60: 151-154

Sjöström E (1993) In: Wood Chemistry Fundamentals and Application, (2nd edn) Academic Press Inc, San Diego, CA, pp 14-15

Srinivasan K, Murakami M, Nakashimada Y, Nishio N (2001) Efficient production of cellulolytic and xylanolytic enzymes by the rumen anaerobic fungus *Neocallimastix frontalis* in a repeated batch culture. J Biosci Bioeng 91: 153-158

Suurnäkki A, Tenkanen M, Buchert J, Viikari L (1997) Hemicellulases in the bleaching of chemical pulps. Adv Biochem Eng Biotechnol 57: 261-287

Techapun C, Poosaran N, Watanabe M, Sasaki K (2003) Optimization of aeration and agitation rates to improve cellulase-free xylanase production by thermotolerant *Streptomyces sp.* Ab106. J. Biosci Bioeng 95: 398–301

Tolan JS, Guenette M (1997) Using enzymes in pulp bleaching: mill applications. Adv. Biochem. Eng. Biotechnol 57: 289-310

Tolan JS, Olson D, Dines RE (1995) Survey of xylanase enzyme usage in bleaching in Canada. Pulp & Paper Canada 96: 107-110

Tolan JS, Vega Canovas R (1992) The use of enzymes to decrease the C12 requirements in pulp bleaching. Pulp Paper Canada 93: 31-36

Viikari L, Ranua M, Kantelinen A, Linko M, Sundquist J (1987) Application of enzymes in bleaching. In: Proc. of 4th Int. Symp. on Wood & Pulping Chem., Paris Vol.1, pp 151

Viikari L, Ranua M, Kantelinen A, Sundquist J, Linko M (1986) Bleaching with enzymes, In: Proc. of 3rd Int. Conference on Biotechnol. in Pulp and Paper Ind., Stockholm, Sweden, pp 67

Wejse PL, Ingversen K, Mortensen KK (2003) Xylanase production by a novel halophilic bacterium increased 20-fold by response surface methodology. Enzyme Microb Technol 32: 721-727

Wenqing L, Defa L, Wu Y (2003) Influence of water activity and temperature on xylanase biosynthesis in pilot-scale solid-state fermentor by *Aspergillus sulphureus*. Enzyme Microb Technol 32: 305-311

Werthemann D (1993) Prebleaching of Pinus radiata pulp using enzymes- technology to reduce AOX. Japanese J Paper Technol 10:15-33

Xiong H, Nyyssölä A, Jänis J, Pastinen O, von Wemarn N, Leisola M, Turumen O (2004) Characterization of the xylanase produced by submerged cultivation of *Thermomyces lanuginosus* DSM 10635. Enzyme Microb Technol 35: 93-99

Xiong H, von Weymarn N, Leisola M, Turunen O (2004) Influence of pH on the production of xylanases by *Trichoderma reesai* Rut C-30. Process Biochem 39: 729-734

Yllner S, Östberg K, Stockman L (1957) Studies of the adsorption of xylan on cellulose fibres during the Sulphate cook. Svensk Paperstidning 60: 795-803

Zheng L, Du Y, Zhang J (2000) Biobleaching effect of xylanase preparation from an alkalophilic *Bacillus* sp. on ramie fibres. Biotechnol.Lett. 22: 1363-1367

Index